The Right Heart

Sean P. Gaine • Robert Naeije
Andrew J. Peacock

Editors

The Right Heart

Second Edition

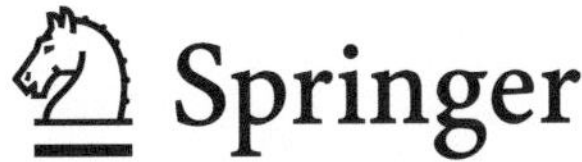

Editors
Sean P. Gaine
National Pulmonary Hypertension Unit
Mater Misericordiae University Hospital
Dublin
Ireland

Robert Naeije
Free University of Brussels
Brussels
Belgium

Andrew J. Peacock
Scottish Pulmonary Vascular Unit
Regional Heart and Lung Centre
Glasgow
UK

ISBN 978-3-030-78257-3   ISBN 978-3-030-78255-9   (eBook)
https://doi.org/10.1007/978-3-030-78255-9

To Francine Schrijen, who taught me to catheterise the right heart, Jack Reeves, who inspired my interest in right ventricular function.

Robert Naeije

To my family as well as to my mentors, colleagues, and patients who have inspired and supported me along my right heart odyssey.

Sean P. Gaine

To my wife Jila and children Leila, Johnnie, and Vita who have always supported my interests in the pulmonary circulation and the right heart even though their interests lay elsewhere.

Andrew J. Peacock

Foreword

Scientific interest in the heart, and particularly the differences between the two sides of the heart, dates back over 2000 years to its earliest depiction by Hippocrates and Galen as a two-sided structure. The description of the pulmonary circulation, accompanied by more accurate speculation regarding its function, however, was only first made over a millennium later by Ibn al-Nafis in 1242. Subsequently, Vesalius performed detailed anatomical studies of the heart and lungs in the mid-sixteenth century, followed by William Harvey's first accurate description of the circulatory system in 1628.

More recent scientific study of the cardiopulmonary system came with the pioneering work by Andre Cournand and his colleagues at Bellevue Hospital in New York City in the mid-twentieth century using the novel technique of catheterisation of the right side of the heart. Their early work included detailed measurements of cardiac function in normal and disease states, particularly conditions that affect both the heart and lungs, such as acute and chronic lung diseases.

As the field of cardiology evolved from primarily observational to interventional, the bulk of cardiovascular scientific study was focused on arteriosclerotic, hypertensive, and valvular heart diseases. Nevertheless, a group of physician-scientists including Al Fishman, Bob Grover, and Jack Reeves made important contributions to our understanding of the cardiopulmonary unit in physiologic conditions such as high altitude and pathologic conditions such as pulmonary hypertension. The development of noninvasive technologies to study the structure and function of the heart and the integrated cardiopulmonary unit, including echocardiography and magnetic resonance imaging, has led to a fuller understanding of right heart function, including important concepts like ventricular interdependence. Indeed, the editors and contributors to this book performed much of this scientific work; their chapters provide the reader with a comprehensive, state-of-the art foundation necessary for both contemporary clinical care and future investigation. For example, the development of specific therapies for pulmonary vascular diseases—pharmacologic, surgical, and interventional—provide the opportunity to study how these approaches affect right heart function and may lead to novel treatments for pulmonary vascular diseases, such as measures directly targeting the diseased right heart.

The global impact of pulmonary vascular disease today remains predominant by age-old conditions such as chronic lung disease, left-sided heart failure, thromboembolic and connective tissue diseases. However, more recently described conditions that affect the pulmonary circulation, such as infectious etiologies like the HIV, hepatitis C, and COVID-19 viruses, are major global health challenges and remain poorly understood. Their emergence underscores the importance of multidisciplinary efforts to further our understanding of the right heart and pulmonary circulation. That the contributors to this volume exemplify this multidisciplinary interest and approach sets the stage for an exciting new era of scientific progress in this field.

New York, NY, USA   Lewis J. Rubin

Preface

The first edition of *The Right Heart* was published in 2014. We believe it was the first book to look exclusively at the normal anatomy and physiology of the right heart as well as the impact of disease on structure and function. It was hoped at the time that the book would take a step towards reversing the historical neglect of the 'lesser circulation' by both pulmonary physicians and cardiologists. The book was very well received with over 22,000 downloads. The growing understanding of the crucial role of the right heart as a fundamental integral component of the cardiopulmonary system has led to significant advances in our understanding since that first edition.

In this second edition, leading right heart experts from around the world have come together to explore the most up-to-date information we have gained over the past decade. The book is divided into sections on physiology, pathology and pathobiology, imaging, as well as sections on the causes of right heart dysfunction and its treatment. Previously, it was accepted that direct treatment of the pulmonary vascular abnormalities was the only way to improve right heart dysfunction by reducing RV afterload, but we realise now that direct treatment of the RV is also possible and indeed desirable.

We do hope that this book will be received with the same enthusiasm as the first edition. The 'lesser circulation' continues to grow in importance to an even wider audience beyond the pulmonologist and cardiologist to include specialists as diverse as the intensivist, radiologist, haematologist, and indeed those involved in transplantation and the development of stents and ventricular assist devices.

In 1989, Jack Reeves invited us to further explore the right heart by remarking that 'One must inquire how increasing pulmonary vascular resistance results in impaired right ventricular function'[1]. We hope after reading this edition that you will agree his invitation has been enthusiastically accepted and that real progress in our understanding of the right heart is now being made.

Dublin, Ireland
Brussels, Belgium
Glasgow, UK

Sean P. Gaine
Robert Naeije
Andrew J. Peacock

---

[1] Reeves JT, Groves BM, Turkevich D, Morrisson DA, Trapp JA. Right ventricular function in pulmonary hypertension. In: Weir EK, Reeves JT, editors. Pulmonary vascular physiology and physiopathology. New York: Marcel Dekker; 1989. p. 325–51. Chap. 10.

Contents

Part I

Physiology, Pathology and Pathobiology

Function of the Right Ventricle

1

Jeroen N. Wessels, Frances S. de Man,
and Anton Vonk Noordegraaf

From Early to Recent Ideas on RV Function

Ideas about right ventricular (RV) function have changed tremendously since the second century when Galen described the RV as merely a conduit, through which part of the blood moves to the lungs for nourishment. The remainder of the blood was thought to go through invisible pores of the septum to the left ventricle for the formation of the vital spirit [1]. It took about ten centuries before Galen's view was opposed. In the thirteenth century, Ibn Nafis disputed the existence of septum pores and stated for the first time in known history that all the blood had to go through the lungs to get from the right to the left ventricle [1, 2]. Ibn Nafis' idea about RV function was also different from Galen's view as he believed that it was responsible for thinning of the blood, making it fit for mixing with air in the lungs [2]. The origin of the idea that the right ventricle is responsible for transmission of blood through the lungs and not for their nourishment has been accredited mostly to William Harvey who described this idea in 1628 in his de Motu Cordis, about three centuries later than Ibn Nafis [3, 4]. Even though Ibn Nafis and Harvey both emphasized the role the right ventricle plays in the pulmonary circulation, centuries passed before the true importance of RV function for both the pulmonary and systemic circulation would be established. The road to this understanding started in the 1940s during which more detailed studies on RV function were performed. Several open-pericardial, open-thorax dog experiments showed that cauterization of the right ventricle did not lead to changes in systemic venous or pulmonary artery pressures [5–7]. Based on these studies it was, still then, concluded that an actively functioning RV was not essential for the maintenance of a normal pressure gradient in the pulmonary and systemic arterial tree. However, several studies conducted between 1950 and 1980 that used experimental models excluding the RV from the circulation concluded that the RV was unquestionably necessary for the maintenance of blood flow and life [8–10]. But because the models used in these studies were far from physiological, the idea of the necessity of the right ventricle for the maintenance of circulation did not gain much support. It took until 1982 to recognize the role of the RV, when it was shown that RV myocardial infarction, this time using an animal model with an intact pericardium, did lead to a reduction in cardiac output [11]. Since then, multiple studies have shown RV function to be of functional and/or prognostic significance in exercising healthy subjects and in disease states [12–15]. Thus at present, we know that the right ventricle is not just a passive conduit for systemic

J. N. Wessels · F. S. de Man · A. Vonk Noordegraaf (✉)
Department of Pulmonary Medicine, Amsterdam
Cardiovascular Sciences, Amsterdam UMC, Vrije
Universiteit Amsterdam, Amsterdam, Netherlands
e-mail: a.vonk@amsterdamumc.nl

S. P. Gaine et al. (eds.), *The Right Heart*, https://doi.org/10.1007/978-3-030-78255-9_1

venous return: the RV plays an important role in maintaining cardiac output in both health and disease.

Physiology of RV Contraction and Relaxation

Myocyte Contraction

In both the left and right ventricles, the structural unit of a cardiomyocyte that is responsible for diastolic muscle properties and cardiac contraction is the sarcomere [16]. The sarcomeric thick (myosin) and thin (actin) filamentous proteins (see Fig. 1.1) determine the contractile properties. The third filament, titin, is responsible for the passive properties of the sarcomere. The myosin filament is composed of a body and cross-bridges. The cross-bridges consist of an "arm and head" and extend outward from the body [17]. The actin filament is made of actin and tropomyosin which form the backbone of the filament. Attached to tropomyosin is the troponin complex (troponin I, T, and C). In a relaxed state, the troponin complex is attached to tropomyosin in a manner that prevents the binding of myosin heads with actin. Cardiomyocyte contraction is initiated by the arrival of the action potential. During the action potential, calcium channels in the cell membrane open, allowing calcium to enter the cell [18]. This event triggers the release of calcium from the sarcoplasmic reticulum, which causes the main increase in the cytosolic calcium concentration (calcium-induced calcium release). The increase in free calcium concentration allows binding of calcium to the myofilamental protein troponin C, thereby changing the confirmation of the troponin complex. The result is exposure of the myosin-binding sites of the actin filament, creating the opportunity for a reaction

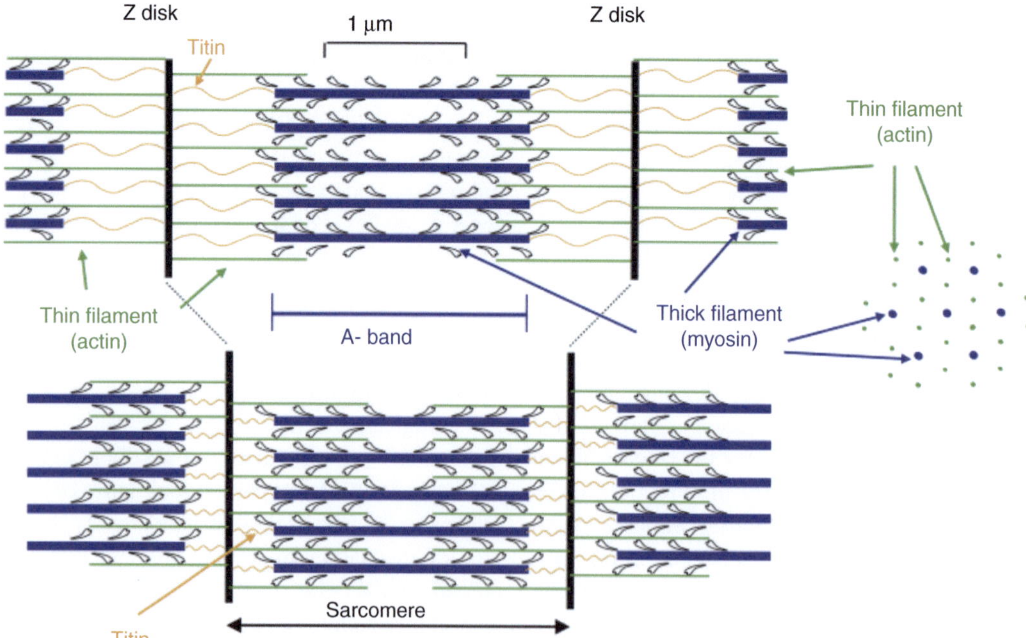

Fig. 1.1 The structural unit of a cardiomyocyte that is responsible for contraction, the sarcomere, is presented at two different muscle lengths. Each sarcomere is bounded at the end by Z-discs. Two types of filaments are shown: (1) the thick filament (blue), with the myosin heads extending from the backbone and connected to the Z-disc by a titin molecule (drawn here is one molecule instead of six), and (2) the thin filament (green), directly attached to the Z-disc. Note that both filaments overlap each other, the extension of which is dependent on muscle length. (Reprinted from Westerhof et al. [17]. With permission from Springer Science)

between actin and myosin heads resulting in sliding of actin along myosin and consequently shortening of the muscle [17, 19].

Myocyte Relaxation

After muscle shortening, calcium ions are pumped out of the cytosol back into the sarcoplasmic reticulum and to the extracellular fluid allowing the sarcomere to relax and lengthen up to its initial diastolic state [17, 18]. The sarcomeric protein that is responsible for the stiffness of the relaxed, diastolic muscle is titin (see Fig. 1.1) [20]. It is the largest protein in the human body and it extends from the Z-disc to the center of the myosin filament. It has several "springlike" regions which determine the stiffness of the protein. Alteration of phosphorylation of these regions or alternative splicing can increase or decrease titin compliance [21]. Myocardial passive tension is also influenced by extracellular collagen, especially at longer sarcomere length. However, titin remains an important contributor to total passive tension, even at large sarcomere lengths [20].

RV Contraction, Ejection, and RV Pressure Curve

That contraction of one single cardiomyocyte leads to shortening of the muscle cell is clear. A more complicated story is how the combined shortening of all the individual RV cardiomyocytes results in the ejection of blood into the pulmonary artery (PA). This is due to the complex geometry and contraction sequence of the RV. The RV is composed of two different anatomical parts, that is, the body (sinus) and the outflow tract (conus or infundibulum). The sinus contains more than 80% of total RV volume [22] and has a different fiber orientation compared to the conus. Also, the timing of contraction during the cardiac cycle is different between these two compartments [22–27]. RV contraction occurs sequentially starting at the apex of the ventricle moving in a peristalsis-like pattern towards the conus [25]. In early systole, the conus even expands before it starts to contract about 20–50 ms later than the body of the ventricle [22, 24, 26]. During early diastole, the conus' tonus partially continues and relaxation may not be seen until atrial contraction [22, 24, 26].

The net result of RV contraction is a chamber volume reduction with propulsion of blood into the pulmonary artery. This is mediated by several mechanisms. The largest contribution to RV volume decrease is shortening of the ventricle in the longitudinal direction, that is, from base to apex [28]. Another mechanism of volume reduction is movement of the RV free wall to the septum (transverse shortening) [4, 29, 30]. Several investigators have mentioned another mechanism of ejection, that is, ejection of blood due to blood momentum [31–33]. Blood momentum refers to the event of continued movement of blood mass under the late-systolic negative pressure gradient (PA > RV pressure) [8, 33]. This mechanism was originally suggested based on LV ejection hemodynamics [33], but similar observations were made on RV ejection hemodynamics. RV ejection, starting when the RV pressure exceeds PA pressure leading to pulmonary valve opening (see Fig. 1.2), continues even when myocardial muscle relaxes and ventricular pressure decreases to values lower than PA pressure. Indeed, RV ejection continues in the presence of declining RV pressure and a negative pressure gradient between the RV and PA [30, 31, 34, 35]. Both observations support the theory of blood momentum. The fact that continued ejection can occur in the course of a declining RV pressure is likely the effect of mass: moving mass continues moving even when a counteracting force exists. Importantly, the disparity between end systole (end of active myocardial shortening) and end ejection makes it necessary to assume equal use of terminology concerning the two events to avoid confusion. However, in pressure-volume analysis end systole is defined as end ejection (see description on pressure-volume analysis below).

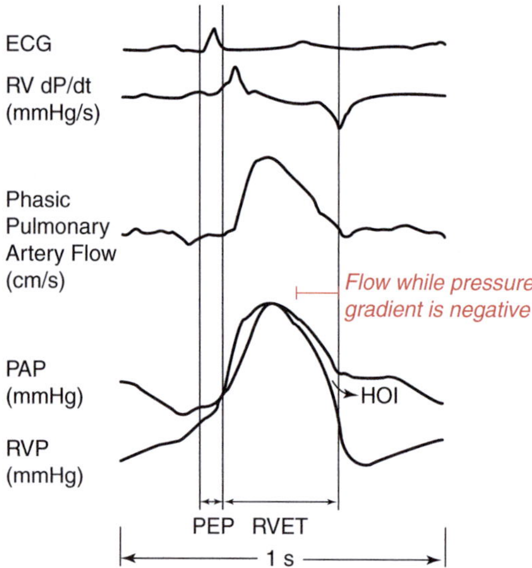

Fig. 1.2 Simultaneously recorded electrocardiogram (ECG), right ventricular (RV) d*P*/d*t*, pulmonary artery (PA) flow, PA and RV pressure. Note the short duration of the pre-ejection time (PEP) and the negative pressure gradient visible during late ejection. *HOI* hangout interval, *RVET* RV ejection time, *PAP* pulmonary artery pressure, *RVP* right ventricular pressure. (Reprinted from Dell'Italia and Walsh [35]. With permission from Elsevier)

Influence of LV Contraction on RV Ejection

The RV is connected in series with the LV; this is called *series* ventricular interaction [36]. As a result, RV stroke volume will greatly determine LV filling and subsequently LV stroke volume. Consequently, factors that influence RV output will also affect LV output. Diseases that affect RV function are described in detail in subsequent chapters in this book.

On top of the indirect *series* interaction, a *direct* ventricular interaction occurs as both ventricles share the interventricular septum, have intertwined muscle bundles, and are enclosed by one single pericardium [8, 36]. Because the pericardium encloses the septum-sharing ventricles and is highly resistant to acute distention, the compliance of one ventricle is influenced by the volume and pressure of the other ventricle [37–39]. Also during systole, ventricular interaction can be observed as LV contraction influences pressure development in

the RV [36, 40]. Approximately 20–40% of the RV systolic pressure development may result from LV contraction [41].

Although ventricular interactions are present in healthy subjects, negative consequences of ventricular interaction manifest only in disease states. For example, in pulmonary arterial hypertension, LV diastolic filling is impaired by both a reduced RV stroke volume resulting from an increased pulmonary vascular resistance (*series* ventricular interaction) and leftward ventricular septum bowing resulting from RV pressure and volume overload (*direct* ventricular interaction) [42].

Description of RV Function

The cardiovascular system has the essential task to provide the tissues in our body with sufficient nutrients and oxygen. Therefore, it is important to maintain cardiac output at an adequate level. Since the left and right ventricles are connected in series, cardiac output is more or less similar for both. Often used methods to determine RV cardiac output are thermodilution or the direct Fick method during a right-heart catheterization [43]. Cardiac output is determined by stroke volume and heart rate. Cardiac magnetic resonance imaging (MRI) is a noninvasive method to assess RV stroke volume. With MRI, aortic and pulmonary flows can be measured. Stroke volume can also be determined by taking the difference between end-systolic and end-diastolic volume. It holds for all methods that both LV and RV measurements can be used to determine stroke volume, since it should be the same for both ventricles. Please note that when valvular insufficiency or a shunt is present, the use of ventricular volumes is not accurate [44]. Despite the fact that stroke volume is the net result of RV contraction, it only gives a limited amount of information about RV function per se. Stroke volume is first of all determined by RV filling (preload). Stroke volume is further determined by RV myocardial function (ventricular contractility) and by the load that opposes RV ejection (arterial system, afterload). Therefore, to understand RV myocardial function, load-independent measures are needed as provided by ventricular pressure-volume analysis.

The Ventricular Pressure-Volume Loop

The first person to describe the cardiac cycle by means of a pressure-volume graph was Otto Frank in 1898 [17, 45]. He described pressure changes during isovolumic (non-ejecting) contractions at various filling volumes and showed maximal pressure increases with increasing diastolic volume. Later, in 1914, Starling described ejection against a constant ejection pressure and found increased stroke volumes with increased filling. The combination of the two findings is what we nowadays call the Frank-Starling mechanism, which will be explained in detail in the section "Regulation of RV Function" below.

A pressure-volume loop describes the changes in ventricular pressure and volume observed during the cardiac cycle (see Fig. 1.3a for a schematic presentation). The cardiac cycle can be divided into four different phases: (1) the filling phase, (2) isovolumic contraction phase, (3) ejection phase, and (4) isovolumic relaxation phase. During the filling phase, RV volume increases considerably while RV pressure only slightly changes [46]. After the onset of contraction, RV pressure increases rapidly. The pulmonary valve opens when RV pressure exceeds PA pressure, thereby ending the isovolumic contraction phase. Normally, this RV isovolumic contraction phase is of short duration due to the low PA pressures (see also Fig. 1.2) [47]. In the ejection phase RV pressure peaks early to subsequently rapid decline during late ejection [48]. During late ejection, a negative pressure gradient between the RV and PA can be observed; this is referred to as the hangout interval (see Fig. 1.2) [35]. The isovolumic relaxation phase starts at pulmonary valve closure and pressure declines back to its initial value.

The information that can be derived from a single pressure-volume loop includes stroke

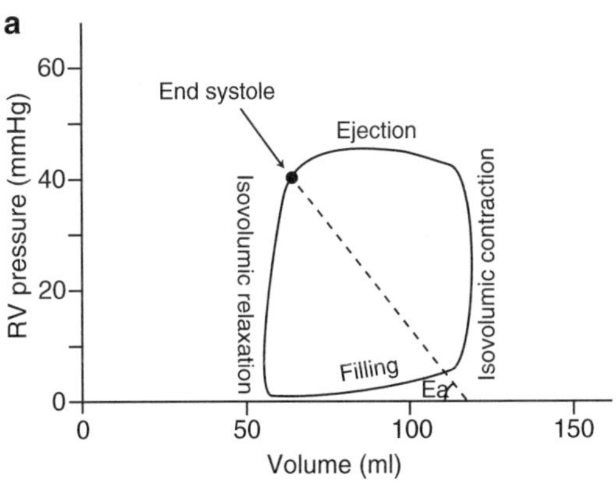

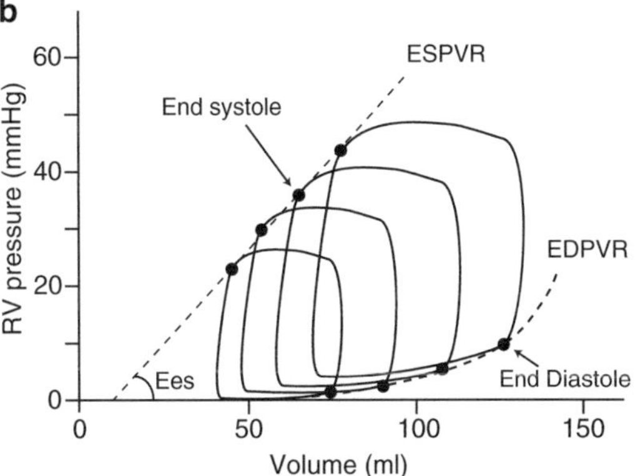

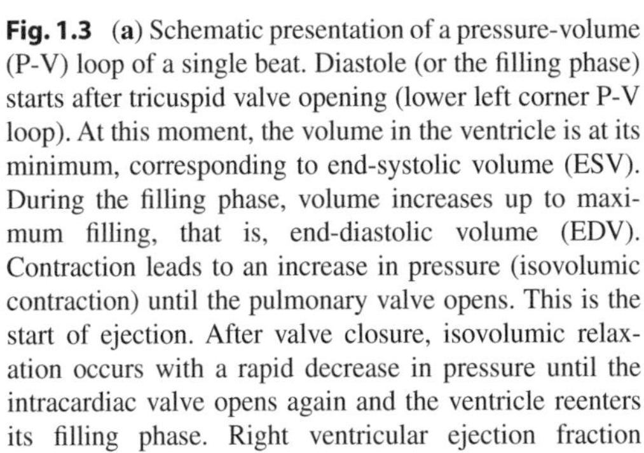

Fig. 1.3 (**a**) Schematic presentation of a pressure-volume (P-V) loop of a single beat. Diastole (or the filling phase) starts after tricuspid valve opening (lower left corner P-V loop). At this moment, the volume in the ventricle is at its minimum, corresponding to end-systolic volume (ESV). During the filling phase, volume increases up to maximum filling, that is, end-diastolic volume (EDV). Contraction leads to an increase in pressure (isovolumic contraction) until the pulmonary valve opens. This is the start of ejection. After valve closure, isovolumic relaxation occurs with a rapid decrease in pressure until the intracardiac valve opens again and the ventricle reenters its filling phase. Right ventricular ejection fraction

(RVEF) can be calculated from a single pressure-volume loop by dividing stroke volume and end-diastolic volume, and then multiplying by 100%. Effective arterial elastance (E_a) is a measure of RV afterload and calculated as the slope of the dotted line from the end-systolic P-V point to the x-intercept at EDV. (**b**) Schematic representation of multiple pressure-volume loops obtained during gradual preload reduction. Note that the end-diastolic pressure-volume points can be connected by a nonlinear line, the end-diastolic pressure volume relation (EDPVR). Also shown is the linear end-systolic pressure volume relation (ESPVR) and its slope E_{es} (end-systolic elastance)

volume, end-diastolic volume, end-systolic volume, and ejection fraction (calculated from end-diastolic volume and stroke volume, see Fig. 1.3a). The information that these parameters give about RV myocardial properties is limited. However, if multiple loops under alteration of loading conditions (preferable preload reduction by vena cava occlusion [17]) are collected, information on both systolic and diastolic properties of the ventricle can be obtained.

Systolic Properties: The End-Systolic Pressure-Volume Relation

Figure 1.3b gives a graphical representation of multiple pressure-volume loops obtained during preload reduction [49]. Although multiple pressure-volume loops can also be acquired by changing afterload, the preferable method is preload reduction, since changes in afterload are more likely to affect the systolic and/or diastolic properties one wishes to measure [50]. When multiple pressure-volume loops are obtained during preload reduction, for example by partial vena cava occlusion using a balloon catheter, both the end-systolic and end-diastolic pressure-volume points can be connected by a line (see Fig. 1.3b). The line connecting the end-systolic pressure-volume points is referred to as the end-systolic pressure-volume relation (ESPVR). This relation is reasonably linear over a physiological range in both the LV and the RV [34, 51, 52]. Therefore, in practice, linearity is assumed for the ESPVR. The slope of the ESPVR is called end-systolic elastance (E_{es}) and due to the assumption of linearity it can be described by the following formula: $E_{es} = P_{es}/(V_{es} - V_0)$, where P_{es} is end-systolic pressure, V_{es} is end-systolic volume, and V_0 is the so called intercept volume of the ESPVR. E_{es} is used as a measure of myocardial contractility for several reasons. First of all, positive and negative inotropic agents such as catecholamines and acute B-blockade, respectively, increase or decrease E_{es} [46, 51–56]. In

addition, E_{es} is assumed independent of pre- or afterload, and therefore considered load independent [34, 56].

In theory, elastance is a measure of stiffness in terms of pressure and volume and the idea that ventricular properties could be described by elastance came from Suga's work on the isolated heart, where the time-varying elastance concept was proposed in the late 1960s [57]. The time-varying ventricular elastance implies that the heart changes its stiffness during the cardiac cycle, with maximal elastance occurring near or at end systole. More extensive information on the theory of time-varying elastance can be found elsewhere [17, 45].

Considerations for the Application of RV ESPVR and E_{es}

For the assessment of changes in contractile state one should consider that the measured ventricular properties, both systolic and diastolic (see below), are influenced by the amount of muscle mass, myocardial properties, and ventricular configuration [45, 50]. Therefore, a shift of the ESPVR in an acute setting (where muscle mass and ventricular configuration are constant) reflects a change in myocardial contractility. However, in a clinical setting muscle mass or ventricular configuration may change over time and an observed shift in the ESPVR can therefore not only be attributed to a change in myocardial contractility [50].

The Cardiopulmonary System

The systolic properties of the right ventricle have to be seen in light of its load [58]. The pulmonary circulation is a low-pressure, high-compliance system in contrast with the systemic circulation. Because the afterload for the right ventricle is low, there is no need for a high E_{es}. However, during exercise, or in disease states in which the afterload increases, the E_{es} has to increase as well [59, 60]. An appropriate measure to describe the afterload is called effective arterial elastance (E_a), which is a measure of total resistance [61]. It can be determined by the ratio of end-systolic pressure to stroke volume (see Fig. 1.3b). In healthy individuals, the transfer of energy from the right ventricle to the pulmonary artery is optimal. In other words, RV contractility is adequately matched to the afterload. This concept is called coupling and is represented by the ratio of E_{es}/E_a. Both E_{es} and E_a describe the function of a subsystem (right ventricle and pulmonary circulation, respectively), independently of each other. The function of the cardiopulmonary system as a whole results from the interaction of these subsystems. Stroke volume, for example, is determined not only by RV function, but also by afterload. Other often used parameters that result from functional interaction include cardiac output, RV ejection fraction, and pulmonary artery pressure [60].

Diastolic Properties: The End-Diastolic Pressure-Volume Relation

In contrast with the rather linear end-systolic pressure-volume relation, the diastolic pressure-volume relation is nonlinear (see Fig. 1.3b) [45, 50]. The end-diastolic pressure-volume relation (EDPVR) shows that at low volumes pressure increases only minimally for a given increase in volume. At higher volumes the pressure rise for an increase in volume is progressively larger, which gives the EDPVR its characteristic nonlinear curve [50]. The sarcomeric structures responsible for the steeper rise in pressure at larger filling volumes are the titin molecules, while outside the sarcomere the extracellular matrix (collagen) resists the further stretching of the myocyte [50, 62]. Diastolic elastance can be measured like systolic elastance with multiple pressure-volume loops under quick alteration of preload and reflects the passive properties of the ventricle

(see Fig. 1.3b) [50]. However, because of the nonlinearity of the EDPVR, nonlinear regression analysis is mandatory to obtain a curve fit and a diastolic stiffness constant [50, 63]. RV diastolic stiffness can be described by the slope of the EDPVR at end-diastolic volume. This measure is called end-diastolic elastance (E_{ed}) [64].

Single-Beat Analysis of E_{es} and E_{ed}

Because the measurement of systolic and diastolic elastances as described above requires simultaneous measurement of RV pressure and volume including an intervention on ventricular loading, this measurement is not easy to apply in a clinical setting and may even be contraindicated in some patients. To overcome these problems, more applicable methods have been developed that do not require multiple pressure-volume loops. These so-called single-beat analyses are available for both the left and right ventricles and for both the systolic [53, 65, 66] and diastolic elastance [63]. Results of the single-beat method to calculate the coupling of E_{es}/E_a are comparable to the multiple-beat method [67].

Regulation of RV Function

The regulation of RV function can best be illustrated by its response to changes in volume and afterload. The RV ventricular response to filling (diastolic) volume is described by the Frank-Starling mechanism and is based on the alteration of the sensitivity of the myofilaments to calcium, as will be described below [18]. The response of the right ventricle to changes in afterload is mediated by neurohormonal mechanisms. Cardiac output can further be altered by changes in heart rate. For mechanisms of subacute and chronic alterations in contractility and diastolic function we refer to the chapters on disease states with altered ventricular loading by volume and/or afterload.

Volume Response: The Frank-Starling Mechanism

The Frank-Starling mechanism refers to the observation that with increasing ventricular end-diastolic volume, stroke volume simultaneously increases. Changes in end-diastolic volume are usually mediated by changes in venous return. Consequently, stroke volume is regulated by venous return in most conditions [19]. At a molecular level the Frank-Starling mechanism refers to the observation that with greater sarcomere length at the start of contraction, a greater force is generated. This is caused by an altered myofilamental sensitivity to calcium by stretching. The proposed mechanism for this altered myofilamental sensitivity has long been the theory of "lattice spacing" [68]. This theory is based on a decrease in spacing between the filaments upon stretching. Consequently, the binding of myosin heads to actin is more likely to occur, thereby increasing force per amount of calcium available. Recently, another explanation has been put forward [68]. It was observed that the stretching of sarcomeres favorably alters the orientation of the myosin heads, making it easier to bind with the actin filament. According to these new findings, the Frank-Starling mechanism may be largely explained by favorable alteration in myosin head orientation, and to a lesser extent by lattice spacing.

Afterload Response: Sympathetic Activation

When the afterload of the right ventricle is acutely increased, stroke volume will decrease if no compensatory mechanisms existed. However, compensatory mechanisms do exist and stroke volume can be maintained to a certain extent under altered loading conditions. One mechanism to maintain stroke volume is by the Frank-Starling mechanism as described above. This occurs when the RV's end-diastolic volume increases as a result of the increased afterload. Another mechanism to maintain stroke volume in an acute setting is through an increase in contractility, facilitated by sympathetic nervous system activation. Sympathetic activation of the heart occurs through B-adrenergic receptors that are localized on cardiomyocytes. Stimulation of B-adrenergic receptors leads to an increase in contractility (inotropy) through increased availability of free intracellular calcium. Sympathetic activation also slightly reduces myofilamental calcium sensitivity. However, the increase in intracellular calcium availability outweighs this reduction [18]. Secondly, sympathetic activation leads to faster relaxation (lusitropy) as a result of a faster reuptake of calcium ions by the sarcoplasmic reticulum and consequently a faster release of calcium from the myofilaments.

A secondary, slower mechanism that increases contractile force has been described by Gleb von Anrep [69]. The so-called Anrep effect refers to the observation that after the initial response, cardiomyocytes further increase their contractile force slowly over the following minutes [69]. The Anrep effect results from autocrine/paracrine mechanisms involving stretch-induced release of angiotensin II and endothelin. More detailed information on the Anrep phenomenon can be found elsewhere [69, 70].

Conclusions

RV function is important in both healthy individuals and disease states. The right ventricle has a complex geometry consisting of two different anatomical parts and RV contraction occurs in a peristaltic-like pattern. In the healthy right ventricle, ejection continues after maximal shortening and in the presence of a negative pressure gradient. Despite the complex hemodynamics, RV systolic and diastolic function can be described by a time-varying elastance. RV output is highly sensitive to changes in filling, which is mediated through the Frank-Starling mechanism, and increases in afterload. An accurate description of RV function incorporates so-called load-independent measurements.

References

1. West JB. Ibn al-Nafis, the pulmonary circulation, and the Islamic Golden Age. J Appl Physiol. 2008;105:1877–80.
2. Haddad SI, Khairallah AA. A forgotten chapter in the history of the circulation of the blood. Ann Surg. 1936;104:1–8.
3. Young RA. The pulmonary circulation-before and after Harvey: Part I. Br Med J. 1940;1:1–5.
4. Haddad F, Hunt SA, Rosenthal DN, Murphy DJ. Right ventricular function in cardiovascular disease, Part I: Anatomy, physiology, aging, and functional assessment of the right ventricle. Circulation. 2008;117:1436–48.
5. Bakos ACP. The question of the function of the right ventricular myocardium: an experimental study. Circulation. 1950;1:724.
6. Kagan A. Dynamic responses of the right ventricle following extensive damage by cauterization. Circulation. 1952;5:816–23.
7. Starr I, Jeffers WA, Mead RH. The absence of conspicuous increments of venous pressure after severe damage to the right ventricle of the dog, with a discussion of the relation between clinical congestive failure and heart disease. Am Heart J. 1943;26:291.
8. Dell'Italia LJ. The right ventricle: anatomy, physiology, and clinical importance. Curr Probl Cardiol. 1991;16:653–720.
9. Puga FJ, McGoon DC. Exclusion of the right ventricle from the circulation: hemodynamic observations. Surgery. 1973;73:607–13.
10. Rose JC, Cosimano SJ Jr, Hufnagel CA, Massullo EA. The effects of exclusion of the right ventricle from the circulation in dogs. J Clin Invest. 1955;34:1625–31.
11. Goldstein JA, Vlahakes GJ, Verrier ED, Schiller NB, Tyberg JV, Ports TA, et al. The role of right ventricular systolic dysfunction and elevated intrapericardial pressure in the genesis of low output in experimental right ventricular infarction. Circulation. 1982;65:513–22.
12. La Gerche A, Gewillig M. What limits cardiac performance during exercise in normal subjects and in healthy Fontan patients? Int J Pediatr. 2010;2010:791291.
13. van Wolferen SA, Marcus JT, Boonstra A, Marques KM, Bronzwaer JG, Spreeuwenberg MD, et al. Prognostic value of right ventricular mass, volume, and function in idiopathic pulmonary arterial hypertension. Eur Heart J. 2007;28:1250–7.
14. Vonk Noordegraaf A, Galie N. The role of the right ventricle in pulmonary arterial hypertension. Eur Respir Rev. 2011;20:243–53.
15. Zehender M, Kasper W, Kauder E, Schonthaler M, Geibel A, Olschewski M, et al. Right ventricular infarction as an independent predictor of prognosis after acute inferior myocardial infarction. N Engl J Med. 1993;328:981–8.
16. Leyton RA, Spotnitz HM, Sonnenblick EH. Cardiac ultrastructure and function: sarcomeres in the right ventricle. Am J Phys. 1971;221:902–10.
17. Westerhof N, Stergiopulos N, Noble MIM, Westerhof BE. Cardiac muscle mechanics. In: Westerhof N, Stergiopulos N, Noble MIM, Westerhof BE, editors. Snapshots of hemodynamics. 3rd ed. New York: Springer; 2019. p. 91–9.
18. Bers DM. Cardiac excitation-contraction coupling. Nature. 2002;415:198–205.
19. Guyton AC, Hall JE. Textbook of medical physiology. 13th ed. Philadelphia: WB Saunders Company; 2016.
20. LeWinter MM, Granzier H. Cardiac Titin. Circulation. 2010;121:2137–45.
21. Methawasin M, Hutchinson KR, Lee EJ, Smith JE, Saripalli C, Hidalgo CG, et al. Experimentally increasing titin compliance in a novel mouse model attenuates the Frank-Starling mechanism but has a beneficial effect on diastole. Circulation. 2014;129:1924–36.
22. Geva T, Powell AJ, Crawford EC, Chung T, Colan SD. Evaluation of regional differences in right ventricular systolic function by acoustic quantification echocardiography and cine magnetic resonance imaging. Circulation. 1998;98:339–45.
23. Armour JA, Pace JB, Randall WC. Interrelationship of architecture and function of the right ventricle. Am J Phys. 1970;218:174–9.
24. March HW, Ross JK, Lower RR. Observations on the behavior of the right ventricular outflow tract, with reference to its developmental origins. Am J Med. 1962;32:835–45.
25. Meier GD, Bove AA, Santamore WP, Lynch PR. Contractile function in canine right ventricle. Am J Phys. 1980;239:H794–804.
26. Raines RA, LeWinter MM, Covell JW. Regional shortening patterns in canine right ventricle. Am J Phys. 1976;231:1395–400.
27. Santamore WP, Meier GD, Bove AA. Effects of hemodynamic alterations on wall motion in the canine right ventricle. Am J Phys. 1979;236:H254–62.
28. Brown SB, Raina A, Katz D, Szerlip M, Wiegers SE, Forfia PR. Longitudinal shortening accounts for the majority of right ventricular contraction and improves after pulmonary vasodilator therapy in normal subjects and patients with pulmonary arterial hypertension. Chest. 2011;140:27–33.
29. Haber I, Metaxas DN, Geva T, Axel L. Three-dimensional systolic kinematics of the right ventricle. Am J Physiol Heart Circ Physiol. 2005;289:H1826–33.
30. Piene H. Pulmonary arterial impedance and right ventricular function. Physiol Rev. 1986;66:606–52.
31. Pouleur H, Lefevre J, Van Mechelen H, Charlier AA. Free-wall shortening and relaxation during ejection in the canine right ventricle. Am J Phys. 1980;239:H601–13.
32. Spencer MP, Greiss FC. Dynamics of ventricular ejection. Circ Res. 1962;10:274–9.
33. Noble MI. The contribution of blood momentum to left ventricular ejection in the dog. Circ Res. 1968;23:663–70.

34. Dell'Italia LJ, Walsh RA. Application of a time varying elastance model to right ventricular performance in man. Cardiovasc Res. 1988;22:864–74.

35. Dell'Italia LJ, Walsh RA. Acute determinants of the hangout interval in the pulmonary circulation. Am Heart J. 1988;116:1289–97.

36. Weber KT, Janicki JS, Shroff S, Fishman AP. Contractile mechanics and interaction of the right and left ventricles. Am J Cardiol. 1981;47:686–95.

37. Frenneaux M, Williams L. Ventricular-arterial and ventricular-ventricular interactions and their relevance to diastolic filling. Prog Cardiovasc Dis. 2007;49:252–62.

38. Laks MM, Garner D, Swan HJ. Volumes and compliances measured simultaneously in the right and left ventricles of the dog. Circ Res. 1967;20:565–9.

39. Taylor RR, Covell JW, Sonnenblick EH, Ross J Jr. Dependence of ventricular distensibility on filling of the opposite ventricle. Am J Phys. 1967;213:711–8.

40. Santamore WP, Lynch PR, Heckman JL, Bove AA, Meier GD. Left ventricular effects on right ventricular developed pressure. J Appl Physiol. 1976;41:925–30.

41. Yamaguchi S, Harasawa H, Li K, Zhu D, Santamore W. Comparative significance in systolic ventricular interaction. Cardiovasc Res. 1991;25:774–83.

42. Marcus JT, Gan CT, Zwanenburg JJ, Boonstra A, Allaart CP, Gotte MJ, et al. Interventricular mechanical asynchrony in pulmonary arterial hypertension: left-to-right delay in peak shortening is related to right ventricular overload and left ventricular underfilling. J Am Coll Cardiol. 2008;51:750–7.

43. Rosenkranz S, Preston IR. Right heart catheterisation: best practice and pitfalls in pulmonary hypertension. Eur Respir Rev. 2015;24:642–52.

44. Mauritz GJ, Marcus JT, Boonstra A, Postmus PE, Westerhof N, Vonk-Noordegraaf A. Non-invasive stroke volume assessment in patients with pulmonary arterial hypertension: left-sided data mandatory. J Cardiovasc Magn Reson. 2008;10:51.

45. Sagawa K, Maughan L, Suga H, Sunagawa K. Cardiac contraction and the pressure-volume relationships. Oxford: Oxford University Press; 1988.

46. Maughan WL, Shoukas AA, Sagawa K, Weisfeldt ML. Instantaneous pressure-volume relationship of the canine right ventricle. Circ Res. 1979;44:309–15.

47. Dell'Italia LJ, Santamore WP. Can indices of left ventricular function be applied to the right ventricle? Prog Cardiovasc Dis. 1998;40:309–24.

48. Dell'Italia LJ. Anatomy and physiology of the right ventricle. Cardiol Clin. 2012;30:167–87.

49. de Man FS, Tu L, Handoko ML, Rain S, Ruiter G, Francois C, et al. Dysregulated renin-angiotensin-aldosterone system contributes to pulmonary arterial hypertension. Am J Respir Crit Care Med. 2012;186:780–9.

50. Burkhoff D, Mirsky I, Suga H. Assessment of systolic and diastolic ventricular properties via pressure-volume analysis: a guide for clinical, translational, and basic researchers. Am J Physiol Heart Circ Physiol. 2005;289:H501–12.

51. Brown KA, Ditchey RV. Human right ventricular end-systolic pressure-volume relation defined by maximal elastance. Circulation. 1988;78:81–91.

52. Suga H. Left ventricular time-varying pressure-volume ratio in systole as an index of myocardial inotropism. Jpn Heart J. 1971;12:153–60.

53. Brimioulle S, Wauthy P, Ewalenko P, Rondelet B, Vermeulen F, Kerbaul F, et al. Single-beat estimation of right ventricular end-systolic pressure-volume relationship. Am J Physiol Heart Circ Physiol. 2003;284:H1625–30.

54. Lafontant RR, Feinberg H, Katz LN. Pressure-volume relationships in right ventricle. Circ Res. 1962;11:699–701.

55. Chemla D, Antony I, Lecarpentier Y, Nitenberg A. Contribution of systemic vascular resistance and total arterial compliance to effective arterial elastance in humans. Am J Physiol Heart Circ Physiol. 2003;285:H614–20.

56. Suga H, Sagawa K, Shoukas AA. Load independence of the instantaneous pressure-volume ratio of the canine left ventricle and effects of epinephrine and heart rate on the ratio. Circ Res. 1973;32:314–22.

57. Suga H. Cardiac energetics: from E(max) to pressure-volume area. Clin Exp Pharmacol Physiol. 2003;30:580–5.

58. Vonk Noordegraaf A, Westerhof BE, Westerhof N. The relationship between the right ventricle and its load in pulmonary hypertension. J Am Coll Cardiol. 2017;69:236–43.

59. Naeije R, Vanderpool R, Peacock A, Badagliacca R. The right heart-pulmonary circulation unit. Heart Fail Clin. 2018;14:237–45.

60. Vonk Noordegraaf A, Chin KM, Haddad F, Hassoun PM, Hemnes AR, Hopkins SR, et al. Pathophysiology of the right ventricle and of the pulmonary circulation in pulmonary hypertension: an update. Eur Respir J. 2019;53:1801900.

61. Chemla D, Hébert JL, Coirault C, Salmeron S, Zamani K, Lecarpentier Y. Matching dicrotic notch and mean pulmonary artery pressures: implication for effective arterial elastance. Am J Physiol Heart Circ Physiol. 1996;271:1287–95.

62. Rain S, Andersen S, Najafi A, Gammelgaard Schultz J, da Silva Gonçalves Bós D, Handoko ML, et al. Right ventricular myocardial stiffness in experimental pulmonary arterial hypertension. Circ Heart Fail. 2016;9:e002636.

63. Rain S, Handoko ML, Trip P, Gan TJ, Westerhof N, Stienen G, et al. Right ventricular diastolic impairment in patients with pulmonary arterial hypertension. Circulation. 2013;128:2016–25.

64. Trip P, Rain S, Handoko ML, van der Bruggen C, Bogaard HJ, Marcus JT, et al. Clinical relevance of right ventricular diastolic stiffness in pulmonary hypertension. Eur Respir J. 2015;45:1603–12.

65. Sunagawa K, Yamada A, Senda Y, Kikuchi Y, Nakamura M, Shibahara T, et al. Estimation of the hydromotive source pressure from ejecting beats

of the left ventricle. IEEE Trans Biomed Eng. 1980;27:299–305.

66. Takeuchi M, Igarashi Y, Tomimoto S, Odake M, Hayashi T, Tsukamoto T, et al. Single-beat estimation of the slope of the end-systolic pressure-volume relation in the human left ventricle. Circulation. 1991;83:202–12.

67. Richter MJ, Peters D, Ghofrani HA, Naeije R, Roller F, Sommer N, et al. Evaluation and prognostic relevance of right ventricular-arterial coupling in pulmonary hypertension. Am J Respir Crit Care Med. 2020;201(1):116–9.

68. Farman GP, Gore D, Allen E, Schoenfelt K, Irving TC, de Tombe PP. Myosin head orientation: a structural determinant for the Frank-Starling relationship. Am J Physiol Heart Circ Physiol. 2011;300:H2155–60.

69. Cingolani HE, Perez NG, Cingolani OH, Ennis IL. The Anrep effect: 100 years later. Am J Physiol Heart Circ Physiol. 2013;304:H175–82.

70. Lamberts RR, Van Rijen MH, Sipkema P, Fransen P, Sys SU, Westerhof N. Coronary perfusion and muscle lengthening increase cardiac contraction: different stretch-triggered mechanisms. Am J Physiol Heart Circ Physiol. 2002;283:H1515–22.

Right Ventricular Pathobiology

Vineet Agrawal, Evan Brittain,
and Anna R. Hemnes

Introduction

Right ventricular (RV) function is a strong, independent prognostic indicator of outcomes in a number of disease states including valvular heart disease, ischemic and nonischemic cardiomyopathy, pulmonary embolism, and pulmonary arterial hypertension (PAH), among others [1–4]. Despite the recognized importance of RV function in these diseases, the underlying pathobiology of RV failure is poorly understood [5]. Global RV function is primarily determined by three dynamic factors: preload, afterload, and myocardial contractility. The primary inputs of RV afterload are pulsatile reflections from the main pulmonary arteries (PA) and early bifurcations, impedance of the proximal PAs, and arteriolar resistance (pulmonary vascular resistance, PVR). RV contractility is a reflection of loading conditions, adrenergic state, heart rate, medications, metabolic status, and ventricular interdependence. How these three facets of RV function alter or are altered by molecular changes in the RV myocardium are in their infancy of mechanistic understanding, but undoubtedly powerfully affect outcomes in situations of RV stress and may be independent targets of therapy. This chapter focuses on the pathobiology of right-heart failure in chronic pulmonary hypertension and highlights areas of recent advances in our molecular understanding of RV function and dysfunction.

RV Functional Decline and Recovery Are Highly Variable

RV failure is a heterogeneous clinical problem. Some patients develop severe RV failure at a given elevation in PA pressure and PVR whereas others maintain long-term preservation of RV function given the same hemodynamic profile. For example, many patients with congenital heart defects who develop Eisenmenger physiology maintain normal RV function for decades despite systemic PA pressures [6]. Relatively good outcomes in Eisenmenger patients are postulated to be related to the development of compensatory RV hypertrophy or persistence of the fetal gene program, but ultimately these mechanisms are not well understood. In many diseases, the RV exhibits a remarkable capacity for functional recovery after insult, for example after RV myocardial infarction or pulmonary thromboendarterectomy [7]. A molecular understanding of

V. Agrawal · E. Brittain
Division of Cardiovascular Medicine, Vanderbilt University Medical Center, Nashville, TN, USA
e-mail: vineet.agrawal@vumc.org;
evan.brittain@vumc.org

A. R. Hemnes (✉)
Division of Allergy, Pulmonary and Critical Care Medicine, Vanderbilt University Medical Center, Nashville, TN, USA
e-mail: anna.r.hemnes@vumc.org

the mechanisms mediating RV decline and recovery will improve our understanding of RV failure and aid in the development of RV-targeted therapy.

RV Failure Is in Part Independent of Pulmonary Hemodynamics

In diseases primarily affecting the pulmonary vasculature such as chronic thromboembolic pulmonary hypertension (CTEPH) and PAH, outcomes more closely mirror RV function and reverse remodeling than improvement in pulmonary hemodynamics [5]. There is increasing recognition that elevated RV afterload is not the sole determinant of RV failure and that RV function often declines despite significant improvement in pulmonary hemodynamics in response to medical therapy. Van de Veerdonk et al. showed that decline in RV function despite a clinically significant decline in PVR was associated with significantly worse survival in patients with PAH [8]. Additional evidence includes the good outcomes of patients with pulmonic valve stenosis and Eisenmenger's syndrome who develop adaptive RVH and the lack of RV failure in experimental models of RV pressure overload using pulmonary artery banding [6, 9]. These findings suggest that the development of RV failure depends not just on elevated afterload from pulmonary vascular resistance and large vessel stiffness but also on additional pathogenic mechanisms. Because RV functional decline is in part independent of pulmonary vascular disease, therapies directed at RV function may lead to improved outcomes. The lack of currently available RV-specific therapies stems from an incomplete understanding of the molecular mechanisms of RV failure.

Pathology of RV Failure

Despite well-characterized pulmonary vascular pathology, the pathology of RV failure has not been well studied. In addition to gross increase in mass, RV myocyte hypertrophy is well described

in the context of PAH [5]. Changes in capillary density or size, role of fibrosis, and differences across the clinically variable causes of RV failure are little described in humans. Several causes of acute RV failure, such as pulmonary embolism and RV infarction, are associated with RV myocardial necrosis [10], but this is not described in chronic causes of RV failure such as PAH. Little comparative information is available about RV pathology in the WHO groups of pulmonary hypertension, but data from humans suggesting that diseases such as scleroderma-associated PAH has disproportionate RV failure [11–13] may point to different patterns of RV pathology in this disease.

On a gross level, it is clear that RV hypertrophy is a key feature of the strained and failing RV. At the time of birth and switch from fetal to adult circulation patterns, the RV undergoes a profound shift from being a high-pressure, high-resistance pump to a low-pressure, high-flow conduit for blood to enter the pulmonary circulation. Mechanical changes including high oxygen tension in the lungs and closure of the patent ductus arteriosus facilitate this switch, but the molecular changes of the RV at this time are unknown. What is clear is that the RV in the adult is a thin-walled structure with a morphology that is described elsewhere in this edition. In situations of acquired increased PVR, the RV increases in size, i.e., hypertrophies, to transition from a flow conduit to a pressure pump. This switch is thought to be required to maintain cardiac output in the face of increased load stress and thus adaptive. However, over time, the RV often fails and thus transitions to maladaptive hypertrophy. In congenital heart disease lesions that include persistent elevations in pulmonary pressure after birth, the RV often retains the capacity to generate high pressures through persistent adaptive hypertrophy. This may underlie the well-described improved survival in congenital heart disease-associated PAH compared with idiopathic PAH in which the elevated pulmonary vascular resistance occurs in the adult circulation [14]. Molecular triggers of this switch from compensated hypertrophy to failing RV are presently unknown and active areas of research.

Molecular Mechanisms of RV Failure

Several molecular mechanisms have been identified to contribute to RV failure in animal models and humans including myocardial ischemia, neurohormonal activation, metabolic dysregulation and mitochondrial dysfunction, sex hormone signaling, and maladaptive myocyte hypertrophy. Ultimately, many of these processes potentiate one another leading to a cycle of worsening myocardial failure (Fig. 2.1). Chronic myocardial ischemia leads to mitochondrial dysfunction and abnormal energy substrate utilization that then fails to provide adequate ATP for efficient myocardial contraction. Ischemia is worsened by the development of maladaptive RVH and a compensatory increase in contractility is compromised by β(beta)-receptor downregulation from chronic neurohormonal stimulation. Much progress has been made in our understanding of these processes in recent years with most available data coming from experimental models of PAH and human cardiac imaging.

Ischemia and Angiogenesis

RV failure has been associated with both macro- and microvascular ischemia. We will touch on macrovascular ischemia first. Patients with PH develop increased myocardial wall stress due to increased RV pressure and dilation resulting in an increased myocardial oxygen demand [15]. A decrease in systemic blood pressure resulting from poor cardiac output combined with an increase in RV pressure augments a decrease in coronary perfusion pressure resulting in ischemia, often manifesting as chest pain in patients with PAH both at rest and with exercise [16]. Right ventricular myocardial ischemia has been documented in PAH using myocardial scintigraphy and correlates directly with increases in RV diastolic pressure [17]. Detailed study of coronary flow patterns in PAH demonstrates a decrease in systolic flow in the right coronary artery compared to healthy controls and a decrease in total flow with increasing RV mass, indicating an imbalance between myocardial supply and demand [18]. Additional factors may contribute to supply/demand mismatch in PAH such as coronary compression from increased wall tension and hypoxemia due to impaired gas exchange.

In addition, there is growing evidence of microvascular dysfunction in the RV as well [19]. Initially noted, capillary loss and failure of new capillary growth in proportion to myocyte hypertrophy were demonstrated to differentiate angio-proliferative models of experimental PAH from RV pressure-overload models. In an experimental

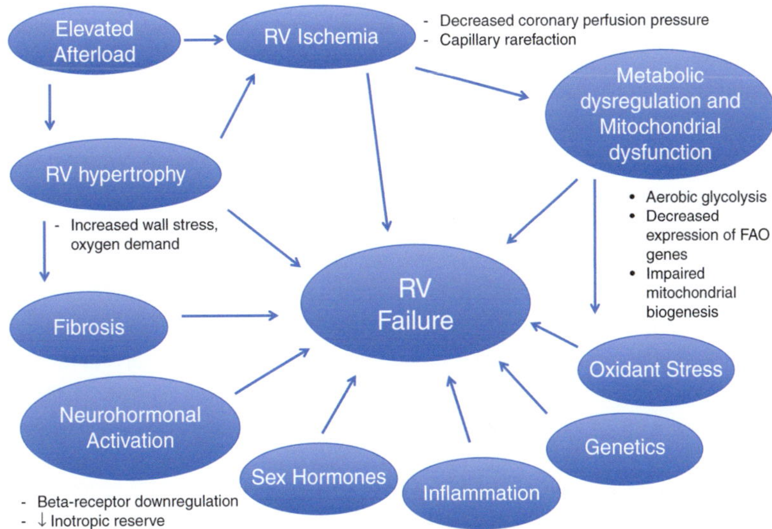

Fig. 2.1 Molecular mechanisms of RV failure. Alone or in combination, the various mechanisms pictured have been implicated in the development of RV failure. Several molecular mechanisms of RV failure such as RV ischemia and hypertrophy occur primarily as a result of elevated RV afterload. However, others such as metabolic dysregulation and mitochondrial dysfunction may be inherent features of PAH

model of PAH using the vascular endothelial growth factor (VEGF) receptor blocker (SuHx), RV failure was associated with decreased RV capillary density accompanied by a reduction in VEGF mRNA and protein transcription [9]. Capillary density and VEGF expression were unchanged in a model of early, adaptive hypertrophy using pulmonary artery banding, providing further evidence that RV failure is not governed solely by elevated afterload and highlighting the potentially critical role of decreased oxygen delivery in the failing right heart. Reductions in both VEGF and capillary density were shown in the monocrotaline model of PAH and genetically engineered reductions in VEGF have been shown to reduce capillary volume in the mouse myocardium. Capillary density is also decreased in RV myocardium from humans with PAH who died of RV failure [20]. These data suggest that VEGF production in PAH may be insufficient to induce adequate angiogenesis relative to cardiac hypertrophy, resulting in RV ischemia. While capillary rarefaction is present in RV failure, it is unknown if reversal of this condition improves RV function. One particular mechanism underlying rarefaction may be miR-126 which is decreased in failing human RVs and mouse models of RV failure, while increased expression of miR-126 was associated with improved vascular density and RV function [21]. Moreover, the relevance to human disease has been called into question by studies using stereology to define RV vascularity in which the failing human PAH RV had an increase in total vascular length [22]. Further study is needed to understand the role of vascular volume in the failing RV.

There is an emerging literature supporting dysregulated angiogenesis, not simply insufficient capillary volume, in the failing RV. There are many regulators of angiogenesis that are relevant to the RV [23] including genetic and epigenetic modulators [24, 25], transcription and growth factors, and immune cells that have been extensively reviewed elsewhere [26]. Perhaps best studied is VEG-F as described above. It is important to note that many studies use VEG-F inhibition in combination with hypoxia (SuHx) to study RV failure and thus there may be, not surprisingly, alterations in angiogenesis genes in this model compared to controls [27]. In addition, it is presently unknown if restoration of normal angiogenesis is beneficial to the RV. In general, animal studies have focused on models of pulmonary vascular disease where independent effects on the RV cannot be discerned [23].

Neurohormonal Activation in RV Failure

Neurohormonal activation is likely both a cause and a consequence of RV failure. Elevated RV afterload results in an increase in norepinephrine to increase inotropy and renal vein hypertension decreases renal perfusion resulting in renin-angiotensin-aldosterone systemic (RAAS) activation. As in left-heart failure, the initial compensatory mechanisms of sympathetic system and RAAS activation ultimately become detrimental in patients with right-heart failure. After prolonged stimulation, this results in downregulation of β(beta)-receptors impairing RV inotropic reserve and worsening RV failure. There is abundant evidence of neurohormonal activation in patients with RV failure: increased heart rate with reduced heart rate variability [28], increased plasma norepinephrine levels [29], decreased β_1-receptor density in the RV in PAH, and increased muscle sympathetic nerve activity [30]. In addition, hyponatremia, an indirect marker of RAAS activation, is associated with reduced survival and RV failure in PAH [31]. Within the RV, there are data that this system is relevant to RV failure. Boehm et al. demonstrated that increase in the pulmonary artery banding model increased mineralocorticoid receptor expression in the RV, though there was no improvement in RV function with eplerenone administration [32]. Focusing on angiotensin II, Friedberg and colleagues did demonstrate that losartan reduces RV hypertrophy and fibrosis in the pulmonary artery banding model, suggesting the relevance of this pathway to RV load stress responses [33].

The role of the sympathetic and parasympathetic nervous system has also been queried in the failing RV and has been recently described in detail [34]. There are limited data on therapeutic interventions to blunt neurohormonal activation in RV failure. In the case of β-blockers, clinical dogma has held that patients with RV failure are heart rate dependent and β-blockers would impair both chronotropic and inotropic reserve [35]. However, evidence from preclinical models of RV failure suggests a potential benefit from β-blockers [36–38]. In the SuHx and monocrotaline PAH models, carvedilol, a $\beta_{1,2}$- and α(alpha)$_1$-blocker with potentially beneficial pleiotropic effects, was found to improve RV function and increase exercise capacity compared to vehicle-treated animals. These effects were associated with an increase in protein kinase G, decreased myocardial fibrosis, and increased RV capillary density [38]. Similarly, the β_1-receptor blocker bisoprolol improved RV function in experimental PAH [23]. Early-phase clinical trials have been published with somewhat conflicting data on the effects of β-blockade in human PAH [39, 40], but they have generally not been adopted in clinical practice as therapy for RV failure. Elevated pulmonary aldosterone expression is present in PAH and correlates directly with endothelin-1 secretion [41]. Treatment with aldosterone antagonists in the SuHx and monocrotaline PAH models reduces pulmonary pressure and PVR without significant systemic side effects [42]; however there are no definitive trials of mineralocorticoid receptor antagonists in RV failure, only demonstrations of their safety [43]. Interestingly, recent data has suggested that impaired parasympathetic nervous system activity is present in PAH-associated RV failure and that drugs to increase activity may be beneficial [44]. Human trials are, however, presently lacking on these interventions.

Right Ventricular Metabolism and Mitochondrial Function

In patients with PH, chronically increased pulmonary pressure and pulmonary vascular resistance result in a stimulus for compensatory RV hypertrophy (RVH), thereby increasing myocardial metabolic demand. Decreased coronary perfusion pressure and capillary rarefaction limit oxygen supply, leading to RV ischemia and oxygen supply/demand mismatch. Evidence from both experimental models and human PAH suggests that the ability of the myocardium to maintain energy substrate flexibility in the setting of RVH and ischemia is an important determinant of RV failure. In the normal adult heart, fatty acid oxidation accounts for the majority of energy supply and metabolic flexibility exists to use glucose as an additional fuel source. Recent evidence suggests that RVH and RV failure is associated with increased utilization of glycolysis for ATP production, even in the setting of abundant oxygen when oxidative metabolism would otherwise be used [45, 46]. This process, well described in cancer cells, is hypothesized to be advantageous because these cells are less reliant on oxygen for energy production and can therefore proliferate in regions of relative hypoxia [47]. Direct measurement of increased RV glycolysis has been demonstrated in the monocrotaline PAH model [48]. Increased glycolysis (and decreased glucose oxidation) in this model is shown to be due to increased pyruvate dehydrogenase kinase (PDK) activity, which inhibits conversion of pyruvate (the product of glycolysis) to acetyl CoA, the substrate for Krebs cycle initiation. Failure to produce additional ATP from glucose oxidation results in decreased oxygen consumption and impaired RV function. Increased RV glucose uptake in human PAH has been shown in several studies using ^{18}F-fluorodeoxyglucose (FDG) positron-emission tomography (PET) [49–51]. Although this suggests an increase in glycolysis given the findings in experimental PAH, it is difficult to draw definitive conclusions because FDG uptake does not directly measure glycolysis but simply glucose uptake. Combination of FDG with other PET tracers measuring oxidative metabolism may help determine the relative activity of glycolysis and fatty acid oxidation in the human RV.

Glucose oxidation and fatty acid oxidation are reciprocating processes in the mitochondria—as one increases the other decreases and vice versa through Randle cycle [52]. This feedback facilitates metabolic flexibility, which is particularly critical for myocardial function in times of nutritional restriction. This cycle has been exploited for therapeutic purposes in experimental PAH in which the PDK inhibitor dichloroacetate and fatty acid oxidation inhibitors trimetazidine and ranolazine have improved RV function [53, 54]. However, recent data from our group and others has shown that impaired fatty acid oxidation may underlie RV failure in PAH [55–58]. Our group first demonstrated that in both human PAH RVs and in a rodent model of BMPR2 mutation with RV failure, there is lipid deposition consistent with lipotoxicity. This lipid accumulation is due to both increased lipid import into cardiomyocytes and impaired mitochondrial fatty acid oxidation, and the net result is increased cytoplasmic triglyceride and ceramide causing lipotoxicity [56, 57]. Others have demonstrated similar findings in the SuHx rodent model [58]. Importantly, lipid deposition is not a unique feature of end-stage RV failure and is demonstrable in humans with early RV strain [55]. Whether lipid deposition is reversible is an unanswered question. There is some preliminary data from a pilot study of metformin, which enhances fatty acid oxidation in addition to increasing glucose sensitivity, that this drug may reduce RV lipid content in humans with PAH [59], but more data is needed. Other approaches to modulating fatty acid oxidation such as PPARγ have shown promise in pre-clinical studies [27, 60, 61] and may be appropriate for further study in humans.

Mitochondrial dysfunction is present in both adaptive and maladaptive RVH and forms the basis for the abnormal energy metabolism observed in RV failure described above. RV failure in the monocrotaline model of PAH is associated with decreased expression of genes required for fatty acid oxidation and mitochondrial biogenesis as well as reduction in mitochondria number per gram of tissue and oxidative capacity [62]. Similar mitochondrial dysfunction was not observed in a pulmonary artery banding model suggesting that mitochondrial metabolic remodeling may be an inherent feature of RV failure in PAH and not simply a consequence of elevated RV afterload. The observation of mitochondrial hyperpolarization in RV tissue from humans with

PH further indicates the presence of mitochondrial dysfunction in RVH [63]. Dysfunction in mitochondria including number, size, and master regulators of biogenesis has been extensively studied and published in PAH and well described elsewhere [23].

There are early trials of metabolic interventions in the failing RV in PAH targeting RV metabolism. The pilot study of metformin was discussed above. Dichloroacetate, an inhibitor of PDK, has been studied in a clinical trial where its effect was primarily in the pulmonary vasculature and appeared to be modulated by sirtuin-3 and uncoupled protein 2 gene variants [64]. Clinical trials of ranolazine, which inhibits fatty acid oxidation, are presently listed in clinicaltrials.gov but have not been published yet. In summary, while it is well accepted that there is metabolic dysfunction in the RV in PAH, many questions remain about how, when, and if intervention on these abnormalities will improve RV function.

Sex Hormones

Although PAH has been known for decades to be female predominant [65, 66], it has recently come to light that males with PAH tend to have worse outcomes than women with PAH [67, 68]. This observation has led to studies of the effects of sex hormones on the RV, as poorer RV function has been identified in males with PAH [68–70]. Not surprisingly, cardiomyocytes express receptors for sex hormones and are capable of sex hormone production and metabolism [71, 72]. Findings of sex hormones in the plasma of patients with PAH have been recently reviewed [23] and there is a growing literature on the molecular underpinnings of these observations. Estrogen (E2) has been recently identified to have RV-protective effects. Using hormone depletion and repletion experiments, Frump et al. showed that E2 reduces RV hypertrophy, improves function, and, on a molecular level, reduces pro-apoptotic signaling, oxidative stress, and mitochondrial dysfunction using rodent models [73–75]. There has been limited research on testosterone in the RV, where it appears to cause increased fibrosis and excess mortality in the pulmonary artery banding model [76]. There are ongoing trials of modulation of estrogen signaling using tamoxifen (clinicaltrials.gov NCT03528902) and anastrozole (clinicaltrials.gov NCT03229499) and the effects of these interventions on RV function will be closely assessed. A pilot study of anastrozole suggested potential safety for the RV [77].

Other Causes of RV Failure

Additional contributing mechanisms for RV failure may include inflammation, oxidant stress, and fibrosis though the relative importance of these processes is not well understood. Myocardial fibrosis is present on cardiac MRI (CMR) in patients with RV failure as well as histology in experimental models of PAH. Fibrosis on CMR correlates with pulmonary hemodynamics and independently predicts clinical worsening in PAH [78]. Whether fibrosis is a consequence of chronic myocardial mechanical strain or myocardial ischemia [46] or an independent pathologic process as a result of endothelial cell dysfunction is not known [79, 80]. Recent work has called into question the hypothesis that all fibrosis is maladaptive as there may be a role for collagen in strengthening the myocardium in an adaptive effort to preserve function in the context of increased load stress [81]. Evidence of RV fibrosis and its molecular origins have been reviewed elsewhere [81].

Genetics of RV Failure

BMPR2

A major hindrance to the study of right-heart failure has been the limitations of currently available animal models. Monocrotaline, SuHx, and pulmonary artery banding all have heterogeneous effects on RV size and function and are of questionable relevance to human diseases. Transgenic models would facilitate a more detailed molecular dissection of the signaling pathways key to the development of RV failure. Archer et al. have used the fawn-hooded rat to identify the key metabolic derangements in RV failure [82]. Our group has described worse survival in patients with heritable PAH compared with idiopathic PAH that may be due to impaired RV compensation in heritable PAH [83]. Heritable PAH is most commonly associated with mutations in the bone morphogenic protein receptor type 2 (BMPR2), for which there are transgenic rodent models [84, 85]. As above, we have found evidence of reduced fatty acid oxidation intermediaries associated with lipid deposition in humans with heritable PAH and in transgenic mice with similar mutation that is universally expressed [55–57]. Moreover, hypertrophic responses in this strain appear to be impaired [86]. The use of transgenic models to study RV failure will facilitate a deeper molecular understanding of the mechanisms that drive the development of this syndrome with particular relevance to humans and potentially point to new, effective therapeutic targets.

RV Failure in Non-group 1 PH

Despite the growing recognition of the importance of RV failure in non-group 1 PH, little is known about the molecular mechanisms underlying RV failure in the absence of PAH. Clinical and translational studies, however, suggest that PAH-related RV failure may share pathophysiologic overlap with PAH-related RV failure, specifically with respect to metabolic dysregulation [23, 87–89]. In the subset of patients with PH due to left-heart disease, patients with concomitant obesity or metabolic syndrome are at the greatest risk for adverse structural RV remodeling and development of RV failure [89, 90]. Supporting the connection between obesity, metabolic syndrome, and RV failure, recent translational studies have also identified that obesity is associated with activation of a unique transcriptional program in myocardial biopsies from patients with heart failure and RV dysfunction, and isolated RV cardiomyocytes from obese patients with heart failure show impaired contractility compared to nonobese patients with heart failure [91]. However, the precise molecular pathways that lead to RV failure from obesity and metabolic syndrome in non-PAH-related conditions are less well understood because relatively few preclinical models have systematically investigated RV function [92–94]. In two models utilizing rodents prone to obesity and insulin resistance in the presence of high-fat diet, RV dysfunction was an early manifestation of heart failure [93, 94], somewhat similar to phenotypes that have been identified in humans [87]. One study identified the natriuretic peptide clearance receptor (NPRC), a gene highly upregulated in the setting of obesity and associated with insulin resistance [95], as the most upregulated gene in the diseased RV [94]. The second study identified both cardiac and extracardiac dysregulation of metabolism by sirtuin-3, an intracellular regulator of mitochondrial function and AMP kinase, as a primary driver of RV dysfunction [93]. Broad metabolic dysregulation and mitochondrial dysfunction have also been reported in multiple studies of diabetic cardiomyopathy-related RV failure (reviewed in [96]).

Future Directions

Preclinical studies of metabolic modulation have shown promise for the treatment of RV failure and pilot clinical trials of metabolic therapy for RV failure in human PAH are underway (metformin and exercise clinicaltrials.gov NCT03617458). If successful, metabolic modulators may represent the first RV-specific heart failure therapies. Whether these therapies will be efficacious in RV failure of other etiologies is unknown. A parallel focus on RV function in addition to pulmonary vascular disease is critical given the strong prognostic power of RV function in PAH. Future clinical trials of pulmonary vasodilator therapies should also include RV-specific functional outcomes [97]. Additional clinical studies are needed to determine the optimal medical management for acute RV failure, including a direct comparison of different inotropic agents.

The current noninvasive evaluation of RV function with echocardiography and CMR is largely descriptive and does not allow for early detection of impending RV failure. Molecular imaging tools that provide a more mechanistic understanding of RV pathophysiology should be expanded and potentially extended into clinical practice. PET imaging with metabolic tracers such as FDG, ^{11}C acetate, and others can provide detailed information about mitochondrial function and metabolic remodeling in the RV. PET may ultimately provide superior biomarkers and clinical trial endpoints of therapeutic efficacy compared to conventional metrics. Finally, given the impact of metabolic dysregulation on RV function, broad metabolite profiling may provide novel insights into the metabolic etiology of both acute and chronic RV failure. Because they are downstream of transcription, translation, and posttranslational modifications, metabolites reflect early alteration in the body's response to disease. A metabolomics approach has previously been used to detect early metabolic changes after myocardial infarction and identify markers of cardiopulmonary fitness [98, 99] and may bear fruit in the study of RV failure.

References

1. Borer JS, Bonow RO. Contemporary approach to aortic and mitral regurgitation. Circulation. 2003;108:2432–8.
2. Ghio S, Gavazzi A, Campana C, et al. Independent and additive prognostic value of right ventricular systolic function and pulmonary artery pressure in patients with chronic heart failure. J Am Coll Cardiol. 2001;37:183–8.
3. Goldhaber SZ, Visani L, De Rosa M. Acute pulmonary embolism: clinical outcomes in the International Cooperative Pulmonary Embolism Registry (ICOPER). Lancet. 1999;353:1386–9.
4. Forfia PR, Fisher MR, Mathai SC, et al. Tricuspid annular displacement predicts survival in pulmonary hypertension. Am J Respir Crit Care Med. 2006;174:1034–41.
5. Voelkel NF, Quaife RA, Leinwand LA, et al. Right ventricular function and failure: report of a National Heart, Lung, and Blood Institute working group on cellular and molecular mechanisms of right heart failure. Circulation. 2006;114:1883–91.

6. Hopkins WE, Ochoa LL, Richardson GW, Trulock EP. Comparison of the hemodynamics and survival of adults with severe primary pulmonary hypertension or Eisenmenger syndrome. J Heart Lung Transplant. 1996;15:100–5.

7. Brittain EL, Hemnes AR, Keebler M, Lawson M, Byrd BF 3rd, Disalvo T. Right ventricular plasticity and functional imaging. Pulm Circ. 2012;2:309–26.

8. van de Veerdonk MC, Kind T, Marcus JT, et al. Progressive right ventricular dysfunction in patients with pulmonary arterial hypertension responding to therapy. J Am Coll Cardiol. 2011;58:2511–9.

9. Bogaard HJ, Natarajan R, Henderson SC, et al. Chronic pulmonary artery pressure elevation is insufficient to explain right heart failure. Circulation. 2009;120:1951–60.

10. Watts JA, Marchick MR, Kline JA. Right ventricular heart failure from pulmonary embolism: key distinctions from chronic pulmonary hypertension. J Card Fail. 2010;16:250–9.

11. Tedford RJ, Mudd JO, Girgis RE, et al. Right ventricular dysfunction in systemic sclerosis-associated pulmonary arterial hypertension. Circ Heart Fail. 2013;6:953–63.

12. Mathai SC, Bueso M, Hummers LK, et al. Disproportionate elevation of N-terminal pro-brain natriuretic peptide in scleroderma-related pulmonary hypertension. Eur Respir J. 2010;35:95–104.

13. Hsu S, Kokkonen-Simon KM, Kirk JA, et al. Right ventricular myofilament functional differences in humans with systemic sclerosis-associated versus idiopathic pulmonary arterial hypertension. Circulation. 2018;137:2360–70.

14. McLaughlin VV, Presberg KW, Doyle RL, et al. Prognosis of pulmonary arterial hypertension: ACCP evidence-based clinical practice guidelines. Chest. 2004;126:78S–92S.

15. Hein S, Arnon E, Kostin S, et al. Progression from compensated hypertrophy to failure in the pressure-overloaded human heart: structural deterioration and compensatory mechanisms. Circulation. 2003;107:984–91.

16. Ross R. Right ventricular hypertension as a cause of precordial pain. Am Heart J. 1961;61:134–5.

17. Gomez A, Bialostozky D, Zajarias A, et al. Right ventricular ischemia in patients with primary pulmonary hypertension. J Am Coll Cardiol. 2001;38:1137–42.

18. van Wolferen SA, Marcus JT, Westerhof N, et al. Right coronary artery flow impairment in patients with pulmonary hypertension. Eur Heart J. 2008;29:120–7.

19. Kajiya M, Hirota M, Inai Y, et al. Impaired NO-mediated vasodilation with increased superoxide but robust EDHF function in right ventricular arterial microvessels of pulmonary hypertensive rats. Am J Physiol Heart Circ Physiol. 2007;292:H2737–44.

20. Ruiter G, Ying Wong Y, de Man FS, et al. Right ventricular oxygen supply parameters are decreased in human and experimental pulmonary hypertension. J Heart Lung Transplant. 2013;32:231–40.

21. Potus F, Ruffenach G, Dahou A, Thebault C, Breuils-Bonnet S, Tremblay E, Nadeau V, Paradis R, Graydon C, Wong R, Johnson I, Paulin R, Lajoie AC, Perron J, Charbonneau E, Joubert P, Pibarot P, Michelakis ED, Provencher S, Bonnet S. Downregulation of miR-126 contributes to the failing right ventricle in pulmonary arterial hypertension. Circulation. 2017; https://doi.org/10.1161/CIRCULATIONAHA.115.016382.

22. Graham BB, Koyanagi D, Kandasamy B, Tuder RM. Right ventricle vasculature in human pulmonary hypertension assessed by stereology. Am J Respir Crit Care Med. 2017;196:1075–7.

23. Agrawal V, Lahm T, Hansmann G, Hemnes AR. Molecular mechanisms of right ventricular dysfunction in pulmonary arterial hypertension: focus on the coronary vasculature, sex hormones, and glucose/lipid metabolism. Cardiovasc Diagn Ther. 2020;10:1522–40.

24. Suen CM, Chaudhary KR, Deng Y, Jiang B, Stewart DJ. Fischer rats exhibit maladaptive structural and molecular right ventricular remodelling in severe pulmonary hypertension: a genetically prone model for right heart failure. Cardiovasc Res. 2019;115:788–99.

25. Reddy S, Zhao M, Hu DQ, et al. Dynamic microRNA expression during the transition from right ventricular hypertrophy to failure. Physiol Genomics. 2012;44:562–75.

26. Frump AL, Bonnet S, de Jesus Perez VA, Lahm T. Emerging role of angiogenesis in adaptive and maladaptive right ventricular remodeling in pulmonary hypertension. Am J Physiol Lung Cell Mol Physiol. 2018;314:L443–L60.

27. Legchenko E, Chouvarine P, Borchert P, et al. PPARgamma agonist pioglitazone reverses pulmonary hypertension and prevents right heart failure via fatty acid oxidation. Sci Transl Med. 2018;10(438):eaao0303.

28. Wensel R, Jilek C, Dorr M, et al. Impaired cardiac autonomic control relates to disease severity in pulmonary hypertension. Eur Respir J. 2009;34:895–901.

29. Nootens M, Kaufmann E, Rector T, et al. Neurohormonal activation in patients with right ventricular failure from pulmonary hypertension: relation to hemodynamic variables and endothelin levels. J Am Coll Cardiol. 1995;26:1581–5.

30. Velez-Roa S, Ciarka A, Najem B, Vachiery JL, Naeije R, van de Borne P. Increased sympathetic nerve activity in pulmonary artery hypertension. Circulation. 2004;110:1308–12.

31. Forfia PR, Mathai SC, Fisher MR, et al. Hyponatremia predicts right heart failure and poor survival in pulmonary arterial hypertension. Am J Respir Crit Care Med. 2008;177:1364–9.

32. Boehm M, Arnold N, Braithwaite A, et al. Eplerenone attenuates pathological pulmonary vascular rather than right ventricular remodeling in pulmonary arterial hypertension. BMC Pulm Med. 2018;18:41.

33. Friedberg MK, Cho MY, Li J, et al. Adverse biventricular remodeling in isolated right ventricular

hypertension is mediated by increased transforming growth factor-beta1 signaling and is abrogated by angiotensin receptor blockade. Am J Respir Cell Mol Biol. 2013;49:1019–28.

34. Maron BA, Leopold JA, Hemnes AR. Metabolic syndrome, neurohumoral modulation, and pulmonary arterial hypertension. Br J Pharmacol. 2020;177:1457–71.

35. Provencher S, Herve P, Jais X, et al. Deleterious effects of beta-blockers on exercise capacity and hemodynamics in patients with portopulmonary hypertension. Gastroenterology. 2006;130:120–6.

36. Okumura K, Kato H, Honjo O, et al. Carvedilol improves biventricular fibrosis and function in experimental pulmonary hypertension. J Mol Med (Berl). 2015;93:663–74.

37. Drake JI, Gomez-Arroyo J, Dumur CI, et al. Chronic carvedilol treatment partially reverses the right ventricular failure transcriptional profile in experimental pulmonary hypertension. Physiol Genomics. 2013;45:449–61.

38. Bogaard HJ, Natarajan R, Mizuno S, et al. Adrenergic receptor blockade reverses right heart remodeling and dysfunction in pulmonary hypertensive rats. Am J Respir Crit Care Med. 2010;182(5):652–60.

39. Farha S, Saygin D, Park MM, et al. Pulmonary arterial hypertension treatment with carvedilol for heart failure: a randomized controlled trial. JCI Insight. 2017;2(16):e95240.

40. van Campen JS, de Boer K, van de Veerdonk MC, et al. Bisoprolol in idiopathic pulmonary arterial hypertension: an explorative study. Eur Respir J. 2016;48:787–96.

41. Maron BA, Opotowsky AR, Landzberg MJ, Loscalzo J, Waxman AB, Leopold JA. Plasma aldosterone levels are elevated in patients with pulmonary arterial hypertension in the absence of left ventricular heart failure: a pilot study. Eur J Heart Fail. 2013;15:277–83.

42. Maron BA, Zhang YY, White K, et al. Aldosterone inactivates the endothelin-B receptor via a cysteinyl thiol redox switch to decrease pulmonary endothelial nitric oxide levels and modulate pulmonary arterial hypertension. Circulation. 2012;126:963–74.

43. Safdar Z, Frost A, Basant A, Deswal A, O'Brian Smith E, Entman M. Spironolactone in pulmonary arterial hypertension: results of a cross-over study. Pulm Circ. 2020;10:2045894019898030.

44. da Silva Goncalves Bos D, Van Der Bruggen CEE, Kurakula K, et al. Contribution of impaired parasympathetic activity to right ventricular dysfunction and pulmonary vascular remodeling in pulmonary arterial hypertension. Circulation. 2018;137:910–24.

45. Piao L, Fang YH, Cadete VJ, et al. The inhibition of pyruvate dehydrogenase kinase improves impaired cardiac function and electrical remodeling in two models of right ventricular hypertrophy: resuscitating the hibernating right ventricle. J Mol Med. 2010;88:47–60.

46. Drake JI, Bogaard HJ, Mizuno S, et al. Molecular signature of a right heart failure program in chronic severe pulmonary hypertension. Am J Respir Cell Mol Biol. 2011;45:1239–47.

47. Vander Heiden MG, Cantley LC, Thompson CB. Understanding the Warburg effect: the metabolic requirements of cell proliferation. Science. 2009;324:1029–33.

48. Piao L, Marsboom G, Archer SL. Mitochondrial metabolic adaptation in right ventricular hypertrophy and failure. J Mol Med. 2010;88:1011–20.

49. Bokhari S, Raina A, Rosenweig EB, et al. PET imaging may provide a novel biomarker and understanding of right ventricular dysfunction in patients with idiopathic pulmonary arterial hypertension. Circ Cardiovasc Imaging. 2011;4:641–7.

50. Oikawa M, Kagaya Y, Otani H, et al. Increased [18F] fluorodeoxyglucose accumulation in right ventricular free wall in patients with pulmonary hypertension and the effect of epoprostenol. J Am Coll Cardiol. 2005;45:1849–55.

51. Mielniczuk LM, Birnie D, Ziadi MC, et al. Relation between right ventricular function and increased right ventricular [18F]fluorodeoxyglucose accumulation in patients with heart failure. Circ Cardiovasc Imaging. 2011;4:59–66.

52. Randle PJ, Garland PB, Hales CN, Newsholme EA. The glucose fatty-acid cycle. Its role in insulin sensitivity and the metabolic disturbances of diabetes mellitus. Lancet. 1963;1:785–9.

53. Archer SL, Fang YH, Ryan JJ, Piao L. Metabolism and bioenergetics in the right ventricle and pulmonary vasculature in pulmonary hypertension. Pulm Circ. 2013;3:144–52.

54. Fang YH, Piao L, Hong Z, et al. Therapeutic inhibition of fatty acid oxidation in right ventricular hypertrophy: exploiting Randle's cycle. J Mol Med (Berl). 2012;90:31–43.

55. Brittain EL, Talati M, Fessel JP, et al. Fatty acid metabolic defects and right ventricular lipotoxicity in human pulmonary arterial hypertension. Circulation. 2016;133(20):1936–44.

56. Talati MH, Brittain EL, Fessel JP, et al. Mechanisms of lipid accumulation in the bone morphogenic protein receptor 2 mutant right ventricle. Am J Respir Crit Care Med. 2016;194(6):719–28.

57. Hemnes AR, Brittain EL, Trammell AW, et al. Evidence for right ventricular lipotoxicity in heritable pulmonary arterial hypertension. Am J Respir Crit Care Med. 2014;189:325–34.

58. Graham BB, Kumar R, Mickael C, et al. Severe pulmonary hypertension is associated with altered right ventricle metabolic substrate uptake. Am J Physiol Lung Cell Mol Physiol. 2015;309:L435–40.

59. Brittain EL, Niswender K, Agrawal V, et al. Mechanistic phase II clinical trial of metformin in pulmonary arterial hypertension. J Am Heart Assoc. 2020;9:e018349.

60. Hansmann G, de Jesus Perez VA, Alastalo TP, et al. An antiproliferative BMP-2/PPARgamma/apoE axis in human and murine SMCs and its role in pulmonary hypertension. J Clin Invest. 2008;118:1846–57.

61. Hansmann G, Wagner RA, Schellong S, et al. Pulmonary arterial hypertension is linked to insulin resistance and reversed by peroxisome proliferator-activated receptor-gamma activation. Circulation. 2007;115:1275–84.

62. Gomez-Arroyo J, Mizuno S, Szczepanek K, et al. Metabolic gene remodeling and mitochondrial dysfunction in failing right ventricular hypertrophy secondary to pulmonary arterial hypertension. Circ Heart Fail. 2013;6:136–44.

63. Nagendran J, Gurtu V, Fu DZ, et al. A dynamic and chamber-specific mitochondrial remodeling in right ventricular hypertrophy can be therapeutically targeted. J Thorac Cardiovasc Surg. 2008;136:168–78, 78.e1–3.

64. Michelakis ED, Gurtu V, Webster L, et al. Inhibition of pyruvate dehydrogenase kinase improves pulmonary arterial hypertension in genetically susceptible patients. Sci Transl Med. 2017;9(413):eaao4583.

65. D'Alonzo GE, Barst RJ, Ayres SM, et al. Survival in patients with primary pulmonary hypertension. Results from a national prospective registry. Ann Intern Med. 1991;115:343–9.

66. Loyd JE, Butler MG, Foroud TM, Conneally PM, Phillips JA III, Newman JH. Genetic anticipation and abnormal gender ratio at birth in familial primary pulmonary hypertension. Am J Respir Crit Care Med. 1995;152:93–7.

67. Humbert M, Sitbon O, Yaici A, et al. Survival in incident and prevalent cohorts of patients with pulmonary arterial hypertension. Eur Respir J. 2010;36(3):549–55.

68. Benza RL, Miller DP, Barst RJ, Badesch DB, Frost AE, McGoon MD. An evaluation of long-term survival from time of diagnosis in pulmonary arterial hypertension from the REVEAL Registry. Chest. 2012;142:448–56.

69. Jacobs W, van de Veerdonk MC, Trip P, et al. The right ventricle explains sex differences in survival in idiopathic pulmonary arterial hypertension. Chest. 2014;145:1230–6.

70. Swift AJ, Capener D, Hammerton C, et al. Right ventricular sex differences in patients with idiopathic pulmonary arterial hypertension characterised by magnetic resonance imaging: pair-matched case controlled study. PLoS One. 2015;10:e0127415.

71. Mendelsohn ME, Karas RH. Molecular and cellular basis of cardiovascular gender differences. Science. 2005;308:1583–7.

72. Thum T, Borlak J. Testosterone, cytochrome P450, and cardiac hypertrophy. FASEB J. 2002;16:1537–49.

73. Frump AL, Goss KN, Vayl A, et al. Estradiol improves right ventricular function in rats with severe angioproliferative pulmonary hypertension: effects of endogenous and exogenous sex hormones. Am J Physiol Lung Cell Mol Physiol. 2015;308:L873–90.

74. Cheng TC, Philip JL, Tabima DM, et al. Estrogen receptor alpha prevents right ventricular diastolic dysfunction and fibrosis in female rats. Am J Physiol Heart Circ Physiol. 2020;319(6):H1459–73.

75. Lahm T, Frump AL, Albrecht ME, et al. 17beta-Estradiol mediates superior adaptation of right ventricular function to acute strenuous exercise in female rats with severe pulmonary hypertension. Am J Physiol Lung Cell Mol Physiol. 2016;311:L375–88.

76. Hemnes AR, Maynard KB, Champion HC, et al. Testosterone negatively regulates right ventricular load stress responses in mice. Pulm Circ. 2012;2:352–8.

77. Kawut SM, Archer-Chicko CL, DeMichele A, et al. Anastrozole in pulmonary arterial hypertension. A randomized, double-blind, placebo-controlled trial. Am J Respir Crit Care Med. 2017;195:360–8.

78. Freed BH, Gomberg-Maitland M, Chandra S, et al. Late gadolinium enhancement cardiovascular magnetic resonance predicts clinical worsening in patients with pulmonary hypertension. J Cardiovasc Magn Reson. 2012;14:11.

79. Zeisberg EM, Ma Q, Juraszek AL, et al. Morphogenesis of the right ventricle requires myocardial expression of Gata4. J Clin Invest. 2005;115:1522–31.

80. Voelkel NF, Gomez-Arroyo J, Abbate A, Bogaard HJ. Mechanisms of right heart failure—a work in progress and a plea for failure prevention. Pulm Circ. 2013;3:137–43.

81. Andersen S, Nielsen-Kudsk JE, Vonk Noordegraaf A, de Man FS. Right ventricular fibrosis. Circulation. 2019;139:269–85.

82. Piao L, Fang YH, Parikh K, Ryan JJ, Toth PT, Archer SL. Cardiac glutaminolysis: a maladaptive cancer metabolism pathway in the right ventricle in pulmonary hypertension. J Mol Med (Berl). 2013;91:1185–97.

83. Brittain EL, Pugh ME, Wheeler LA, et al. Shorter survival in familial versus idiopathic pulmonary arterial hypertension is associated with hemodynamic markers of impaired right ventricular function. Pulm Circ. 2013;3:589–98.

84. Johnson JA, Hemnes AR, Perrien DS, et al. Cytoskeletal defects in Bmpr2-associated pulmonary arterial hypertension. Am J Physiol Lung Cell Mol Physiol. 2012;302:L474–84.

85. West J, Fagan K, Steudel W, et al. Pulmonary hypertension in transgenic mice expressing a dominant-negative BMPRII gene in smooth muscle. Circ Res. 2004;94:1109–14.

86. West J, Niswender KD, Johnson JA, et al. A potential role for insulin resistance in experimental pulmonary hypertension. Eur Respir J. 2013;41:861–71.

87. Obokata M, Reddy YNV, Pislaru SV, Melenovsky V, Borlaug BA. Evidence supporting the existence of a distinct obese phenotype of heart failure with preserved ejection fraction. Circulation. 2017;136:6–19.

88. Assad TR, Hemnes AR, Larkin EK, et al. Clinical and biological insights into combined post- and pre-capillary pulmonary hypertension. J Am Coll Cardiol. 2016;68:2525–36.

89. Gopal DM, Santhanakrishnan R, Wang YC, et al. Impaired right ventricular hemodynamics indi-

cate preclinical pulmonary hypertension in patients with metabolic syndrome. J Am Heart Assoc. 2015;4:e001597.

90. Obokata M, Reddy YNV, Melenovsky V, Pislaru S, Borlaug BA. Deterioration in right ventricular structure and function over time in patients with heart failure and preserved ejection fraction. Eur Heart J. 2019;40:689–97.

91. Aslam MI, Hahn VS, Jani V, Hus S, Sharma K, Kass DA. Reduced right ventricular sarcomere contractility in HFpEF with severe obesity. Circulation. 2020;143(9):965–7.

92. Meng Q, Lai YC, Kelly NJ, et al. Development of a mouse model of metabolic syndrome, pulmonary hypertension, and heart failure with preserved ejection fraction. Am J Respir Cell Mol Biol. 2017;56:497–505.

93. Lai YC, Tabima DM, Dube JJ, et al. SIRT3-AMP-activated protein kinase activation by nitrite and metformin improves hyperglycemia and normalizes pulmonary hypertension associated with heart failure with preserved ejection fraction. Circulation. 2016;133:717–31.

94. Agrawal V, Fortune N, Yu S, et al. Natriuretic peptide receptor C contributes to disproportionate right ventricular hypertrophy in a rodent model of obesity-induced heart failure with preserved ejection fraction with pulmonary hypertension. Pulm Circ. 2019;9:2045894019878599.

95. Wu W, Shi F, Liu D, et al. Enhancing natriuretic peptide signaling in adipose tissue, but not in muscle, protects against diet-induced obesity and insulin resistance. Sci Signal. 2017;10(489):eaam6870.

96. Kang Y, Wang S, Huang J, Cai L, Keller BB. Right ventricular dysfunction and remodeling in diabetic cardiomyopathy. Am J Physiol Heart Circ Physiol. 2019;316:H113–H22.

97. Archer SL. Riociguat for pulmonary hypertension—a glass half full. N Engl J Med. 2013;369:386–8.

98. Lewis GD, Farrell L, Wood MJ, et al. Metabolic signatures of exercise in human plasma. Sci Transl Med. 2010;2:33ra7.

99. Lewis GD, Wei R, Liu E, et al. Metabolite profiling of blood from individuals undergoing planned myocardial infarction reveals early markers of myocardial injury. J Clin Invest. 2008;118:3503–12.

Mario Boehm, Ralph Theo Schermuly,
and Baktybek Kojonazarov

Abbreviations

COPD	Chronic obstructive pulmonary disease
CTEPH	Chronic thromboembolic pulmonary hypertension
CYP3A4	Cytochrome P450
FDG	^{18}F-fluorodeoxyglucose
FHR	Fawn-hooded rat
HFD	High-fat diet
LAD	Left anterior descending
LHD	Left-heart disease
LV	Left ventricular
MCT	Monocrotaline
MCTP	Dehydromonocrotaline
MI	Myocardial infarction
MMP	Matrix metalloproteinase
MS	Metabolic syndrome
OSA	Obstructive sleep apnea
PA AcT	Pulmonary artery acceleration time
PAB	Pulmonary artery banding
PAH	Pulmonary arterial hypertension
PAP	Pulmonary artery pressure
PH	Pulmonary hypertension
PVR	Pulmonary vascular resistance
RV	Right ventricle
SUHx	Sugen plus hypoxia
TAC	Transverse aortic constriction
TUNEL	Terminal deoxynucleotidyl transferase dUTP nick end labeling
VEGF	Vascular endothelial growth factor

M. Boehm · R. T. Schermuly (✉)
Department of Pulmonary Pharmacotherapy,
Excellence Cluster Cardio-Pulmonary Institute,
Justus-Liebig University of Giessen, German Center
for Lung Research, Giessen, Germany
e-mail: Mario.boehm@innere.med.uni-giessen.de;
ralph.schermuly@innere.med.uni-giessen.de

B. Kojonazarov
Department of Pulmonary Pharmacotherapy,
Excellence Cluster Cardio-Pulmonary Institute,
Justus-Liebig University of Giessen, German Center
for Lung Research, Giessen, Germany

Department of Small Animal Imaging, Institute for
Lung Health, Justus-Liebig University of Giessen,
Giessen, Germany
e-mail: baktybek.kojonazarov@innere.med.uni-giessen.de

Introduction

The ability of the right ventricle to adapt to changes in load is the most important determinant of survival in patients suffering from pulmonary arterial hypertension (PAH), despite a predominant occlusive pulmonary vasculopathy of pulmonary arteries [1–4]. Our knowledge of the molecular physiology and pathophysiology of RV adaptation and the transition towards failure in response to pressure or volume overload are still limited, and most data are derived from research on the left heart, with increasing efforts and studies focusing on the right ventricle of the heart [5]. However, molecular mechanisms

S. P. Gaine et al. (eds.), *The Right Heart*, https://doi.org/10.1007/978-3-030-78255-9_3

involved in left ventricular (LV) remodeling cannot be generalized to the right ventricle because the ventricles differ substantially in their developmental origin, morphology, and function. Furthermore, despite recent advances in the treatment of PAH which relieve symptoms, prognosis and long-term survival of patients are still poor [6]. Currently approved therapies act primarily through vasodilation of pulmonary vessels, leaving processes that drive the progressive narrowing of pulmonary vessels unchecked [7–9].

Therefore, novel, safe, and efficacious therapies are warranted that directly halt disease progression either by blocking fundamental disease-causing processes in the pulmonary vascular compartment or by intrinsically strengthening RV adaptation to an increased afterload burden in order to prevent or delay RV decompensation, failure, and death [10]. The development of such therapies requires testing of putative therapeutics in animal models that resemble key features of the human situation. Since pulmonary vascular and RV remodeling are multifaceted processes and, at least in part, dependent on each other, focused investigations into several animal models that reflect different angles of the disease-causing processes are often necessary to allow meaningful and clinically relevant conclusions [5, 11]. Scientists frequently combine knowledge acquired from different models to uncover key pathophysiological mechanisms of RV remodeling.

Numerous studies have demonstrated the benefits of large-animal pulmonary hypertension (PH) models by recapitulating humanlike PH lung phenotypes, in species including primates [12], calves [13], sheep [14], pigs [15], and dogs [16]. In addition, large animals occasionally allow modeling of mechanisms that are technically challenging in smaller animals such as rodents, due to size constraints. However, large-scale therapeutic testing in large animal models is economically and technically challenging, and increasingly perceived as inacceptable for ethical reasons [17]. The practical advantages of rodents over many large animals include their short gestation period and low breeding and housing costs.

In addition, deciphering of the rodent genome together with the possibility of specific transgene insertion to generate custom genetically modified mouse and rat strains allows for detailed pharmacological as well as molecular-mechanistic studies with a clear focus on the cardiopulmonary system, aiming to better understand the physiology and pathology of human disease. The optimal phenotyping of such cardiopulmonary rodent animal models includes adequate longitudinal noninvasive imaging approaches (e.g., echocardiography or magnetic resonance imaging) of a single animal during disease progression combined with invasive intracardiac hemodynamic characterization of cardiopulmonary function. Technological advancements allow for such phenotyping approaches even in juvenile mice [5, 11]. Therefore, scientists increasingly take advantage of these techniques to closely monitor disease progression and gain a deeper understanding of the underlying disease mechanisms.

PH in small animal models is broadly defined as a chronic increase in PA/RV pressure, and PH rodent models are classified—in analogy to humans—according to the World Health Organization nomenclature (Table 3.1). This is important as some models are used across different classifications (such as the hypoxia mouse model), while others are difficult to assign to the given categories (such as genetically modified mice). Disease-related changes in RV structure and function are often a direct consequence of changes in pre- and/or afterload (Table 3.2), and therefore it is difficult to decipher whether therapeutic interventions primarily interfere with the pulmonary or with the cardiac compartment. Novel models, such as the pulmonary artery banding model, in which changes in RV structure and function can be studied without interfering afterload alterations, have already assisted scientists to decipher afterload-dependent and -independent effects of putative therapeutics (Fig. 3.1).

Although our understanding of RV adaptation and maladaptation has significantly improved over the years, detailed knowledge of the relevance of several (patho-) physiological features underlying the RV response to pressure overload, such as RV fibrosis, cardiomyocyte hypertrophy,

Table 3.1 World Health Organization classification of PH and small animal models

Group of PH	Animal models
Group 1 PAH	MCT-induced PAH in rats
	MCT + pneumonectomy in rats
	Sugen + hypoxia in rats and mice
	Fawn-hooded rat
	Schistosomiasis in mice
Group 2 PH due to left-heart disease	TAC in mice and rats
	Acute MI model
	Metabolic syndrome in mice and rats
Group 3 PH due to lung disease and/or hypoxia	Hypoxia-induced PH in mice and rats
	Chronic intermittent hypoxia in mice
	COPD models or smoke exposure model in mice
	Bleomycin-induced pulmonary fibrosis
	Lung cancer-associated PH in mice
Group 4 CTEPH	Repeated microembolization with microspheres in rats
Group 5 PH with unclear and/or multifactorial mechanism	–

COPD chronic obstructive pulmonary disease, *CTEPH* chronic thromboembolic pulmonary hypertension, *MCT* monocrotaline, *MI* myocardial infarction, *PAH* pulmonary arterial hypertension, *PH* pulmonary hypertension, *TAC* transaortic constriction

Table 3.2 Animal models and the right ventricle

Animal model	Precapillary arteriopathy	Plexiform-like lesions	RVSP	RVH	RV function	RV fibrosis	RV vascularization
MCT rat model	↑+	–	↑+	↑+	↓+	↑+	↓+
MCT + pneumonectomy	↑+	↑+	↑+	↑+	↓+	NA	NA
Chronic hypoxia in rats	↑+	–	↑+	↑+	↓+	↑+	NA
Chronic hypoxia in mice	↑+	–	↑+	↑+	↓+	↑+	NA
SUHx in rats	↑+	↑+	↑+	↑+	↓+	↑+	↓
SUHx in mice	↑+	↑+	↑+	↑+	↓+	NA	NA
Lung cancer-associated PH in mice	↑+	–	↑+	↑+	↓+	↑+	NA
PAB in rats	–	–	↑+	↑+	↓ or ↔	↑ or ↔	↓ or ↔
PAB in mice	–	–	↑+	↑+	↓+	↑+	NA
Schistosomiasis	↑+	↑+	↑+	↑+	↓+	NA	NA
TAC	↑+	–	↑+	↑+	↓+	↑+	NA
MI	↑+	–	↑+ or ↔	↑ or ↔	↓+	↑+	NA
Metabolic syndrome SAB + HFD + olanzapine	↑+	–	↑	NA	↓+	–	–
Smoke exposure model	↑+	–	↑+	↑+	NA	NA	NA
Intermittent hypoxia	↑+	–	↑+	↑+	NA	NA	NA

MCT monocrotaline-induced pulmonary arterial hypertension, *MI* myocardial infarction, *NA* data not available, *PAB* pulmonary artery banding, *RV* right ventricular, *RVH* right ventricular hypertrophy, *RVSP* right ventricular systolic pressure, *SUHx* Sugen + hypoxia model of pulmonary arterial hypertension, *TAC* transaortic constriction, *SAB* supracoronary artery banding, *HFD* high-fat diet, ↑+ present and increased, ↔ no change, ↓+ present and decreased, – not present

or decreased RV capillarization, is still lacking [5]. A better understanding of the mechanisms that underlie the transition from RV adaptation towards maladaptation, decompensation, and failure is a strong focus of current research [18]. Below, we focus on the right ventricle in rodent animal models and discuss mechanisms that affect the right ventricle and pulmonary

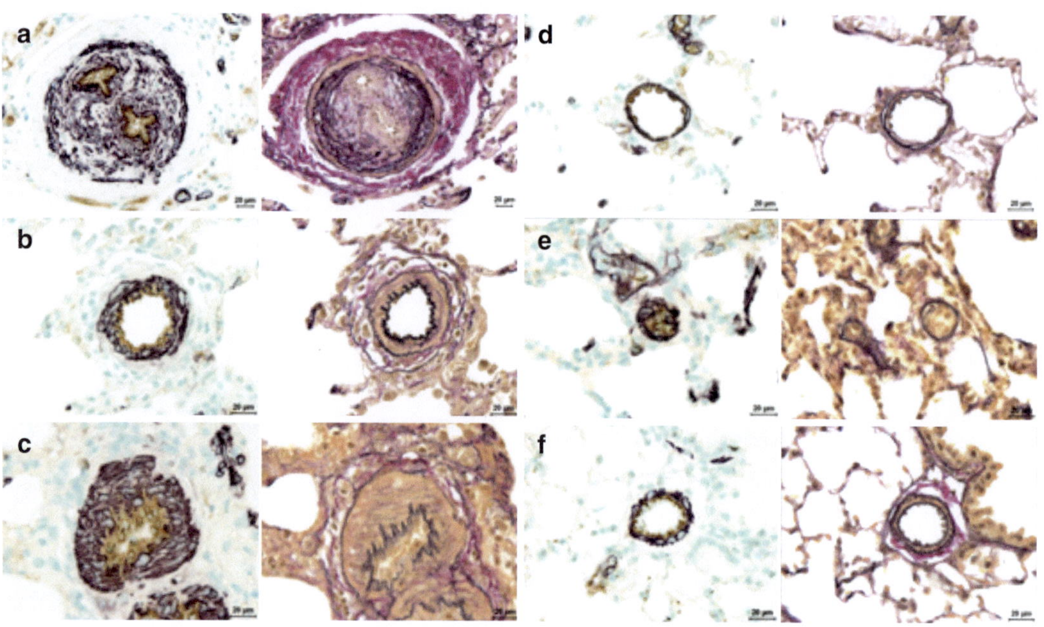

Fig. 3.1 Pulmonary vascular changes in animal models of pulmonary hypertension. Representative images of lung vessels from human idiopathic pulmonary arterial hypertension (PAH) (**a**) and different models of PH: monocrotaline-induced PAH (**b**); monocrotaline + pneumonectomy (**c**); hypoxia-induced pulmonary hypertension in rats (**d**); Sugen + hypoxia (SUHx)-induced pulmonary arterial hypertension in rats (**e**); hypoxia-induced pulmonary hypertension in mice (**f**)

vasculature in response to a variety of chemical (e.g., monocrotaline [MCT]) and environmental (e.g., hypoxia) stimuli.

MCT-Induced PAH

MCT-induced PAH remains a frequently investigated model. MCT is an 11-membered macrocyclic pyrrolizidine alkaloid derived from the seeds of the *Crotalaria spectabilis* plant. After a single subcutaneous or intraperitoneal injection of MCT, the alkaloid is converted in the liver by cytochrome P450 (CYP3A4) to the reactive pyrrole metabolite dehydromonocrotaline (MCTP) [19–21], which in turn causes endothelial cell injury in the pulmonary vasculature with subsequent remodeling of the precapillary vessels (medial thickening and de novo muscularization of small pulmonary arterioles) and progressive PH and RV failure [22, 23].

The response to MCT is variable among species, strains, and even individual animals due to differences in the hepatic metabolism by cytochrome P450 [24]. While MCT injection leads to severe PAH in rats, the injection or oral application of MCT in mice causes liver damage [25], modest pulmonary fibrosis [26–28], and immunotoxicity [29, 30], but not PH. This phenomenon can be explained by the fact that the liver metabolism of MCT to MCTP by the cytochrome P450 system may differ between rats and mice [20, 31]. However, our group has recently demonstrated that after MCTP injection, mice develop a typical early-phase acute lung injury characterized by lung edema, neutrophil influx, hypoxemia, reduced lung compliance, and high mortality. In the late phase, MCTP injection resulted in limited lung fibrosis and no obvious PH [32]. Therefore, the MCT rat model of PH remains a model favored by many investigators.

Although the MCT model has been in use for several decades, the basic mechanisms that underlie the induction of PH in this model remain unclear. It is known that the active MCTP rapidly causes pulmonary artery endothelial cell injury, pulmonary arterial medial hyperplasia, interstitial edema, adventitial inflammation, hemorrhage, and fibrosis [24, 33–35]. As a result, pulmonary vascular resistance (PVR) increases and RV hypertrophy and failure occur. Several investigators demonstrated that a single MCT injection leads to time- and dose-dependent abnormalities in the pulmonary vasculature and RV hypertrophy as well as abnormalities in function. It was shown that a single exposure of rats to MCT at a dose of 60–100 mg/kg results in PH and RV hypertrophy, dilatation, and failure in 3 or 4 weeks, and leads to mortality in most rats within 4–8 weeks [36–39]. In contrast, MCT at a dose of 30 mg/kg induces compensatory RV hypertrophy without signs of RV systolic dysfunction, but with diastolic dysfunction [38, 40], 4 weeks after injection. Recently, Ruiter et al. published an interesting observation [41]: the authors demonstrated that an injection of 40 mg/kg of MCT induces acute muscularization of the smallest pulmonary arterioles, together with high PVR, RV hypertrophy, and diminished RV function, as measured by echocardiography and confirmed by invasive hemodynamic measurement. However, 8 and 12 weeks after MCT administration, pulmonary arteriolar abnormalities were resolved, accompanied by normalization of RV function, although cardiomyocyte hypertrophy was maintained. The authors concluded that MCT-induced PH is reversible after 4 weeks and does not resemble the progressive nature of human PH [41]. This observation needs to be confirmed in a larger cohort of animals.

Nevertheless, numerous published reports have proposed that subcutaneous injection of 30–60 mg/kg of MCT in rats is appropriate to study compensatory and maladaptive RV remodeling. Many factors such as neurohormonal activation, oxidative and nitrosative stress, immune activation, myocardial ischemia, and cardiomyocyte apoptosis are involved in reprogramming the heart from adaptive to maladaptive remodeling. The underlying mechanisms of RV hypertrophy and failure in MCT rats are extremely complex and still not well defined. Several studies demonstrate that despite a similar degree of pulmonary artery pressure (PAP) or RV systolic pressure in rats treated with MCT and rats subjected to PAB or Sugen plus hypoxia (SUHx), the severity of RV failure and mortality in MCT rats remains extremely high [42–45]. It is still not clear whether RV failure is associated with heart inflammation/myocarditis due to direct effects of MCT on the RV myocardium [46, 47], or if it is a secondary effect due to pulmonary vascular injury and release of mediators which can increase stress on the right ventricle and lead to maladaptive RV hypertrophy.

Histomorphological evaluation of RV tissue demonstrated that MCT rats exhibit increased levels of RV interstitial and perivascular collagen deposition levels [43], which continuously increase throughout RV disease progression, being highest during RV failure [48]. In contrast, serial noninvasive measurements by scintigraphy with ^{99m}Tc-annexin, also confirmed by autoradiography and terminal deoxynucleotidyl transferase dUTP nick end labeling (TUNEL) assay, show that in right ventricles of MCT rats, cardiomyocyte apoptosis occurs at the early compensatory disease stage and declines, while still remaining significantly increased, when RV failure has occurred [48, 49].

Few reports have addressed the role of inflammation in RV remodeling in MCT-induced PH. It has been shown that progressive RV failure is associated with an increased number of leukocytes in the right but not the left ventricle [50]. However, in rats subjected to a low dose of MCT (40 mg/kg) the number of CD45-positive leukocyte cells was comparable with that in healthy control animals [41, 47]. Additionally, it was reported that inflammation, assessed noninvasively by ^{67}Ga (an agent that binds to transferrin, leukocyte lactoferrin, bacterial siderophores, inflammatory proteins, and cell membranes in neutrophils), is elevated at an early compensatory stage of RV hypertrophy, reaches its highest levels at the stage of RV dilatation, and remains elevated compared with baseline throughout disease progression to RV failure [51]. In parallel, high immunoreactivity and elevated levels of matrix metalloproteinase (MMP)-2 and MMP-9 were found in RV tissue of MCT rats [52].

Electrophysiological studies revealed that in MCT rats, all of the abovementioned changes in the failing heart can lead to RV electrical remodeling, arrhythmias, and even spontaneous ventricular fibrillation, which may be considered to be the main reasons for high mortality in this model [53–55].

Additionally, there is growing evidence that an oxygen supply/demand mismatch and metabolic changes in the right ventricle play an important role in adaptive or maladaptive RV remodeling [56]. RV capillary rarefaction is one phenomenon that leads to maladaptive RV remodeling. Interestingly, some studies examining capillary density in MCT rats demonstrated reduced numbers of capillaries and downregulated vascular endothelial growth factor (VEGF) expression in advanced MCT-induced RV failure [50, 56, 57]. In parallel, it was suggested that the failing right ventricle is characterized by abnormal metabolism due to the pressure overload. It was demonstrated that ^{18}F-fluorodeoxyglucose (FDG) uptake in the lungs of MCT animals increases with progression of the disease, and MCT treatment also leads to reduction of oxygen consumption and increased glycolysis as well as FDG uptake in the failing right ventricle [44, 58]. Similar findings were observed in patients with idiopathic PAH and congenital heart disease [59]. These studies indicate that increased FDG uptake by the lung and the right ventricle reflects the metabolic state of the small pulmonary arteries and the pressure-overloaded right ventricle, and therefore can be used as an early diagnostic marker of disease severity and might be useful for PAH monitoring.

Although several studies demonstrate the role of long noncoding RNAs (LncRNAs) in cardiovascular diseases, including PAH [60–62], the contribution of LncRNAs in RV adaptation in response to pressure overload still needs to be elucidated. A recently published report suggested that LncRNA, specifically H19, is upregulated in the decompensated RV from PAH patients and monocrotaline-induced PH and correlates with biochemical and histological markers of maladaptive RV remodeling. The authors demonstrate that the silencing of H19 limits pathological RV hypertrophy, fibrosis, and capillary rarefaction, thus preserving RV function in monocrotaline and pulmonary artery banding rats without affecting pulmonary vascular remodeling, suggesting that circulating H19 might be a useful biomarker for the assessment of the severity of the disease and prognosis [63].

Thus, as mentioned above, MCT-induced PH in rats is still a suitable model in which to study compensatory and maladaptive RV remodeling.

MCT Plus Pneumonectomy

As mentioned above, the MCT rat model is the most frequently used model in which animals develop PAH with endothelial damage, vascular smooth muscle hypertrophy, and severe RV failure. However, in this model the plexiform-like vascular lesions that are found in human PAH do not occur. Since the MCT model does not fully reflect the clinical or pathological picture seen in human PAH, efforts have been made to modify this model to induce progressive pulmonary vascular disease with neointimal changes. Thus, Okada et al. established a new animal model in which MCT administration is followed by unilateral pneumonectomy [64]. The authors compared the changes in pulmonary vasculature in MCT plus pneumonectomy animals with the changes in those receiving MCT or pneumonectomy alone. They found that neointimal changes developed in more than 90% of all right-lung intra-acinar vessels in rats subjected to MCT injection plus pneumonectomy, but not in animals receiving either MCT or pneumonectomy alone. Additionally, they demonstrated that animals with a neointimal pattern of remodeling developed more severe RV hypertrophy compared with animals receiving MCT or pneumonectomy alone [64, 65]. Importantly, other investigators were able to reproduce this observation [65–67]. Despite the fact that the exact mechanisms that lead to neointimal formation in this model are still unknown, it is clear that the combination of MCT-induced endothelial lung injury and increased vascular shear stress and blood flow to the remaining lung due to pneumonectomy is necessary to produce neointimal formation.

White et al. administered MCT to young rats following pneumonectomy and found that younger animals develop a more severe phenotype and die earlier than in previously reported models [64, 68]. This more severe phenotype was associated with plexiform-like lesions, severe vascular pruning, and networks of disorganized capillaries. Unfortunately, none of these studies investigated the RV histomorphological changes and function in detail, and therefore additional studies are required to distinguish the mechanisms involved in the formation of occlusive and plexiform-like lesions in this model.

Hypoxia-Induced PH

Chronic hypoxia is the most commonly used physiological stimulus for PH development in animal models. This experimental model of PH represents group 3 of the WHO PH classification. Exposure of animals to normobaric or hypobaric hypoxia for 2 weeks or longer induces PH in a wide variety of animal species including rats, mice, guinea pigs, dogs, cows, pigs, and sheep. The most commonly used species in laboratory models of PH are rats and mice. The hypoxia model is useful because it is very predictable and reproducible within the selected animal species as well as strain. However, there is a great variability in responses to chronic hypoxia between species [24]. The most common pathological findings are muscularization of previously nonmuscularized vessels and a moderate medial thickening of muscular resistance vessels. Both pulmonary smooth muscle cells and adventitial fibroblasts proliferate under hypoxia [24, 69, 70]. These features are largely reversible on return to normoxic conditions.

Chronic Hypoxia in Mice

The mouse is a widely used species for the investigation of a growing number of disease states. In particular, the availability of knockout and transgenic mouse strains allows us to understand the molecular mechanisms of diseases more precisely. Chronic exposure of mice to a hypoxic environment leads to pulmonary vasoconstriction, endothelial dysfunction, extracellular matrix deposition, muscularization of previously nonmuscularized vessels, medial thickening of muscular resistance vessels, and subsequently an elevation in PAP, PVR, and RV hypertrophy [71–74].

Despite the fact that many investigators have extensively studied the mechanisms of hypoxia-induced pulmonary vascular remodeling in rodents, the mechanisms underlying RV hypertrophy and failure in hypoxic models remain largely elusive. Recent advances in noninvasive high-resolution imaging techniques allow us to characterize heart function in rodent models of PH more precisely. Basic parameters such as RV internal diameter, pulmonary artery acceleration time (PAAcT), or ratio of PAAcT to pulmonary artery ejection time, cardiac output, and tricuspid annular plane systolic excursion have been described and validated in humans and rodents [75–79].

The results of hemodynamic and echocardiographic studies in hypoxic mice showed that mice developed mild or moderate PH with shortened PAAcT, and RV hypertrophy with preserved systolic function [77, 80, 81], or in some cases mild systolic dysfunction [73, 82–84]. Only one study quantified collagen content in the right ventricle by immunohistochemistry, and in this study the authors showed increased collagen content in hypoxic mice [74]. However, it should be mentioned that responses to hypoxia in mice are strain specific, and that intraspecies comparisons could vary significantly depending on the strains compared. For example, in a recently published article, the authors demonstrated that Ras association domain family 1A (RASSF1A) might play a significant role in hypoxia-induced PH and RV function. The authors demonstrate that RASSF1A is significantly upregulated in the lungs of mice exposed to hypoxia compared to normoxic mice, while RASSF1A inactivation protected mice against chronic hypoxia-evoked right-heart abnormalities such as enlargement of

RV, increase of end-diastolic and end-systolic volumes, and augmentation of RV mass [85].

Chronic Hypoxia in Rats

Hypoxic rats develop more severe PH than hypoxic mice. However, there is considerable variability in the magnitude of the response to chronic hypoxia exposure in different rat strains due to genetic origin. For example, the fawn-hooded rat (FHR) is a strain in which PH occurs spontaneously [86], and it appears to be more susceptible to the development of more severe PH than control rats even after exposure to only mild hypoxia [87]. FHRs show increased endothelin levels, enhanced serotonin-induced vasoconstriction, a platelet storage pool deficiency, excessive pulmonary artery smooth muscle cell proliferation, and mitochondrial dysfunction [87, 88]. FHRs have been described as having normal PAP until 20 weeks of age, but by 40 weeks, despite normal systemic blood pressure and oxygen partial pressure, they develop PAH and RV hypertrophy. Moreover, normoxic FHRs show a leftward shift in the pulmonary vascular pressure–flow relationship, which is similar to that shown by Sprague-Dawley rats exposed to chronic hypoxia, and they display medial hypertrophy of resistance pulmonary arteries in a comparable manner [88]. In contrast, the Fischer 344 rat strain is relatively well protected from hypoxia-induced pulmonary vascular and cardiac responses compared with the Wistar Kyoto rat strain [89, 90]. However, the major limitation of the abovementioned animal models of PH is that they do not develop occlusive neointimal and plexiform lesions, even in rats exposed to longer periods of hypoxia [91].

Sugen 5416 Plus Chronic Hypoxia in Rats

A rat model that more closely mimics the pulmonary vascular changes seen in human PAH is the combination of a single subcutaneous injection of the VEGF receptor inhibitor Sugen (SU5416) with exposure to chronic hypoxia (SUHx) for 3–5 weeks [92, 93] followed by re-exposure to normoxia [92, 94]. SU5416 is a multikinase inhibitor which acts on VEGFR2 (vascular endothelial growth factor receptor [FLK1/KDR]; half-maximal inhibitory concentration [IC_{50}] = 1 μM), PDGFR (platelet-derived growth factor receptor; IC_{50} = 20 μM), c-Kit (stem cell factor receptor; IC_{50} = 30 nM), RET (tyrosine kinase receptor encoded by the ret proto-oncogene; IC_{50} = 170 nM), FLT3 (fms-like tyrosine kinase-3; IC_{50} = 160 nM), ABL (Abelson murine leukemia viral oncogene homolog 1; IC_{50} = 1 μM), and ALK (anaplastic lymphoma kinase; IC_{50} = 1.2 μM) [95].

It has been shown that SUHx rats develop progressive PH and vascular remodeling even after being re-exposed to normoxia [92, 96]. By 5 weeks (3 weeks of hypoxia and 2 weeks of re-exposure to normoxia) after the SU5416 injection, the rats had developed severe PH and RV hypertrophy accompanied by proliferation of apoptosis-resistant endothelial cells and occlusive neointimal but not plexiform-like lesions in precapillary pulmonary arterioles. Abe et al. demonstrated that rats receiving a single injection of SU5416 followed by exposure to 3 weeks of hypoxia and an additional 10–11 weeks of re-exposure to normoxia (13–14 weeks after the SU5416 injection) developed severe PAH accompanied by pulmonary arteriopathy, strikingly similar to that observed in severe human PAH. In this study, the authors found that at a much later stage (13–14 weeks after the SU5416 injection) the rats developed complex plexiform lesions [94]. Interestingly, the irreversible progression of the pulmonary vascular disease and RV failure in this model led to death in some but not all animals, and at different time courses [94]. However, longitudinal monitoring of the RVSP by telemetry reveals a partial reversibility of pulmonary hypertension in SUHx rats, despite progressive remodeling of the pulmonary vascular wall, in particular the intima layer [97].

Nevertheless, our recently published study demonstrates the presence of pulmonary emphysema in SUHx Wistar Kyoto rats injected by SU5416 and exposed to 3 weeks of hypoxia and an additional 2 weeks of re-exposure to normoxia [98]. In another study it was demonstrated that Sprague-Dawley rats obtained from Harlan developed mild lung emphysema, while Sprague-Dawley rats obtained from Charles River laboratories did not develop lung emphysema in response to SUHx [99]. Le Cras and Abman suggested that early disruption of angiogenesis in neonatal rats by SU5416 not only impairs alveolar growth throughout infancy but can also extend into adult life, which likely increases susceptibility for chronic lung disease [100]. All of these data suggest that the alveolar and vascular changes in the SUHx model might depend on the strain and different times of normoxic re-exposure [101].

Indeed, SUHx rats develop severe RV hypertrophy, dysfunction, and failure. A noninvasive evaluation of cardiac function by echocardiography or microscopic computed tomographic (μCT) showed that SUHx rats developed severe RV hypertrophy with deteriorated systolic and diastolic functions, which progressively worsened from day 21 to day 35 [102]. However, it was well described that there are strain-dependent differences in the severity of PH phenotype in rats exposed either to a single injection of the SU5416 or to a combination with a 3-week chronic hypoxic exposure [103]. The authors showed that Fischer rats exhibited very high mortality in the SUHx model of severe PAH by 7 weeks, whereas Sprague-Dawley (SD) rats showed excellent survival for up to 14 weeks in the same model [103]. In the follow-up study, the authors showed that a high rate of mortality due to severe RV failure in Fischer rats can be explained by a lack of adequate microvascular angiogenesis, together with metabolic and immunological responses in the hypertrophied RV [104].

RV failure in SUHx rats is accompanied by fibrosis, capillary rarefaction, cardiomyocyte apoptosis, and furthermore by decreased expression of genes encoding angiogenesis factors such as VEGF, insulin-like growth factor 1, apelin, and angiopoeitin-1, and by increased expression of genes encoding a set of glycolytic enzymes [89, 92, 93]. A recently published study revealed that cyclin-dependent kinase (CDK) family members play a significant role in the pathobiology of the pulmonary vascular as well as RV remodeling in animal models of PH. The authors demonstrate that targeted CDK 4 and 6 inhibition leads to improvement of pulmonary vascular remodeling and RV function in SUHx as well as in MCT-induced PH and RV pressure overload [105]. It seems that the SUHx rat model may be useful for addressing the etiological mechanisms involved in endothelial cell hyperproliferation, which is a distinctive plexogenic arteriopathy characteristic in humans with severe PAH.

Sugen 5416 Plus Chronic Hypoxia in Mice

Recently, Ciuclan et al. established a mouse model in which PH is induced by the abovementioned combination of VEGF receptor-focused multikinase inhibition and chronic hypoxic exposure [84]. Compared with normobaric chronic hypoxia alone, treatment with SU5416 resulted in markedly increased RV systolic pressure, increased RV hypertrophy, and increased muscularization of small pulmonary vessels. In addition, the authors found occlusive neointimal lesions of small vessels in SUHx mice, which do not occur in mice under hypoxia alone. The vascular remodeling process induced by a combined application of hypoxia and SU5416 was paralleled by an increased caspase activity and an increased proliferation of endothelial cells. The authors also demonstrated that SUHx mice developed more severe RV dilatation and cardiac dysfunction compared with mice exposed to hypoxia alone. The authors addressed the question of whether the PAH pathologies in SUHx mice are reversible after returning mice to normoxic conditions. Thus, 10 days after normoxic exposure SUHx mice showed slight decreases in hemodynamic parameters, indicating that this model of PH is less severe than the one in rats.

Two follow-up studies in SUHx mice confirmed this observation [106, 107]. Combined with the obvious ease of gene manipulation in mice, this new model of PH may prove to be useful in deciphering specific mechanisms and designing targeted therapies [108].

Schistosomiasis

Schistosomiasis is one of the most common causes of PAH: of the more than 200 million individuals chronically infected worldwide, 2–5% have PAH [109]. Approximately 10% of people chronically infected with *Schistosoma mansoni* develop hepatosplenic schistosomiasis, a syndrome of periportal fibrosis, and portocaval shunting [110]. Approximately 10–20% of those patients with hepatosplenic disease, or 2–5 million people worldwide, develop PAH [111, 112]. Patients who develop schistosomiasis-associated PAH have the signs and symptoms of this condition, primarily resulting from progressive right-heart failure. The pulmonary histopathology of schistosomiasis-associated PAH has both similarities to and differences from other forms of PAH that are more common in the developed world, most classically idiopathic PAH [113]. Analysis of pulmonary tissues from patients who died from schistosomiasis-associated PAH revealed that all lung samples showed evidence of pulmonary vascular remodeling, arterial medial thickening, and plexiform-like lesions [114, 115].

It was demonstrated that up to 20 weeks after infection with *S. mansoni* in mice, a time-dependent increase in liver and lung egg burden resulted in extensive pulmonary vascular remodeling and development of plexiform-like vascular lesions but only mild increases in RV pressures (PH) and RV hypertrophy [116]. This finding was accompanied by heterogeneity in the lung egg burden among individual animals. In individual animals the authors found a significant correlation between lung egg burden and ratio of RV weight to LV plus septum weight, indicating that the RV index was higher in animals with a greater density of eggs in the lung. In another study,

Crosby et al. demonstrated that at a later time point (25 weeks), chronic infection with *S. mansoni* leads to significant elevation of the RV systolic pressure and RV hypertrophy [117].

The pathogenic mechanism by which the combination of the parasite's effect on the host and the host's immune response to the parasite results in PAH remains unclear. However, local inflammation may contribute to the process of pulmonary vascular remodeling [117–119]. Further preclinical investigations are needed to uncover the pathophysiological mechanisms involved in the development of severe pulmonary vascular remodeling and RV hypertrophy.

PH Due to Left-Heart Disease

PH due to left-heart disease (PH-LHD) is the most prevalent form of PH worldwide [120, 121] and is associated with impaired exercise capacity, increased risk for hospitalization, and reduced survival [122]. Therefore, PH-LHD represents a high socioeconomic burden and the development of specific therapies would represent a breakthrough.

In these patients, LHD such as ischemic heart failure and heart failure with reduced or preserved ejection fraction causes LV systolic and/or diastolic abnormalities that lead to elevation in left atrial filling pressures and subsequent retrograde increases in pulmonary venous, capillary, and arterial pressures [123]. Over time, this hindrance of pulmonary venous outflow initiates remodeling events in the pulmonary vasculature with increases in pulmonary vascular resistance (PVR), further augmenting the RV afterload with subsequent RV hypertrophy, increased risk for HF hospitalization, and ultimately RV failure [124–126]. Based on their hemodynamic profile, PH-LHD patients are subcategorized into patients with isolated postcapillary PH (Ipc-PH), defined by a mean pulmonary artery pressure ≥25 mmHg combined with a mean pulmonary artery wedge pressure (PAWP) >15 mmHg and PVR ≤3 Wood units, suggesting that these patients suffer from a sole passive postcapillary disease component, and patients with combined post- and precapillary PH (Cpc-PH), defined by a mean PAP

≥25 mmHg, a mean PAWP >15 mmHg, and PVR >3 Wood units, suggesting that there is an additional precapillary component adding to disease development [125, 127].

Despite the high medical need, there are currently no specific clinically approved therapeutic options available for the treatment of PH-LHD patients. International guidelines inform management of LHD and volume status of these patients and treatment of underlying comorbidities, such as diabetes mellitus. Importantly, the European Society of Cardiology and European Respiratory Society guidelines discourage the use of PAH drugs for the treatment of PH-LHD patients, since clinical evidence for a favorable risk-to-benefit ratio is missing [125, 128, 129]. Therefore, further PH-LHD-tailored research is needed that employs animal models with clinically relevant endpoints to identify novel therapeutic targets and study pharmacological concepts.

As the cause for PH-LHD development is often multifactorial and involves multiple comorbidities (such as heart failure, systemic hypertension, diabetes mellitus, obesity) [125, 126], animal models that recapitulate different features of the disease were developed. The most commonly employed models involve either surgical interventions that alter cardiac mechanics to mimic the multimodal effects of LV heart failure [130] or single or combinations of systemic stimuli that model frequent comorbidities, such as systemic hypertension, metabolic syndrome, or aging [131, 132]. Importantly, PH-LHD often develops rapidly after disease induction, especially in surgical models, whereas human disease is often a manifestation of different stimuli that promote disease development over a long period of time, often in combination with age-related systemic alterations.

Myocardial Infarction (MI)

The left and right ventricles are affected by compensatory mechanisms after an acute MI. RV hypertrophy may even develop in the long run in experimental models of MI in which the right ventricle is initially spared [133]. In addition, substantial myocardial damage can also be caused by RV infarction, leading to heart failure, shock, arrhythmias, and death of the patient [134]. The chronic MI model was first described in rats by Pfeffer et al. in 1979 [135]. It resembles the pathophysiological changes of remodeling and deterioration of systolic and diastolic cardiac function in patients with ischemia-induced heart failure. The animals develop myocardial hypertrophy, inflammation, and fibrosis resulting in LV systolic and diastolic dysfunction with reduced contractility and increased LV end-diastolic pressure [80]. Since then, the murine model of MI and ischemia-reperfusion has been described widely in the literature, and a detailed experimental protocol was published by Michael et al. in 1995 [136]. The most common approach is to ligate the left anterior descending (LAD) coronary artery, the major vessel for left ventricular blood supply [137]. Once the LAD artery is occluded, MI of the anterior wall of the left ventricle and the anterior portion of the interventricular septum is observed [138]. The infarction size and site are crucially dependent on the ligation position and individual anatomy of the rat/mouse: for most studies, the LAD artery is ligated below the tip of the left auricle, which induces roughly 40–50% ischemia of the left ventricle.

A number of studies focused on the effects of MI-dependent left-heart failure on PH and RV function. In 2000, Nguyen et al. reported that an early intervention with endothelin receptor antagonists following coronary artery ligation in male Wistar rats reduced the development of PH as reflected by a significant decrease in RV systolic pressure, despite an unaltered LV dysfunction [139]. Ben Driss and colleagues showed that in compensated left-heart failure induced by small MI in male Wistar rats, hemodynamics, vascular wall function, and structure were altered in the pulmonary artery but preserved in the thoracic aorta. They concluded that the pulmonary vascular bed is an early target of regional circulatory alterations in left-heart failure [140]. Later, in 2003, Jasmin et al. found that rats with large MIs developed progressive PH and right-heart hypertrophy due to important pulmonary structural remodeling, which was already apparent 2 weeks after surgery [141]. They measured marked elevations in the RV systolic and diastolic pressures as well as an increased ratio of RV weight to LV plus septum weight in rats with MIs, changes that were completely reversed by therapy with an angiotensin II receptor antagonist [141]. In 2010, Jiang et al. studied the applicability of a single measurement of troponin T for early prediction of infarct size, congestive heart failure, and PH in an animal model of MI. They concluded that an early single plasma cardiac troponin T measurement correlated with the infarct size in rats, and provided sensitivity and specificity to predict congestive heart failure with secondary PH [142]. In 2011 the same working group investigated the effects of statins on PH and RV function in ischemic congestive heart failure. The authors reported that statins reduced lung remodeling and dysfunction associated with heart failure, with prevention of RV hypertrophy and PH [143]. In the same year, Toldo et al. reported that acute MI led to hypertrophy and induced a significant acute decline in RV systolic function even in the absence of PH [144]. They concluded that RV dysfunction also develops independently of changes in RV afterload [144].

More recently, Philip and colleagues investigated the mechanical consequences of MI-induced left-heart failure on the pulmonary vasculature and right ventricle by invasive measures [145]. The authors reported pulmonary hypertension 12 weeks post-MI, along with RV contractile dysfunction and decreased coupling of the pulmonary vascular-right ventricular unit. On a structural level, these impairments were linked to fibrotic remodeling, recapitulating an important feature of human PH-LHD. Similarly, Dayeh et al. demonstrated via noninvasive echocardiography that MI-caused left-heart failure causes PH and identified noninvasive indices that may help in the future to improve efficiency and design of preclinical studies focusing on PH in the setting of heart failure with reduced ejection fraction [146].

Transverse Aortic Constriction (TAC)

Numerous LV pressure overload models have been developed in rodents in recent decades, whereas the TAC model remains the most widely used version. First described by Rockmann et al. in 1994 [147], the aortic banding model induces a pressure overload physiology similar to disease pathology observed in patients with aortic stenosis, systemic hypertension, or coarctation of the aorta. Initially, TAC leads to compensated hypertrophy of the heart (left ventricle), which is often accompanied by increased cardiac contractility. However, during disease progression, TAC-induced chronic pressure overload causes left ventricular decompensation characterized by severe dilatation and functional decline [148]. Within 2 weeks after TAC surgery, an approximate 50% increase in LV mass is observed, allowing studies of pharmacological interventions that affect hypertrophy, fibrosis pathogenesis, and/or functional decline [149]. Several locations of the aortic arch may be banded to induce pressure overload: by positioning a needle next to the ascending or transverse aorta, tying a thread around artery and the needle, and pulling back the needle, the aorta is constricted in the size of the needle diameter [137]. Once constricted, the increased vascular resistance causes chronic LV pressure overload with subsequent pathological LV remodeling of structure and function. The dominant drawback of this animal model is the acute disease onset directly after banding which immediately mimics severe hypertension and LV overloading, more similar to an acute aortic stenosis than to chronic and progressive pressure overload. In addition, there is significant heterogeneity in the LV response to aortic constriction: For instance, C57BL6 mice develop rapid LV dilation after TAC which may not develop in other strains [150, 151]. However, this model is frequently used to identify and modify novel therapeutic targets in the area of left-heart failure.

Increasing evidence suggests that chronic LV pressure overload after TAC induces PH, potentially via increased backward transmission of blood into the lung. In 2012, Chen et al. reported that male C57BL/6J mice present with RV hypertrophy and RV fibrosis, increased RV end-diastolic pressure, and right atrial hypertrophy 8 weeks after TAC [152]. Similarly, the effects of sGC stimulation with Riociguat and PDE5 inhibition with sildenafil on TAC-induced PH were studied 6 weeks after disease induction and were linked to reduced cardiopulmonary remodeling [153]. Therefore, this model may represent a tool for studies focusing on PH-LHD associated with heart failure caused by chronic LV pressure overload.

Metabolic Syndrome

PH-LHD patients frequently present with a number of comorbidities that cause metabolic alterations in the body and are summarized as metabolic syndrome which includes central obesity, systemic hypertension, type 2 diabetes mellitus, and dyslipidemia [125, 126]. Therefore, an increasing number of studies recently focused on PH development and RV functional characterization in animals that resemble such comorbidities, either as a single stimulus or in combination. For example, Meng and colleagues screened 36 mouse strains for their response to develop high-fat diet (HFD)-induced pulmonary hypertension and identified significant heterogeneity in PH disease severity at 20 weeks after disease induction [154]. They further reported glucose intolerance in the 129S1/SvlmJ strain after HFD—the top responder in this study—suggesting that metabolic syndrome and aging contribute to PH manifestation in this model. Along this line, Ranchoux et al. combined supracoronary aortic banding to induce diastolic LV impairments with HFD and olanzapine treatment to induce metabolic syndrome and PH in rats [132]. Treatment with the metabolic modulator metformin improved RV function and reduced PH, further supporting a concept in which metabolic syndrome is a driver of PH disease progression in this context. Additional evidence arises from aged genetically modified female mice that lack

apolipoprotein E (ApoE) protein on HFD and develop severe PH [155, 156]. However, PH-LHD is likely a manifestation of different disease stimuli with rather complicated mechanics involving the arterial and venous pulmonary vascular compartment as well as the left and right sides of the heart. To better understand these complex disease-causing mechanisms and mechanics and to develop novel, efficacious, and safe therapies, more studies focusing on disease-relevant aspects with clinically meaningful endpoints are warranted.

Chronic Thromboembolic PH (CTEPH)

CTEPH is a form of PH caused by unresolved thromboemboli from sites of venous thrombosis, which undergo fibrotic organization in the lung. Incomplete thromboembolic resolution results in endothelialized residua that obstruct or significantly narrow major pulmonary arteries [157]. Once lodged in the lung arteries, these residua can cause more clots to form (thrombosis) and add more resistance to the blood flow through the lung, thereby increasing the pressure inside the lung. This obstruction of proximal pulmonary arteries leads to an increased PVR, development of PH, and progressive RV remodeling and failure. Pulmonary endarterectomy, a surgical method that removes the obstruction from pulmonary vessels, is the treatment of choice for patients with CTEPH [158].

Much effort has been made to generate appropriate animal models for this disease in order to better understand the pathophysiology of CTEPH and to test new therapeutic approaches. In contrast to CTEPH, acute pulmonary embolism is easily reproduced in several animal models: to study the pathophysiological mechanisms or drug effects within the first hour following embolization, various different materials including autologous blood clots have been employed [159–161]. The development of a chronic CTEPH model turned out to be extremely challenging because of very efficient endogenous fibrinolytic systems in the employed animal species [162, 163]. Additionally, Mitzner et al. reported that the systemic vascular response to chronic pulmonary vascular obstruction varies from species to species, with proliferation of bronchial arteries into the intraparenchymal airways in large animals or, in contrast, with proliferation of intercostal arteries into the pleural space in mice [162, 164]. CTEPH can be generated in dogs by repeated microembolizations of microspheres (e.g., Sephadex) [165, 166]. The vascular lesions can be targeted to vessels of different sizes based upon the size of the injected microspheres. Repeated administration can lead to a sustained rise in pulmonary pressure [166]. High PVR is the result of primary vascular mechanical obstruction and vasoconstriction [46, 167]. In pigs, Weimann et al. generated a different model employing three repeated embolizations with polydextran microspheres, which led to sustained PH with sustained elevation in PAP as well as RV hypertrophy [166]. Another chronic model of CTEPH in dogs was described by Moser et al., who employed a combination approach: pulmonary emboli were released from autologous venous thrombi, and the endogenous fibrinolytic system was inhibited by administration of tranexamic acid [168] or plasminogen activator inhibitor type 1 [169]. Unfortunately, these attempts did not result in stabilization of the thrombus, but resulted in its resolution at the latest by 1 week. In 2013, Li et al. reported that this method was also efficient in Sprague-Dawley rats and induced a stable increase in RV systolic pressure, right-heart hypertrophy, and fibrosis [170]. Other authors used a surgical approach, the unilateral PAB model, to mimic CTEPH in pigs [171]. Naturally, a partial stenosis of the right or left pulmonary artery leads to an increased pressure in the right ventricle with development of RV hypertrophy and fibrosis, but this type of model does not reproduce distal vascular remodeling in the non-obstructed pulmonary arterial bed as seen in the human disease situation, which finally leads to the development of PH. Recently, Mercier et al. developed a CTEPH piglet model, which consists of a primary left pulmonary artery ligation via a sternotomy followed by weekly transcatheter embolizations, under fluoroscopic control, of the tissue adhesive enbucrilate (Histoacryl) into the right lower lobe for a duration of 5 weeks [172]. The authors asserted that this model reproduced all the features of human CTEPH: increased PVR, increased mean PAP, increased medial thickness of distal pulmonary arteries in both obstructed and unobstructed territories, increased systemic blood supply through the bronchial arteries in the obstructed territories, RV hypertrophy, RV enlargement, and paradoxical septal motion [172].

To conclude, over recent decades several animal models for CTEPH have been developed, which have provided valuable insights into some aspects of the pathophysiology of CTEPH. Animal models that represent more closely the human situation need to be developed in future.

Pulmonary Artery Banding (PAB)

Many animal models have been studied to assess the anatomical, pathophysiological, and molecular mechanisms underlying RV adaptation processes and disease progression. These models frequently involve direct modifications to the pulmonary vasculature (such as chronic hypoxia exposure or MCT injection) that result in an increased pulmonary vascular resistance and therefore elevated RV afterload. The RV has to work against this increased afterload burden to maintain cardiac output, and introduces intrinsic changes in RV structure and function as a direct consequence (Fig. 3.2). Pharmacological studies in these models fail to inform whether improvements in RV structure and function are caused secondarily through a decrease in pulmonary vascular resistance and RV unloading or by direct beneficial cardiac effects [5]. In this context, the PAB model is superior to the abovementioned models as a partial stenosis of the main pulmonary artery generates an immediate fixed increase in resistance that is independent from changes in the pulmonary vasculature, thereby allowing for distinguishing between direct cardiac and afterload-dependent treatment effects. The PAB model was first established in

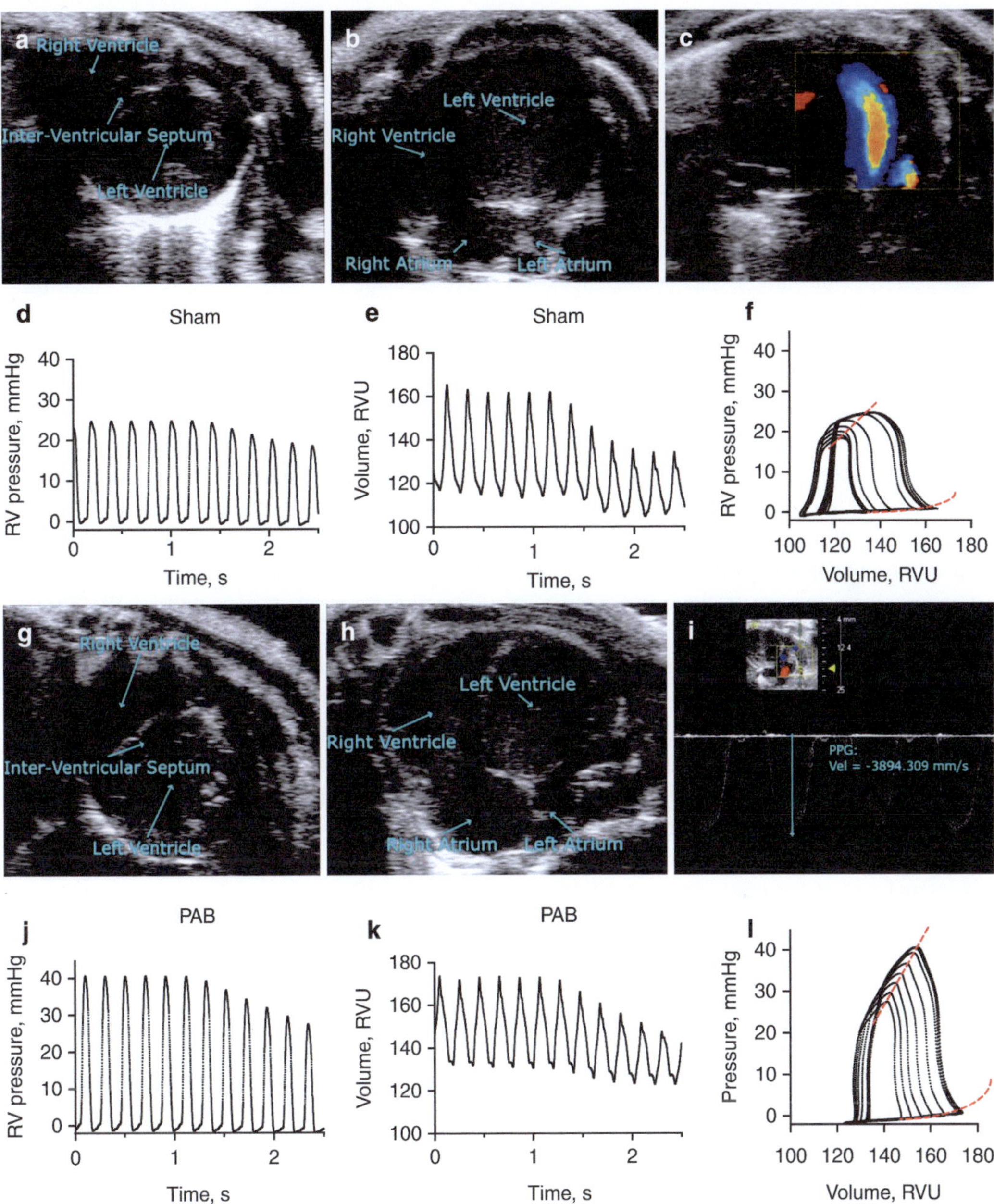

Fig. 3.2 Noninvasive and invasive measures of the healthy and pressure-overloaded rat heart. Representative echocardiographic short-axis view on the level of papillary muscles (**a**) and four-chamber view of the healthy rat heart (**b**). Pulsed-wave Doppler echocardiography visualizes pulmonary artery blood flow (**c**). Intracardiac catheter-derived RV pressure (**d**) and simultaneous volume (**e**) traces during vena cava inferior (IVC) occlusion for preload reduction and pressure-volume loop characterization (**f**). Lanes indicate end-systolic pressure-volume (ESPVR) and end-diastolic pressure-volume relationships (EDPVR) for end-systolic elastance (Ees) and end-diastolic elastance (Eed) quantification. Seven days of pressure overload after PAB causes RV dilatation and RV hypertrophy as demonstrated in short-axis (**g**) and four-chamber view (**h**) of the rat heart. Peak pressure gradient (PPG) is measured at the PA constriction side via pulsed-wave Doppler echocardiography (**i**) to quantify the degree of PAB-induced PA stenosis. Representative RV pressure (**j**) and volume (**k**) traces demonstrate increases in RV pressures and a shift in RV volumes caused by PAB, along with changes in ESPVR and EDPVR, representing increased RV contractility and stiffness (**l**)

dogs and piglets and transferred to rodents with advancements in microsurgical techniques [173, 174]. In 1994 Rockmann et al. successfully performed PAB in mice [147], yet the first comprehensive publication by Tarnavski et al. appeared in 2004 [137]. Technically, a needle is positioned next to the main pulmonary artery in proximity to the first bifurcation, a thread is placed around the artery and needle and tied, and the needle is subsequently removed, leaving a constriction loop with the needle diameter. Other groups modified this method and used a metal clip instead of needle and thread [175, 176], which offers several advantages: (1) the hemoclip can be applied quickly; (2) a complete constriction of the pulmonary artery is avoided; and (3) a constriction with a non-deformable clip as compared with the deformable thread provides more stability at the constriction site for reproducible results.

On a functional level, a rapid immediate decline upon PA constriction is followed by adaptation and recovery, and a maintained RV ejection fraction for 7–14 days, as well as a transition phase towards uncoupling and failure [177–179]. Subsequently, RV function declines and structural changes manifest: These include (1) an increase of the right ventricular free wall diameter through thickening of individual cardiomyocytes; (2) RV chamber dilatation to reduce RV wall stress; (3) abnormalities in cardiac capillarization; and (4) an increase in RV collagen content [176–181]. RV fibrosis is experimentally and clinically associated with a decrease in RV ejection fraction [182] and diastolic heart failure [183], and is used as a predictor of diastolic and systolic dysfunction during exercise in hypertrophic cardiomyopathic patients who successfully underwent surgery [184]. A reduced compliance of the (right) side of the heart can be the result of the pathological increase in collagen levels that leads to increased myocardial stiffness [185, 186]. Additionally, nutrient supply of the contractile cardiomyocytes may be impaired by excessive perivascular fibrosis, whereas interstitial ECM components may interfere with the well-coordinated excitation–contraction coupling, which in turn reduces cardiac pumping function [183]. Importantly, the left ventricle is likewise affected by RV changes as ventricular interdependency causes a reduction in LV mass through septal bowing and molecular changes that impair the left ventricle to expand to its original volume, causing reductions in LV stroke volume and therefore decreased function [187]. Compression of the left ventricle is a direct result of increased pressure in the right ventricle, which in turn exerts pressure on the left ventricle, reflected by an elevated LV eccentricity index.

The degree of RV structural and functional remodeling is dependent on the constriction severity. For example, rats with a mild constriction fail to transition towards failure [42] while increasing the constriction severity promotes RV functional decline with a decreased RV pumping function, RV dilatation, RV fibrosis, RV capillary rarefaction, and a metabolic switch from glucose oxidation to glycolysis [43, 188–190]. In a modified version of the PAB model, which applies absorbable sutures to constrict the PA, an initial functional decline is followed by functional and structural recovery once the PA band dissolves and the afterload burden is relieved [191]. This model allows studies focused on RV recovery processes from chronic pressure overload. In addition, models vary among species and strains. As an example, evidence suggests that in some instances rats react with more severe hemodynamic changes to stimuli as compared to mice (e.g., in the SUHx model [97, 192]). The major drawback of the PAB model in general is the immediate fixed increase in resistance after surgery that—to some extent—rather reflects an acute pulmonary embolism than the progressive gradual increase in resistance associated with PH and the transition from RV adaption towards decompensation and failure. As alternative models that more closely reflect the human situation are missing, the PAB model remains the gold standard when addressing direct RV treatment effects. In summary, the PAB model represents a reproducible animal model of right-sided heart hypertrophy and failure caused by RV-selective chronic pressure overload.

Other Models

Smoke-Induced PH

Cigarette smoke is the main preventable cause for chronic obstructive pulmonary disease (COPD), resulting in progressive proteolytic, inflammatory, and vasoactive responses that lead to emphysema, small-airway obstruction, and PH. Originally, it was believed that the increase in PAP is secondary to the lung pathology associated with COPD, as a result of hypoxia, emphysema, and loss of the vascular bed [193]. However, a recently published observation revealed that pulmonary vascular dysfunction, vascular remodeling, and PH precede the development of alveolar destruction [194]. In this paper the authors demonstrated that smoke exposure for up to 8 months resulted in the development of emphysema after 6 months in mice. Within 3 months, tobacco-smoke exposure caused increases in RV systolic pressure and ratio of the absolute numbers of alveoli to the number of vessels, followed by RV hypertrophy: i.e., development of PH preceded the development of lung emphysema [194]. Also, guinea pigs exposed to cigarette smoke develop PH and RV hypertrophy at levels similar to those seen in animals exposed to hypoxia [195]. Although it has been shown that tobacco smoke leads to PH and RV hypertrophy, the effects of smoke exposure on the right ventricle still need to be elucidated.

Intermittent Hypoxia

Obstructive sleep apnea (OSA) is a highly prevalent sleep-related breathing disorder and contributes to the emergence of systemic arterial hypertension, peripheral vascular disease, stroke, PH, and sudden cardiac death [196–198]. Based on human research, sympathetic activation, inflammation, and oxidative stress are thought to play major roles in the pathophysiology of OSA-related cardiovascular diseases. Exposure of rodents to brief episodes of hypoxia mimics the hypoxia and cardiovascular and metabolic effects observed in patients with OSA. Animal models of OSA have shown that endothelial dysfunction, vascular remodeling, systemic and pulmonary arterial hypertension, and heart failure can develop in response to chronic intermittent hypoxia. It was shown that 20–30% of untreated OSA patients suffer from PAH. It was first thought that this phenomenon is restricted to patients with pulmonary comorbidities such as COPD, but it is now widely accepted that OSA can itself lead to PH [199]. A histomorphometric study showed that mice exposed to chronic intermittent hypoxia develop characteristic features of PH such as elevated PAP, RV hypertrophy, and muscularization of small pulmonary arteries [200, 201]. Further research of chronic intermittent hypoxia in animal models is needed to enhance our understanding of the pathogenesis of OSA-related cardiovascular disease and PH and RV remodeling.

Lung Cancer-Associated PH

Lung cancer remains the most common cause of death worldwide, but some of the biology underlying the symptoms of this disease is still not well understood. In a recently published paper, Pullamsetti and co-authors described presence of vascular remodeling, PH, and perivascular inflammatory cell accumulation in three mouse models (LLC1, *KRas^{LA2}*, and *cRaf-BxB*) of lung cancer [202]. In this study the authors demonstrated that PH in these mice was accompanied by RV hypertrophy, dilatation, RV systolic and diastolic dysfunction, and fibrosis [202]. In a follow-up study in patients with lung cancer, the authors demonstrated that PH is present in a significant proportion of lung cancer patients. Moreover, they showed that the presence of PH has a marked impact on the clinical outcome of lung cancer patients, including survival [203].

Summary

There is no preclinical model that accurately recapitulates all features and heterogeneity of human disease, including right ventricular adaptation and transition towards failure in the context of pulmonary hypertension. Therefore, studies that employ a combination of different models which mimic key features of the disease tailored to a specific research question are necessary to advance our current understanding of disease development and progression. Animal models are very valuable scientific tools that, when applied in the correct context with strong, reliable, and clinically relevant endpoints, are crucial to the development of novel therapeutic concepts, elucidate pathophysiological disease-causing mechanisms, and uncover load dependencies in PH research.

References

1. van Wolferen SA, Marcus JT, Boonstra A, Marques KM, Bronzwaer JG, Spreeuwenberg MD, Postmus PE, Vonk-Noordegraaf A. Prognostic value of right ventricular mass, volume, and function in idiopathic pulmonary arterial hypertension. Eur Heart J. 2007;28:1250–7.
2. Champion HC, Michelakis ED, Hassoun PM. Comprehensive invasive and noninvasive approach to the right ventricle-pulmonary circulation unit: state of the art and clinical and research implications. Circulation. 2009;120:992–1007.
3. Huez S, Vachiery JL, Unger P, Brimioulle S, Naeije R. Tissue Doppler imaging evaluation of cardiac adaptation to severe pulmonary hypertension. Am J Cardiol. 2007;100:1473–8.
4. Schermuly RT, Ghofrani HA, Wilkins MR, Grimminger F. Mechanisms of disease: pulmonary arterial hypertension. Nat Rev Cardiol. 2011;8:443–55.
5. Lahm T, Douglas IS, Archer SL, Bogaard HJ, Chesler NC, Haddad F, Hemnes AR, Kawut SM, Kline JA, Kolb TM, et al. Assessment of right ventricular function in the research setting: knowledge gaps and pathways forward. An Official American Thoracic Society Research Statement. Am J Respir Crit Care Med. 2018;198:e15–43.
6. Humbert M, Sitbon O, Chaouat A, Bertocchi M, Habib G, Gressin V, Yaici A, Weitzenblum E, Cordier JF, Chabot F, et al. Pulmonary arterial hypertension in France: results from a national registry. Am J Respir Crit Care Med. 2006;173:1023–30.
7. Naeije R, Huez S. Expert opinion on available options treating pulmonary arterial hypertension. Expert Opin Pharmacother. 2007;8:2247–65.
8. Galie N, Hoeper MM, Humbert M, Torbicki A, Vachiery JL, Barbera JA, Beghetti M, Corris P, Gaine S, Gibbs JS, et al. Guidelines for the diagnosis and treatment of pulmonary hypertension: the Task Force for the Diagnosis and Treatment of Pulmonary Hypertension of the European Society of Cardiology (ESC) and the European Respiratory Society (ERS), endorsed by the International Society of Heart and Lung Transplantation (ISHLT). Eur Heart J. 2009;30:2493–537.
9. Peacock AJ, Naeije R, Galie N, Rubin L. Endpoints and clinical trial design in pulmonary arterial hypertension: have we made progress? Eur Respir J. 2009;34:231–42.
10. Borgdorff MA, Dickinson MG, Berger RM, Bartelds B. Right ventricular failure due to chronic pressure load: what have we learned in animal models since the NIH working group statement? Heart Fail Rev. 2015;20:475–91.
11. Humbert M, Guignabert C, Bonnet S, Dorfmüller P, Klinger JR, Nicolls MR, Olschewski AJ, Pullamsetti SS, Schermuly RT, Stenmark KR, Rabinovitch M. Pathology and pathobiology of pulmonary hypertension: state of the art and research perspectives. Eur Respir J. 2019;53(1):1801887.
12. Chesney CF, Allen JR. Endocardial fibrosis associated with monocrotaline-induced pulmonary hypertension in nonhuman primates (Macaca arctoides). Am J Vet Res. 1973;34:1577–81.
13. Stenmark KR, Fasules J, Hyde DM, Voelkel NF, Henson J, Tucker A, Wilson H, Reeves JT. Severe pulmonary hypertension and arterial adventitial changes in newborn calves at 4,300 m. J Appl Physiol. 1987;62:821–30.
14. Villamor E, Le Cras TD, Horan MP, Halbower AC, Tuder RM, Abman SH. Chronic intrauterine pulmonary hypertension impairs endothelial nitric oxide synthase in the ovine fetus. Am J Phys. 1997;272:L1013–20.
15. Rondelet B, Dewachter C, Kerbaul F, Kang X, Fesler P, Brimioulle S, Naeije R, Dewachter L. Prolonged overcirculation-induced pulmonary arterial hypertension as a cause of right ventricular failure. Eur Heart J. 2012;33:1017–26.
16. Hubloue I, Rondelet B, Kerbaul F, Biarent D, Milani GM, Staroukine M, Bergmann P, Naeije R, Leeman M. Endogenous angiotensin II in the regulation of hypoxic pulmonary vasoconstriction in anaesthetized dogs. Crit Care. 2004;8:R163–71.
17. Ryan J, Bloch K, Archer SL. Rodent models of pulmonary hypertension: harmonisation with the World Health Organisation's categorisation of human PH. Int J Clin Pract Suppl. 2011:15–34.
18. Tello K, Gall H, Richter M, Ghofrani A, Schermuly R. Right ventricular function in pulmonary (arterial) hypertension. Herz. 2019;44:509–16.
19. Wilson DW, Segall HJ, Pan LC, Lame MW, Estep JE, Morin D. Mechanisms and pathology of monocrotaline pulmonary toxicity. Crit Rev Toxicol. 1992;22:307–25.
20. Reid MJ, Lame MW, Morin D, Wilson DW, Segall HJ. Involvement of cytochrome P450 3A in the metabolism and covalent binding of

14C-monocrotaline in rat liver microsomes. J Biochem Mol Toxicol. 1998;12:157–66.

21. Kasahara Y, Kiyatake K, Tatsumi K, Sugito K, Kakusaka I, Yamagata S, Ohmori S, Kitada M, Kuriyama T. Bioactivation of monocrotaline by P-450 3A in rat liver. J Cardiovasc Pharmacol. 1997;30:124–9.

22. Rosenberg HC, Rabinovitch M. Endothelial injury and vascular reactivity in monocrotaline pulmonary hypertension. Am J Phys. 1988;255:H1484–91.

23. Schermuly RT, Kreisselmeier KP, Ghofrani HA, Yilmaz H, Butrous G, Ermert L, Ermert M, Weissmann N, Rose F, Guenther A, et al. Chronic sildenafil treatment inhibits monocrotaline-induced pulmonary hypertension in rats. Am J Respir Crit Care Med. 2004;169:39–45.

24. Stenmark K, Meyrick B, Galie N, Mooi WJ, Mcmurtry IF. Animal models of pulmonary arterial hypertension: the hope for etiological discovery and pharmacological cure. Am J Physiol Lung Cell Mol Physiol. 2009;297:L1013–32.

25. Miranda CL, Henderson MC, Schmitz JA, Buhler DR. Protective role of dietary butylated hydroxyanisole against chemical-induced acute liver damage in mice. Toxicol Appl Pharmacol. 1983;69:73–80.

26. Yasuhara K, Mitsumori K, Shimo T, Onodera H, Takahashi M, Hayashi Y. Mice with focal pulmonary fibrosis caused by monocrotaline are insensitive to urethane induction of lung tumorigenesis. Toxicol Pathol. 1997;25:574–81.

27. Molteni A, Ward WF, Ts'ao CH, Solliday NH. Monocrotaline pneumotoxicity in mice. Virchows Arch B Cell Pathol Incl Mol Pathol. 1989;57:149–55.

28. Hayashi S, Mitsumori K, Imaida K, Imazawa T, Yasuhara K, Uneyama C, Hayashi Y. Establishment of an animal model for pulmonary fibrosis in mice using monocrotaline. Toxicol Pathol. 1995;23:63–71.

29. Deyo JA, Kerkvliet NI. Immunotoxicity of the pyrrolizidine alkaloid monocrotaline following subchronic administration to C57Bl/6 mice. Fundam Appl Toxicol. 1990;14:842–9.

30. Deyo JA, Kerkvliet NI. Tier-2 studies on monocrotaline immunotoxicity in C57BL/6 mice. Toxicology. 1991;70:313–25.

31. Deyo JA, Reed RL, Buhler DR, Kerkvliet NI. Role of metabolism in monocrotaline-induced immunotoxicity in C57BL/6 mice. Toxicology. 1994;94:209–22.

32. Dumitrascu R, Koebrich S, Dony E, Weissmann N, Savai R, Pullamsetti SS, Ghofrani HA, Samidurai A, Traupe H, Seeger W, et al. Characterization of a murine model of monocrotaline pyrrole-induced acute lung injury. BMC Pulm Med. 2008;8:25.

33. Pak O, Janssen W, Ghofrani HA, Seeger W, Grimminger F, Schermuly RT, Weissmann N. Animal models of pulmonary hypertension: role in translational research. Drug Disc Today Dis Models. 2010;7:89–97.

34. Todorovich-Hunter L, Johnson DJ, Ranger P, Keeley FW, Rabinovitch M. Altered elastin and collagen synthesis associated with progressive pulmonary hypertension induced by monocrotaline. A biochemical and ultrastructural study. Lab Investig. 1988;58:184–95.

35. Schermuly RT, Pullamsetti SS, Kwapiszewska G, Dumitrascu R, Tian X, Weissmann N, Ghofrani HA, Kaulen C, Dunkern T, Schudt C, et al. Phosphodiesterase 1 upregulation in pulmonary arterial hypertension: target for reverse-remodeling therapy. Circulation. 2007;115:2331–9.

36. Kay JM, Harris P, Heath D. Pulmonary hypertension produced in rats by ingestion of Crotalaria spectabilis seeds. Thorax. 1967;22:176–9.

37. Schermuly RT, Dony E, Ghofrani HA, Pullamsetti S, Savai R, Roth M, Sydykov A, Lai YJ, Weissmann N, Seeger W, Grimminger F. Reversal of experimental pulmonary hypertension by PDGF inhibition. J Clin Invest. 2005;115:2811–21.

38. Buermans HP, Redout EM, Schiel AE, Musters RJ, Zuidwijk M, Eijk PP, van Hardeveld C, Kasanmoentalib S, Visser FC, Ylstra B, Simonides WS. Microarray analysis reveals pivotal divergent mRNA expression profiles early in the development of either compensated ventricular hypertrophy or heart failure. Physiol Genomics. 2005;21:314–23.

39. Daicho T, Yagi T, Abe Y, Ohara M, Marunouchi T, Takeo S, Tanonaka K. Possible involvement of mitochondrial energy-producing ability in the development of right ventricular failure in monocrotaline-induced pulmonary hypertensive rats. J Pharmacol Sci. 2009;111:33–43.

40. Hessel MH, Steendijk P, den Adel B, Schutte CI, van der Laarse A. Characterization of right ventricular function after monocrotaline-induced pulmonary hypertension in the intact rat. Am J Physiol Heart Circ Physiol. 2006;291:H2424–30.

41. Ruiter G, de Man FS, Schalij I, Sairras S, Grunberg K, Westerhof N, van der Laarse WJ, Vonk-Noordegraaf A. Reversibility of the monocrotaline pulmonary hypertension rat model. Eur Respir J. 2013;42:553–6.

42. Bogaard HJ, Natarajan R, Henderson SC, Long CS, Kraskauskas D, Smithson L, Ockaili R, McCord JM, Voelkel NF. Chronic pulmonary artery pressure elevation is insufficient to explain right heart failure. Circulation. 2009;120:1951–60.

43. Kojonazarov B, Sydykov A, Pullamsetti SS, Luitel H, Dahal BK, Kosanovic D, Tian X, Majewski M, Baumann C, Evans S, et al. Effects of multikinase inhibitors on pressure overload-induced right ventricular remodeling. Int J Cardiol. 2012;167(6):2630–7.

44. Piao L, Fang YH, Cadete VJ, Wietholt C, Urboniene D, Toth PT, Marsboom G, Zhang HJ, Haber I, Rehman J, et al. The inhibition of pyruvate dehydrogenase kinase improves impaired cardiac function and electrical remodeling in two models of right ventricular hypertrophy: resuscitating the hibernating

right ventricle. J Mol Med (Berl). 2010;88:
47–60.

45. Kosanovic D, Kojonazarov B, Luitel H, Dahal BK,
Sydykov A, Cornitescu T, Janssen W, Brandes RP,
Davie N, Ghofrani HA, et al. Therapeutic efficacy
of TBC3711 in monocrotaline-induced pulmonary
hypertension. Respir Res. 2011;12:87.

46. Campian ME, Hardziyenka M, Michel MC, Tan
HL. How valid are animal models to evaluate
treatments for pulmonary hypertension? Naunyn
Schmiedebergs Arch Pharmacol. 2006;373:
391–400.

47. Handoko ML, Lamberts RR, Redout EM, de Man
FS, Boer C, Simonides WS, Paulus WJ, Westerhof
N, Allaart CP, Vonk-Noordegraaf A. Right ventricular pacing improves right heart function in experimental pulmonary arterial hypertension: a study in
the isolated heart. Am J Physiol Heart Circ Physiol.
2009;297:H1752–9.

48. Campian ME, Verberne HJ, Hardziyenka M, de
Bruin K, Selwaness M, van den Hoff MJ, Ruijter
JM, van Eck-Smit BL, de Bakker JM, Tan HL. Serial
noninvasive assessment of apoptosis during right
ventricular disease progression in rats. J Nucl Med.
2009;50:1371–7.

49. Ecarnot-Laubriet A, Assem M, Poirson-Bichat F,
Moisant M, Bernard C, Lecour S, Solary E, Rochette
L, Teyssier JR. Stage-dependent activation of cell
cycle and apoptosis mechanisms in the right ventricle by pressure overload. Biochim Biophys Acta.
2002;1586:233–42.

50. de Man FS, Handoko ML, van Ballegoij JJ, Schalij
I, Bogaards SJ, Postmus PE, van der Velden J,
Westerhof N, Paulus WJ, Vonk-Noordegraaf
A. Bisoprolol delays progression towards right heart
failure in experimental pulmonary hypertension.
Circ Heart Fail. 2012;5:97–105.

51. Campian ME, Hardziyenka M, de Bruin K, van Eck-
Smit BL, de Bakker JM, Verberne HJ, Tan HL. Early
inflammatory response during the development of
right ventricular heart failure in a rat model. Eur J
Heart Fail. 2010;12:653–8.

52. Umar S, Hessel M, Steendijk P, Bax W, Schutte C,
Schalij M, van der Wall E, Atsma D, van der Laarse
A. Activation of signaling molecules and matrix
metalloproteinases in right ventricular myocardium
of rats with pulmonary hypertension. Pathol Res
Pract. 2007;203:863–72.

53. Benoist D, Stones R, Drinkhill M, Bernus O, White
E. Arrhythmogenic substrate in hearts of rats with
monocrotaline-induced pulmonary hypertension and
right ventricular hypertrophy. Am J Physiol Heart
Circ Physiol. 2011;300:H2230–7.

54. Benoist D, Stones R, Drinkhill MJ, Benson AP,
Yang Z, Cassan C, Gilbert SH, Saint DA, Cazorla
O, Steele DS, et al. Cardiac arrhythmia mechanisms in rats with heart failure induced by pulmonary hypertension. Am J Physiol Heart Circ Physiol.
2012;302:H2381–95.

55. Umar S, Lee JH, de Lange E, Iorga A, Partow-Navid
R, Bapat A, van der Laarse A, Saggar R, Ypey DL,
Karagueuzian HS, Eghbali M. Spontaneous ventric-
ular fibrillation in right ventricular failure secondary
to chronic pulmonary hypertension. Circ Arrhythm
Electrophysiol. 2012;5:181–90.

56. Archer SL, Fang YH, Ryan JJ, Piao L. Metabolism
and bioenergetics in the right ventricle and pulmonary vasculature in pulmonary hypertension. Pulm
Circ. 2013;3:144–52.

57. Partovian C, Adnot S, Eddahibi S, Teiger E, Levame
M, Dreyfus P, Raffestin B, Frelin C. Heart and lung
VEGF mRNA expression in rats with monocrota-
line- or hypoxia-induced pulmonary hypertension.
Am J Phys. 1998;275:H1948–56.

58. Marsboom G, Wietholt C, Haney CR, Toth PT, Ryan
JJ, Morrow E, Thenappan T, Bache-Wiig P, Piao L,
Paul J, et al. Lung (1)(8)F-fluorodeoxyglucose posi-
tron emission tomography for diagnosis and moni-
toring of pulmonary arterial hypertension. Am J
Respir Crit Care Med. 2012;185:670–9.

59. Fang W, Zhao L, Xiong CM, Ni XH, He ZX, He
JG, Wilkins MR. Comparison of 18F-FDG uptake
by right ventricular myocardium in idiopathic pulmonary arterial hypertension and pulmonary arterial
hypertension associated with congenital heart disease. Pulm Circ. 2012;2:365–72.

60. Zehendner CM, Valasarajan C, Werner A, Boeckel
JN, Bischoff FC, John D, Weirick T, Glaser SF,
Rossbach O, Jaé N, et al. Long noncoding RNA
TYKRIL plays a role in pulmonary hypertension
via the p53-mediated regulation of PDGFRβ. Am J
Respir Crit Care Med. 2020;202:1445–57.

61. Liu Y, Sun Z, Zhu J, Xiao B, Dong J, Li X. LncRNA-
TCONS_00034812 in cell proliferation and apoptosis of pulmonary artery smooth muscle cells and its
mechanism. J Cell Physiol. 2018;233:4801–14.

62. Lei S, Peng F, Li ML, Duan WB, Peng CQ, Wu
SJ. LncRNA-SMILR modulates RhoA/ROCK signaling by targeting miR-141 to regulate vascular
remodeling in pulmonary arterial hypertension. Am
J Physiol Heart Circ Physiol. 2020;319:H377–91.

63. Omura J, Habbout K, Shimauchi T, Wu WH,
Breuils-Bonnet S, Tremblay E, Martineau S, Nadeau
V, Gagnon K, Mazoyer F, et al. Identification of
long noncoding RNA H19 as a new biomarker
and therapeutic target in right ventricular failure
in pulmonary arterial hypertension. Circulation.
2020;142:1464–84.

64. Okada K, Tanaka Y, Bernstein M, Zhang W, Patterson
GA, Botney MD. Pulmonary hemodynamics modify
the rat pulmonary artery response to injury. A neointimal model of pulmonary hypertension. Am J
Pathol. 1997;151:1019–25.

65. Nishimura T, Faul JL, Berry GJ, Vaszar LT, Qiu D,
Pearl RG, Kao PN. Simvastatin attenuates smooth
muscle neointimal proliferation and pulmonary
hypertension in rats. Am J Respir Crit Care Med.
2002;166:1403–8.

66. Nishimura T, Faul JL, Berry GJ, Veve I, Pearl RG, Kao PN. 40-O-(2-hydroxyethyl)-rapamycin attenuates pulmonary arterial hypertension and neointimal formation in rats. Am J Respir Crit Care Med. 2001;163:498–502.

67. Homma N, Nagaoka T, Karoor V, Imamura M, Taraseviciene-Stewart L, Walker LA, Fagan KA, McMurtry IF, Oka M. Involvement of RhoA/Rho kinase signaling in protection against monocrotaline-induced pulmonary hypertension in pneumonectomized rats by dehydroepiandrosterone. Am J Physiol Lung Cell Mol Physiol. 2008;295:L71–8.

68. Faul JL, Nishimura T, Berry GJ, Benson GV, Pearl RG, Kao PN. Triptolide attenuates pulmonary arterial hypertension and neointimal formation in rats. Am J Respir Crit Care Med. 2000;162:2252–8.

69. Welsh DJ, Peacock AJ, MacLean M, Harnett M. Chronic hypoxia induces constitutive p38 mitogen-activated protein kinase activity that correlates with enhanced cellular proliferation in fibroblasts from rat pulmonary but not systemic arteries. Am J Respir Crit Care Med. 2001;164:282–9.

70. Weerackody RP, Welsh DJ, Wadsworth RM, Peacock AJ. Inhibition of p38 MAPK reverses hypoxia-induced pulmonary artery endothelial dysfunction. Am J Physiol Heart Circ Physiol. 2009;296:H1312–20.

71. Zhao L, Mason NA, Morrell NW, Kojonazarov B, Sadykov A, Maripov A, Mirrakhimov MM, Aldashev A, Wilkins MR. Sildenafil inhibits hypoxia-induced pulmonary hypertension. Circulation. 2001;104:424–8.

72. Dahal BK, Heuchel R, Pullamsetti SS, Wilhelm J, Ghofrani HA, Weissmann N, Seeger W, Grimminger F, Schermuly RT. Hypoxic pulmonary hypertension in mice with constitutively active platelet-derived growth factor receptor-beta. Pulm Circ. 2011;1:259–68.

73. Kwapiszewska G, Markart P, Dahal BK, Kojonazarov B, Marsh LM, Schermuly RT, Taube C, Meinhardt A, Ghofrani HA, Steinhoff M, et al. PAR-2 inhibition reverses experimental pulmonary hypertension. Circ Res. 2012;110:1179–91.

74. Pullamsetti SS, Doebele C, Fischer A, Savai R, Kojonazarov B, Dahal BK, Ghofrani HA, Weissmann N, Grimminger F, Bonauer A, et al. Inhibition of microRNA-17 improves lung and heart function in experimental pulmonary hypertension. Am J Respir Crit Care Med. 2012;185:409–19.

75. Kitabatake A, Inoue M, Asao M, Masuyama T, Tanouchi J, Morita T, Mishima M, Uematsu M, Shimazu T, Hori M, Abe H. Noninvasive evaluation of pulmonary hypertension by a pulsed Doppler technique. Circulation. 1983;68:302–9.

76. Kojonazarov BK, Imanov BZ, Amatov TA, Mirrakhimov MM, Naeije R, Wilkins MR, Aldashev AA. Noninvasive and invasive evaluation of pulmonary arterial pressure in highlanders. Eur Respir J. 2007;29:352–6.

77. Scherrer-Crosbie M, Steudel W, Hunziker PR, Foster GP, Garrido L, Liel-Cohen N, Zapol WM, Picard MH. Determination of right ventricular structure and function in normoxic and hypoxic mice: a transesophageal echocardiographic study. Circulation. 1998;98:1015–21.

78. Thibault HB, Kurtz B, Raher MJ, Shaik RS, Waxman A, Derumeaux G, Halpern EF, Bloch KD, Scherrer-Crosbie M. Noninvasive assessment of murine pulmonary arterial pressure: validation and application to models of pulmonary hypertension. Circ Cardiovasc Imaging. 2010;3:157–63.

79. Tournoux F, Petersen B, Thibault H, Zou L, Raher MJ, Kurtz B, Halpern EF, Chaput M, Chao W, Picard MH, Scherrer-Crosbie M. Validation of non-invasive measurements of cardiac output in mice using echocardiography. J Am Soc Echocardiogr. 2011;24:465–70.

80. Lutgens E, Daemen MJ, de Muinck ED, Debets J, Leenders P, Smits JF. Chronic myocardial infarction in the mouse: cardiac structural and functional changes. Cardiovasc Res. 1999;41:586–93.

81. Mouraret N, Marcos E, Abid S, Gary-Bobo G, Saker M, Houssaini A, Dubois-Rande JL, Boyer L, Boczkowski J, Derumeaux G, et al. Activation of lung p53 by Nutlin-3a prevents and reverses experimental pulmonary hypertension. Circulation. 2013;127:1664–76.

82. Tabima DM, Hacker TA, Chesler NC. Measuring right ventricular function in the normal and hypertensive mouse hearts using admittance-derived pressure-volume loops. Am J Physiol Heart Circ Physiol. 2010;299:H2069–75.

83. Hameed AG, Arnold ND, Chamberlain J, Pickworth JA, Paiva C, Dawson S, Cross S, Long L, Zhao L, Morrell NW, et al. Inhibition of tumor necrosis factor-related apoptosis-inducing ligand (TRAIL) reverses experimental pulmonary hypertension. J Exp Med. 2012;209:1919–35.

84. Ciuclan L, Bonneau O, Hussey M, Duggan N, Holmes AM, Good R, Stringer R, Jones P, Morrell NW, Jarai G, et al. A novel murine model of severe pulmonary arterial hypertension. Am J Respir Crit Care Med. 2011;184:1171–82.

85. Dabral S, Muecke C, Valasarajan C, Schmoranzer M, Wietelmann A, Semenza GL, Meister M, Muley T, Seeger-Nukpezah T, Samakovlis C, et al. A RASSF1A-HIF1α loop drives Warburg effect in cancer and pulmonary hypertension. Nat Commun. 2019;10:2130.

86. Sato K, Webb S, Tucker A, Rabinovitch M, O'Brien RF, McMurtry IF, Stelzner TJ. Factors influencing the idiopathic development of pulmonary hypertension in the fawn hooded rat. Am Rev Respir Dis. 1992;145:793–7.

87. Nagaoka T, Muramatsu M, Sato K, McMurtry I, Oka M, Fukuchi Y. Mild hypoxia causes severe pulmonary hypertension in fawn-hooded but not in Tester Moriyama rats. Respir Physiol. 2001;127:53–60.

88. Bonnet S, Michelakis ED, Porter CJ, Andrade-Navarro MA, Thebaud B, Haromy A, Harry G, Moudgil R, McMurtry MS, Weir EK, Archer SL. An abnormal mitochondrial-hypoxia inducible factor-1alpha-Kv channel pathway disrupts oxygen sensing and triggers pulmonary arterial hypertension in fawn hooded rats: similarities to human pulmonary arterial hypertension. Circulation. 2006;113:2630–41.

89. Aguirre JI, Morrell NW, Long L, Clift P, Upton PD, Polak JM, Wilkins MR. Vascular remodeling and ET-1 expression in rat strains with different responses to chronic hypoxia. Am J Physiol Lung Cell Mol Physiol. 2000;278:L981–7.

90. Zhao L, Sebkhi A, Nunez DJ, Long L, Haley CS, Szpirer J, Szpirer C, Williams AJ, Wilkins MR. Right ventricular hypertrophy secondary to pulmonary hypertension is linked to rat chromosome 17: evaluation of cardiac ryanodine Ryr2 receptor as a candidate. Circulation. 2001;103:442–7.

91. Herget J, Suggett AJ, Leach E, Barer GR. Resolution of pulmonary hypertension and other features induced by chronic hypoxia in rats during complete and intermittent normoxia. Thorax. 1978;33:468–73.

92. Taraseviciene-Stewart L, Kasahara Y, Alger L, Hirth P, McMahon G, Waltenberger J, Voelkel NF, Tuder RM. Inhibition of the VEGF receptor 2 combined with chronic hypoxia causes cell death-dependent pulmonary endothelial cell proliferation and severe pulmonary hypertension. FASEB J. 2001;15:427–38.

93. Lang M, Kojonazarov B, Tian X, Kalymbetov A, Weissmann N, Grimminger F, Kretschmer A, Stasch JP, Seeger W, Ghofrani HA, Schermuly RT. The soluble guanylate cyclase stimulator riociguat ameliorates pulmonary hypertension induced by hypoxia and SU5416 in rats. PLoS One. 2012;7:e43433.

94. Abe K, Toba M, Alzoubi A, Ito M, Fagan KA, Cool CD, Voelkel NF, McMurtry IF, Oka M. Formation of plexiform lesions in experimental severe pulmonary arterial hypertension. Circulation. 2010;121:2747–54.

95. Fong TA, Shawver LK, Sun L, Tang C, App H, Powell TJ, Kim YH, Schreck R, Wang X, Risau W, et al. SU5416 is a potent and selective inhibitor of the vascular endothelial growth factor receptor (Flk-1/KDR) that inhibits tyrosine kinase catalysis, tumor vascularization, and growth of multiple tumor types. Cancer Res. 1999;59:99–106.

96. Oka M, Homma N, Taraseviciene-Stewart L, Morris KG, Kraskauskas D, Burns N, Voelkel NF, McMurtry IF. Rho kinase-mediated vasoconstriction is important in severe occlusive pulmonary arterial hypertension in rats. Circ Res. 2007;100:923–9.

97. de Raaf MA, Schalij I, Gomez-Arroyo J, Rol N, Happé C, de Man FS, Vonk-Noordegraaf A, Westerhof N, Voelkel NF, Bogaard HJ. SuHx rat model: partly reversible pulmonary hypertension and progressive intima obstruction. Eur Respir J. 2014;44:160–8.

98. Kojonazarov B, Hadzic S, Ghofrani HA, Grimminger F, Seeger W, Weissmann N, Schermuly RT. Severe emphysema in the SU5416/hypoxia rat model of pulmonary hypertension. Am J Respir Crit Care Med. 2019;200:515–8.

99. Bogaard HJ, Legchenko E, Chaudhary KR, Sun XQ, Stewart DJ, Hansmann G. Emphysema is-at the most-only a mild phenotype in the Sugen/hypoxia rat model of pulmonary arterial hypertension. Am J Respir Crit Care Med. 2019;200:1447–50.

100. Le Cras TD, Abman SH. Early disruption of VEGF receptor signaling and the risk for adult emphysema. Am J Respir Crit Care Med. 2020;201:620–1.

101. Kojonazarov B, Hadzic S, Ghofrani HA, Grimminger F, Seeger W, Weissmann N, Schermuly RT. Reply to Bogaard et al.: Emphysema is-at the most-only a mild phenotype in the Sugen/hypoxia rat model of pulmonary arterial hypertension. Am J Respir Crit Care Med. 2019;200:1450–2.

102. Kojonazarov B, Belenkov A, Shinomiya S, Wilchelm J, Kampschulte M, Mizuno S, Ghofrani HA, Grimminger F, Weissmann N, Seeger W, Schermuly RT. Evaluating systolic and diastolic cardiac function in rodents using microscopic computed tomography. Circ Cardiovasc Imaging. 2018;11:e007653.

103. Jiang B, Deng Y, Suen C, Taha M, Chaudhary KR, Courtman DW, Stewart DJ. Marked strain-specific differences in the SU5416 rat model of severe pulmonary arterial hypertension. Am J Respir Cell Mol Biol. 2016;54:461–8.

104. Suen CM, Chaudhary KR, Deng Y, Jiang B, Stewart DJ. Fischer rats exhibit maladaptive structural and molecular right ventricular remodelling in severe pulmonary hypertension: a genetically prone model for right heart failure. Cardiovasc Res. 2019;115:788–99.

105. Weiss A, Neubauer MC, Yerabolu D, Kojonazarov B, Schlueter BC, Neubert L, Jonigk D, Baal N, Ruppert C, Dorfmuller P, et al. Targeting cyclin-dependent kinases for the treatment of pulmonary arterial hypertension. Nat Commun. 2019;10:2204.

106. White K, Johansen AK, Nilsen M, Ciuclan L, Wallace E, Paton L, Campbell A, Morecroft I, Loughlin L, McClure JD, et al. Activity of the estrogen-metabolizing enzyme cytochrome P450 1B1 influences the development of pulmonary arterial hypertension. Circulation. 2012;126:1087–98.

107. Ciuclan L, Hussey MJ, Burton V, Good R, Duggan N, Beach S, Jones P, Fox R, Clay I, Bonneau O, et al. Imatinib attenuates hypoxia-induced pulmonary arterial hypertension pathology via reduction in 5-hydroxytryptamine through inhibition of tryptophan hydroxylase 1 expression. Am J Respir Crit Care Med. 2013;187:78–89.

108. Weissmann N. VEGF receptor inhibition as a model of pulmonary hypertension in mice. Am J Respir Crit Care Med. 2011;184:1103–5.

109. Butrous G, Ghofrani HA, Grimminger F. Pulmonary vascular disease in the developing world. Circulation. 2008;118:1758–66.

110. Warren KS. Hepatosplenic schistosomiasis: a great neglected disease of the liver. Gut. 1978;19:572–7.

111. de Cleva R, Herman P, Pugliese V, Zilberstein B, Saad WA, Rodrigues JJ, Laudanna AA. Prevalence of pulmonary hypertension in patients with hepatosplenic mansonic schistosomiasis—prospective study. Hepatogastroenterology. 2003;50:2028–30.

112. Lapa M, Dias B, Jardim C, Fernandes CJ, Dourado PM, Figueiredo M, Farias A, Tsutsui J, Terra-Filho M, Humbert M, Souza R. Cardiopulmonary manifestations of hepatosplenic schistosomiasis. Circulation. 2009;119:1518–23.

113. Tuder RM. Pathology of pulmonary arterial hypertension. Semin Respir Crit Care Med. 2009;30:376–85.

114. Graham BB, Chabon J, Bandeira A, Espinheira L, Butrous G, Tuder RM. Significant intrapulmonary Schistosoma egg antigens are not present in schistosomiasis-associated pulmonary hypertension. Pulm Circ. 2011;1:456–61.

115. Kolosionek E, Graham BB, Tuder RM, Butrous G. Pulmonary vascular disease associated with parasitic infection—the role of schistosomiasis. Clin Microbiol Infect. 2011;17:15–24.

116. Crosby A, Jones FM, Southwood M, Stewart S, Schermuly R, Butrous G, Dunne DW, Morrell NW. Pulmonary vascular remodeling correlates with lung eggs and cytokines in murine schistosomiasis. Am J Respir Crit Care Med. 2010;181:279–88.

117. Crosby A, Jones FM, Kolosionek E, Southwood M, Purvis I, Soon E, Butrous G, Dunne DE, Morrell NW. Praziquantel reverses pulmonary hypertension and vascular remodeling in murine schistosomiasis. Am J Respir Crit Care Med. 2011;184:467–73.

118. Graham BB, Chabon J, Kumar R, Kolosionek E, Gebreab L, Debella E, Edwards M, Diener K, Shade T, Bifeng G, et al. Protective role of IL6 in vascular remodeling in schistosoma-pulmonary hypertension. Am J Respir Cell Mol Biol. 2013;49(6):951–9.

119. Graham BB, Mentink-Kane MM, El-Haddad H, Purnell S, Zhang L, Zaiman A, Redente EF, Riches DW, Hassoun PM, Bandeira A, et al. Schistosomiasis-induced experimental pulmonary hypertension: role of interleukin-13 signaling. Am J Pathol. 2010;177:1549–61.

120. Wijeratne DT, Lajkosz K, Brogly SB, Lougheed MD, Jiang L, Housin A, Barber D, Johnson A, Doliszny KM, Archer SL. Increasing incidence and prevalence of World Health Organization groups 1 to 4 pulmonary hypertension: a population-based cohort study in Ontario, Canada. Circ Cardiovasc Qual Outcomes. 2018;11:e003973.

121. Vachiéry JL, Tedford RJ, Rosenkranz S, Palazzini M, Lang I, Guazzi M, Coghlan G, Chazova I, De Marco T. Pulmonary hypertension due to left heart disease. Eur Respir J. 2019;53(1):1801897.

122. Lam CS, Roger VL, Rodeheffer RJ, Borlaug BA, Enders FT, Redfield MM. Pulmonary hypertension in heart failure with preserved ejection fraction: a community-based study. J Am Coll Cardiol. 2009;53:1119–26.

123. Fayyaz AU, Edwards WD, Maleszewski JJ, Konik EA, DuBrock HM, Borlaug BA, Frantz RP, Jenkins SM, Redfield MM. Global pulmonary vascular remodeling in pulmonary hypertension associated with heart failure and preserved or reduced ejection fraction. Circulation. 2018;137:1796–810.

124. Tedford RJ, Hassoun PM, Mathai SC, Girgis RE, Russell SD, Thiemann DR, Cingolani OH, Mudd JO, Borlaug BA, Redfield MM, et al. Pulmonary capillary wedge pressure augments right ventricular pulsatile loading. Circulation. 2012;125:289–97.

125. Gorter TM, van Veldhuisen DJ, Bauersachs J, Borlaug BA, Celutkiene J, Coats AJS, Crespo-Leiro MG, Guazzi M, Harjola VP, Heymans S, et al. Right heart dysfunction and failure in heart failure with preserved ejection fraction: mechanisms and management. Position statement on behalf of the Heart Failure Association of the European Society of Cardiology. Eur J Heart Fail. 2018;20:16–37.

126. Leung CC, Moondra V, Catherwood E, Andrus BW. Prevalence and risk factors of pulmonary hypertension in patients with elevated pulmonary venous pressure and preserved ejection fraction. Am J Cardiol. 2010;106:284–6.

127. Gorter TM, van Veldhuisen DJ, Voors AA, Hummel YM, Lam CSP, Berger RMF, van Melle JP, Hoendermis ES. Right ventricular-vascular coupling in heart failure with preserved ejection fraction and pre- vs. post-capillary pulmonary hypertension. Eur Heart J Cardiovasc Imaging. 2018;19:425–32.

128. Hoeper MM, Barberà JA, Channick RN, Hassoun PM, Lang IM, Manes A, Martinez FJ, Naeije R, Olschewski H, Pepke-Zaba J, et al. Diagnosis, assessment, and treatment of non-pulmonary arterial hypertension pulmonary hypertension. J Am Coll Cardiol. 2009;54:S85–96.

129. Guazzi M, Borlaug BA. Pulmonary hypertension due to left heart disease. Circulation. 2012;126:975–90.

130. Breitling S, Ravindran K, Goldenberg NM, Kuebler WM. The pathophysiology of pulmonary hypertension in left heart disease. Am J Physiol Lung Cell Mol Physiol. 2015;309:L924–41.

131. Xiong PY, Potus F, Chan W, Archer SL. Models and molecular mechanisms of World Health Organization group 2 to 4 pulmonary hypertension. Hypertension. 2018;71:34–55.

132. Ranchoux B, Nadeau V, Bourgeois A, Provencher S, Tremblay É, Omura J, Coté N, Abu-Alhayja'a R, Dumais V, Nachbar RT, et al. Metabolic syndrome exacerbates pulmonary hypertension due to left heart disease. Circ Res. 2019;125:449–66.

133. Patten RD, Aronovitz MJ, Deras-Mejia L, Pandian NG, Hanak GG, Smith JJ, Mendelsohn ME, Konstam MA. Ventricular remodeling in a mouse model of myocardial infarction. Am J Phys. 1998;274:H1812–20.

134. de Groote P, Millaire A, Foucher-Hossein C, Nugue O, Marchandise X, Ducloux G, Lablanche JM. Right ventricular ejection fraction is an

independent predictor of survival in patients with moderate heart failure. J Am Coll Cardiol. 1998;32:948–54.

135. Pfeffer MA, Pfeffer JM, Fishbein MC, Fletcher PJ, Spadaro J, Kloner RA, Braunwald E. Myocardial infarct size and ventricular function in rats. Circ Res. 1979;44:503–12.

136. Michael LH, Entman ML, Hartley CJ, Youker KA, Zhu J, Hall SR, Hawkins HK, Berens K, Ballantyne CM. Myocardial ischemia and reperfusion: a murine model. Am J Phys. 1995;269:H2147–54.

137. Tarnavski O, McMullen JR, Schinke M, Nie Q, Kong S, Izumo S. Mouse cardiac surgery: comprehensive techniques for the generation of mouse models of human diseases and their application for genomic studies. Physiol Genomics. 2004;16:349–60.

138. Wang J, Bo H, Meng X, Wu Y, Bao Y, Li Y. A simple and fast experimental model of myocardial infarction in the mouse. Texas Heart Inst J. 2006;33:290–3.

139. Nguyen QT, Colombo F, Rouleau JL, Dupuis J, Calderone A. LU135252, an endothelin(A) receptor antagonist did not prevent pulmonary vascular remodelling or lung fibrosis in a rat model of myocardial infarction. Br J Pharmacol. 2000;130:1525–30.

140. Ben Driss A, Devaux C, Henrion D, Duriez M, Thuillez C, Levy BI, Michel JB. Hemodynamic stresses induce endothelial dysfunction and remodeling of pulmonary artery in experimental compensated heart failure. Circulation. 2000;101:2764–70.

141. Jasmin JF, Calderone A, Leung TK, Villeneuve L, Dupuis J. Lung structural remodeling and pulmonary hypertension after myocardial infarction: complete reversal with irbesartan. Cardiovasc Res. 2003;58:621–31.

142. Jiang BH, Nguyen QT, Tardif JC, Shi Y, Dupuis J. Single measurement of troponin T for early prediction of infarct size, congestive heart failure, and pulmonary hypertension in an animal model of myocardial infarction. Cardiovasc Pathol. 2011;20:e85–9.

143. Jiang BH, Tardif JC, Sauvageau S, Ducharme A, Shi Y, Martin JG, Dupuis J. Beneficial effects of atorvastatin on lung structural remodeling and function in ischemic heart failure. J Card Fail. 2010;16:679–88.

144. Toldo S, Bogaard HJ, Van Tassell BW, Mezzaroma E, Seropian IM, Robati R, Salloum FN, Voelkel NF, Abbate A. Right ventricular dysfunction following acute myocardial infarction in the absence of pulmonary hypertension in the mouse. PLoS One. 2011;6:e18102.

145. Philip JL, Murphy TM, Schreier DA, Stevens S, Tabima DM, Albrecht M, Frump AL, Hacker TA, Lahm T, Chesler NC. Pulmonary vascular mechanical consequences of ischemic heart failure and implications for right ventricular function. Am J Physiol Heart Circ Physiol. 2019;316:H1167–77.

146. Dayeh NR, Tardif JC, Shi Y, Tanguay M, Ledoux J, Dupuis J. Echocardiographic validation of pulmonary hypertension due to heart failure with reduced ejection fraction in mice. Sci Rep. 2018;8:1363.

147. Rockman HA, Ono S, Ross RS, Jones LR, Karimi M, Bhargava V, Ross J Jr, Chien KR. Molecular and physiological alterations in murine ventricular dysfunction. Proc Natl Acad Sci U S A. 1994;91:2694–8.

148. de Almeida AC, van Oort RJ, Wehrens XH. Transverse aortic constriction in mice. J Vis Exp. 2010;(38):1729.

149. Patten RD, Hall-Porter MR. Small animal models of heart failure: development of novel therapies, past and present. Circ Heart Fail. 2009;2:138–44.

150. Barrick CJ, Rojas M, Schoonhoven R, Smyth SS, Threadgill DW. Cardiac response to pressure overload in 129S1/SvImJ and C57BL/6J mice: temporal- and background-dependent development of concentric left ventricular hypertrophy. Am J Phys Heart Circ Phys. 2007;292:H2119–30.

151. Patten RD, Pourati I, Aronovitz MJ, Alsheikh-Ali A, Eder S, Force T, Mendelsohn ME, Karas RH. 17 Beta-estradiol differentially affects left ventricular and cardiomyocyte hypertrophy following myocardial infarction and pressure overload. J Card Fail. 2008;14:245–53.

152. Chen Y, Guo H, Xu D, Xu X, Wang H, Hu X, Lu Z, Kwak D, Xu Y, Gunther R, et al. Left ventricular failure produces profound lung remodeling and pulmonary hypertension in mice: heart failure causes severe lung disease. Hypertension. 2012;59:1170–8.

153. Pradhan K, Sydykov A, Tian X, Mamazhakypov A, Neupane B, Luitel H, Weissmann N, Seeger W, Grimminger F, Kretschmer A, et al. Soluble guanylate cyclase stimulator riociguat and phosphodiesterase 5 inhibitor sildenafil ameliorate pulmonary hypertension due to left heart disease in mice. Int J Cardiol. 2016;216:85–91.

154. Meng Q, Lai YC, Kelly NJ, Bueno M, Baust JJ, Bachman TN, Goncharov D, Vanderpool RR, Radder JE, Hu J, et al. Development of a mouse model of metabolic syndrome, pulmonary hypertension, and heart failure with preserved ejection fraction. Am J Respir Cell Mol Biol. 2017;56:497–505.

155. Umar S, Partow-Navid R, Ruffenach G, Iorga A, Moazeni S, Eghbali M. Severe pulmonary hypertension in aging female apolipoprotein E-deficient mice is rescued by estrogen replacement therapy. Biol Sex Differ. 2017;8:9.

156. Lawrie A, Hameed AG, Chamberlain J, Arnold N, Kennerley A, Hopkinson K, Pickworth J, Kiely DG, Crossman DC, Francis SE. Paigen diet-fed apolipoprotein E knockout mice develop severe pulmonary hypertension in an interleukin-1-dependent manner. Am J Pathol. 2011;179:1693–705.

157. Fedullo P, Kerr KM, Kim NH, Auger WR. Chronic thromboembolic pulmonary hypertension. Am J Respir Crit Care Med. 2011;183:1605–13.

158. Mayer E, Klepetko W. Techniques and outcomes of pulmonary endarterectomy for chronic thromboembolic pulmonary hypertension. Proc Am Thorac Soc. 2006;3:589–93.

159. Bottiger BW, Motsch J, Dorsam J, Mieck U, Gries A, Weimann J, Martin E. Inhaled nitric oxide selectively decreases pulmonary artery pressure and pulmonary vascular resistance following acute massive pulmonary microembolism in piglets. Chest. 1996;110:1041–7.

160. Malik AB, van der Zee H. Time course of pulmonary vascular response to microembolization. J Appl Physiol Respir Environ Exerc Physiol. 1977;43:51–8.

161. Palevsky HI, Fishman AP. Chronic cor pulmonale. Etiology and management. JAMA. 1990;263:2347–53.

162. Delcroix M, Vonk Noordegraaf A, Fadel E, Lang I, Simonneau G, Naeije R. Vascular and right ventricular remodelling in chronic thromboembolic pulmonary hypertension. Eur Respir J. 2013;41: 224–32.

163. Lang IM, Marsh JJ, Konopka RG, Olman MA, Binder BR, Moser KM, Schleef RR. Factors contributing to increased vascular fibrinolytic activity in mongrel dogs. Circulation. 1993;87: 1990–2000.

164. Mitzner W, Wagner EM. Vascular remodeling in the circulations of the lung. J Appl Physiol. 2004;97:1999–2004.

165. Shelub I, van Grondelle A, McCullough R, Hofmeister S, Reeves JT. A model of embolic chronic pulmonary hypertension in the dog. J Appl Physiol Respir Environ Exerc Physiol. 1984;56:810–5.

166. Weimann J, Zink W, Schnabel PA, Jakob H, Gebhard MM, Martin E, Motsch J. Selective vasodilation by nitric oxide inhalation during sustained pulmonary hypertension following recurrent microembolism in pigs. J Crit Care. 1999;14:133–40.

167. Dantzker DR, Bower JS. Partial reversibility of chronic pulmonary hypertension caused by pulmonary thromboembolic disease. Am Rev Respir Dis. 1981;124:129–31.

168. Moser KM, Cantor JP, Olman M, Villespin I, Graif JL, Konopka R, Marsh JJ, Pedersen C. Chronic pulmonary thromboembolism in dogs treated with tranexamic acid. Circulation. 1991;83:1371–9.

169. Marsh JJ, Konopka RG, Lang IM, Wang HY, Pedersen C, Chiles P, Reilly CF, Moser KM. Suppression of thrombolysis in a canine model of pulmonary embolism. Circulation. 1994;90:3091–7.

170. Li C-y, Deng W, Liao X-q, Deng J, Zhang Y-k, Wang D-x. The effects and mechanism of ginsenoside Rg1 on myocardial remodeling in an animal model of chronic thromboembolic pulmonary hypertension. Eur J Med Res. 2013;18(1):16.

171. Fadel E, Mazmanian GM, Chapelier A, Baudet B, Detruit H, de Montpreville V, Libert JM, Wartski M, Herve P, Dartevelle P. Lung reperfusion injury after chronic or acute unilateral pulmonary artery occlusion. Am J Respir Crit Care Med. 1998;157:1294–300.

172. Mercier O, Tivane A, Raoux F, Decante B, Eddahibi S, Dartevelle PG, Fadel E. A reliable piglet model of chronic thrombo-embolic pulmonary hypertension. Am J Respir Crit Care Med. 2011;183:A2415.

173. Bär H, Kreuzer J, Cojoc A, Jahn L. Upregulation of embryonic transcription factors right ventricular hypertrophy. Basic Res Cardiol. 2003;98:285–94.

174. Faber MJ, Dalinghaus M, Lankhuizen IM, Steendijk P, Hop WC, Schoemaker RG, Duncker DJ, Lamers JM, Helbing WA. Right and left ventricular function after chronic pulmonary artery banding in rats assessed with biventricular pressure-volume loops. Am J Phys Heart Circ Phys. 2006;291:H1580–6.

175. Kreymborg K, Uchida S, Gellert P, Schneider A, Boettger T, Voswinckel R, Wietelmann A, Szibor M, Weissmann N, Ghofrani AH, et al. Identification of right heart-enriched genes in a murine model of chronic outflow tract obstruction. J Mol Cell Cardiol. 2010;49:598–605.

176. Janssen W, Schymura Y, Novoyatleva T, Kojonazarov B, Boehm M, Wietelmann A, Luitel H, Murmann K, Krompiec DR, Tretyn A, et al. 5-HT2B receptor antagonists inhibit fibrosis and protect from RV heart failure. Biomed Res Int. 2015;2015:438403.

177. Boehm M, Lawrie A, Wilhelm J, Ghofrani HA, Grimminger F, Weissmann N, Seeger W, Schermuly RT, Kojonazarov B. Maintained right ventricular pressure overload induces ventricular-arterial decoupling in mice. Exp Physiol. 2017;102:180–9.

178. Kojonazarov B, Novoyatleva T, Boehm M, Happe C, Sibinska Z, Tian X, Sajjad A, Luitel H, Kriechling P, Posern G, et al. p38 MAPK inhibition improves heart function in pressure-loaded right ventricular hypertrophy. Am J Respir Cell Mol Biol. 2017;57: 603–14.

179. Budas GR, Boehm M, Kojonazarov B, Viswanathan G, Tian X, Veeroju S, Novoyatleva T, Grimminger F, Hinojosa-Kirschenbaum F, Ghofrani HA, et al. ASK1 inhibition halts disease progression in preclinical models of pulmonary arterial hypertension. Am J Respir Crit Care Med. 2018;197:373–85.

180. Boehm M, Arnold N, Braithwaite A, Pickworth J, Lu C, Novoyatleva T, Kiely DG, Grimminger F, Ghofrani HA, Weissmann N, et al. Eplerenone attenuates pathological pulmonary vascular rather than right ventricular remodeling in pulmonary arterial hypertension. BMC Pulm Med. 2018;18:41.

181. Boehm M, Novoyatleva T, Kojonazarov B, Veit F, Weissmann N, Ghofrani HA, Seeger W, Schermuly RT. Nitric oxide synthase 2 induction promotes right ventricular fibrosis. Am J Respir Cell Mol Biol. 2019;60:346–56.

182. Giardini A, Lovato L, Donti A, Formigari R, Oppido G, Gargiulo G, Picchio FM, Fattori R. Relation between right ventricular structural alterations and markers of adverse clinical outcome in adults

with systemic right ventricle and either congenital complete (after Senning operation) or congenitally corrected transposition of the great arteries. Am J Cardiol. 2006;98:1277–82.

183. Berk BC, Fujiwara K, Lehoux S. ECM remodeling in hypertensive heart disease. J Clin Invest. 2007;117:568–75.

184. Mundhenke M, Schwartzkopff B, Stark P, Schulte HD, Strauer BE. Myocardial collagen type I and impaired left ventricular function under exercise in hypertrophic cardiomyopathy. Thorac Cardiovasc Surg. 2002;50:216–22.

185. Jalil JE, Doering CW, Janicki JS, Pick R, Shroff SG, Weber KT. Fibrillar collagen and myocardial stiffness in the intact hypertrophied rat left ventricle. Circ Res. 1989;64:1041–50.

186. Wu Y, Cazorla O, Labeit D, Labeit S, Granzier H. Changes in titin and collagen underlie diastolic stiffness diversity of cardiac muscle. J Mol Cell Cardiol. 2000;32:2151–62.

187. Kheyfets VO, Dufva MJ, Boehm M, Tian X, Qin X, Tabakh JE, Truong U, Ivy D, Spiekerkoetter E. The left ventricle undergoes biomechanical and gene expression changes in response to increased right ventricular pressure overload. Physiol Rep. 2020;8:e14347.

188. Piao L, Fang YH, Parikh K, Ryan JJ, Toth PT, Archer SL. Cardiac glutaminolysis: a maladaptive cancer metabolism pathway in the right ventricle in pulmonary hypertension. J Mol Med (Berl). 2013;91:1185–97.

189. Piao L, Marsboom G, Archer SL. Mitochondrial metabolic adaptation in right ventricular hypertrophy and failure. J Mol Med (Berl). 2010;88: 1011–20.

190. Borgdorff MA, Koop AM, Bloks VW, Dickinson MG, Steendijk P, Sillje HH, van Wiechen MP, Berger RM, Bartelds B. Clinical symptoms of right ventricular failure in experimental chronic pressure load are associated with progressive diastolic dysfunction. J Mol Cell Cardiol. 2015;79:244–53.

191. Boehm M, Tian X, Mao Y, Ichimura K, Dufva MJ, Ali K, Dannewitz Prosseda S, Shi Y, Kuramoto K, Reddy S, et al. Delineating the molecular and histological events that govern right ventricular recovery using a novel mouse model of pulmonary artery debanding. Cardiovasc Res. 2020;116:1700–9.

192. Penumatsa KC, Warburton RR, Hill NS, Fanburg BL. CrossTalk proposal: the mouse SuHx model is a good model of pulmonary arterial hypertension. J Physiol. 2019;597:975–7.

193. Wright JL, Levy RD, Churg A. Pulmonary hypertension in chronic obstructive pulmonary disease: cur-

rent theories of pathogenesis and their implications for treatment. Thorax. 2005;60:605–9.

194. Seimetz M, Parajuli N, Pichl A, Veit F, Kwapiszewska G, Weisel FC, Milger K, Egemnazarov B, Turowska A, Fuchs B, et al. Inducible NOS inhibition reverses tobacco-smoke-induced emphysema and pulmonary hypertension in mice. Cell. 2011;147: 293–305.

195. Ferrer E, Peinado VI, Castañeda J, Prieto-Lloret J, Olea E, González-Martín MC, Vega-Agapito MV, Díez M, Domínguez-Fandos D, Obeso A, et al. Effects of cigarette smoke and hypoxia on pulmonary circulation in the guinea pig. Eur Respir J. 2011;38:617–27.

196. Marin JM, Carrizo SJ, Vicente E, Agusti AG. Long-term cardiovascular outcomes in men with obstructive sleep apnoea-hypopnoea with or without treatment with continuous positive airway pressure: an observational study. Lancet. 2005;365:1046–53.

197. Shahar E, Whitney CW, Redline S, Lee ET, Newman AB, Nieto FJ, O'Connor GT, Boland LL, Schwartz JE, Samet JM. Sleep-disordered breathing and cardiovascular disease: cross-sectional results of the Sleep Heart Health Study. Am J Respir Crit Care Med. 2001;163:19–25.

198. Dumitrascu R, Heitmann J, Seeger W, Weissmann N, Schulz R. Obstructive sleep apnea, oxidative stress and cardiovascular disease: lessons from animal studies. Oxidative Med Cell Longev. 2013;2013: 234631.

199. Sajkov D, McEvoy RD. Obstructive sleep apnea and pulmonary hypertension. Prog Cardiovasc Dis. 2009;51:363–70.

200. Fagan KA. Selected contribution: Pulmonary hypertension in mice following intermittent hypoxia. J Appl Physiol (1985). 2001;90:2502–7.

201. Campen MJ, Shimoda LA, O'Donnell CP. Acute and chronic cardiovascular effects of intermittent hypoxia in C57BL/6J mice. J Appl Physiol (1985). 2005;99:2028–35.

202. Pullamsetti SS, Kojonazarov B, Storn S, Gall H, Salazar Y, Wolf J, Weigert A, El-Nikhely N, Ghofrani HA, Krombach GA, et al. Lung cancer-associated pulmonary hypertension: role of microenvironmental inflammation based on tumor cell-immune cell cross-talk. Sci Transl Med. 2017;9(416):eaai9048.

203. Eul B, Cekay M, Pullamsetti SS, Tello K, Wilhelm J, Gattenlöhner S, Sibelius U, Grimminger F, Seeger W, Savai R. Non-invasive surrogate markers of PH are associated with poor survival in lung cancer patients. Am J Respir Crit Care Med. 2021; https://doi.org/10.1164/rccm.202005-2023LE.

Mechanical and Functional Interdependence Between the RV and LV

4

Mark K. Friedberg

Introduction

Although the left (LV) and right (RV) ventricles have different embryological origins, they are bound together through epicardial myofibers that encircle them, through myofibers that form a common apex, through the interventricular septum, their attachment to each other at the septal hinge points, the common pericardial space, the in-series configuration of the pulmonary and systemic circulation, and the coronary circulation [1, 2]. As a result, the RV and LV are anatomically and functionally connected. This tight coupling between the ventricles affects RV and LV function in health and disease. In normal physiology, RV and LV cardiac cycle events such as the onset of contraction, aortic and pulmonary flow, and RV and LV filling are closely aligned. In various conditions, such as adverse loading, electromechanical dyssynchrony, and ventricular failure, the alignment of these events is disrupted, further contributing to dysfunction and adverse ventricular-ventricular interactions. The impact of events and function in one ventricle on the contralateral ventricle is clinically important as in various diseases, RV and LV systolic functions are linearly related [3, 4]. Moreover, coexisting LV dysfunction is a key risk factor for functional decline and mortality in diseases characterized by RV dysfunction [5], and concomitant RV failure is a risk factor for death in diseases primarily characterized by LV failure [6, 7].

Physiology of RV-LV Interactions

Over the past decades, fundamental experimental work has been instrumental in delineating the importance of ventricular-ventricular interactions to cardiac function and its mechanisms (Fig. 4.1). These experiments first delineated the contribution of the LV to normal RV function. In open-chest experiments, the RV was completely electrically separated from the LV by a full-thickness RV ventriculotomy, but then sewed together to restore mechanical continuity [8]. Thus, electrical stimulation of each ventricle individually, without activation of the entire heart, could delineate the hemodynamic effects of one ventricle on developed pressure in the ipsilateral and contralateral ventricle [8]. In this experiment, stimulating the LV led to almost normal RV pressure development and pulmonary blood flow. In fact, two waveforms for RV pressure and pulmonary arterial blood flow delineated the direct contribution of RV free-wall contraction, versus LV and septal contraction, to RV developed pressure. For RV pressure and pulmonary arterial blood flow, the LV and septal

M. K. Friedberg (✉)
Division of Cardiology, The Labatt Family Heart Center, Hospital for Sick Children,
Toronto, ON, Canada
e-mail: mark.friedberg@sickkids.ca

© The Author(s), under exclusive license to Springer Nature Switzerland AG 2021
S. P. Gaine et al. (eds.), *The Right Heart*, https://doi.org/10.1007/978-3-030-78255-9_4

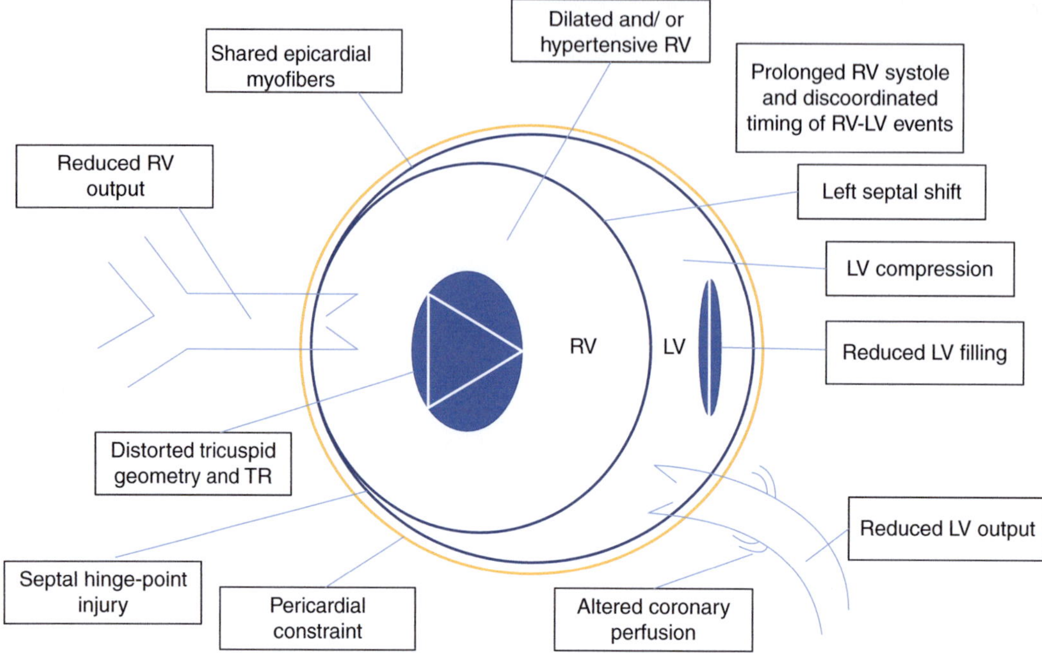

Fig. 4.1 Schematic representation of key mechanisms underlying adverse right ventricular (RV)-left ventricular (LV) interactions. Schematically depicted is a dilated RV with leftward septal shift, typical of severe pulmonary hypertension. These mechanisms manifest in other conditions as well as are detailed in the text. Within the constraints of the relatively fixed pericardial space, the hypertensive dilated RV compresses the LV and impedes its filling. Prolonged RV systolic duration and incoordinate timing of events contribute to this interaction and may impact RV and LV coronary filling and ischemia, thereby worsening dysfunction. RV dilatation predisposes to tricuspid regurgitation, which may further impede effective RV output. Decreased RV output further reduces LV filling and LV output, with a resultant decrease in cardiac output. The distorted RV and LV geometry and septal shift increase wall stress in the septum and septal hinge-point regions which triggers molecular fibrosis signaling and fibrosis. These further worsen the function of the ischemic, metabolically challenged RV. Distorted septal and ventricular geometry further impairs the function of common myofibers in the septum and superficial epicardial layers contributing to RV and LV dysfunction. Several of these mechanisms can be targeted or leveraged therapeutically to improve contralateral ventricular function

contribution were larger than the RV free-wall component. In contrast, stimulating the RV to contract led to normal RV developed pressure, but minimal developed pressure in the LV [8]. Taking these experiments further by surgically disrupting the LV free wall, to prevent it from generating any force, further confirmed these observations, with a dramatic decrease of around 45% in the systolic pressure generated by the RV [9]. The differential influence of RV and LV contraction to RV developed pressure and output has also been shown in human subjects using preexcitation of the RV by pacing or measuring hemodynamics during extrasystolic beats [10]. As in the experimental models, measurement of LV pressures during these events revealed the signifi-cant contribution of LV contraction to pressure development in the human RV [10].

Consequently, modulating LV contractile force, for example by changing LV volume, or by occlusion of the left coronary artery, impedes RV developed pressure [9]. Indeed, these studies showed that over 50% of the mechanical work of the normal RV may be generated by LV contraction and that the LV free wall plays a pivotal role in RV function [9]. Moreover, even when the RV free wall is entirely replaced with a noncontractile prosthesis, so that there is a total lack of RV free-wall contraction, there is still near-normal RV pressure generation, as a consequence of normal LV shortening [11]. In some experiments, the change in RV developed force in response to modulation of LV contraction, or loading, correlated with the degree of septal bulging into the RV cavity during systole, suggesting that the septum plays an important role in mediating these physiologic ventricular-ventricular interactions. Interestingly, however, surgically disrupting the septum did not affect RV developed pressure, but was associated with a dramatic decrease in LV developed pressure [12]. In contrast, injecting glutaraldehyde to the septum affected developed pressure in both ventricles [12]. The timing of contraction of the RV and LV further contributes to these interactions with LV contribution to RV developed pressure and pulmonary artery blood flow starting in the LV isovolumic contraction period [13].

These experiments show that under normal physiological conditions, the LV has enormous impact on RV pressure development and pulmonary arterial blood flow. This raises the question of what is the impact of the RV on normal LV function. The experiments above show that, under normal circumstances, RV contraction has little impact on developed pressure in the LV or on aortic blood flow. Even experimental ischemia of the RV free wall has minimal impact on LV developed pressure [12], and replacing the RV free wall with a noncontractile prosthesis had little effect on LV developed pressure and flow [11]. This may lead one to think that the RV has little effect on LV function, but this assumption would not be true. Firstly, the in-series configuration of the RV and LV determines that the flow generated by the RV through the pulmonary bed forms the LV preload. Additionally, changes in RV volume can profoundly affect LV contractile function. Indeed, in the aforementioned experiments that replaced the RV free wall with a noncontractile prosthesis, progressive enlargement of the noncontractile RV, by progressively repositioning a clamp along the prosthesis to increase RV cavity volume, led to progressive reduction in LV pressure development and stroke work [11]. In fact, changes in RV volume are associated with changes in the LV pressure-volume relation, which is a fundamental property and descriptor of ventricular function [10]. For example, experimental coronary artery ligation to induce acute

RV ischemia causes acute RV dilatation and reduced LV end-systolic elastance, a pressure-volume measure of contractility [14]. The change in LV function and output cannot be attributed solely to reduced LV volume secondary to RV dilatation as end-systolic elastance is a load-independent measure of LV contractility [14]. Interestingly, decreased LV end-systolic elastance secondary to RV ischemia could be reversed by creation of a superior vena cava to pulmonary artery shunt which "bypasses" the RV and reduces RV volume loading to restore more normal LV geometry [14]. This experimental observation has clinical implications in the treatment of complex congenital heart disease where placement of a superior vena cava to pulmonary artery shunt is commonly performed. The clinically important impact of RV volumes on LV stroke volume is also clinically evident during mechanical ventilation [15].

Compression of the LV during RV dilatation is dependent on the confined pericardial space that the ventricles share. In this situation, dilation of one ventricle in a confined space causes compression of the contralateral ventricle. Consequently, releasing the pericardium can normalize LV contractility even when the ischemic RV remains dilated [16]. In essence, this overlaps with the pathophysiology of cardiac tamponade where respiratory-dependent changes in RV and LV filling cause enlargement of one chamber, at the expense of the other, when the pericardial restraint or pressures are high.

RV-LV Interactions When the RV Is Hypertensive

The impact of a dilated RV on LV function becomes critical when the RV is additionally hypertensive. In patients with severe pulmonary arterial hypertension (PAH), RV dilatation compresses the LV within the confines of the relatively fixed, noncompliant, pericardial space, while high RV pressures displace the interventricular septum leftward [17]. The compressed LV and small LV volumes are further exacerbated by reduced preload due to RV dysfunction and the resulting decreased stroke volume is ejected into the pulmonary bed [17]. The combination of these factors leads to reduced LV filling while the distorted LV geometry may impede its normal contractility [18–23]. The importance of these LV geometrical changes is demonstrated by the finding that in PAH, LV, more than RV, end-diastolic volume is linearly related to cardiac output [19]. The importance of the interaction between the dilated hypertensive RV and compressed LV is further confirmed by the LV eccentricity index being linked to catheter-measured hemodynamics as well as death or lung transplantation in children with PAH [24–27]. Although perhaps most emphasized in PAH, this pathophysiological mechanism is relevant to any condition with severe RV hypertension. For example, in patients with repaired tetralogy of Fallot with severe RV hypertension from RV-pulmonary artery conduit stenosis, prolonged septal shift and prolonged RV contraction produce reduced LV filling as the septum bulges into the LV during LV diastole [28]. Consequently, alleviating stenosis of the RV-PA conduit reduces RV hypertension and normalizes septal curvature and RV contraction time, which synchronizes LV and RV contraction and relaxation [28]. The restoration of normal RV-LV interactions increases LV diastolic filling and improves exercise capacity, which is an important clinical outcome in this population [28]. Impaired LV systolic function during RV hypertension induced by pulmonary artery constriction can partly be attributed to changed LV geometry and alterations at the septal insertion points where the RV and LV connect [23]. These alterations at the septal hinge points will be further detailed later in the chapter.

As these observations suggest, the temporal disparity between RV and LV cardiac cycle events compounds the geometrical interactions induced by left septal shift. In the hypertensive RV, be it from severe conduit stenosis or PAH, RV contraction and systolic time prolong because of prolonged isovolumic contraction and relaxation [29]. Prolongation of RV systole in the dysfunctional hypertensive RV causes peak RV myocardial shortening and persistence

of elevated RV pressures into early LV diastole, at the same time that LV pressures are rapidly falling during isovolumic relaxation and rapid filling [20, 30]. This causes an abrupt leftward shift of the interventricular septum exactly as the LV is rapidly relaxing and the mitral valve is opening, impeding the dominant phase of LV filling in early LV diastole [30]. Consequently children with PAH exhibit impaired LV diastolic filling and function [26]. These adverse geometrical-temporal RV-LV interactions worsen with increasing heart rate, as diastole, and the time available for ventricular filling, is disproportionately shortened versus systole by heart rate [29]. The systolic to diastolic duration ratio, as measured from the duration of tricuspid regurgitation spectral Doppler [29], or strain imaging [20, 31], is a marker of RV systolic prolongation and decreased RV and LV filling, associated with death or lung transplantation [29]. The result of shortened RV diastolic duration and impaired LV filling is clinically important reduced stroke volume and cardiac output [19, 32–34]. The compromised hemodynamics are further worsened by inefficient RV pump function, as even though RV contraction (systolic duration) is prolonged, the short RV ejection time due to the high pulmonary vascular resistance compromises RV output, LV preload, and consequently LV filling and cardiac output [34]. These adverse interactions translate into clinical outcomes as left septal shift, LV filling, and RV systolic to diastolic duration ratio are linked to clinical outcome [29, 35].

As mentioned above, RV hypertension, dilation, and septal displacement further compromise efficient RV pump function and RV-LV interactions as they lead to incoordinate RV contraction between the septum and lateral wall and between the RV and LV lateral walls [34, 36–39]. An interventricular mechanical delay, that can occur in both RV and LV dysfunction, may further worsen LV function as well as increase the risk of arrhythmia and decrease exercise tolerance [40, 41]. The pathophysiological effect of incoordinate RV and LV cardiac cycle events also becomes evident during support of the LV by an assist device. LV assist devices are associated with shortening of LV systolic duration, disparity between LV and RV filling, and reduction in LV stroke volume secondary to reduced preload [42]. These experimental findings translate into clinical decision-making, as the speed setting in the LV assist device impacts LV sphericity, rightward septal bulge, LV-RV interactions, and RV filling, all of which ultimately affect cardiac output [43]. While the above observations emphasize RV systolic interactions, diastolic RV-LV interactions are also important. During lower body suction in patients with heart failure, decreased RV end-diastolic volume results in increased LV end-diastolic volume despite reduced pulmonary capillary wedge pressure [44, 45]. Experimentally, RV free-wall stiffening, which occurs when the RV is hypertensive [46], leads to increased septal diastolic length and increased LV stiffness, even when LV volume is constant [47]. This interaction may be mediated by the common myocardial tracts encircling the two ventricles.

Mediation of ventricular-ventricular interactions through the common myocardial tracts is also invoked as LV geometrical-temporal interactions do not account for all the adverse RV-LV interactions described above. When the RV acutely dilates secondary to right coronary obstruction and ischemia within the pericardium, there is a compression of the LV, but also impaired LV contractility that is independent of loading conditions [16]. Although leftward septal displacement within the constraints of the noncompliant pericardium is crucial in mediating ventricular interactions [48], release of the pericardium leads to restoration of LV contractility that is not solely attributable to reduced LV volume or distorted LV geometry [16]. These load-independent changes in LV contractility may stem from changed contractility in the shared superficial myofiber tracts running between the ventricles [18, 49, 50].

These shared myocardial tracts can be leveraged for therapeutic benefit. It had previously been established that acutely constricting the aorta during acute increases in RV afterload leads to increased stroke volume [51]. Although changed coronary flow patterns may explain beneficial effects of supra-aortic banding in RV pressure loading, these experiments kept coronary flow constant, so that the effects occurred independent of right coronary artery perfusion [51]. This demonstrates that, under these circumstances, there are additional factors that contribute to RV-LV interactions, most likely the shared epicardial and septal fibers [52, 53].

Increasing of the contralateral ventricle's afterload to improve ipsilateral ventricular function is also used in patients who have congenitally corrected transposition of the great arteries and tricuspid regurgitation. In this congenital heart disease, the RV is the systemic ventricle and the tricuspid valve is often malformed ("Ebstein-like") and regurgitant [54]. Often, the dilated, systemic RV and interventricular septum bulge towards the LV, further distorting the tricuspid annulus with progressively worsening tricuspid regurgitation and RV dilation [55]. Pulmonary artery banding can be used in these patients to increase LV afterload and pressure, so that the septum shifts towards the RV, into a more neutral position, thereby improving TV annular configuration and reducing TR [55]. In this condition, pulmonary artery banding may also increase contractility of the sub-pulmonary LV, leading to increased contractility of the systemic RV through the shared myocardial fibers. However, in practice, placing an adequately tight band to induce LV pressure load on the one hand, while avoiding LV failure from excessive pressure loading on the other, is a delicate balance and one not easily assessed. Increasing the contralateral ventricle's afterload has also been harnessed in children with severe dilated LV cardiomyopathy and left-heart failure, where pulmonary artery banding in carefully selected patients can lead to reduced LV dilatation, decreased mitral regurgitation, and increased LVEF [56].

The systolic interactions between the RV and LV are mediated not only by changes in septal position, and the common superficial myocardial tracts, but also by the oblique orientation of the myofibers in the interventricular septum [57]. In left-heart failure, as the LV remodels and progressively becomes more spherical, the septal fibers lose their oblique angle, thereby reducing their mechanical efficiency to reduce not only LV, but also RV contractile function. The decrease in RV function can lead to increasing tricuspid regurgitation and further RV dilatation, and a viscous cycle of additional reduction in the oblique angle of the septal myofibers [57].

Mechanical-Molecular RV-LV Interactions in RV Hypertension

Our group's experiments in a more chronic rabbit model of RV hypertension from pulmonary artery banding further extended the potential therapeutic effects of harnessing common myocardial fibers discussed above in regard to the benefits of acute aortic constriction on RV function during acute RV hypertension [52]. We found that RV hypertension leads to RV and LV dysfunction and impaired contractile function in association with myocyte hypertrophy and development of interstitial fibrosis [52]. By adding a mildly constricting aortic band, we obtained an increase in RV contractility without compromising LV contractility (indeed there was even a small increase in LV contractility) [52]. This functional benefit was associated with improved histological findings including decreased extracellular matrix remodeling, decreased biventricular fibrosis, and decreased profibrotic molecular signaling through the transforming growth factor beta (TGFβ1) and endothelin (ET)-1 pathways [52, 58, 59]. Similarly, in juvenile rabbits with RV hypertension and pulmonary artery banding, septal apoptosis, fibrosis, and reduced capillary density develop and extend to the LV free wall [60]. The improved RV and LV function with addition of a mild aortic band in the pulmonary artery band rabbit model may also stem from partial reversal of leftward septal displacement, improved RV and LV geometry, and increased LV contractility secondary to the increased LV load. The development of RV and LV fibrosis secondary to RV hypertension can also be ameliorated by pharmacological therapy including angiotensin receptor and ET-1 receptor blockade which reduce TGFβ1 signaling [58, 59, 61].

RV-LV Interactions at the Septal Hinge-Point Regions

The geometrical-temporal RV-LV cross talk in RV hypertension occurs, at least in part, at the septal hinge-point regions where increased shear stress and regional injury occur [21, 62, 63]. Indeed, LV circumferential and RV longitudinal shortening at the RV septal insertion regions contribute to increased stress, shear forces, and fibrosis [21, 64, 65]. These increased mechanical stresses trigger mechanotransduction and molecular signaling through integrins to upregulate transforming growth factor beta (TGFβ) signaling that ultimately is associated with extracellular matrix remodeling and fibrosis [66]. This mechanotransduction signaling is most prominent in the hypertensive RV and septal hinge-point regions [63, 66]. However, effects may not all be detrimental, as concomitantly with increased fibrosis, we also found increased elastin deposition at the septal hinge points [66]. Elastin, a more compliant material than stiff fibrillar collagen, may serve to increase compliance in these septal connecting regions, thereby partially buffering the LV from adverse myocardial RV-LV interactions [66].

The high-stress septal hinge-point areas also manifest clinically in human PAH patients, where MRI delayed gadolinium enhancement fibrosis imaging is increased at the RV septal insertion points in relation to the severity of RV afterload [64, 67, 68]. Thus, septal hinge-point fibrosis may be clinically important as it is associated with reduced RV function and increased mortality [64, 67]. In children with PAH, we found that decreased LV myocardial shortening was most prominent at the septum, consistent with the experimental and clinical findings at the septal hinge-point regions [69].

Similar to findings in rat and rabbit PAB models, mice with PAB demonstrate impaired RV and LV systolic function along with decreased LV stroke work, torsion and torsion rate, and mildly increased LV fibrosis, attributed to increased myocardial stress [70]. The LV histological and functional changes and fibrosis were accompanied by increased β-MHC expression and decreased expression of Ca^{2+}-handling proteins [70]. The changes in α- and β-MHC expression were in turn associated with the changes in LV mechanics. Interestingly, the association between increased RV pressure loading and decreased LV torsion mechanics is in contrast to findings from acute experiments where the LV responded to an acute increase in RV pressure loading and decreased RV stroke volume by an acute increase in torsion and untwist rate [71]. The differences between these results may possibly be explained by the development of myocardial hypertrophy and fibrosis in the chronic models and by differences in volume loading, coronary perfusion, and different myocardial mechanics in acute versus chronic conditions. Indeed, acute RV pressure loading can lead to acute decreases in LV contractility, developed pressure, diastolic volume, and cardiac output that correlate with decreased LV and septal circumferential strain, LV untwisting, and apical rotation [72]. The septal circumferential strain, which likely correlates with septal oblique myofibers described above, was the most important factor associated with reduced LV performance [72].

Therapeutic Targeting of Molecular-Tissue RV-LV Interactions in RV Hypertension

Increasing the pressure load of the contralateral ventricle through aortic or pulmonary artery banding may be effective in changing ventricular geometry, septal position, and contralateral ventricular contractility. However, this invasive approach may be difficult to apply clinically in fragile patients. Consequently, pharmacologically inhibiting the adverse molecular signaling in the RV and the septal hinge-point regions leading to tissue injury and increased fibrosis may be a therapeutic option to address the molecular-tissue effects of adverse RV-LV interactions. As detailed above, in PAB rabbit models, we showed that angiotensin and endothelin-receptor blockades, both of which decrease TGFβ signaling, lead to decreased biventricular fibrosis and improved biventricular function [58, 59, 61].

Pharmacological therapy to reduce heart rate may also be beneficial in certain circumstances to address the temporal aspects of adverse RV-LV interactions in RV pressure loading and PAH. In rat models of PAH and pulmonary artery banding, we showed that slowing heart rate using the beta-adrenergic receptor antagonist carvedilol, or the non-adrenergic agent ivabradine, improves RV and LV function through alignment of RV and LV events [73–75]. We attributed this realignment in RV-LV events to improved RV diastolic relaxation, possibly due to improved Ca^{2+} cycling [73–75]. Importantly, the improved biventricular function was associated with reduced fibrosis and cardiomyocyte hypertrophy, even though RV systolic pressures and RV-LV geometry and compression were unchanged, showing that heart rate-reducing agents were not acting through alleviation of pulmonary arterial or RV pressures [73–75].

RV-LV Interactions in Congenital Heart Disease

Because of pressure and/or volume loading and distorted ventricular structure and geometry, various congenital heart diseases can demonstrate the physiological and clinical importance of ventricular-ventricular interactions. An intriguing example is when one of the ventricles is severely hypoplastic. Functionally single ventricles have markedly altered myocardial mechanics including myocardial shortening, twist, and radial motion. While these may be impacted by multiple factors, the lack of a contralateral ventricle may constitute one of these factors. An example of such adverse interactions can be seen in hypoplastic left-heart syndrome, where the direct and indirect impacts of an underdeveloped LV may alter RV and TV annular configuration and worsen TR, which increases the risk for death or need for heart transplant [76]. The presence of a small LV can also distort RV geometry and cause RV apical bulging, which we found to be associated with impaired RV mechanics and increased risk for heart transplant or death [77]. We further found diminished septal strain in

HLHS patients with a moderately hypoplastic LV (and hence relatively larger LV) versus a diminutive (and hence almost absent) LV, in association with asymmetric RV mechanics and worse clinical outcome [78]. Thus, the presence of a hypoplastic LV may be worse than having no discernable LV, as RV geometry appears to be adversely affected.

A maldeveloped RV can also impact LV function, as occurs in Ebstein's anomaly of the tricuspid valve. In this condition, the tricuspid septal and inferior leaflets are displaced and rotated apically and towards the RV outflow tract. This yields a variable length of the interventricular septum as part of functional right atrium, a small "functional" RV distal to the displaced tricuspid leaflets, that has impaired myocardial function, and variable but often severe TR. In these children, we found that an early diastolic leftward interventricular shift is found in most patients and associated with decreased LV filling and with more TR [79]. Moreover, reduced pulmonary artery antegrade flow was associated with lower LV filling, LV volumes, LVEF, and output. Importantly, from a clinical perspective, impaired LV systolic and diastolic volumes and performance were associated with reduced exercise capacity [79]. We hypothesized that prolonged RV systole and increased TR may impede LV filling, whereas decreased LVEF, SV, systolic strain, and delayed aortic and atrioventricular valve opening and closure suggest impaired contractile force development, possibly related to enlargement and dysfunction of the "functional" RV (the portion of the RV that remains distal to the displaced tricuspid valve). We also hypothesized that early rightward IVS motion may impede LV systolic function, and an ineffective leftward systolic septal shift may impede pressure development [79]. Thus, although the pathophysiology is completely different from PAH, some of the adverse RV-LV interactions have similar features stemming from impaired RV contractile function and disparate RV and LV events and geometry. Indeed, severe Ebstein's anomaly that manifests clinically in the early neonatal period can be very difficult to manage, even if the LV functions well. Thus, the RV is clearly central to cardiac function and clinical outcomes in these situations.

The effects of an abnormal RV on the LV are also apparent in repaired tetralogy of Fallot. Tetralogy of Fallot is a cyanotic congenital heart disease characterized by RV outflow tract obstruction and a large ventricular septal defect. After surgical "repair" in infancy, which patch-closes the ventricular septal defect and relieves RV outflow tract obstruction, there is often pulmonary regurgitation due to disruption of the pulmonary valve [80]. Consequently, chronic RV volume loading and dilatation impact both RV and LV filling, function, and mechanics [81]. RV dilatation is associated with impaired LV intracavitary flow patterns, specifically, LV diastolic flow and flow of the residual blood volume that is retained in the ventricle after ejection [82]. These impaired LV flow patterns correlate with reduced LV circumferential shortening and ejection fraction [82]. These abnormal flow patterns are likely associated with impaired LV kinetic energy [83]. Reduced LV twist and strain have also been found in this population, in relation to RV dilatation [4, 84–88]. The common apical myofibers, which determine to a large extent LV twist-untwist, may be responsible for the decrease in LV torsion, and consequently decreases in LV intraventricular pressure gradients and diastolic suction [89, 90]. Indeed, even though tetralogy of Fallot is thought to be a "right-heart" disease, both RV and LV diastolic functions are impaired after tetralogy of Fallot surgical repair, in part due to the effects of adverse ventricular-ventricular interactions [91–93]. The association between RV and LV function in repaired tetralogy of Fallot is also found at the myocardial level [94]. Our group showed that reduced LV early diastolic deformation is associated with RV dilatation and pulmonary regurgitation [91]. However, LV dysfunction in repaired tetralogy of Fallot may not only stem from RV abnormalities. Aortic dilatation is very common after tetralogy of Fallot repair and may be associated with increased aortic shear stress, stiffness, and abnormal flow that may directly impact LV function [95, 96].

Summary

In summary, the RV and LV are tightly linked. Consequently, function and events in one ventricle can profoundly impact the contralateral ventricle. These adverse interactions are found in diverse acquired and congenital heart diseases and seem to be critical in severe RV hypertension, most importantly PAH. The challenge is often to determine which outcomes are due to adverse RV-LV interactions versus ipsilateral effects. Answering this question will assist in designing therapies that can leverage beneficial ventricular-ventricular interactions while reducing the effects of adverse RV-LV interactions.

References

1. Appleyard RF, Glantz SA. Pulmonary model to predict the effects of series ventricular interaction. Circ Res. 1990;67(5):1225–37.
2. Slinker BK, Glantz SA. End-systolic and end-diastolic ventricular interaction. Am J Physiol. 1986;251(5 Pt 2):H1062–75.
3. Davlouros PA, Kilner PJ, Hornung TS, Li W, Francis JM, Moon JC, et al. Right ventricular function in adults with repaired tetralogy of Fallot assessed with cardiovascular magnetic resonance imaging: detrimental role of right ventricular outflow aneurysms or akinesia and adverse right-to-left ventricular interaction. J Am Coll Cardiol. 2002;40(11):2044–52.
4. Kempny A, Diller GP, Orwat S, Kaleschke G, Kerckhoff G, Bunck A, et al. Right ventricular-left ventricular interaction in adults with tetralogy of Fallot: a combined cardiac magnetic resonance and echocardiographic speckle tracking study. Int J Cardiol. 2012;154(3):259–64.
5. Ghai A, Silversides C, Harris L, Webb GD, Siu SC, Therrien J. Left ventricular dysfunction is a risk factor for sudden cardiac death in adults late after repair of tetralogy of Fallot. J Am Coll Cardiol. 2002;40(9):1675–80.
6. Gulati A, Ismail TF, Jabbour A, Alpendurada F, Guha K, Ismail NA, et al. The prevalence and prognostic significance of right ventricular systolic dysfunction in nonischemic dilated cardiomyopathy. Circulation. 2013;128(15):1623–33.
7. Alhamshari YS, Alnabelsi T, Mulki R, Cepeda-Valery B, Figueredo VM, Romero-Corral A. Right ventricular function measured by TAPSE in obese subjects at the time of acute myocardial infarction and 2 year outcomes. Int J Cardiol. 2017;232:181–5.
8. Damiano RJ Jr, La Follette P Jr, Cox JL, Lowe JE, Santamore WP. Significant left ventricular contribution to right ventricular systolic function. Am J Physiol. 1991;261(5 Pt 2):H1514–24.
9. Santamore WP, Lynch PR, Heckman JL, Bove AA, Meier GD. Left ventricular effects on right ventricular developed pressure. J Appl Physiol. 1976;41(6):925–30.
10. Feneley MP, Gavaghan TP, Baron DW, Branson JA, Roy PR, Morgan JJ. Contribution of left ventricular contraction to the generation of right ventricular systolic pressure in the human heart. Circulation. 1985;71(3):473–80.
11. Hoffman D, Sisto D, Frater RW, Nikolic SD. Left-to-right ventricular interaction with a noncontracting right ventricle. J Thorac Cardiovasc Surg. 1994;107(6):1496–502.
12. Li KS, Santamore WP. Contribution of each wall to biventricular function. Cardiovasc Res. 1993;27(5):792–800.
13. Schertz C, Pinsky MR. Effect of the pericardium on systolic ventricular interdependence in the dog. J Crit Care. 1993;8(1):17–23.
14. Danton MH, Byrne JG, Flores KQ, Hsin M, Martin JS, Laurence RG, et al. Modified Glenn connection for acutely ischemic right ventricular failure reverses secondary left ventricular dysfunction. J Thorac Cardiovasc Surg. 2001;122(1):80–91.
15. Mitchell JR, Whitelaw WA, Sas R, Smith ER, Tyberg JV, Belenkie I. RV filling modulates LV function by direct ventricular interaction during mechanical ventilation. Am J Physiol Heart Circ Physiol. 2005;289(2):H549–57.
16. Brookes C, Ravn H, White P, Moeldrup U, Oldershaw P, Redington A. Acute right ventricular dilatation in response to ischemia significantly impairs left ventricular systolic performance. Circulation. 1999;100(7):761–7.
17. Friedberg MK. Imaging right-left ventricular interactions. JACC Cardiovasc Imaging. 2018;11(5):755–71.
18. Moulopoulos SD, Sarcas A, Stamatelopoulos S, Arealis E. Left ventricular performance during bypass or distension of the right ventricle. Circ Res. 1965;17(6):484–91.
19. Gan C, Lankhaar JW, Marcus JT, Westerhof N, Marques KM, Bronzwaer JG, et al. Impaired left ventricular filling due to right-to-left ventricular interaction in patients with pulmonary arterial hypertension. Am J Physiol Heart Circ Physiol. 2006;290(4):H1528–33.
20. Marcus JT, Vonk Noordegraaf A, Roeleveld RJ, Postmus PE, Heethaar RM, Van Rossum AC, et al. Impaired left ventricular filling due to right ventricular pressure overload in primary pulmonary hypertension: noninvasive monitoring using MRI. Chest. 2001;119(6):1761–5.
21. Nelson GS, Sayed-Ahmed EY, Kroeker CA, Sun YH, Keurs HE, Shrive NG, et al. Compression of interventricular septum during right ventricular

pressure loading. Am J Physiol Heart Circ Physiol. 2001;280(6):H2639–48.

22. Roeleveld RJ, Marcus JT, Faes TJ, Gan TJ, Boonstra A, Postmus PE, et al. Interventricular septal configuration at MR imaging and pulmonary arterial pressure in pulmonary hypertension. Radiology. 2005;234(3):710–7.

23. Visner MC, Arentzen CE, O'Connor MJ, Larson EV, Anderson RW. Alterations in left ventricular three-dimensional dynamic geometry and systolic function during acute right ventricular hypertension in the conscious dog. Circulation. 1983;67(2):353–65.

24. Burkett DA, Patel SS, Mertens L, Friedberg MK, Ivy DD. Relationship between left ventricular geometry and invasive hemodynamics in pediatric pulmonary hypertension. Circ Cardiovasc Imaging. 2020;13(5):e009825.

25. Kassem E, Humpl T, Friedberg MK. Prognostic significance of 2-dimensional, M-mode, and Doppler echo indices of right ventricular function in children with pulmonary arterial hypertension. Am Heart J. 2013;165(6):1024–31.

26. Burkett DA, Slorach C, Patel SS, Redington AN, Ivy DD, Mertens L, et al. Impact of pulmonary hemodynamics and ventricular interdependence on left ventricular diastolic function in children with pulmonary hypertension. Circ Cardiovasc Imaging. 2016;9(9):e004612.

27. Jone PN, Hinzman J, Wagner BD, Ivy DD, Younoszai A. Right ventricular to left ventricular diameter ratio at end-systole in evaluating outcomes in children with pulmonary hypertension. J Am Soc Echocardiogr. 2014;27(2):172–8.

28. Lurz P, Puranik R, Nordmeyer J, Muthurangu V, Hansen MS, Schievano S, et al. Improvement in left ventricular filling properties after relief of right ventricle to pulmonary artery conduit obstruction: contribution of septal motion and interventricular mechanical delay. Eur Heart J. 2009;30(18):2266–74.

29. Alkon J, Humpl T, Manlhiot C, McCrindle BW, Reyes JT, Friedberg MK. Usefulness of the right ventricular systolic to diastolic duration ratio to predict functional capacity and survival in children with pulmonary arterial hypertension. Am J Cardiol. 2010;106(3):430–6.

30. Driessen MM, Hui W, Bijnens BH, Dragulescu A, Mertens L, Meijboom FJ, et al. Adverse ventricular-ventricular interactions in right ventricular pressure load: insights from pediatric pulmonary hypertension versus pulmonary stenosis. Physiol Rep. 2016;4(11):e12833.

31. Hui W, Slorach C, Iori S, Dragulescu A, Mertens L, Friedberg MK. The right ventricular myocardial systolic-to-diastolic duration ratio in children after surgical repair of tetralogy of Fallot. J Appl Physiol (1985). 2020;128(6):1677–83.

32. Taylor RR, Covell JW, Sonnenblick EH, Ross J Jr. Dependence of ventricular distensibility on filling of the opposite ventricle. Am J Physiol. 1967;213(3):711–8.

33. Duffels MG, Hardziyenka M, Surie S, de Bruin-Bon RH, Hoendermis ES, van Dijk AP, et al. Duration of right ventricular contraction predicts the efficacy of bosentan treatment in patients with pulmonary hypertension. Eur J Echocardiogr. 2009;10(3):433–8.

34. Gurudevan SV, Malouf PJ, Auger WR, Waltman TJ, Madani M, Raisinghani AB, et al. Abnormal left ventricular diastolic filling in chronic thromboembolic pulmonary hypertension: true diastolic dysfunction or left ventricular underfilling? J Am Coll Cardiol. 2007;49(12):1334–9.

35. Mahmud E, Raisinghani A, Hassankhani A, Sadeghi HM, Strachan GM, Auger W, et al. Correlation of left ventricular diastolic filling characteristics with right ventricular overload and pulmonary artery pressure in chronic thromboembolic pulmonary hypertension. J Am Coll Cardiol. 2002;40(2):318–24.

36. Kalogeropoulos AP, Georgiopoulou VV, Howell S, Pernetz MA, Fisher MR, Lerakis S, et al. Evaluation of right intraventricular dyssynchrony by two-dimensional strain echocardiography in patients with pulmonary arterial hypertension. J Am Soc Echocardiogr. 2008;21(9):1028–34.

37. Lopez-Candales A, Dohi K, Rajagopalan N, Suffoletto M, Murali S, Gorcsan J, et al. Right ventricular dyssynchrony in patients with pulmonary hypertension is associated with disease severity and functional class. Cardiovasc Ultrasound. 2005;3:23.

38. Vonk-Noordegraaf A, Marcus JT, Gan CT, Boonstra A, Postmus PE. Interventricular mechanical asynchrony due to right ventricular pressure overload in pulmonary hypertension plays an important role in impaired left ventricular filling. Chest. 2005;128(6 Suppl):628S–30S.

39. Marcus JT, Gan CT, Zwanenburg JJ, Boonstra A, Allaart CP, Gotte MJ, et al. Interventricular mechanical asynchrony in pulmonary arterial hypertension: left-to-right delay in peak shortening is related to right ventricular overload and left ventricular underfilling. J Am Coll Cardiol. 2008;51(7):750–7.

40. D'Andrea A, Caso P, Sarubbi B, D'Alto M, Giovanna Russo M, Scherillo M, et al. Right ventricular myocardial activation delay in adult patients with right bundle branch block late after repair of tetralogy of Fallot. Eur J Echocardiogr. 2004;5(2):123–31.

41. Hui W, Slorach C, Friedberg MK. Apical transverse motion is associated with interventricular mechanical delay and decreased left ventricular function in children with dilated cardiomyopathy. J Am Soc Echocardiogr. 2018;31(8):943–50.

42. Shimamura J, Nishimura T, Mizuno T, Takewa Y, Tsukiya T, Inatomi A, et al. Quantification of interventricular dyssynchrony during continuous-flow left ventricular assist device support. J Artif Organs. 2019;22(4):269–75.

43. Addetia K, Uriel N, Maffessanti F, Sayer G, Adatya S, Kim GH, et al. 3D morphological changes in LV and RV during LVAD ramp studies. JACC Cardiovasc Imaging. 2018;11(2 Pt 1):159–69.

44. Tyberg JV, Belenkie I, Manyari DE, Smith ER. Ventricular interaction and venous capacitance modulate left ventricular preload. Can J Cardiol. 1996;12(10):1058–64.

45. Atherton JJ, Moore TD, Lele SS, Thomson HL, Galbraith AJ, Belenkie I, et al. Diastolic ventricular interaction in chronic heart failure. Lancet. 1997;349(9067):1720–4.

46. Rain S, Andersen S, Najafi A, Gammelgaard Schultz J, da Silva Goncalves Bos D, Handoko ML, et al. Right ventricular myocardial stiffness in experimental pulmonary arterial hypertension: relative contribution of fibrosis and myofibril stiffness. Circ Heart Fail. 2016;9(7):e002636.

47. Shirakabe M, Yamaguchi S, Tamada Y, Baniya G, Fukui A, Miyawaki H, et al. Impaired distensibility of the left ventricle after stiffening of the right ventricle. J Appl Physiol (1985). 2001;91(1):435–40.

48. Kroeker CA, Shrive NG, Belenkie I, Tyberg JV. Pericardium modulates left and right ventricular stroke volumes to compensate for sudden changes in atrial volume. Am J Physiol Heart Circ Physiol. 2003;284(6):H2247–54.

49. Sanchez-Quintana D, Climent V, Ho SY, Anderson RH. Myoarchitecture and connective tissue in hearts with tricuspid atresia. Heart. 1999;81(2):182–91.

50. Smerup M, Nielsen E, Agger P, Frandsen J, Vestergaard-Poulsen P, Andersen J, et al. The three-dimensional arrangement of the myocytes aggregated together within the mammalian ventricular myocardium. Anat Rec (Hoboken). 2009;292(1):1–11.

51. Belenkie I, Horne SG, Dani R, Smith ER, Tyberg JV. Effects of aortic constriction during experimental acute right ventricular pressure loading. Further insights into diastolic and systolic ventricular interaction. Circulation. 1995;92(3):546–54.

52. Apitz C, Honjo O, Humpl T, Li J, Assad RS, Cho MY, et al. Biventricular structural and functional responses to aortic constriction in a rabbit model of chronic right ventricular pressure overload. J Thorac Cardiovasc Surg. 2012;144(6):1494–501.

53. Apitz C, Honjo O, Friedberg MK, Assad RS, Van Arsdell G, Humpl T, et al. Beneficial effects of vasopressors on right ventricular function in experimental acute right ventricular failure in a rabbit model. Thorac Cardiovasc Surg. 2012;60(1):17–23.

54. Prieto LR, Hordof AJ, Secic M, Rosenbaum MS, Gersony WM. Progressive tricuspid valve disease in patients with congenitally corrected transposition of the great arteries. Circulation. 1998;98(10):997–1005.

55. Kral Kollars CA, Gelehrter S, Bove EL, Ensing G. Effects of morphologic left ventricular pressure on right ventricular geometry and tricuspid valve regurgitation in patients with congenitally corrected transposition of the great arteries. Am J Cardiol. 2010;105(5):735–9.

56. Schranz D, Rupp S, Muller M, Schmidt D, Bauer A, Valeske K, et al. Pulmonary artery banding in infants and young children with left ventricular dilated cardiomyopathy: a novel therapeutic strategy before heart transplantation. J Heart Lung Transplant. 2013;32(5):475–81.

57. Schwarz K, Singh S, Dawson D, Frenneaux MP. Right ventricular function in left ventricular disease: pathophysiology and implications. Heart Lung Circ. 2013;22(7):507–11.

58. Ramos SR, Pieles G, Sun M, Slorach C, Hui W, Friedberg MK. Early versus late cardiac remodeling during right ventricular pressure load and impact of preventive versus rescue therapy with endothelin-1 receptor blockers. J Appl Physiol (1985). 2018;124(5):1349–62.

59. Nielsen EA, Sun M, Honjo O, Hjortdal VE, Redington AN, Friedberg MK. Dual endothelin receptor blockade abrogates right ventricular remodeling and biventricular fibrosis in isolated elevated right ventricular afterload. PLoS One. 2016;11(1):e0146767.

60. Kitahori K, He H, Kawata M, Cowan DB, Friehs I, Del Nido PJ, et al. Development of left ventricular diastolic dysfunction with preservation of ejection fraction during progression of infant right ventricular hypertrophy. Circ Heart Fail. 2009;2(6):599–607.

61. Friedberg MK, Cho MY, Li J, Assad RS, Sun M, Rohailla S, et al. Adverse biventricular remodeling in isolated right ventricular hypertension is mediated by increased transforming growth factor-beta1 signaling and is abrogated by angiotensin receptor blockade. Am J Respir Cell Mol Biol. 2013;49(6):1019–28.

62. Gold J, Akazawa Y, Sun M, Hunter KS, Friedberg MK. Relation between right ventricular wall stress, fibrosis, and function in right ventricular pressure loading. Am J Physiol Heart Circ Physiol. 2020;318(2):H366–H77.

63. Nielsen EA, Okumura K, Sun M, Hjortdal VE, Redington AN, Friedberg MK. Regional septal hinge-point injury contributes to adverse biventricular interactions in pulmonary hypertension. Physiol Rep. 2017;5(14):e13332.

64. McCann GP, Gan CT, Beek AM, Niessen HW, Vonk Noordegraaf A, van Rossum AC. Extent of MRI delayed enhancement of myocardial mass is related to right ventricular dysfunction in pulmonary artery hypertension. AJR Am J Roentgenol. 2007;188(2):349–55.

65. Beyar R, Dong SJ, Smith ER, Belenkie I, Tyberg JV. Ventricular interaction and septal deformation: a model compared with experimental data. Am J Phys. 1993;265(6 Pt 2):H2044–56.

66. Sun M, Ishii R, Okumura K, Krauszman A, Breitling S, Gomez O, et al. Experimental right ventricular hypertension induces regional beta1-integrin-mediated transduction of hypertrophic and profibrotic right and left ventricular signaling. J Am Heart Assoc. 2018;7(7):e007928.

67. Shehata ML, Lossnitzer D, Skrok J, Boyce D, Lechtzin N, Mathai SC, et al. Myocardial delayed enhancement

in pulmonary hypertension: pulmonary hemodynamics, right ventricular function, and remodeling. AJR Am J Roentgenol. 2011;196(1):87–94.

68. Sanz J, Dellegrottaglie S, Kariisa M, Sulica R, Poon M, O'Donnell TP, et al. Prevalence and correlates of septal delayed contrast enhancement in patients with pulmonary hypertension. Am J Cardiol. 2007;100(4):731–5.

69. Burkett DA, Slorach C, Patel SS, Redington AN, Ivy DD, Mertens L, et al. Left ventricular myocardial function in children with pulmonary hypertension: relation to right ventricular performance and hemodynamics. Circ Cardiovasc Imaging. 2015;8(8):e003260.

70. Kheyfets VO, Dufva MJ, Boehm M, Tian X, Qin X, Tabakh JE, et al. The left ventricle undergoes biomechanical and gene expression changes in response to increased right ventricular pressure overload. Physiol Rep. 2020;8(9):e14347.

71. Cho EJ, Jiamsripong P, Calleja AM, Alharthi MS, McMahon EM, Chandrasekaran K, et al. The left ventricle responds to acute graded elevation of right ventricular afterload by augmentation of twist magnitude and untwist rate. J Am Soc Echocardiogr. 2011;24(8):922–9.

72. Chua J, Zhou W, Ho JK, Patel NA, Mackensen GB, Mahajan A. Acute right ventricular pressure overload compromises left ventricular function by altering septal strain and rotation. J Appl Physiol (1985). 2013;115(2):186–93.

73. Gomez O, Okumura K, Honjo O, Sun M, Ishii R, Bijnens B, et al. Heart rate reduction improves biventricular function and interactions in experimental pulmonary hypertension. Am J Physiol Heart Circ Physiol. 2018;314(3):H542–H51.

74. Ishii R, Okumura K, Akazawa Y, Malhi M, Ebata R, Sun M, et al. Heart rate reduction improves right ventricular function and fibrosis in pulmonary hypertension. Am J Respir Cell Mol Biol. 2020;63(6): 843–55.

75. Okumura K, Kato H, Honjo O, Breitling S, Kuebler WM, Sun M, et al. Carvedilol improves biventricular fibrosis and function in experimental pulmonary hypertension. J Mol Med (Berl). 2015;93(6):663–74.

76. Takahashi K, Inage A, Rebeyka IM, Ross DB, Thompson RB, Mackie AS, et al. Real-time 3-dimensional echocardiography provides new insight into mechanisms of tricuspid valve regurgitation in patients with hypoplastic left heart syndrome. Circulation. 2009;120(12):1091–8.

77. Rosner A, Bharucha T, James A, Mertens L, Friedberg MK. Impact of right ventricular geometry and left ventricular hypertrophy on right ventricular mechanics and clinical outcomes in hypoplastic left heart syndrome. J Am Soc Echocardiogr. 2019;32(10): 1350–8.

78. Forsha D, Li L, Joseph N, Kutty S, Friedberg MK. Association of left ventricular size with regional right ventricular mechanics in hypoplastic left heart syndrome. Int J Cardiol. 2020;298:66–71.

79. Fujioka T, Kuhn A, Sanchez-Martinez S, Bijnens BH, Hui W, Slorach C, et al. Impact of interventricular interactions on left ventricular function, stroke volume, and exercise capacity in children and adults with Ebstein's anomaly. JACC Cardiovasc Imaging. 2019;12(5):925–7.

80. Hickey EJ, Veldtman G, Bradley TJ, Gengsakul A, Manlhiot C, Williams WG, et al. Late risk of outcomes for adults with repaired tetralogy of Fallot from an inception cohort spanning four decades. Eur J Cardiothorac Surg. 2009;35(1):156–64; discussion 64.

81. Larios G, Friedberg MK. Imaging in repaired tetralogy of Fallot with a focus on recent advances in echocardiography. Curr Opin Cardiol. 2017;32(5): 490–502.

82. Schafer M, Browne LP, Jaggers J, Barker AJ, Morgan GJ, Ivy DD, et al. Abnormal left ventricular flow organization following repair of tetralogy of Fallot. J Thorac Cardiovasc Surg. 2020;160(4): 1008–15.

83. Sjoberg P, Bidhult S, Bock J, Heiberg E, Arheden H, Gustafsson R, et al. Disturbed left and right ventricular kinetic energy in patients with repaired tetralogy of Fallot: pathophysiological insights using 4D-flow MRI. Eur Radiol. 2018;28(10):4066–76.

84. Li SN, Yu W, Lai CT, Wong SJ, Cheung YF. Left ventricular mechanics in repaired tetralogy of Fallot with and without pulmonary valve replacement: analysis by three-dimensional speckle tracking echocardiography. PLoS One. 2013;8(11):e78826.

85. Dragulescu A, Friedberg MK, Grosse-Wortmann L, Redington A, Mertens L. Effect of chronic right ventricular volume overload on ventricular interaction in patients after tetralogy of Fallot repair. J Am Soc Echocardiogr. 2014;27(8):896–902.

86. Fernandes FP, Manlhiot C, Roche SL, Grosse-Wortmann L, Slorach C, McCrindle BW, et al. Impaired left ventricular myocardial mechanics and their relation to pulmonary regurgitation, right ventricular enlargement and exercise capacity in asymptomatic children after repair of tetralogy of Fallot. J Am Soc Echocardiogr. 2012;25(5):494–503.

87. Cheung EW, Liang XC, Lam WW, Cheung YF. Impact of right ventricular dilation on left ventricular myocardial deformation in patients after surgical repair of tetralogy of fallot. Am J Cardiol. 2009;104(9):1264–70.

88. Li Y, Xie M, Wang X, Lu Q, Zhang L, Ren P. Impaired right and left ventricular function in asymptomatic children with repaired tetralogy of Fallot by two-dimensional speckle tracking echocardiography study. Echocardiography. 2015;32(1):135–43.

89. Firstenberg MS, Smedira NG, Greenberg NL, Prior DL, McCarthy PM, Garcia MJ, et al. Relationship between early diastolic intraventricular pressure gradients, an index of elastic recoil, and improvements in systolic and diastolic function. Circulation. 2001;104(12 Suppl 1):I330–5.

90. Kobayashi M, Takahashi K, Yamada M, Yazaki K, Matsui K, Tanaka N, et al. Assessment of early diastolic intraventricular pressure gradient in the left ventricle among patients with repaired tetralogy of Fallot. Heart Vessel. 2017;32(11):1364–74.

91. Friedberg MK, Fernandes FP, Roche SL, Grosse-Wortmann L, Manlhiot C, Fackoury C, et al. Impaired right and left ventricular diastolic myocardial mechanics and filling in asymptomatic children and adolescents after repair of tetralogy of Fallot. Eur Heart J Cardiovasc Imaging. 2012;13(11):905–13.

92. Cullen S, Shore D, Redington A. Characterization of right ventricular diastolic performance after complete repair of tetralogy of Fallot. Restrictive physiology predicts slow postoperative recovery. Circulation. 1995;91(6):1782–9.

93. Liang XC, Cheung EW, Wong SJ, Cheung YF. Impact of right ventricular volume overload on three-dimensional global left ventricular mechanical dyssynchrony after surgical repair of tetralogy of Fallot. Am J Cardiol. 2008;102(12):1731–6.

94. Li VW, Yu CK, So EK, Wong WH, Cheung YF. Ventricular myocardial deformation imaging of patients with repaired tetralogy of Fallot. J Am Soc Echocardiogr. 2020;33(7):788–801.

95. Grotenhuis HB, Dallaire F, Verpalen IM, van den Akker MJE, Mertens L, Friedberg MK. Aortic root dilatation and aortic-related complications in children after tetralogy of Fallot repair. Circ Cardiovasc Imaging. 2018;11(12):e007611.

96. Schafer M, Browne LP, Morgan GJ, Barker AJ, Fonseca B, Ivy DD, et al. Reduced proximal aortic compliance and elevated wall shear stress after early repair of tetralogy of Fallot. J Thorac Cardiovasc Surg. 2018;156(6):2239–49.

MRI of the Right Ventricle in Normal Subjects and Those with Pulmonary Hypertension

5

Andrew J. Peacock and Melanie J. Brewis

Abbreviations

BMI	Body mass index
BSA	Body surface area
CMR	Cardiac magnetic resonance imaging
LV	Left ventricular
MESA-RV	Multi-ethnic study of atherosclerosis right ventricle study
RV	Right ventricular
RVEDV	Right ventricular end-diastolic volume
RVEF	Right ventricular ejection fraction
RVESV	Right ventricular end-systolic volume
RVM	Right ventricular mass
RVSV	Right ventricular stroke volume
SENC	Strain encoding
SSFP	Steady-state free procession
TAPSE	Tricuspid annular plane excursion

Introduction

The role of cardiac magnetic resonance (CMR) imaging is well established in the evaluation of a wide range of cardiovascular diseases, both acquired and congenital. It is non-invasive, does not need favourable acoustic windows and does not involve the use of ionising radiation. Determination of ventricular volumes and function can be obtained by steady-state free procession (SSFP) bright blood cine MRI without the need for contrast administration. Over the last two decades CMR has become recognised as the gold standard for determining left and right ventricular structure and function with accuracy demonstrated in a broad range of diseases [1–6] and in comparison to anatomical specimens [7]. It is particularly suited to the morphology of the right ventricle (RV) because the RV has a complex structure and contractile pattern which makes accurate assessment by 2D methods such as standard echocardiography more difficult. The high-resolution, three-dimensional images obtainable by CMR (Fig. 5.1) avoid the need for any geometrical assumptions and have been shown to have superior interstudy reproducibility for right ventricular volume and mass when compared with echocardiography. CMR is therefore an attractive modality for monitoring ventricular function in disease states [8–10].

More recently three-dimensional echocardiography has also emerged as a promising tool for the assessment of RV volumes.

A. J. Peacock (✉) · M. J. Brewis
Scottish Pulmonary Vascular Unit,
Golden Jubilee National Hospital, Glasgow, UK
e-mail: andrew.peacock@glasgow.ac.uk;
melanie.brewis5@nhs.scot

© The Author(s), under exclusive license to Springer Nature Switzerland AG 2021
S. P. Gaine et al. (eds.), *The Right Heart*, https://doi.org/10.1007/978-3-030-78255-9_5

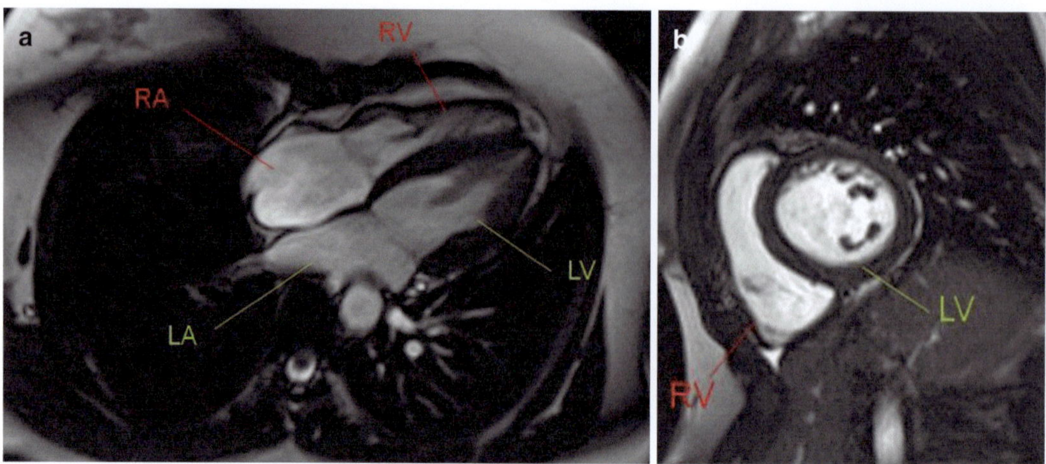

Fig. 5.1 Cardiac MRI images of a normal subject. (**a**) Four-chamber long-axis view showing right and left atria (RA and LA, respectively) and right and left ventricle (RV, LV, respectively). (**b**) Short-axis view

Accurate volumetric data has been reported in a variety of disease states including pulmonary hypertension (PH) and congenital heart disease. However reported accuracy in the literature has varied [11–15]. Challenges remain in acquiring good-quality 3D data sets in patients with poor imaging windows and accuracy tends to decrease with increasing RV dilatation potentially limiting the use of 3D echocardiography in more advanced RV disease [16].

It is now clear that, for patients with pulmonary hypertension, the extent of right ventricular adaptation to an increased afterload is the main determinant of outcome. What is also clear is that there is not a linear relationship between pulmonary vascular resistance and right ventricular function; the right ventricle is coupled to the pulmonary circulation but it is possible for there to be an improvement in pulmonary vascular resistance but a deterioration in right ventricular function and it is the right ventricular function that determines prognosis.

CMR also provides information on RV performance in the context of loading conditions through the assessment of both global and regional ventricular function, interventricular interdependence and right ventricular-pulmonary circulatory coupling. Finally damage to the ventricle such as myocardial scarring and fibrosis can be determined from late gadolinium enhancement or T1 mapping.

CMR is not without limitation. It is less suitable for haemodynamic measurements than echocardiography due to more limited temporal resolution and, though accurate measurements can be made of flow, CMR cannot be used to measure pressure. It should be noted however that pulmonary artery pressure (PAH) alone does not define right ventricular function but the many variables that can be measured by CMR do estimate RV function and we know that it is right ventricular function not pressure that determines survival in pulmonary hypertension. CMR is expensive and less widely available in clinical practice. Incompatibilities with some ferrous implants such as cardiac pacemakers or aneurysm clips exist [17]. Claustrophobia, body habitus, long scan times and need for repetitive breath-holds for acquisition of images to reduce respiratory motion artefact may limit tolerance in some patients. However with advancing technology it is now possible to perform both single breath-hold techniques and real-time acquisitions with adequate resolution [18, 19]. One of the main reasons for the lack of widespread use of CMR in the evaluation of patients with pulmonary hypertension is that CMR has not been used in clinical trials. This is now changing (see later) and we can expect that the unique advantages of CMR will become more apparent.

In this chapter we describe the CMR variables that can be recorded in the normal right ventricle and then examine the effects of pulmonary hypertension and the effects of treatment of pulmonary hypertension on these variables.

Measuring Ventricular Volumes, Mass and Global Function

Ventricular volume is determined using a "stack" of contiguous short-axis slices 5–10 mm thick acquired during breath-hold (typically in regions of 5–18 s), ECG-gated cine "bright" blood sequences (Fig. 5.2). This sequence gives good blood-myocardial contrast to allow tracing of endocardial and epicardial contours either manually or with the use of semi-automated software on end-diastolic and end-systolic frames. Ventricular volume is calculated as the sum of individual slice volumes (Simpson's rule). Ventricular mass is determined by multiplying

myocardial volume by the muscle-specific density for myocardial tissue 1.05 g/cm^3 (Fig. 5.3). Inclusion or exclusion of the RV trabeculations as either mass or volume is the source of inter-study variability and standardised approach is recommended [20]. Geometric shortening can be determined in both longitudinal and transverse planes. In the normal subject most of the RV contraction is longitudinal and is well described by echocardiogram-derived tricuspid annular plane systolic excursion (TAPSE). However, transverse plane shortening has been shown to be superior to echo-derived TAPSE as a surrogate for right ventricular ejection fraction (RVEF) in RV disease [21] and a potential tool for monitoring RV performance [22]. Isovolumetric relaxation time can also be a marker of RV diastolic dysfunction which has been related to the severity of disease in pulmonary arterial hypertension [23].

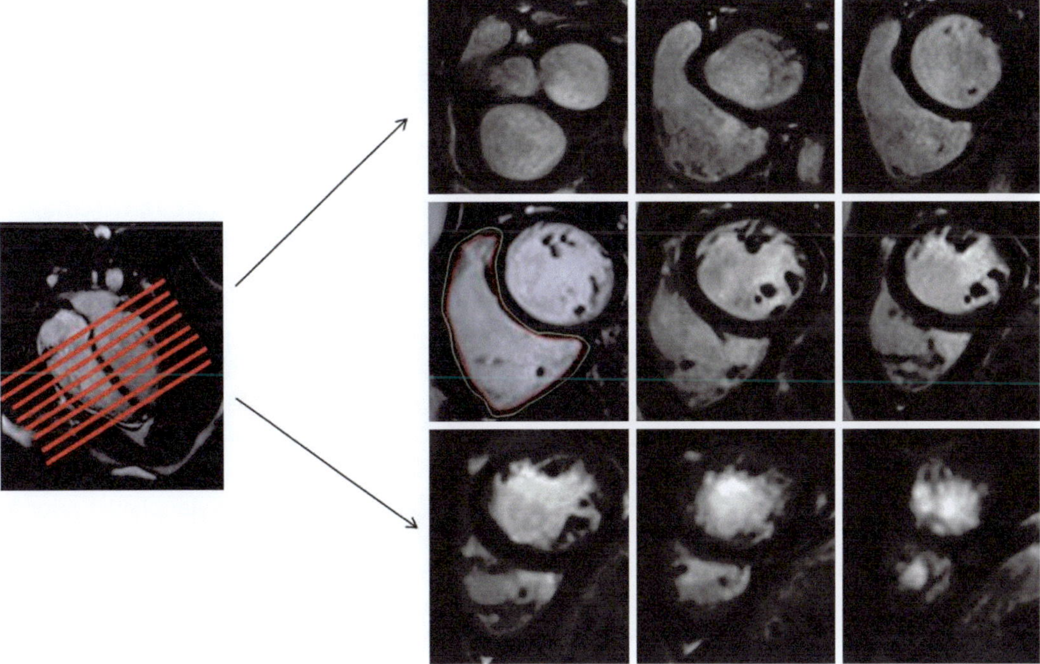

Fig. 5.2 Ventricular volume is determined using a "stack" of contiguous short-axis slices 5–10 mm thick. Endocardial (shown in red) and epicardial contours (in green) are then traced on end-diastolic and end-systolic frames. Ventricular volume is calculated as the sum of individual slice volumes (Simpson's rule). Ventricular mass is determined by multiplying myocardial volume by the muscle-specific density for myocardial tissue (1.05 g/cm^3). Ejection fraction is then calculated by end-diastolic volume–end-systolic volume (i.e. stroke volume) divided by end-diastolic volume

Fig. 5.3 Measurement of RV mass and ventricular mass index (VMI). The ventricle (RV or LV) is sliced up and then the volume of each slice calculated and this is multiplied by myocardial density of 1.05 g/ml to calculate mass. To calculate ventricular mass index the mass of the right ventricle is divided by the mass of the left ventricle

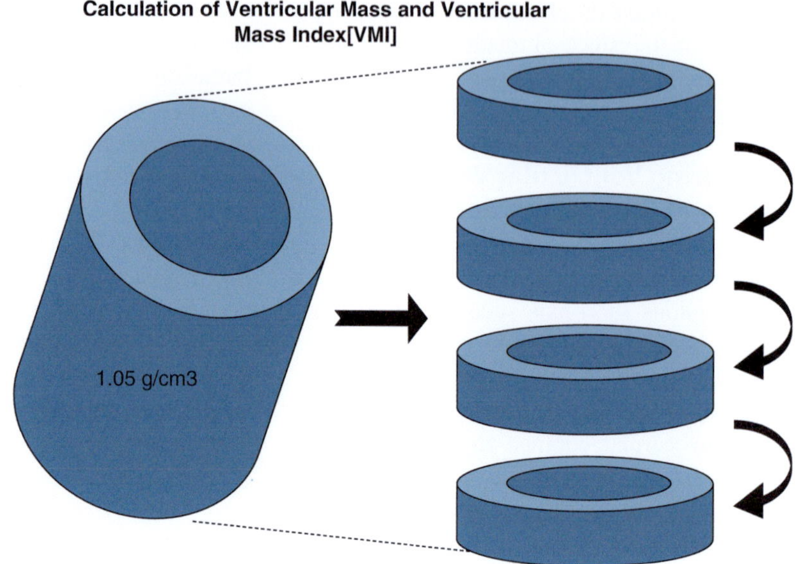

Interventricular interaction is another important consideration in RV dysfunction. In pulmonary hypertension, increased trans-septal pressure gradient causes bowing of the interventricular septum towards the LV (LVSB) [24]. Furthermore the two ventricles become dyssynchronous. CMR studies in PH, using myocardial tagging techniques (discussed below), have shown ventricular asynchrony with a left-to-right delay in myocardial peak shortening due to prolonged RV shortening [25]. This is likely related to increased RV wall tension, and is a probable explanation of LVSB seen in PH due to ongoing RV contraction during the LV relaxation phase.

Encoding the CMR signal phase for velocity (phase velocity mapping) allows determination of flow velocities and volume. By multiplying blood velocity by the cross-sectional area of chosen vessel, such as the main pulmonary artery, volumetric flow such as stroke volume (SV) can be calculated [26]. In addition this method can be used to quantify valvular regurgitant fractions and ventricular ejection fraction; determine ventricular diastolic filling patterns; and, by comparing aortic and pulmonary arterial flow, provide a measure of intra-cardiac shunt [27]. Flow assessment by CMR has an advantage over echocardiography because it can be conducted in any orientation or plane whereas accurate echocar-

diographic assessment requires the flow to be parallel to the echocardiographic plane. Additionally, CMR is better suited to interrogate eccentric regurgitant jets in valvular disease [17, 28, 29]. Phase-contrast flow is however less accurate in the presence of cardiac arrhythmia or turbulent blood flow.

Measuring Regional Right Ventricular Function: Myocardial Tagging and Strain Mapping

The CMR equivalent to echocardiographic tissue Doppler techniques to demonstrate regional myocardial defects is myocardial tagging which can be used to determine three-dimensional motion and deformation in the heart [30]. Tags are regions of tissue which are altered prior to acquisition so that they appear as dark regions in a grid-like pattern on CMR images. Changes of these dark areas during contraction provide information about myocardial shortening. *Strain* is defined as a relative change in tissue length, expressed as a percentage. Longitudinal strain is measured from a four-chamber tagged slice. Radial and circumferential strains are determined from short-axis images [31, 32]. *Strain rate* (change in strain per unit time) can also be determined and give clues to diastolic RV dysfunction [33]. In addition to quantitative strain maps, direct visual assessment of myocardial contractility is possible using *strain encoding* (SENC) imaging which provides colour-coded, high-resolution map of plane strain [34]. Tissue tagging in the RV in comparison to the left ventricle (LV) is challenging due to reduced RV wall thickness (normally 2–6 mm) which limits the number of tag lines for strain analysis. However, improving techniques have demonstrated good inter- and intra-observer variability [35–38]. In particular feature tracking appears to be a major advance and regional motion in both the RV and LV can be determined at the same sitting (Fig. 5.4).

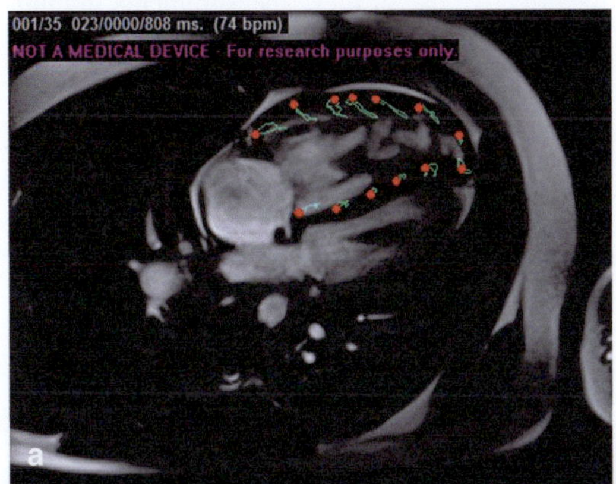

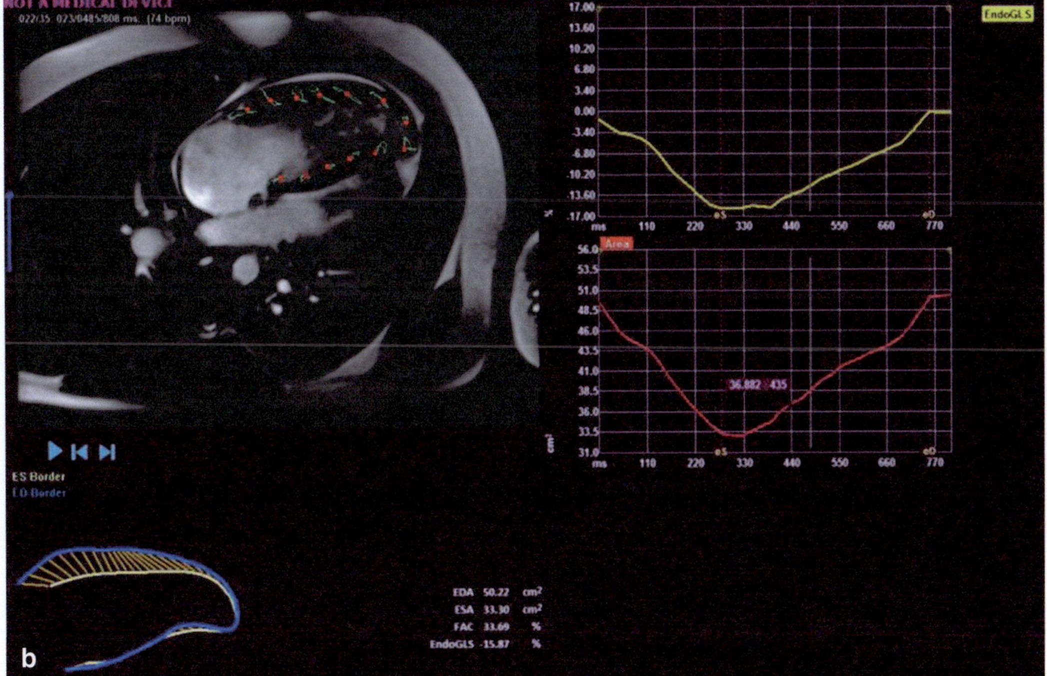

Fig. 5.4 Strain by feature tracking. Features are placed along the endocardium that correspond to unique anatomical structures. These structures can be followed through the cardiac cycle. Green loops are tracks of movement of that segment during contraction and relaxation. (**a**) RV strain by feature tracking. (**b**) Calculation of regional RV strain from images in (**a**)

CMR-Guided Right-Heart Catheterisation

CMR is ideally suited for the determination of RV pump function but cannot be used to determine the cardiovascular pressures which are required for the assessment of more load-independent variables such as myocardial contractility. Pressure-volume (PV) relationships derived from RV PV loops provide additional information on RV pump function, mechanical interaction of the RV with its pulmonary vascular load (RV-PA coupling—see below) and its contractile state. Recent advances in CMR have enabled a hybrid technique of real-time imaging CMR-guided endovascular catheterisation (magnetic resonance fluoroscopy) which has allowed generation of RV pressure-volume loops with derivation of RV afterload and myocardial contractility allowing determination of RV-PA coupling, the interaction between the two variables [39]. Experiences described in the literature are limited to single-centre experience but demonstrated reproducible assessment of PVR in patients with pulmonary hypertension (PH) [40]. Inefficient RV coupling in comparison to six control subjects has been shown in PH patients by this method despite higher myocardial contractility [41]. At present the technique of CMR-guided catheterisation is a research tool only and has significant limitations due to costs and availability of CMR-compatible equipment which may restrict eventual clinical applications.

A simplified method—known as the *volume method*—for determining RV-PA coupling non-invasively by CMR using the ratio of stroke volume to end-systolic volume (SV/ESV) has been shown to be preserved initially in mild PH, which then falls with increasing disease severity [42]. This surrogate measure potentially evaluates RV systolic function in a less preload-dependent fashion than the traditional RVEF. However, this ratio assumes in its derivation that the volume intercept of the end-systolic pressure-volume slope is zero. Recent report in literature in PH has suggested that this may not be true [43]. SV/ESV therefore required further evaluation of its clinical application and this has been done (see later).

Defining Normal Values for Right Ventricular Mass and Volume

Accurate quantification of ventricular dimensions and function is crucial in distinguishing disease states from the normal. It has been shown that the development of CMR has improved the measurement accuracy of RV variables. Establishing what constitutes a "normal range" of RV volumes, mass and function is essential for the effective use of these measurements in clinical practice. LV mass and volumes are known to vary by age, sex and race and are typically adjusted for body surface area (BSA) [44–46]. Echocardiography and autopsy studies have demonstrated significant age- and sex-related differences in both cardiac function and mass in healthy subjects [47–49]. Autopsy studies have also shown that cardiac mass is related to subject weight, height and BSA [49, 50]. Establishing CMR RV mass, volume (RV end-diastolic volume (RVEDV) and RV end-systolic volume (RVESV)) and function (RVEF) reference ranges therefore requires consideration of both absolute and "normalised" values in a diverse healthy reference database. Over the last decade a number of studies have reported normal values for right ventricular structure and function but have been limited by small sample size over a narrow age range with varying acquisition techniques [9, 51–53]. More recently, the multi-ethnic study of atherosclerosis (MESA)-right ventricle study, a multicentre prospective cohort study of over 4000 participants without evidence of clinical cardiovascular disease at baseline [54], has evaluated a number of patient demographics that should be considered in CMR value interpretation, including body size, age, sex and race, physical activity and obesity.

Factors Affecting Normal Values: Scaling Right Ventricular Size and Function for Body Size

Extensive evidence exists from both the animal kingdom and human autopsy studies which showed that cardiac size and function vary with body size and scaling of functional cardiac variables such as cardiac output is a common clinical practice. Conventional cardiovascular scaling approach uses a ratiometric method of dividing indices such as RV mass by a measure of body size such as height or BSA.

Ratiometric scaling relies on linear relationship between RV variables and body size variables. This method has been proposed to have several limitations for cardiovascular scaling and allometric scaling, where the cardiovascular variable divided by the body size variable raised to a scalar exponent is suggested as a superior alternative [55, 56]. This has been modelled in LV parameters of cavity dimensions and mass where the relationship between BSA and LV volume and mass was better described by the allometric method [57, 58]. Currently scaling methods for the RV are uncertain and a subject of research.

Ageing and the Right Ventricle

In autopsy studies, increasing age is associated with myocyte loss and decreases in LV mass and volume in males but not females [50]. Absolute and indexed CMR-derived RV mass and volumes have also been shown to be lower with increasing age [59–62].

Sex

In large population studies of healthy individuals free from cardiovascular disease absolute right ventricular volumes are consistently greater in men than women [59, 63]. RV mass has been reported as up to 8–15% lower and RV volumes 10–25% lower in females [59, 60]. These differences have been shown to persist despite adjustment for the larger BSA seen in men [62]. In general no sex differences have been reported in RVEF, with the exception of the larger MESA-RV study where males had 4% lower RVEF after adjustment for age and ethnicity [59]. These sex differences are likely hormonal related [64–66]. Higher levels of estradiol are associated with better RV systolic function in healthy postmenopausal women taking hormone replacement and higher levels of androgens in both males and postmenopausal women are associated with greater RV mass, higher stroke volume and larger RV volumes [67].

Race

The influence of ethnicity on CMR RV variables has been less well studied. MESA-RV has reported lower RV mass in African Americans and higher RV mass in Hispanics in comparison to Caucasians in a population free of cardiovascular disease [59]. After adjustment for LV mass, only lower RV mass in African Americans remained significant suggesting a RV-specific effect.

Physical Activity (in the Non-athlete)

Long-term high-intensity exercise in elite athletes is well documented to cause adaptive changes in cardiac structure characterised by increases in LV mass, volume and wall thickness with a small number of CMR studies showing increases in RV mass and volume, the so-called athlete's heart which will be discussed in Chap. 6 [68–71]. Levels of physical activity in nonathletes however have also been shown to influence RV mass and volumes. The MESA-RV cohort has been used to interrogate levels and intensity of activity from household chores, gardening and walking to sports and leisure activities [72]. Higher levels of moderate and vigorous physical activity were associated with greater RV mass and volumes after age, body size and sex adjustment, although the absolute value was low (1 g of RV mass from lowest to highest quintile of activity, and 7% increase in RVEDV) which remained significant after adjusting for LV size.

Obesity

RV mass and volumes determined by CMR are higher in obese individuals even after adjustment for the corresponding LV variable and demographics. Chahal et al. demonstrated a 14% absolute and 8% LV-adjusted higher RV mass, 16% higher RVSV, larger RVEDV and slightly lower RVEF in healthy obese individuals without reported symptoms suggestive of a sleep disorder [73, 74]. Persistence of greater RV mass and volumes after adjustment for LV variables or height suggests that these increases could not be attributed to increased body size alone.

Normative Equations for RV Variables

MESA-RV study has derived sex-specific reference equations for RV mass, RV volumes and

RVEF from a subset of 441 healthy, non-obese, never smokers which incorporate age, height and weight adjustment [59]. While these equations need to be validated before clinical use they may in future serve as reference values in defining abnormal RV morphology and function. Three large cohort studies including MESA-RV have now published age- and sex-specific CMR right ventricular reference ranges for mass, volume and function [59, 60, 62].

monary hypertension rather than the cause of pulmonary hypertension [74–76] (Table 5.1).

The exceptions to this rule are the diagnosis of PH in association with congenital heart disease and the diagnosis of PH associated with diastolic dysfunction of the left ventricle (Hf-PEF) where the size of the left atrium—easily determined by CMR—tells us whether a patient is suffering from pulmonary arterial hypertension or pulmonary venous hypertension [77] (Fig. 5.6).

Role of CMR in the Diagnosis and Management of Patients with Pulmonary Hypertension

Diagnosis of Pulmonary Hypertension

As the afterload (PVR) increases in patients with pulmonary hypertension the RV initially compensates (homeometric/adaptive hypertrophy) and then as the condition progresses starts to decompensate with asymmetrical hypertrophy, dilatation and loss of ventriculo-arterial coupling (Fig. 5.5). The main use of CMR in PH is to determine this right ventricular response to pul-

Effects of Pulmonary Hypertension on Cardiac Structure: Measurements by CMR

RV (and LV) Mass/Volumes/Damage

With the rise in primary vascular resistance there is an associated increase in right ventricular *mass*. What is unclear is whether this increase in *mass* is a good thing or a bad thing. It certainly seems that compensatory increase in mass is a good thing (e.g. in congenital heart disease) but too much or asymmetric increase in *mass* is a bad thing. *Mass* can be best estimated using CMR by measurement of ventricular mass index VMI [78] where the RV mass is divided by the LV mass. As

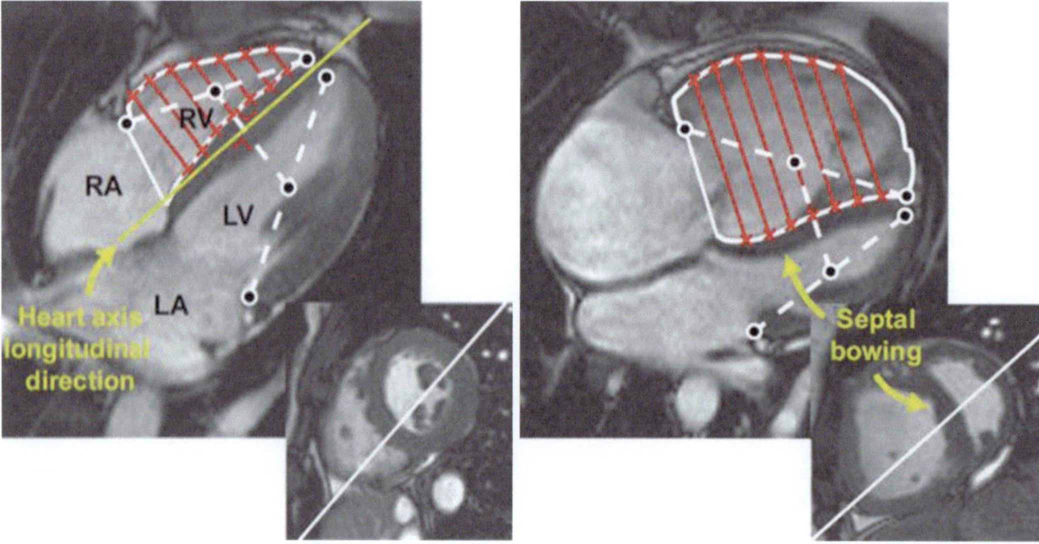

Fig. 5.5 Cardiac MRI in a healthy subject and one with severe PAH. Four-chamber and short-axis views show the abnormalities seen in pulmonary hypertension. (Kind T. et al. *J Cardiovasc Magn Reson* 2010;12:35)

Table 5.1 Cardiac magnetic resonance imaging (CMRI) variables that have prognostic value in pulmonary hypertension

RVEF%	<35
Stroke volume index (ml/m²)	<25
Ventricular mass index	>0.56
LV end-diastolic volume index (ml/m²)	<40
RV end-diastolic volume index (ml/m²)	>84
LV end-systolic volume index (ml/m²)	15 ± 9
RV end-systolic volume index (ml/m²)	47 ± 21

the RV mass rises the LV mass falls in PH because of decreased filling pressure of the LV and there is a very good relationship between VMI and PA pressure. However, RV mass change is probably not an important variable when monitoring response to treatment for pulmonary hypertension [79].

CMR can be used to measure the following *volumes*: end-systolic volume (ESV),

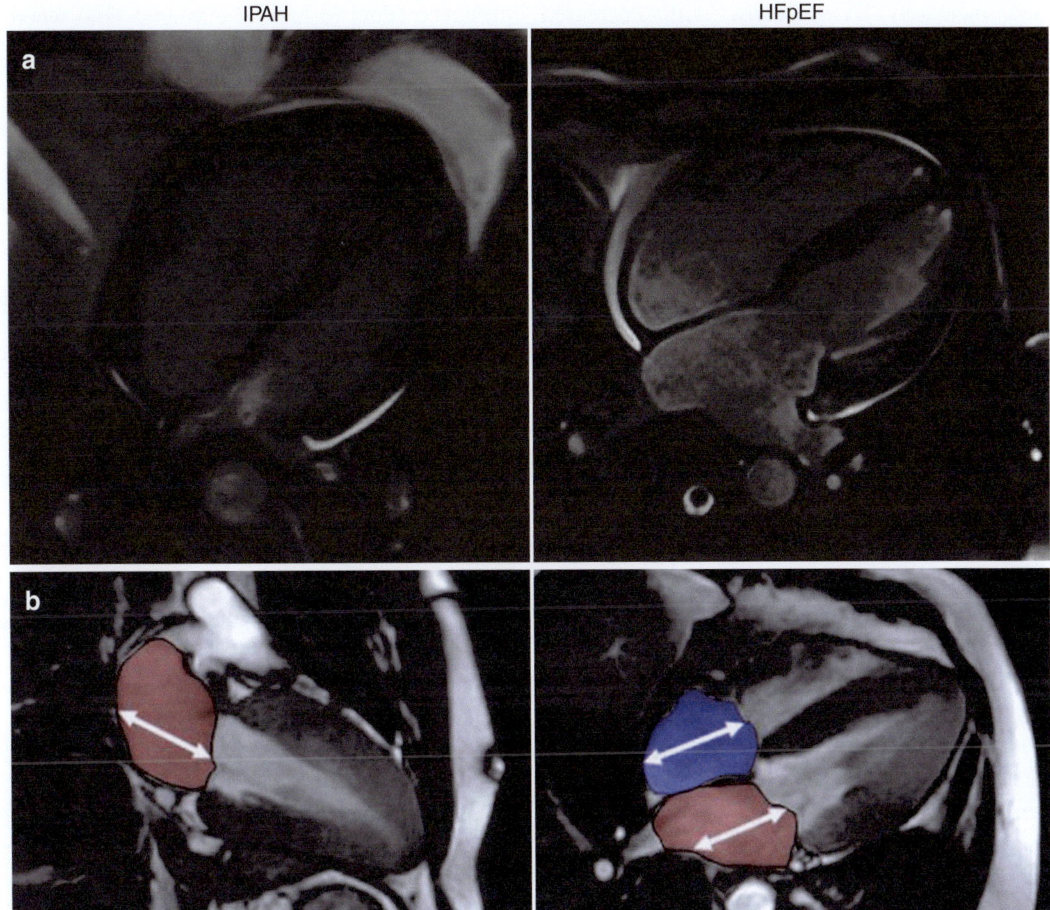

- Biplane Area-length Method

- Left Atrial Volume
      = (0.848 x area4ch x area2ch/[(length4ch x length2ch)/2]

- Left Atrial Volume (LAV) then indexed to Body Surface Area

Fig. 5.6 Distinguishing pulmonary venous hypertension (HFpEF) from pulmonary arterial hypertension. Four-chamber view shows enlargement of right atrium and right ventricle in both patients but in the patient with HFpEF there is enlargement of the left atrium (Fig. 5.4a); this is measured (Fig. 5.4b) by the biplane method and if enlarged reliably excludes PAH. (Crawley et al. JACC Imaging 2013)

end-diastolic volume (EDV), stroke volume (SV) and ejection fraction (EF) [75, 80]. Clearly all these variables can be measured in both the RV and the LV at the same sitting and it is very interesting that often the LV variables, because they are surrogates for RV function, are as important and are easier to measure [81]. Of these probably the most important variables in the determination of RV function are the RVEF and the RVSV (LVSV).

The presence of reduced SV, reduced RVEF and increased RV volumes with decreased LVEDV all point to a poor prognosis [74]. Global RV systolic function is probably best measured by right ventricular ejection fraction but the *volume* measure of ventriculo-arterial coupling SV over ESV has been shown to be even more significant than RVEF in some studies [82, 83] (see below).

The best way to measure right ventricular *damage* in the face of pulmonary hypertension is by late gadolinium enhancement. Gadolinium is a contrast agent used in CMR and when there is damage to the myocardium the gadolinium does not clear from the damaged tissue so outlines that tissue. It has been shown that in pulmonary hypertension there is late gadolinium enhancement in the interventricular septum but also particularly at the insertion points of the right ventricle into the left ventricle. The mass of late gadolinium enhancement which is believed to be due to cardiac fibrosis (Fig. 5.7, [84]) corresponds with a number of measures of RV function [85]. Gadolinium is nephrotoxic so there has been research into ways of getting the same imaging without the use of the injected contrast; this can be provided by T1 mapping using CMR.

Effects of Pulmonary Hypertension on Cardiac Function: Measurements by CMR

RV-PA Coupling

The gold standard measure of RV systolic functional adaptation to changes in afterload is to measure end-systolic elastance (Ees), which is derived by dividing end-systolic pressure (ESP) by end-systolic volume (ESV), corrected for arterial elastance (Ea) (stroke volume/ESP). This load-independent measure of RV-PA coupling defines matching of RV contractility to afterload. This calculation requires instantaneous measurement of RV pressure and volume which is not practical; this can be simplified for pressure and expressed as the SV/ESV ratio (the *volume* method).

The mathematical formulation is as follows:

RV-PA coupling is the ratio of RV end-systolic elastance (Ees) to arterial elastance (Ea) where Ees = end-systolic pressure (ESP)/end-systolic volume (ESV) and Ea = ESP/stroke volume (SV).

We can solve for ESP which gives us RV-PA coupling = ESV/SV.

In a study of 140 treatment-naïve patients by Brewis et al. [82] RV-PA coupling measurements by volume method (SV/ESV) predicted outcome even better than RVEF, and there were no added benefits of RV-PA coupling measurements by the invasive pressure method [42].

Global vs. Regional Cardiac Function in PH

Clearly, *global* RV function can be well described by ventricular volumes and volume change as noted above but *regional* cardiac function measurement which can be measured by MRI tagging techniques such as feature tracking is becoming increasingly important in our investigation of changes in cardiac function with pulmonary hypertension. These analyses by *strain* and *strain rate* allow us to examine regional distortion of ventricular shape and function, e.g. longitudinal vs. circumferential (Fig. 5.4) and interventricular dyssynchrony.

Myocardial Perfusion

Myocardial perfusion can be determined by CMR after intravenous injection of agents such as adenosine. It has been shown that myocardial perfusion indices are reduced in patients with pulmonary arterial hypertension and the perfusion is inversely related to RV work or PAP. Studies continue into the use of this measurement but at present we do not know whether

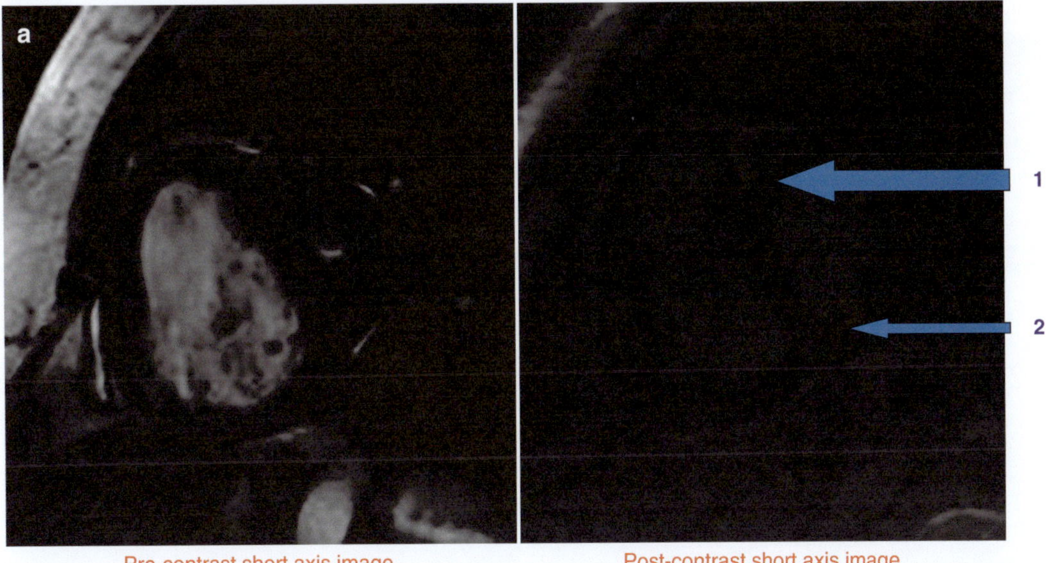

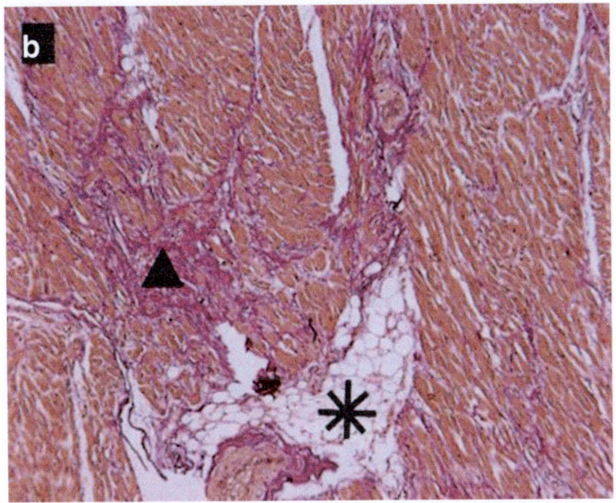

Fig. 5.7 Imaging of right ventricular myocardial damage in a patient with pulmonary hypertension; there is (**a**) late gadolinium enhancement related to the interventricular septum and right ventricular insertion points. (**b**) Histology of an area of late gadolinium enhancement in an animal model showing fibrosis at the site. (McCann AJR 2007)

the reduced perfusion is a cause or a consequence of the reduced RV function.

Treatment of Pulmonary Hypertension: Efficacy Measured by CMR

It is clear that the purpose of treatment of pulmonary hypertension is not simply a reduction in pressure or even in PVR but an improvement in RV function (Fig. 5.8). The dissociation between RV function and PVR was shown by van de Veerdonk [86]. The use of CMR to measure the efficacy of treatment for pulmonary hypertension was suggested a number of years ago by the Euro-MR study [81], which was the largest study ever conducted on the treatment effect in PAH measured by CMR. The study examined patients from Glasgow, Rome, Amsterdam and Graz. The

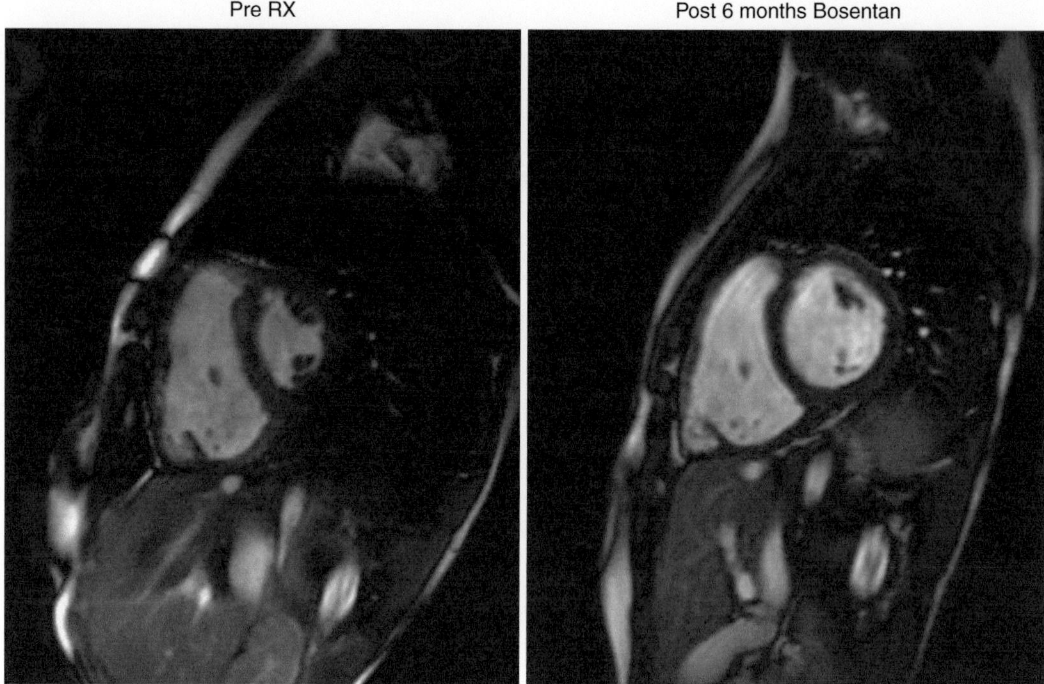

Fig. 5.8 MR as an end point showing the benefits of treatment in a patient with a PAH measured by cross-sectional MR. The patient was a 16-year-old boy with PAH. Images are at baseline and after 6-month treatment with bosentan. Post-treatment the RV looks similar but there is a marked improvement in the LV due to increase in filling pressures from the recovered RV function

investigators found that CMR-derived variables measured at baseline, 4 months and 12 months following approved PAH treatment not only improved early on (i.e. <4 months) but the improvement was maintained at 12 months. This improvement was best measured by improvements in RV volumes and left ventricular function (due to the increased filling by the recovering RV). It has been shown [87] that a significant improvement in the clinical state of pulmonary hypertension requires at least a 10 ml improvement in SV measured by CMR.

That study was not a clinical trial. In a recent editorial we heard a cry of distress from the Amsterdam group [88]; their cry, in relation to the use of MRI in pulmonary hypertension, was "Why are we still waiting?" Their answer which is probably correct was that clinicians do not take notice of a measurement until it has been used in clinical trials. CMR-derived changes in RV variables are now being used in clinical trials and for the first time being used as a primary end point in the REPLACE and REPAIR studies [89, 90].

Conclusion

CMR is well suited for the determination of RV variables because the complex configuration of the RV is better described by three-dimensional volume acquisition. CMR has shown excellent accuracy and reproducibility for RV measurements and is superior to echocardiography. It is important to characterise normal variants in order to establish healthy reference ranges which can be compared with disease states and in serial studies adjust for confounders. The normal range of RV mass and volume varies with age, sex, race, body size, levels of physical activity and obesity. Interpretation of CMR RV variables should be considered in the context of patient demographics.

CMR is particularly suited for looking at right ventricular (and left ventricle) variables in the context of pulmonary hypertension. These variables can be used to distinguish types of pulmonary hypertension, e.g. LV-PH versus pulmonary arterial hypertension, and also to determine the effects of pulmonary hypertension on RV (and LV function) in terms of cardiac structure and function both global and regional, and damage to the myocardium by the increased pressures and deformation. Lastly CMR is likely to prove useful in the evaluation of right-heart function in response to the treatment for pulmonary hypertension. We hope that this image modality will be used increasingly in clinical trials of new therapies for this devastating disease.

References

1. Katz J, Whang J, Boxt LM, Barst RJ. Estimation of right ventricular mass in normal subjects and in patients with primary pulmonary hypertension by nuclear magnetic resonance imaging. J Am Coll Cardiol. 1993;21(6):1475–81.
2. Boxt LM, Katz J, Kolb T, Czegledy FP, Barst RJ. Direct quantitation of right and left ventricular volumes with nuclear magnetic resonance imaging in patients with primary pulmonary hypertension. J Am Coll Cardiol. 1992;19(7):1508–15.
3. Doherty NE III, Fujita N, Caputo GR, Higgins CB. Measurement of right ventricular mass in normal and dilated cardiomyopathic ventricles using cine magnetic resonance imaging. Am J Cardiol. 1992;69(14):1223–8.
4. Pattynama PM, Willems LN, Smit AH, van der Wall EE, de Roos A. Early diagnosis of cor pulmonale with MR imaging of the right ventricle. Radiology. 1992;182(2):375–9.
5. Bottini PB, Carr AA, Prisant LM, Flickinger FW, Allison JD, Gottdiener JS. Magnetic resonance imaging compared to echocardiography to assess left ventricular mass in the hypertensive patient. Am J Hypertens. 1995;8(3):221–8.
6. McLure LER, Peacock AJ. Cardiac magnetic resonance imaging for the assessment of the heart and pulmonary circulation in pulmonary hypertension. Eur Respir J. 2009;33(6):1454–66.
7. Calverley PM, Howatson R, Flenley DC, Lamb D. Clinicopathological correlations in cor pulmonale. Thorax. 1992;47(7):494–8.
8. Grothues F, Smith GC, Moon JC, Bellenger NG, Collins P, Klein HU, et al. Comparison of interstudy reproducibility of cardiovascular magnetic resonance with two-dimensional echocardiography in normal subjects and in patients with heart failure or left ventricular hypertrophy. Am J Cardiol. 2002;90(1):29–34.
9. Grothues F, Moon JC, Bellenger NG, Smith GS, Klein HU, Pennell DJ. Interstudy reproducibility of right ventricular volumes, function, and mass with cardiovascular magnetic resonance. Am Heart J. 2004;147(2):218–23.
10. Vonk-Noordegraaf A, van Wolferen SA, Marcus JT, Boonstra A, Postmus PE, Peeters JWL, et al. Noninvasive assessment and monitoring of the pulmonary circulation. Eur Respir J. 2005;25(4):758–66.
11. van der Zwaan HB, Geleijnse ML, McGhie JS, Boersma E, Helbing WA, Meijboom FJ, et al. Right ventricular quantification in clinical practice: two-dimensional vs. three-dimensional echocardiography compared with cardiac magnetic resonance imaging. Eur J Echocardiogr. 2011;12(9):656–64.
12. Fang F, Chan A, Lee AP, Sanderson JE, Kwong JS, Luo XX, et al. Variation in right ventricular volumes assessment by real-time three-dimensional echocardiography between dilated and normal right ventricle: comparison with cardiac magnetic resonance imaging. Int J Cardiol. 2013;168(4):4391–3.
13. Shimada YJ, Shiota M, Siegel RJ, Shiota T. Accuracy of right ventricular volumes and function determined by three-dimensional echocardiography in comparison with magnetic resonance imaging: a meta-analysis study. J Am Soc Echocardiogr. 2010;23(9):943–53.
14. Grewal J, Majdalany D, Syed I, Pellikka P, Warnes CA. Three-dimensional echocardiographic assessment of right ventricular volume and function in adult patients with congenital heart disease: comparison with magnetic resonance imaging. J Am Soc Echocardiogr. 2010;23(2):127–33.
15. van der Zwaan HB, Geleijnse ML, Soliman OI, McGhie JS, Wiegers-Groeneweg EJ, Helbing WA, et al. Test-retest variability of volumetric right ventricular measurements using real-time three-dimensional echocardiography. J Am Soc Echocardiogr. 2011;24(6):671–9.
16. Crean AM, Maredia N, Ballard G, Menezes R, Wharton G, Forster J, et al. 3D Echo systematically underestimates right ventricular volumes compared to cardiovascular magnetic resonance in adult congenital heart disease patients with moderate or severe RV dilatation. J Cardiovasc Magn Reson. 2011;13:78.
17. Pennell DJ, Sechtem UP, Higgins CB, Manning WJ, Pohost GM, Rademakers FE, et al. Clinical indications for cardiovascular magnetic resonance (CMR): Consensus Panel report. J Cardiovasc Magn Reson. 2004;6(4):727–65.
18. Muthurangu V, Lurz P, Critchely JD, Deanfield JE, Taylor AM, Hansen MS. Real-time assessment of right and left ventricular volumes and function in patients with congenital heart disease by using high spatio-temporal resolution radial k-t SENSE. Radiology. 2008;248(3):782–91.
19. Zhang H, Wahle A, Johnson RK, Scholz TD, Sonka M. 4-D cardiac MR image analysis: left and right

ventricular morphology and function. IEEE Trans Med Imaging. 2010;29(2):350–64.

20. Winter MM, Bernink FJ, Groenink M, Bouma BJ, van Dijk AP, Helbing WA, et al. Evaluating the systemic right ventricle by CMR: the importance of consistent and reproducible delineation of the cavity. J Cardiovasc Magn Reson. 2008;10:40.

21. Kind T, Mauritz GJ, Marcus JT, van de Veerdonk M, Westerhof N, Vonk-Noordegraaf A. Right ventricular ejection fraction is better reflected by transverse rather than longitudinal wall motion in pulmonary hypertension. J Cardiovasc Magn Reson. 2010;12:35.

22. Mauritz GJ, Kind T, Marcus JT, Bogaard HJ, van de Veerdonk M, Postmus PE, et al. Progressive changes in right ventricular geometric shortening and long-term survival in pulmonary arterial hypertension. Chest. 2011;141(4):935–43.

23. Gan CTJ, Holverda S, Marcus JT, Paulus WJ, Marques KM, Bronzwaer JGF, et al. Right ventricular diastolic dysfunction and the acute effects of sildenafil in pulmonary hypertension patients. Chest. 2007;132(1):11–7.

24. Gan CT, Lankhaar JW, Marcus JT, Westerhof N, Marques KM, Bronzwaer JG, et al. Impaired left ventricular filling due to right-to-left ventricular interaction in patients with pulmonary arterial hypertension. Am J Physiol Heart Circ Physiol. 2006;290(4):H1528–33.

25. Marcus JT, Gan CT, Zwanenburg JJ, Boonstra A, Allaart CP, Gotte MJ, et al. Interventricular mechanical asynchrony in pulmonary arterial hypertension: left-to-right delay in peak shortening is related to right ventricular overload and left ventricular underfilling. J Am Coll Cardiol. 2008;51(7):750–7.

26. Nayler GL, Firmin DN, Longmore DB. Blood flow imaging by cine magnetic resonance. J Comput Assist Tomogr. 1986;10(5):715–22.

27. Beerbaum P, Korperich H, Barth P, Esdorn H, Gieseke J, Meyer H. Noninvasive quantification of left-to-right shunt in pediatric patients: phase-contrast cine magnetic resonance imaging compared with invasive oximetry. Circulation. 2001;103(20):2476–82.

28. Benza R, Biederman R, Murali S, Gupta H. Role of cardiac magnetic resonance imaging in the management of patients with pulmonary arterial hypertension. J Am Coll Cardiol. 2008;52(21):1683–92.

29. Biederman RWW. Cardiovascular magnetic resonance imaging as applied to patients with pulmonary arterial hypertension. Int J Clin Pract. 2009;63:20–35.

30. Zerhouni EA, Parish DM, Rogers WJ, Yang A, Shapiro EP. Human heart: tagging with MR imaging—a method for noninvasive assessment of myocardial motion. Radiology. 1988;169(1):59–63.

31. Osman NF, Kerwin WS, McVeigh ER, Prince JL. Cardiac motion tracking using CINE harmonic phase (HARP) magnetic resonance imaging. Magn Reson Med. 1999;42(6):1048–60.

32. Osman NF, Sampath S, Atalar E, Prince JL. Imaging longitudinal cardiac strain on short-axis images using strain-encoded MRI. Magn Reson Med. 2001;46(2):324–34.

33. Ibrahim el SH, White RD. Cardiovascular magnetic resonance for the assessment of pulmonary arterial hypertension: toward a comprehensive CMR exam. Magn Reson Imaging. 2012;30(8):1047–58.

34. Shehata ML, Basha TA, Tantawy WH, Lima JA, Vogel-Claussen J, Bluemke DA, et al. Real-time single-heartbeat fast strain-encoded imaging of right ventricular regional function: normal versus chronic pulmonary hypertension. Magn Reson Med. 2010;64(1):98–106.

35. Youssef A, Ibrahim el SH, Korosoglou G, Abraham MR, Weiss RG, Osman NF. Strain-encoding cardiovascular magnetic resonance for assessment of right-ventricular regional function. J Cardiovasc Magn Reson. 2008;10:33.

36. Hamdan A, Thouet T, Kelle S, Paetsch I, Gebker R, Wellnhofer E, et al. Regional right ventricular function and timing of contraction in healthy volunteers evaluated by strain-encoded MRI. J Magn Reson Imaging. 2008;28(6):1379–85.

37. Menteer J, Weinberg PM, Fogel MA. Quantifying regional right ventricular function in tetralogy of Fallot. J Cardiovasc Magn Reson. 2005;7(5):753–61.

38. Kukulski T, Hubbert L, Arnold M, Wranne B, Hatle L, Sutherland GR. Normal regional right ventricular function and its change with age: a Doppler myocardial imaging study. J Am Soc Echocardiogr. 2000;13(3):194–204.

39. Lederman RJ. Cardiovascular interventional magnetic resonance imaging. Circulation. 2005;112(19):3009–17.

40. Kuehne T, Yilmaz S, Schulze-Neick I, Wellnhofer E, Ewert P, Nagel E, et al. Magnetic resonance imaging guided catheterisation for assessment of pulmonary vascular resistance: in vivo validation and clinical application in patients with pulmonary hypertension. Heart. 2005;91(8):1064–9.

41. Kuehne T, Yilmaz S, Steendijk P, Moore P, Groenink M, Saaed M, et al. Magnetic resonance imaging analysis of right ventricular pressure-volume loops: in vivo validation and clinical application in patients with pulmonary hypertension. Circulation. 2004;110(14):2010–6.

42. Sanz J, Garcia-Alvarez A, Fernandez-Friera L, Nair A, Mirelis JG, Sawit ST, et al. Right ventriculo-arterial coupling in pulmonary hypertension: a magnetic resonance study. Heart. 2012;98(3):238–43.

43. Trip P, Kind T, van de Veerdonk MC, Marcus JT, de Man FS, Westerhof N, et al. Accurate assessment of load-independent right ventricular systolic function in patients with pulmonary hypertension. J Heart Lung Transplant. 2013;32(1):50–5.

44. Salton CJ, Chuang ML, O'Donnell CJ, Kupka MJ, Larson MG, Kissinger KV, et al. Gender differences and normal left ventricular anatomy in an adult population free of hypertension. A cardiovascular magnetic resonance study of the Framingham

Heart Study Offspring cohort. J Am Coll Cardiol. 2002;39(6):1055–60.

45. Natori S, Lai S, Finn JP, Gomes AS, Hundley WG, Jerosch-Herold M, et al. Cardiovascular function in multi-ethnic study of atherosclerosis: normal values by age, sex, and ethnicity. AJR Am J Roentgenol. 2006;186(6 Suppl 2):S357–65.

46. Cheng S, Fernandes VR, Bluemke DA, McClelland RL, Kronmal RA, Lima JA. Age-related left ventricular remodeling and associated risk for cardiovascular outcomes: the Multi-Ethnic Study of Atherosclerosis. Circ Cardiovasc Imaging. 2009;2(3):191–8.

47. Slotwiner DJ, Devereux RB, Schwartz JE, Pickering TG, de Simone G, Ganau A, et al. Relation of age to left ventricular function in clinically normal adults. Am J Cardiol. 1998;82(5):621–6.

48. Hangartner JR, Marley NJ, Whitehead A, Thomas AC, Davies MJ. The assessment of cardiac hypertrophy at autopsy. Histopathology. 1985;9(12):1295–306.

49. Kitzman DW, Scholz DG, Hagen PT, Ilstrup DM, Edwards WD. Age-related changes in normal human hearts during the first 10 decades of life. Part II (Maturity): A quantitative anatomic study of 765 specimens from subjects 20 to 99 years old. Mayo Clin Proc. 1988;63(2):137–46.

50. Olivetti G, Giordano G, Corradi D, Melissari M, Lagrasta C, Gambert SR, et al. Gender differences and aging: effects on the human heart. J Am Coll Cardiol. 1995;26(4):1068–79.

51. Lorenz CH, Walker ES, Morgan VL, Klein SS, Graham TP Jr. Normal human right and left ventricular mass, systolic function, and gender differences by cine magnetic resonance imaging. J Cardiovasc Magn Reson. 1999;1(1):7–21.

52. Sandstede J, Lipke C, Beer M, Hofmann S, Pabst T, Kenn W, et al. Age- and gender-specific differences in left and right ventricular cardiac function and mass determined by cine magnetic resonance imaging. Eur Radiol. 2000;10(3):438–42.

53. Danias PG, Tritos NA, Stuber M, Kissinger KV, Salton CJ, Manning WJ. Cardiac structure and function in the obese: a cardiovascular magnetic resonance imaging study. J Cardiovasc Magn Reson. 2003;5(3):431–8.

54. Bild DE, Bluemke DA, Burke GL, Detrano R, Diez Roux AV, Folsom AR, et al. Multi-ethnic study of atherosclerosis: objectives and design. Am J Epidemiol. 2002;156(9):871–81.

55. Dewey FE, Rosenthal D, Murphy DJ Jr, Froelicher VF, Ashley EA. Does size matter? Clinical applications of scaling cardiac size and function for body size. Circulation. 2008;117(17):2279–87.

56. de Simone G, Kizer JR, Chinali M, Roman MJ, Bella JN, Best LG, et al. Normalization for body size and population-attributable risk of left ventricular hypertrophy: the Strong Heart Study. Am J Hypertens. 2005;18(2 Pt 1):191–6.

57. de Simone G, Daniels SR, Devereux RB, Meyer RA, Roman MJ, de Divitiis O, et al. Left ventricular mass and body size in normotensive children and adults: assessment of allometric relations and impact of overweight. J Am Coll Cardiol. 1992;20(5):1251–60.

58. George K, Sharma S, Batterham A, Whyte G, McKenna W. Allometric analysis of the association between cardiac dimensions and body size variables in 464 junior athletes. Clin Sci (Lond). 2001;100(1):47–54.

59. Kawut SM, Lima JA, Barr RG, Chahal H, Jain A, Tandri H, et al. Sex and race differences in right ventricular structure and function: the multi-ethnic study of atherosclerosis-right ventricle study. Circulation. 2011;123(22):2542–51.

60. Hudsmith LE, Petersen SE, Francis JM, Robson MD, Neubauer S. Normal human left and right ventricular and left atrial dimensions using steady state free precession magnetic resonance imaging. J Cardiovasc Magn Reson. 2005;7(5):775–82.

61. Fiechter M, Fuchs TA, Gebhard C, Stehli J, Klaeser B, Stahli BE, et al. Age-related normal structural and functional ventricular values in cardiac function assessed by magnetic resonance. BMC Med Imaging. 2013;13:6.

62. Maceira AM, Prasad SK, Khan M, Pennell DJ. Reference right ventricular systolic and diastolic function normalized to age, gender and body surface area from steady-state free precession cardiovascular magnetic resonance. Eur Heart J. 2006;27(23):2879–88.

63. Tandri H, Daya SK, Nasir K, Bomma C, Lima JA, Calkins H, et al. Normal reference values for the adult right ventricle by magnetic resonance imaging. Am J Cardiol. 2006;98(12):1660–4.

64. Rominger MB, Bachmann GF, Pabst W, Rau WS. Right ventricular volumes and ejection fraction with fast cine MR imaging in breath-hold technique: applicability, normal values from 52 volunteers, and evaluation of 325 adult cardiac patients. J Magn Reson Imaging. 1999;10(6):908–18.

65. Skavdahl M, Steenbergen C, Clark J, Myers P, Demianenko T, Mao L, et al. Estrogen receptor-beta mediates male-female differences in the development of pressure overload hypertrophy. Am J Physiol Heart Circ Physiol. 2005;288(2):H469–76.

66. Mendelsohn ME, Karas RH. The protective effects of estrogen on the cardiovascular system. N Engl J Med. 1999;340(23):1801–11.

67. Ventetuolo CE, Ouyang P, Bluemke DA, Tandri H, Barr RG, Bagiella E, et al. Sex hormones are associated with right ventricular structure and function: the MESA-right ventricle study. Am J Respir Crit Care Med. 2011;183(5):659–67.

68. Pluim BM, Zwinderman AH, van der Laarse A, van der Wall EE. The athlete's heart. A meta-analysis of cardiac structure and function. Circulation. 2000 25;101(3):336–44.

69. Scharhag J, Schneider G, Urhausen A, Rochette V, Kramann B, Kindermann W. Athlete's heart: right and left ventricular mass and function in male endurance athletes and untrained individuals determined

by magnetic resonance imaging. J Am Coll Cardiol. 2002;40(10):1856–63.

70. Perseghin G, De Cobelli F, Esposito A, Lattuada G, Terruzzi I, La Torre A, et al. Effect of the sporting discipline on the right and left ventricular morphology and function of elite male track runners: a magnetic resonance imaging and phosphorus 31 spectroscopy study. Am Heart J. 2007;154(5):937–42.

71. Erol MK, Karakelleoglu S. Assessment of right heart function in the athlete's heart. Heart Vessel. 2002;16(5):175–80.

72. Aaron CP, Tandri H, Barr RG, Johnson WC, Bagiella E, Chahal H, et al. Physical activity and right ventricular structure and function. The MESA-Right Ventricle Study. Am J Respir Crit Care Med. 2011;183(3):396–404.

73. Chahal H, McClelland RL, Tandri H, Jain A, Turkbey EB, Hundley WG, et al. Obesity and right ventricular structure and function: the MESA-Right Ventricle Study. Chest. 2012;141(2):388–95.

74. vonk Noordegraaf A, Haddad F, Bogaard H, Hassoun PM. Non-invasive imaging in the assessment of the cardiopulmonary vascular unit. Circulation. 2015;131:899–913.

75. Crowe T, Jayasekera G, Peacock AJ. Non-invasive imaging of global and regional cardiac function in pulmonary hypertension. Pulmonary Circ. 2017;8:1–20.

76. Grunig E, Peacock AJ. Imaging the heart in pulmonary hypertension: an update. Eur Respir Rev. 2015;24:653–64.

77. Crawley SF, Johnson MK, Dargie HJ, et al. LA volume by CMR distinguishes idiopathic from pulmonary hypertension due to HfPEF. JACC Cardiovasc Imaging. 2013;6:1120–1.

78. Saba TS, Foster J, Cockburn M, et al. Ventricular mass index using magnetic resonance imaging accurately estimate pulmonary artery pressure. Eur Respir J. 2002;20:1519–24.

79. Naeije R, Ghio S. More on the right ventricle in primary hypertension. Eur Respir J. 2015;45:33–5.

80. Aryal SR, Sharifov OF, Lloyd SG. Emerging role of cardiovascular magnetic resonance imaging in the management of pulmonary hypertension. Eur Respir Rev. 2020;29:190138–2019.

81. Peacock AJ, Crawley S, McClure L. Changes in right ventricular function measured by cardiac magnetic resonance imaging in patients receiving pulmonary arterial hypertension targeted therapy: the EURO-MR study. Circ Cardiovasc Imaging. 2014;7:107–14.

82. Brewis MJ, et al. Imaging right ventricular function to predict outcome in pulmonary arterial hypertension. Int J Cardiol. 2016;218:206–2011.

83. Vanderpool RR, et al. RV—pulmonary arterial coupling predicts outcome in patients referred for pulmonary hypertension. Heart. 2015;101:37–43.

84. McCann GP, Gan CT, Beek AM, et al. Extent of MRI delayed enhancement of myocardial mass is related to right ventricular dysfunction in primary arterial hypertension. Am J Roentgenol. 2007;188:349–55.

85. Blyth K, Groenning BA, Martin TN, et al. Contrast enhanced cardiovascular magnetic resonance imaging in patients with pulmonary hypertension. Eur Heart J. 2005;26:1993–9.

86. Van de Veerdonk MC, Kind T, Marcus JT, et al. Progressive right ventricular dysfunction in patients with pulmonary arterial hypertension responding to therapy. J Am Coll Cardiol. 2011;58:2511–9.

87. Van Wolferen SA, van de Verdonk MC, Mauritz GJ, et al. Clinically significant change in stroke volume in pulmonary hypertension. Chest. 2011;139:1003–9.

88. Wessels JN, de Man FS, vonk Noordegraaf A. The use of magnetic resonance imaging in pulmonary hypertension: why are we still waiting? Eur Respir Rev. 2020;26:200139–20.

89. REPLACE clinical trials.gov NCT02829034. REPLACE Riociguat replacing phosphodiesterase 5 inhibitor (PDE5i) therapy evaluated against continued PDE5i therapy in patients with pulmonary arterial hypertension (PAH).

90. Vonk Noordegraaf A, Channick R, Cottreel E, Kiely DG, Marcus JT, Martin N, Moiseeva O, Peacock A, Swift AJ, Tawakol A, Torbicki A, Rosenkranz S, Galiè N. Effects of macitentan on right ventricular remodelling and function in pulmonary arterial hypertension: results from the REPAIR study REPAIR Right Ventricular Remodeling in Pulmonary Arterial Hypertension. (In Press).

Right Ventricular Structure and Function During Exercise

André La Gerche

Introduction: Why Is Right Ventricular Function Important During Exercise?

In health and disease, exercise capacity is limited by the extent to which the working muscles receive and utilise oxygen. With the exception of patients with severe pulmonary disease, the most important factor in the supply of oxygen to the muscles is cardiac output (CO). Traditionally, investigators have sought to explain exercise-induced increases in CO (often termed "cardiac reserve") by means of increases in heart rate, augmentation in the left ventricular (LV) function and vasodilation of the systemic circulation [1, 2]. Often overlooked is the fact that *cardiac output is only as good as your worst ventricle*. This statement grossly simplifies important ventricular-arterial and ventricular-ventricular interactions but nonetheless it is important to realise that overall cardiac performance is determined by two circulations in series. If, for example, the systemic ventricle only receives 3 L/min of input due to limitations in the pre-systemic

circulation then, at best, it can only deliver 3 L/min. This highlights the fact that dysfunction of the pre-systemic circulation can impair overall CO and that a more holistic approach to cardiac function needs to consider the entire circulation. This chapter highlights the complex interaction between the RV and its vascular load and how their interdependence means that any increase in pulmonary vascular pressures results in increased work for the RV. Moreover, we discuss how in most situations the work of the RV increases disproportionately during exercise such that the RV contributes little to the maintenance of CO at rest but is critical to cardiac reserve during exercise.

The consideration of RV function during exercise is of prime clinical relevance. The majority of our patients experience breathlessness with exertion rather than at rest, and yet the majority of assessments are made in the resting state. Thus, resting measures may be a poor surrogate measure of cardiac dysfunction. The slogan "to assess exertional breathlessness, you must exert the breathless" serves to remind us that the functional characteristics of the resting heart and circulation may change dramatically during exercise. In Fig. 6.1, the importance of exercise testing is illustrated in two patients who had no symptoms at rest but developed severe breathlessness and pre-syncope with exercise. Only mild changes were evident at rest but marked RV dysfunction and resulting impairment in LV filling occurred with exercise—correlating with the onset of symptoms.

A. La Gerche (✉)
Clinical Research Domain, Baker Heart and Diabetes Institute, Melbourne, VIC, Australia

National Centre for Sports Cardiology, St Vincent's Hospital Melbourne, Fitzroy, VIC, Australia

Department of Cardiometabolic Health, University of Melbourne, Parkville, VIC, Australia
e-mail: andre.lagerche@baker.edu.au;
Andre.LAGERCHE@svha.org.au

© The Author(s), under exclusive license to Springer Nature Switzerland AG 2021
S. P. Gaine et al. (eds.), *The Right Heart*, https://doi.org/10.1007/978-3-030-78255-9_6

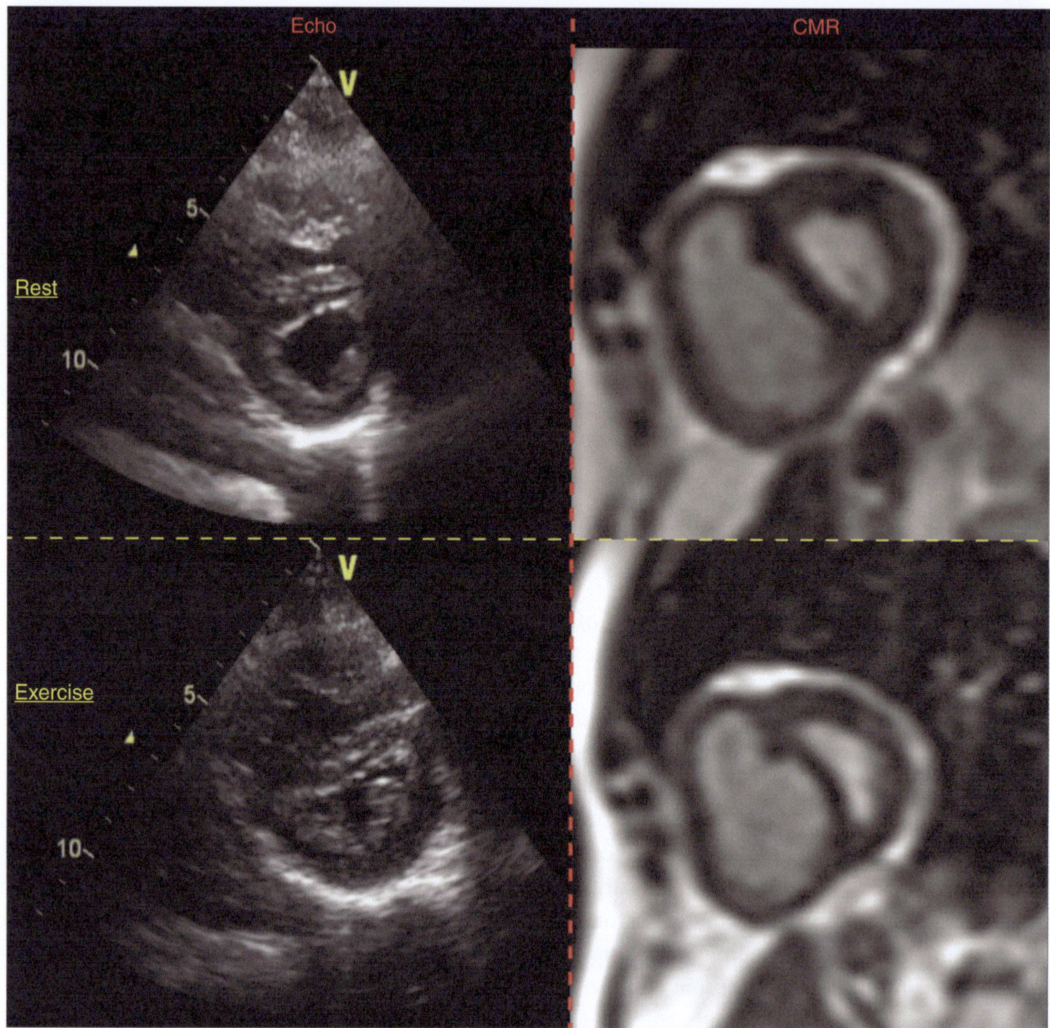

Fig. 6.1 Two patients with exertional symptoms correlating with exercise-induced right ventricular dysfunction. Patient 1 underwent exercise echocardiography to investigate severe exertional breathlessness. Resting examination suggested mild pulmonary hypertension. Exercise CMR was performed in patient 2 who had mild chronic thromboembolic pulmonary hypertension and was limited by pre-syncope on relatively mild exercise. In a similar manner, short-axis images acquired at a mid-ventricular level during early diastole demonstrate only mild RV dilation and septal flattening at rest. However, during exercise the RV becomes more dilated and there is prominent septal shift which greatly impairs LV filling during early diastole. As a result of the reduced RV ejection and reduced LV filling, cardiac output is markedly impaired. Thus, as compared with rest, the exercise pathophysiology better explains the severity of the symptoms

In addition to diagnostic insights, the study of RV function has important implications for prognosis. It has been repeatedly demonstrated that RV functional measures are independent predictors of outcome in various cardiac pathologies such as valvular heart disease, myocardial infarction and congestive heart failure [3–7]. However, of even greater intrigue is the finding that RV reserve is perhaps an even more important determinant of clinical outcomes [8–15] and exercise capacity [16–18], even amongst the very fittest of athletes [19–21].

This chapter reviews the physiological rationale underpinning the assertion that the

RV and pulmonary circulation are critical determinants of exercise performance in health and disease. We will discuss established and evolving techniques for the assessment of RV function during exercise and clinical situations in which RV functional capacity may be insufficient to meet the metabolic demands of exercise. Finally, the promise and limitations of maximising exercise capacity via therapies targeting the RV and pulmonary circulation are discussed.

Physiology of the RV and Pulmonary Circulation and Its Relevance to Exercise

In order to understand ventricular function, one must consider the venous preload which facilitates output by means of elastic recoil (Starling effect) and the arterial load against which it must pump. In the resting circulation the healthy RV has slightly lower preload [22] and substantially lower afterload [23] than the LV. In fact, in the resting state, the afterload against which the RV must work is so slight that a near-normal CO can be maintained by means of venous preload and increase in RV pressure resulting from ventricular interdependence. This has been demonstrated by animal studies in which the RV has been electrically isolated [24], replaced by a non-contractile patch [25], or by the Fontan palliation in which surgical "bypass" directly connecting the venous circulation to the pulmonary arteries is compatible with near-normal resting haemodynamics [26]. Although the ventricular work required may be sufficient to maintain trans-pulmonary blood flow in the healthy resting circulation, this does not apply when there is an increase in afterload [4] or during exercise when an increase in pulmonary artery pressures mandates an increase in cardiac work [27]. Whilst the Fontan circulation is often cited as evidence of the RV's limited role in generating cardiac output, it must be remembered that a circulation without a sub-pulmonary pump has grossly inadequate reserve during exercise.

Although the pulmonary circulation shares much in common with the systemic circulation there are also some important differences. The pulmonary circulation receives the entire cardiac output but has a pressure of approximately one-fifth that of the systemic circulation, a figure which is remarkably consistent across mammalian species [28]. The relationship between pressure (P), flow (F) and resistance (R) can be simplified as $F \propto P/R$ which is a simile of Ohm's law for electric circuits and is often referred to as the simplified Poiseuille's law in vascular circuits. Thus, the lower pressure pulmonary system equates to a lower resistance system. This lower resistance is a product of a number of unique features: firstly, there is rapid and prolific branching of vessels in the pulmonary circulation. Total vascular resistance may be quantified as the sum of the reciprocal of the resistance of each branch (i.e. $1/R_{total} = 1/R_1 + 1/R_2 + 1/R_3 \ldots$) such that the greater the number of parallel branches the lower the total resistance. Also, the pulmonary arteries and arterioles are thinner walled than their systemic counterparts. This has a very important implication in that the thinner walled vessels are more compliant and this results in further reductions in resistance and pressure. This concept is summarised in the Windkessel model of vascular flow [29, 30]. This model predicts that compliance is inversely proportional to resistance and thus the "stretching" of compliant vessels with pulsatile flow serves to decrease the resistance and blunt pressure rises. Therefore, the differences between the pulmonary and systemic circulations are that the former forms a more extensive and earlier parallel circuit and is more compliant, both serving to make RV afterload low.

Another difference between the pulmonary and systemic circulations is the effect of venous pressure on ventricular afterload. The high arteriolar pressures in the systemic circulation mean that systemic venous pressures would need to be very high before exerting a significant "back-pressure effect". In the pulmonary vasculature, however, there is much greater back-pressure effect such that increases in left atrial pressure have a strong bearing on pulmonary artery pressures. It has been suggested that left atrial pressures explain approximately 80% of the variance in pulmonary artery pressures in the absence of pulmonary vascular disease [22, 31]. This may be of particular importance during exercise. Descriptions of heart failure are often dichotomised into those with abnormalities in lusitropic and contractile dysfunction in whom left atrial pressures increase during exercise and those with healthy heart function in whom filling pressures do not increase [32]. Augmentation in CO during exercise requires increasing filling volumes within shorter diastolic filling times. This can be achieved by means of greater ventricular suction, greater atrial pressures or both. Nonogi et al. demonstrated that early diastolic ventricular suction increases during exercise [33]. They demonstrated that active ventricular relaxation (time constant of relaxation—tau) improved and that early-diastolic and mid-diastolic ventricular pressures were lower during exercise as compared with rest. However, these differences were relatively modest and it would seem unlikely that this degree of "suck" could generate the massive outputs (in excess of 40 L/min [34, 35]) generated by well-trained athletes during exercise. Rather, it is most likely that an increase in atrial pressure is also required to "push" blood across the atrioventricular valve during exercise. Relatively few studies have assessed left atrial pressures during exercise in healthy subjects and those studies that exist have used pulmonary artery balloon occlusion ("wedge") catheters as a surrogate of left atrial pressure, a method that has potential limitations during vigorous exercise. Nonetheless, existing data supports the premise that exercise-induced increases in cardiac output require an increase in left atrial pressure [36]. Reeves et al. measured right atrial and pulmonary artery occlusion pressures (PAOP) in eight healthy volunteers during intense exercise and found a fairly strong correlation between these measures and CO [22]. Interestingly, the four subjects with the highest oxygen consumption (VO$_2$max) had PAOPs between 19 and 35 mmHg. More recently, Lewis et al. also observed a strong correlation between PAOP and CO in control subjects and determined

the relationship PAOP (mmHg) = 1.1 × CO (L/min), albeit within a group with substantially more modest exercise capacity [14]. However, if one were to extrapolate the relationship derived by Lewis et al. to the athletes studied by Reeves, there is considerable agreement in the range of values. Stickland et al. compared young healthy subjects of low fitness to highly trained athletes and observed increases in PAOP in both cohorts to similar values but at a much higher cardiac output in the athletes. Similar observations were made by Pandey et al. in a large cohort of healthy subjects across a wide age range [37]. They observed an increase in PAOP with exercise with a peak pressure that was relatively stable across all ages. In contrast, peak exercise cardiac output reduced with age. Thus, the following consistent findings can be gleaned: (1) left atrial pressures increase with exercise in proportion to increases in cardiac output and (2) steepness of this relationship increases with reduced fitness, heart failure and age.

Thus, one cannot focus on ventricular filling pressures without context. The heart failure patient may have elevated left atrial pressures whilst walking up a flight of stairs whilst an athlete may have similar left atrial pressures whilst running at a record pace. In both cases, the subjects are breathless, ventricular filling pressures increase, and CO is close to maximal and is insufficient for the metabolic demands of the working muscles. The difference is the work level and cardiac output at which cardiac function is maximised. "Heart failure" represents a continuum in which relatively arbitrary clinical cut-offs are set to distinguish normal cardiac performance from failure.

The concept of exercise-induced LV filling pressures is extremely relevant to the further discussion regarding the performance of the pulmonary circulation and RV during exercise. The increased LV filling pressures are relayed "upstream" and contribute to the afterload against which the RV must pump. Thus, during exercise the RV is faced with the increased afterload of the sum of LV filling pressures and any additional flow-induced increase in pulmonary artery pressures (Fig. 6.2).

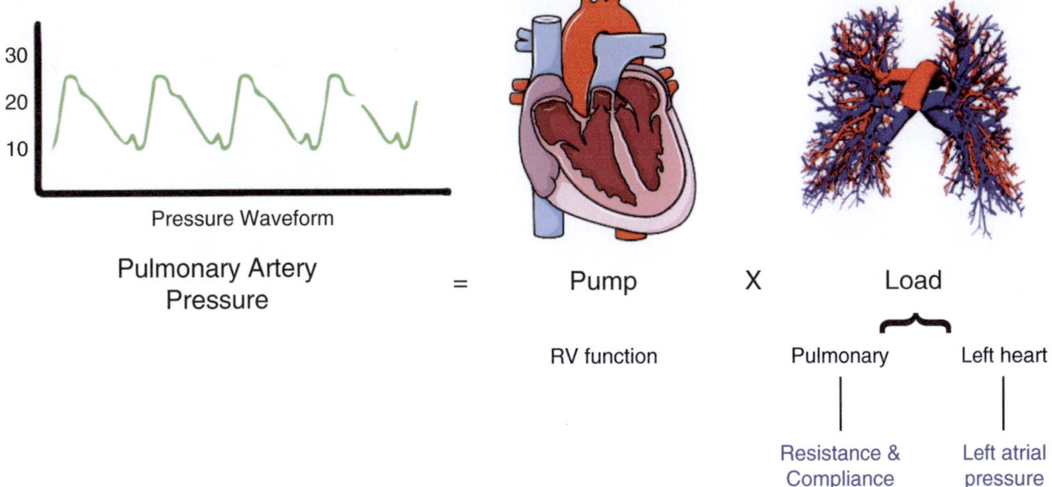

Fig. 6.2 The relationship between pulmonary artery pressures, right ventricular function and vascular load. Pulmonary artery pressures are determined by both the ability of the RV pump to generate pressure and the load against which this pump must push. The RV afterload is determined by pulmonary vascular factors (resistance, compliance and impedance) and by left atrial pressures

Exercise Causes a Disproportionate Increase in RV Pressures, Wall Stress and Work

There are differences between the RV and LV in the arterial load imposed by exercise and in the ventricular capacity to counter that load (i.e. maintain ventricular arterial coupling). As illustrated in Fig. 6.3, at rest the LV contracts against a systemic circulation with moderate resistance and compliance as compared with the low resistance and high compliance of the pulmonary circulation. During exercise, CO increases manyfold (as much as eightfold in well-trained athletes [34, 35]) and therefore vascular pressures would be expected to increase unless sufficiently counterbalanced by decreases in resistance and increases in compliance. However, the pulmonary vasculature has very low resistance at rest and it has somewhat limited capacity for further decreases [38, 39]. Recruitment of upper lobe vessels in combination with flow-mediated and neurohormonal vasodilation affects a reduction in PVR of approximately 20–50% [38]. Such changes are limited compared with the profound reductions in systemic vascular resistance which is enabled by the greater capacity for redistribution to vascular territories of low resistance. The moderating effect of vascular compliance may also be less than anticipated. During exercise, the vasculature is distended by the high flow rates meaning that compliance (the ability to further distend the vessels with any given change in pressure) is reduced [7, 40, 41]. Therefore, vascular pressures increase and, these increases are greater for the pulmonary circulation than for the systemic circulation [42, 43].

Several studies have reported substantial increases in pulmonary artery pressures during exercise using echocardiographic estimates [42–46] and direct invasive measures [14, 39, 47]. Figure 6.4a summarises data from these studies that demonstrate remarkable consistency in the linear regression derived for the relationship between mean pulmonary artery pressure (mPAP) and CO with normal values approximating 1 mmHg of increase in mean pulmonary artery pressure for every litre increase in cardiac output and any relationship >3 mmHg/L being considered abnormal. Using direct catheter measures, Lewis et al. [14] observed an increase of 1.5 mmHg in mean pulmonary artery pressure for each litre increase in CO. Less steep mPAP/CO relationship has been observed in the younger

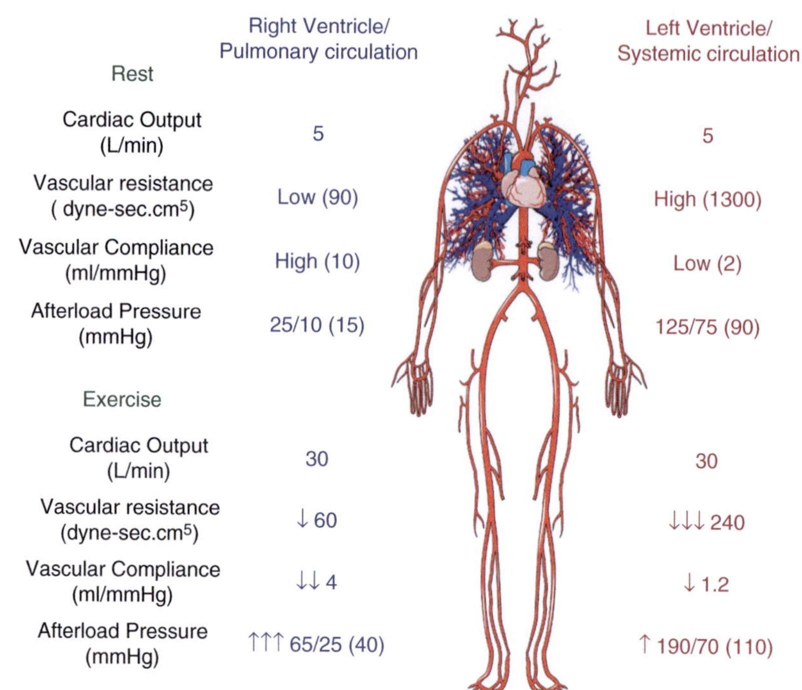

Fig. 6.3 Comparison between the load and function of the pre-systemic and systemic ventricles at rest and during exercise. Relative to the LV, the RV is a low-pressure chamber subject to low afterload at rest. However, during exercise, pressures in the RV increase disproportionately due to relatively less capacity for the pulmonary circulation to dilate, distend and recruit new vascular territories

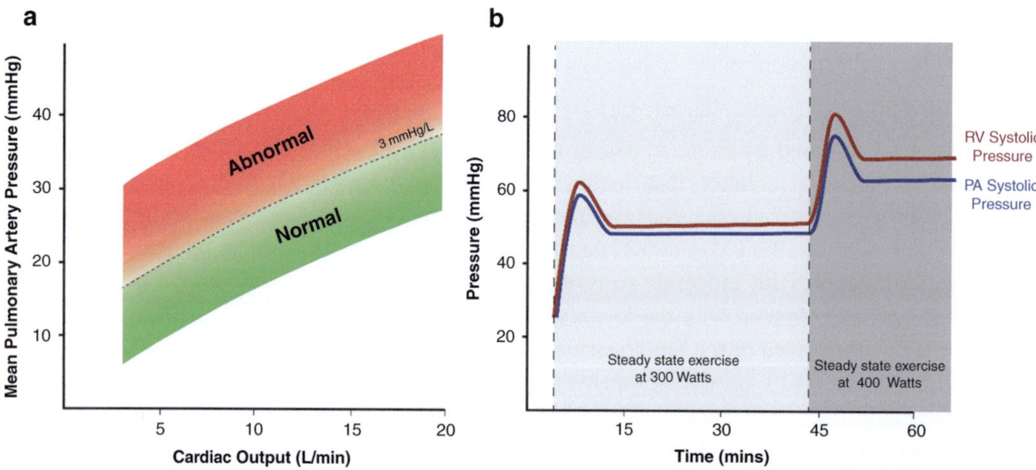

Fig. 6.4 A consistent near-linear relationship between increases in pulmonary artery pressures and cardiac output during exercise. Data from several studies have enabled us to define a healthy relationship between mean pulmonary artery pressures and cardiac output with >3 mmHg/L signifying an abnormal increase in pulmonary artery pressures during exercise (panel **a**). Steady-state exercise results in an initial increase in pulmonary artery pressures that then attenuate somewhat if exercise is maintained (here exemplified by two steady-state bouts of exercise). Also notable is the increasing gap between RV and pulmonary artery systolic pressures due to an increasing exercise gradient across the RV outflow tract and pulmonary valve (panel **b**)

and fitter cohorts of Argiento et al. [45] and La Gerche et al. [43] Other potential confounders such as the postural effects on pulmonary vascular recruitment [38] and differences in both pulmonary artery estimates (echocardiographic vs. catheter) and CO estimates (thermodilution vs. echo Doppler vs. exercise MRI) may explain the variance in the mPAP/CO relationships observed.

Despite this, there is considerable consistency in these results which predict significant increases in pulmonary artery pressures during intense exercise. For example, an increase in CO of 30 L/min would equate to a mean pulmonary artery pressure exceeding 50 mmHg—representing an increase of threefold or more from rest. Furthermore, the relationship between pulmonary artery pressures and CO appears similar regardless of athletic conditioning. However, because athletes have greater exercise capacity they are able to generate higher outputs and higher pulmonary artery pressures [43]. This represents a disproportionately large increase in RV afterload compared with mean arterial pressure increases which rarely exceed 50% in the LV. It is also important to note that there is a rapid recovery of pulmonary artery pressures after the completion of exercise [48]. This is of critical importance in clinical assessments where there is a tendency to resort to post-exercise measures. The considerable variance in the rate of recovery is an important confounder in this setting.

Two potentially important observations have advanced our understanding of the behaviour of right-heart pressures during exercise. Firstly, researchers from Toronto, Canada, challenged the view that there is a linear increase in pulmonary artery pressures relative to cardiac output by demonstrating that there is a degree of accommodation that results in a reduction in pulmonary artery pressures when a steady state in exercise intensity and cardiac output is achieved. In other words, pulmonary artery pressures increase with exercise intensity initially but then moderate when workload is kept constant [49, 50]. This is of considerable importance when one contrasts the ramp design of many experimental exercise protocols to the "real world" in which people rarely undertake exercise with a continuously increasing exercise intensity. In short, pulmonary artery pressures may not be quite as high during normal exercise activities as those that we measure in the lab. Secondly, with simultaneous right ventricular and pulmonary artery catheter measures during exercise, two independent research groups have identified an increasing ventricular-arterial gradient in the right heart [51, 52]. At rest, RV and pulmonary artery peak systolic pressures were the same but during exercise the RV pressure increased more than the pulmonary artery systolic pressure (54 ± 10 vs. 37 ± 9 mmHg at moderate exercise intensity) suggesting the emergence of a pressure gradient during exercise across the RV outflow tract or pulmonary valve. This might explain why echocardiographic measures, that use the tricuspid regurgitant signal to estimate RV systolic pressure, tend to slightly overestimate pulmonary artery systolic pressures when measured invasively during exercise [53]. These two concepts are illustrated in Fig. 6.4b.

Therefore, it is evident that during exercise there is an increase in left atrial pressures leading to an increase in pulmonary artery pressures and an increase in RV pressures. This "backing up of pressure" imposes a relatively greater load on the RV during exercise.

We sought to assess this seemingly disproportionate ventricular load using a combination of magnetic resonance and echocardiographic imaging at rest and during exercise to quantify RV systolic wall stress, as compared with that of the LV [42]. Using the simple construct of the LaPlace relationship, we found that during exercise, increases in both pressures and volumes were greater for the RV, whilst increases in wall thickness were relatively less than those for the LV. As a result, RV wall stress estimates increased 125% during exercise as compared with a modest 14% increase in LV wall stress [42]. Thus, it may be contended that the stress, work and metabolic demands placed on the RV during exercise are relatively greater than those of the LV (Fig. 6.5).

Such substantive afterload would seem a significant burden for the contractile reserve of the RV and raises the possibility that in the extremes of exercise the RV/pulmonary vascular unit may limit the output just as it does in some disease states [16, 17]. At rest, RV measures of mass and contractility are one-third to one-fifth those of the LV and this appropriately matches the pressure requirements of each [54, 55]. This lesser myocardial mass of the RV suggests that it may have a diminished contractile reserve and may be less able to accommodate marked changes in loading. This is supported by studies which demonstrate

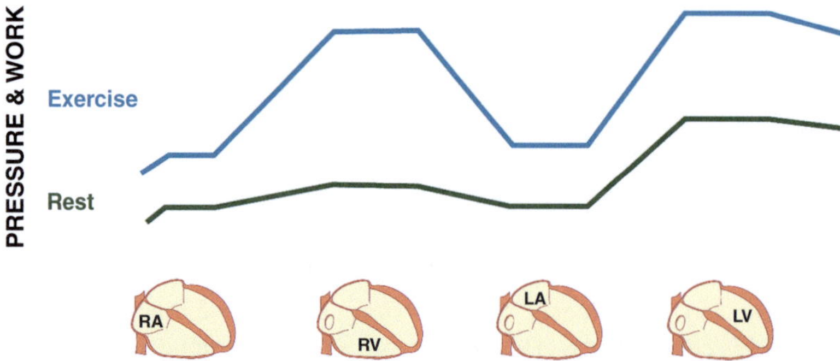

Fig. 6.5 Disproportionate right-heart pressure and workload with exercise. There is an increase in left ventricular (LV) pressure and work during exercise relative to rest. The relative increase in left atrial (LA) pressure is more significant due to the flow-related build-up of pressure whilst the mitral valve is closed (representing an increasingly large proportion of the cardiac cycle during exercise). This increase in LA pressure translates to an increase in pulmonary artery pressures and a large increase in right ventricular (RV) pressure and work. The increase in RV work during exercise exceeds that of the LV

that afterload increases result in a marked reduction in RV stroke volume but only a slight decrease in LV stroke volume [56, 57]. MacNee et al. quantified the relative reductions in stroke volume in either ventricle at rest with increasing afterload. The ~30% reduction in RV stroke volume compared with ~10% fall in LV stroke volume suggests that the RV has less contractile reserve to accommodate afterload increases. Given the potential limitations in RV reserve and the far greater increases in RV afterload relative to the LV, one might hypothesise that the RV could limit CO during intense exercise. This hypothesis has been raised previously [58–60], but has not been actively pursued over the last three decades, perhaps due to limitations in imaging the RV during exercise.

How Can RV Function Be Assessed During Exercise?

One of the major issues in attempting to appraise the hypothesis that the RV may serve as an important limitation to CO during exercise is the difficulty in assessing the RV during exercise. The RV has complex geometry and relatively heterogeneous regional function and is situated behind the sternum, thereby limiting echocardiographic windows. Of perhaps greatest importance, particularly during exercise, is the profound influence of loading conditions on the RV and thus it is important for functional measures to either be load independent or incorporate an assessment of load.

The earliest attempts to define the RV response to exercise utilised radionuclide ventriculography. Morrison et al. used radiolabelled red cells and acquired steady-state data over 2 min during four stages of exercise of increasing intensity [61]. In nine healthy volunteers, they observed a progressive increase in RV ejection fraction (EF%) and an inverse relationship between RVEF% and pulmonary vascular resistance (PVR), thereby concluding that RVEF is strongly influenced by afterload. Hirata et al. advanced this hypothesis further by examining radionuclide RVEF in subjects with variable pulmonary vascular resistance as a result of atrial septal defects or rheumatic mitral stenosis. They also reported a strong inverse relationship between the change in RVEF% during exercise and PVR [62]. Radionuclide ventriculography was well suited to the investigation of RV function given that the technique relies on geometry-independent count-based techniques. However, limitations include overlap of counts from the atria and LV, lack of detail in regard to RV morphology and need for a prolonged steady state for gated acquisitions. Moreover, there is substantial radiation exposure involved, particularly when repeated measures are acquired.

Echocardiography is a readily accessible, safe and adaptable imaging technique but RV imaging presents some unique challenges given the irregular geometry and retrosternal positioning of the RV. Nonetheless, a number of investigators have sought to assess RV function during exercise. Given the considerable load dependency of the RV, investigators have sought to evaluate RV contractility using relatively load-independent measures. RV strain rate measures the speed of myocardial deformation and has been quantified during intense exercise using vector imaging, 2D tracking and tissue Doppler techniques [20, 21, 63]. However, these remain specialised measures with high variability and are exquisitely dependent upon the quality and temporal resolution of the data set. Perhaps of greater appeal is the concept of combining functional and load measures in a manner akin to pressure-volume analyses. This can be achieved with 2D echocardiographic measures with the assumption that an area/volume relationship approximates the gold standard pressure-volume measures. Indeed, this seems to be a reasonable assumption with Claessen et al. demonstrating that a totally non-invasive approximation using RV areas and approximates of pulmonary artery pressures using tricuspid regurgitant velocity is robust and quite an accurate estimate of gold standard measures using invasive catheter measures of pressure and real-time exercise RV volumes using exercise-magnetic resonance imaging (ex-CMR) [53]. These hybrid pressure-volume techniques have been used for varied important clinical questions (see below).

Cardiac magnetic resonance Imaging (CMR) is ideally suited to the assessment of the RV during exercise. Unlike with echocardiography, RV volumes can be accurately quantified during intense exercise in all subjects regardless of body habitus [34, 64]. Technical advances have enabled real-time CMR acquisitions in which ECG gating is not required and respiratory translation can be accounted for post hoc such that biventricular volume quantification compares favourably with invasive standards [34]. Temporal resolution remains a constraint (approximately 7–8 frames/cardiac cycle during maximal exercise tachycardia) although the use of parallel processing and improved retrospective gating of respiratory motion may facilitate improved image quality, automated quantification of volumes and shorter processing times [65].

Even with technical advances to enable wider use of exercise CMR, its use is currently largely limited to research settings. Whilst offering superb insights into the mechanics and quantification of impaired cardiac reserve, simpler tests are necessary to identify those patients in whom RV functional reserve is reduced due to either RV dysfunction or pathological increases in pulmonary vascular load. To this end, indirect measures show promise. Lewis et al. elegantly demonstrated that ventilator efficiency (VE/VCO$_2$) on cardiopulmonary testing correlated well with pulmonary vascular resistance, determined by a combination of invasive pressure estimates and nuclear ventriculography [66]. Furthermore, they demonstrated a reduction in VE/VCO$_2$ following treatment with a pulmonary vasodilator but not in those receiving placebo suggesting that this non-invasive measure may reflect RV/pulmonary vascular coupling during exercise.

Can the Healthy RV Cope with the Increased Pulmonary Vascular Load of Exercise?

As discussed in the section "Exercise Causes a Disproportionate Increase in RV Pressures, Wall Stress and Work", there is a significant increase in RV afterload during exercise which increases RV wall stress and work. The question that arises, therefore, is whether the RV can generate the increased work that is required against the accumulating load of intense exercise. In healthy subjects during exercise of short duration, it would seem that the answer is yes. Using echocardiography and CMR during exercise, several studies have demonstrated that RV area progressively decreases as pulmonary artery pressures increase (using echocardiography) and that RV end-systolic volume decreases with exercise intensity (CMR) [20, 21, 34, 67, 68]—see Fig. 6.6. This is perhaps not surprising given the near-linear

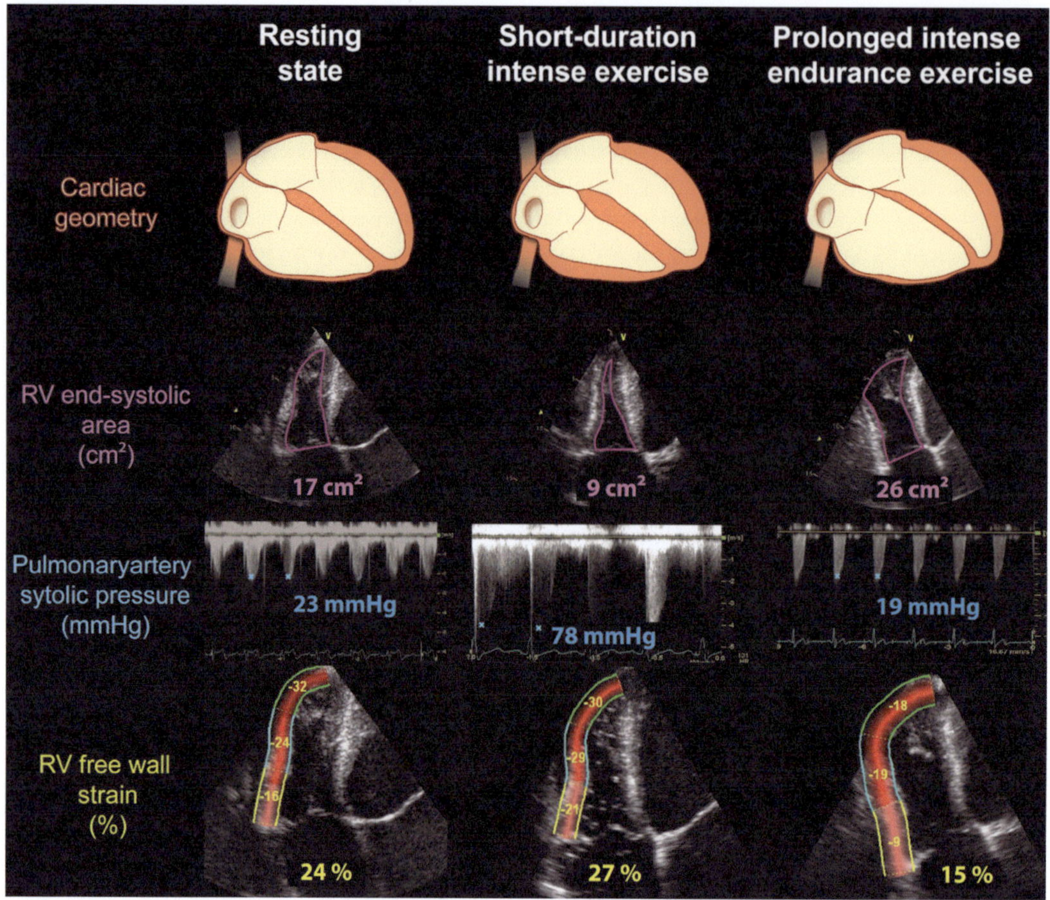

Fig. 6.6 Summary of right ventricular structural and functional changes during exercise of different durations. Typical changes in RV function at rest (left), during short-duration intense exercise (middle) and immediately following an ultra-endurance triathlon (right) are demonstrated using the example of a professional triathlete. At rest, the RV is moderately enlarged with normal pulmonary artery pressures and deformation. During exercise, large increases in cardiac output result in proportional increases in pulmonary artery pressures. RV function is able to match demand with systolic augmentation evidenced by a reduction in systolic area and a small increase in strain (larger increases in strain rate not shown here). After prolonged exercise it seems that these substantial RV work demands result in RV fatigue/injury reflected by RV dilation and systolic dysfunction as evidenced by an increase in systolic area and a reduction in strain

relationship that exists between cardiac output and exercise intensity suggesting that ventricular ejection augments despite increases in vascular load. The athlete's heart represents the extremes of physiology with marked changes in right ventricular volumes during exercise that also change according to respiration such that the respiratory pump of exercise causes an increase in RV volumes that combines with the increases in RV pressure to affect a flattening of the interventricular septum [69]. Figure 6.7 illustrates some similarities between an athlete's heart and that of a patient with pulmonary hypertension during exercise.

However, multiple recent studies have observed a decrement in RV function after more prolonged intense exercise suggesting that whilst the RV can maintain function against the disproportionate increase in vascular load during exercise of short duration, there is a point at which the RV fatigues. Given the observation that RV load, wall stress and work increase to a relatively greater extent than in the LV, it is perhaps not surprising that the RV fatigue precedes

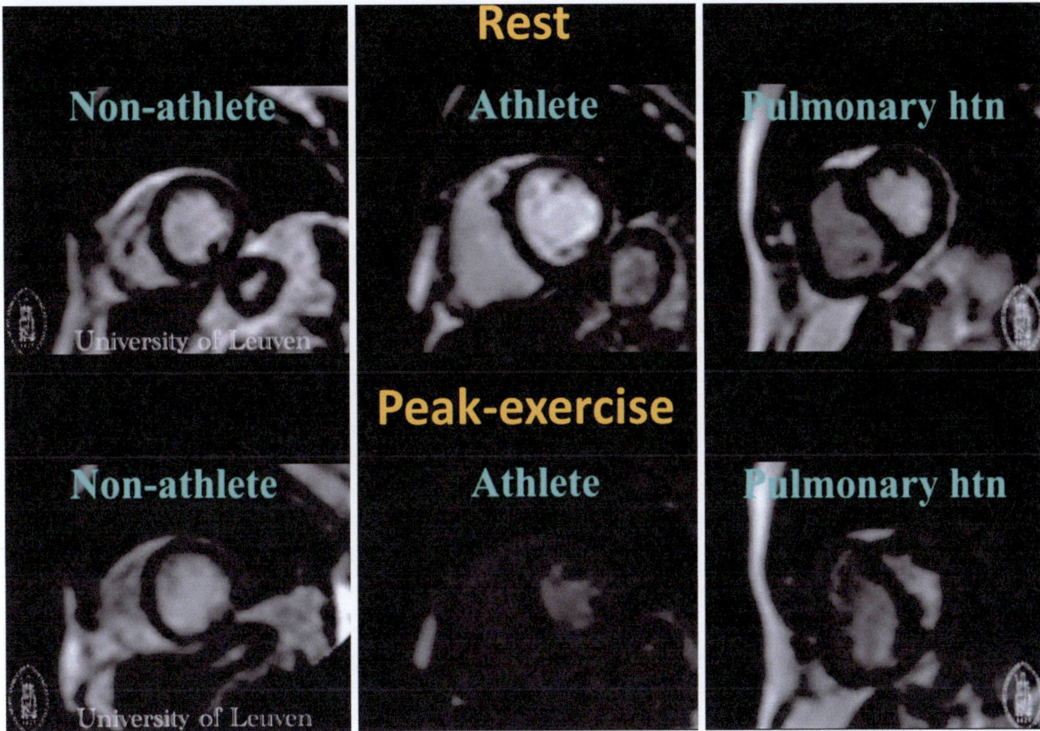

Fig. 6.7 Exercise cardiac magnetic resonance imaging providing an improved insight into pathophysiological changes in right ventricular function during exercise. Early diastolic mid-ventricular short-axis CMR images acquired at rest provide a comparison between a healthy non-athlete, an athlete and a patient with pulmonary hypertension. The RV:LV ratio increases and there is greater ventricular interaction (right-to-left septal shift) in the athlete, as compared with the non-athlete and even more so in the patient. However, these changes are far more obvious during exercise. In the athlete the RV is slightly more dilated and the septal shift becomes appreciable. In the pulmonary hypertension patient, these changes become marked

that of the LV. Studies in relatively amateur marathon runners [70–72] as well as well-trained ultra-endurance runners [73] and triathletes [74, 75] have consistently demonstrated significant decrements in RV function immediately following exercise, whereas LV function is preserved.

Figure 6.6 summarises the changes in RV function during exercise in the healthy person or healthy athlete. During short intense exercise there is an increase in RV pressures and systolic function but when this exercise becomes protracted the RV can fatigue in response to working against a sustained increase in load. The exact mechanism of this fatigue is not known—substrate deficiency, beta-receptor desensitisation, inflammation or neurohormonal dysregulation are all potential candidates [76].

Clinical Settings in Which the Assessment of RV Function During Exercise May Be Important

Athletes

Assessment of the RV during exercise is important in athletes for two reasons: (1) resting measures can be difficult to interpret and (2) athletes regularly place significant stress on the RV and appear to be at risk of adverse remodelling and arrhythmias. It has been well demonstrated that resting measures of RV function are frequently reduced in athletes [77, 78] and that resting measures of RV function do not adequately discriminate between disease and pathology [21, 68]. Echocardiographic assessment of the RV area/pressure relationship was used to demonstrate an appropriate augmentation of contractility in athletes despite low resting functional measures [20, 21] and this finding has been repeatedly validated using more intensive hybrid methods of invasive catheterisation and ex-CMR [68]. Of greater importance, RV contractile reserve has been shown to be impaired in athletes with complex ventricular arrhythmias [21, 68]. This suggests that athletes presenting with ventricular arrhythmias may have evidence of subtle RV injury (either genetic or acquired) that may only be evident with novel imaging techniques and exercise [79].

Chronic Pulmonary Disease

Exercise CMR has provided some important insights into RV limitations to cardiac performance in patients with pulmonary vascular pathology. Holverda et al. observed that whilst RV end-systolic volume decreased with exercise in healthy control subjects, it remained unchanged or even increased in patients with pulmonary hypertension and patients with chronic obstructive airway disease [16, 17]. Thus, a lack of augmentation in RV stroke volume limits overall cardiac performance such that oxygen delivery to the working muscles is insufficient, resulting in premature anaerobic metabolism, breathlessness and fatigue. Rozenbaum et al. recently validated these findings using exercise echocardiography noting a reduction in RV contractile reserve resulting in flattening of the interventricular septum causing impairment in early filling of the LV [80]. Thus, a vicious circle develops in which diastolic filling impairment further increases RV load and dysfunction. Similar findings have also been observed in interstitial lung disease [81].

Pulmonary Vascular Pathology

In the patient with a pathology of the RV and pulmonary circulation, elegant studies of the Vonk Noordegraaf group were the first to illustrate how RV failure could be accentuated during exercise [16, 17]. Grunig et al. demonstrated that RV contractile reserve (measured indirectly as augmen-

tation of pulmonary artery pressures) was a key determinant of outcomes in patients with pulmonary arterial hypertension, suggesting that failure of the RV to meet the increased afterload during exercise was a key indicator of a failure of adaptation [10]. This concept has been developed with implications in milder forms of pulmonary vascular disease. Claeys et al. compared RV contractile reserve in healthy subjects, patients with chronic thromboembolic disease (CTED—defined by persistent perfusion defects in the absence of pulmonary hypertension at rest) and patients with chronic thromboembolic pulmonary hypertension. Although RV function was similar between healthy subjects and those with CTED at rest, during exercise, RV contractile reserve was reduced in CTED patients with a phenotype in between health and pulmonary hypertension [67]. In perhaps the subtlest form of pulmonary vascular disease, Claessen et al. demonstrated slight abnormalities in the relationship between pulmonary artery pressures and cardiac output during exercise in patients with a genetic predisposition to pulmonary hypertension (BMPR2 mutation) but preserved RV contractile reserve [82]. Finally, augmentation of RV contractile reserve has been demonstrated following the administration of pulmonary vasodilator therapy in patients with chronic thromboembolic pulmonary hypertension before [83], and after [84], pulmonary endarterectomy. These measures not only serve to provide novel insights into the pathophysiology underpinning patients' symptoms but also provide a potential measure of short-term efficacy for new therapies in these conditions.

Heart Failure

There is intense interest in the need for better characterisation of heart failure patients in order to best individualise therapies and improve outcomes. Plehn et al. demonstrated that RV end-systolic volume reduced during exercise in healthy controls but not in patients with hypertrophic and dilated cardiomyopathies, and this attenuation in systolic performance did not seem to be accounted for by the slightly greater increases in pulmonary artery pressures [85]. Guazzi et al. demonstrated a relationship between reduced RV contractile reserve and ventilatory inefficiency in patients with heart failure and reduced ejection fraction, thereby raising the possibility that some patients may benefit from specific pulmonary vasodilator therapy in addition to traditional heart failure treatment, although this hypothesis is yet to be validated in a clinical trial [86, 87]. Of greater potential importance are the patients with heart failure and preserved ejection fraction (HFPEF) in whom there are few proven efficacious therapies. In an elegant comparison of healthy subjects and two groups of HFPEF patients (those with and without evidence of pulmonary vascular disease in addition to raised LV filling pressures during exercise), Gorter et al. identified a failure in RV augmentation with exercise as an important limitation in the overall cardiovascular performance [88]. The concept that pulmonary vasodilator therapy may assist in attenuating RV afterload and enhancing RV performance during exercise in HFPEF patients was interrogated by Huang et al. who used inhaled prostacyclin therapy to improve RV and overall myocardial function during exercise [89]. Whilst these results are cause for some optimism, clinical trials have largely failed to demonstrate a benefit from pulmonary vasodilators [90, 91].

Valvular Heart Disease

An increase in pulmonary artery pressures during exercise is a recognised adverse prognostic sign in valvular heart disease. However, the failure of RV function to augment during exercise to meet the demands of an increase in afterload has been demonstrated to be a particularly important prognostic indictor for post-surgical outcomes [8, 92].

Congenital Heart Disease

Intriguing insights into RV function can be extrapolated from the unique patient group with congenitally corrected transposition of the great arteries (TGA) in whom the RV is subjected to systemic afterload and has a tendency to decompensate with time. Van der Bom et al. demonstrated that a combination of RV end-diastolic volume and peak exercise blood pressure was the strongest determinant of clinical events such as worsening heart failure [11]. Helsen et al. dissected this physiology further with the demonstration that contractile reserve (RV end-systolic pressure/volume relationship) was impaired in both congenitally corrected and surgically corrected TGA patients and that this, combined with a reduction in chronotropic reserve, limited cardiac output and exercise capacity [93].

Can Pulmonary Vasodilators Improve Exercise Tolerance?

The preceding sections detail a disproportionate increase in RV load during exercise and a predisposition for RV failure during exercise, either early in those with a pathology of the pulmonary circulation or only after very prolonged exercise in those with a normal RV and pulmonary circulation. This assertion that the pre-systemic circulation may limit cardiac performance during exercise would imply that pulmonary vasodilators may improve exercise performance by means of attenuating the disproportionate increase in RV load. Pulmonary vasodilators have proven efficacy in improving exercise tolerance in those patients with pulmonary arterial hypertension [40, 94] due to their ability to attenuate the pathological increases in RV load, thereby improving RV function during exercise. However, taking this one step further, one may even anticipate that these agents could improve exercise capacity in those with a normal pulmonary circulation.

Ghofrani et al. performed a randomised, double-blind placebo-controlled trial assessing the efficacy of sildenafil in improving exercise haemodynamics in 14 healthy subjects during normobaric hypoxia (10% O_2) and at altitude (Mount Everest base camp, 5245 m above sea level). As compared with placebo, sildenafil resulted in a decrease in pulmonary artery pressures and an increase in exercise workload and cardiac output in both the hypoxic and high-altitude settings [95]. Further studies using both PDE5 receptor and endothelin antagonists have been consistent in demonstrating improvements in haemodynamics and exercise performance in hypoxic conditions but have failed to show any benefit in normoxia [96–98]. There are a number of reasons why pulmonary vasodilators may have limited efficacy in healthy subjects at sea level. One of the more likely hypotheses is that the pulmonary circulation is maximally dilated during exercise and there is little capacity for further decreases in pulmonary vascular resistance. This would perhaps explain why pulmonary vasodilators do not seem to improve exercise capacity at sea level whilst increases in basal pulmonary vascular tone (with hypoxia and/or altitude) provide an opportunity for pulmonary vasodilators to reduce resistance, aid RV ejection and improve exercise parameters.

Conclusions

The RV appears to be a potential "Achilles' heel" for the exercising heart. The RV is subject to disproportionate increases in load during exercise and, as compared with the LV, impairment in function develops earlier and more significantly when exercise is prolonged. Separating and comparing the function of various elements of the circulation ignore complex interactions and a comprehensive understanding of exercise physiology needs a more holistic approach to cardiac function than has been previously considered. The importance of the RV and pulmonary circulation should not be overlooked. It may be an important component of exercise limitation and may even be the "weak link" in some settings. Fortunately, we now have methodologies capable of quantifying RV function during exercise with utility demonstrated in multiple clinical settings.

References

1. Epstein SE, Beiser GD, Stampfer M, Robinson BF, Braunwald E. Characterization of the circulatory response to maximal upright exercise in normal subjects and patients with heart disease. Circulation. 1967;35:1049–62.

2. Guyton AC. Regulation of cardiac output. N Engl J Med. 1967;277:805–12.

3. Nagel E, Stuber M, Hess OM. Importance of the right ventricle in valvular heart disease. Eur Heart J. 1996;17:829–36.

4. Le Tourneau T, Deswarte G, Lamblin N, Foucher-Hossein C, Fayad G, Richardson M, Polge AS, Vannesson C, Topilsky Y, Juthier F, Trochu JN, Enriquez-Sarano M, Bauters C. Right ventricular systolic function in organic mitral regurgitation: impact of biventricular impairment. Circulation. 2013;127:1597–608.

5. Miszalski-Jamka T, Klimeczek P, Tomala M, Krupinski M, Zawadowski G, Noelting J, Lada M, Sip K, Banys R, Mazur W, Kereiakes DJ, Zmudka K, Pasowicz M. Extent of RV dysfunction and myocardial infarction assessed by CMR are independent outcome predictors early after STEMI treated with primary angioplasty. JACC Cardiovasc Imaging. 2010;3:1237–46.

6. Ghio S, Gavazzi A, Campana C, Inserra C, Klersy C, Sebastiani R, Arbustini E, Recusani F, Tavazzi L. Independent and additive prognostic value of right ventricular systolic function and pulmonary artery pressure in patients with chronic heart failure. J Am Coll Cardiol. 2001;37:183–8.

7. Otsuki T, Maeda S, Iemitsu M, Saito Y, Tanimura Y, Ajisaka R, Miyauchi T. Systemic arterial compliance, systemic vascular resistance, and effective arterial elastance during exercise in endurance-trained men. Am J Physiol Regul Integr Comp Physiol. 2008;295:R228–35.

8. Vitel E, Galli E, Leclercq C, Fournet M, Bosseau C, Corbineau H, Bouzille G, Donal E. Right ventricular exercise contractile reserve and outcomes after early surgery for primary mitral regurgitation. Heart. 2018;104:855–60.

9. Blumberg FC, Arzt M, Lange T, Schroll S, Pfeifer M, Wensel R. Impact of right ventricular reserve on exercise capacity and survival in patients with pulmonary hypertension. Eur J Heart Fail. 2013;15(7):771–5.

10. Grunig E, Tiede H, Enyimayew EO, Ehlken N, Seyfarth HJ, Bossone E, D'Andrea A, Naeije R, Olschewski H, Ulrich S, Nagel C, Halank M, Fischer C. Assessment and prognostic relevance of right ventricular contractile reserve in patients with severe pulmonary hypertension. Circulation. 2013;128(18):2005–15.

11. van der Bom T, Winter MM, Groenink M, Vliegen HW, Pieper PG, van Dijk AP, Sieswerda GT, Roos-Hesselink JW, Zwinderman AH, Mulder BJ, Bouma BJ. Right ventricular end-diastolic volume combined with peak systolic blood pressure during exercise identifies patients at risk for complications in adults with a systemic right ventricle. J Am Coll Cardiol. 2013;62:926–36.

12. Hanft LM, Korte FS, McDonald KS. Cardiac function and modulation of sarcomeric function by length. Cardiovasc Res. 2008;77:627–36.

13. Troisi F, Greco S, Brunetti ND, Di Biase M. Right heart dysfunction assessed with echography, B-type

natriuretic peptide and cardiopulmonary test in patients with chronic heart failure. J Cardiovasc Med (Hagerstown). 2008;9:672–6.

14. Lewis GD, Murphy RM, Shah RV, Pappagianopoulos PP, Malhotra R, Bloch KD, Systrom DM, Semigran MJ. Pulmonary vascular response patterns during exercise in left ventricular systolic dysfunction predict exercise capacity and outcomes. Circ Heart Fail. 2011;4:276–85.

15. Tran T, Muralidhar A, Hunter K, Buchanan C, Coe G, Hieda M, Tompkins C, Zipse M, Spotts MJ, Laing SG, Fosmark K, Hoffman J, Ambardekar AV, Wolfel EE, Lawley J, Levine B, Kohrt WM, Pal J, Cornwell WK 3rd. Right ventricular function and cardiopulmonary performance among patients with heart failure supported by durable mechanical circulatory support devices. J Heart Lung Transplant. 2021;40:128–37.

16. Holverda S, Gan CT, Marcus JT, Postmus PE, Boonstra A, Vonk-Noordegraaf A. Impaired stroke volume response to exercise in pulmonary arterial hypertension. J Am Coll Cardiol. 2006;47:1732–3.

17. Holverda S, Rietema H, Westerhof N, Marcus JT, Gan CT, Postmus PE, Vonk-Noordegraaf A. Stroke volume increase to exercise in chronic obstructive pulmonary disease is limited by increased pulmonary artery pressure. Heart. 2009;95:137–41.

18. Kinoshita M, Inoue K, Higashi H, Akazawa Y, Sasaki Y, Fujii A, Uetani T, Inaba S, Aono J, Nagai T, Nishimura K, Ikeda S, Yamaguchi O. Impact of right ventricular contractile reserve during low-load exercise on exercise intolerance in heart failure. ESC Heart Fail. 2020;7(6):3810–20.

19. Haskell WL, Lee IM, Pate RR, Powell KE, Blair SN, Franklin BA, Macera CA, Heath GW, Thompson PD, Bauman A. Physical activity and public health - updated recommendation for adults from the American College of Sports Medicine and the American Heart Association. Circulation. 2007;116:1081–93.

20. La Gerche A, Burns AT, D'Hooge J, Macisaac AI, Heidbuchel H, Prior DL. Exercise strain rate imaging demonstrates normal right ventricular contractile reserve and clarifies ambiguous resting measures in endurance athletes. J Am Soc Echocardiogr. 2012;25:253–262.e1.

21. Claeys M, Claessen G, Claus P, De Bosscher R, Dausin C, Voigt JU, Willems R, Heidbuchel H, La Gerche A. Right ventricular strain rate during exercise accurately identifies male athletes with right ventricular arrhythmias. Eur Heart J Cardiovasc Imaging. 2020;21:282–90.

22. Reeves JT, Groves BM, Cymerman A, Sutton JR, Wagner PD, Turkevich D, Houston CS. Operation Everest II: cardiac filling pressures during cycle exercise at sea level. Respir Physiol. 1990;80:147–54.

23. Jurcut R, Giusca S, La Gerche A, Vasile S, Ginghina C, Voigt JU. The echocardiographic assessment of the right ventricle: what to do in 2010? Eur J Echocardiogr. 2010;11:81–96.

24. Damiano RJ Jr, La Follette P Jr, Cox JL, Lowe JE, Santamore WP. Significant left ventricular contribu-

tion to right ventricular systolic function. Am J Phys. 1991;261:H1514–24.

25. Hoffman D, Sisto D, Frater RW, Nikolic SD. Left-to-right ventricular interaction with a noncontracting right ventricle. J Thorac Cardiovasc Surg. 1994;107:1496–502.

26. Gewillig M, Brown SC, Eyskens B, Heying R, Ganame J, Budts W, La Gerche A, Gorenflo M. The Fontan circulation: who controls cardiac output? Interact Cardiovasc Thorac Surg. 2010;10:428–33.

27. La Gerche A, Gewillig M. What limits cardiac performance during exercise in normal subjects and in healthy Fontan patients? Int J Pediatr. 2010;2010:791291.

28. West JB, Watson RR, Fu Z. Major differences in the pulmonary circulation between birds and mammals. Respir Physiol Neurobiol. 2007;157:382–90.

29. Lankhaar JW, Westerhof N, Faes TJ, Gan CT, Marques KM, Boonstra A, van den Berg FG, Postmus PE, Vonk-Noordegraaf A. Pulmonary vascular resistance and compliance stay inversely related during treatment of pulmonary hypertension. Eur Heart J. 2008;29:1688–95.

30. Slife DM, Latham RD, Sipkema P, Westerhof N. Pulmonary arterial compliance at rest and exercise in normal humans. Am J Phys. 1990;258:H1823–8.

31. Tedford RJ, Hassoun PM, Mathai SC, Girgis RE, Russell SD, Thiemann DR, Cingolani OH, Mudd JO, Borlaug BA, Redfield MM, Lederer DJ, Kass DA. Pulmonary capillary wedge pressure augments right ventricular pulsatile loading. Circulation. 2012;125:289–97.

32. Borlaug BA, Nishimura RA, Sorajja P, Lam CS, Redfield MM. Exercise hemodynamics enhance diagnosis of early heart failure with preserved ejection fraction. Circ Heart Fail. 2010;3:588–95.

33. Nonogi H, Hess OM, Ritter M, Krayenbuehl HP. Diastolic properties of the normal left ventricle during supine exercise. Br Heart J. 1988;60:30–8.

34. La Gerche A, Claessen G, Van de Bruaene A, Pattyn N, Van Cleemput J, Gewillig M, Bogaert J, Dymarkowski S, Claus P, Heidbuchel H. Cardiac MRI: a new gold standard for ventricular volume quantification during high-intensity exercise. Circ Cardiovasc Imaging. 2013;6:329–38.

35. Levine BD. VO2max: what do we know, and what do we still need to know? J Physiol. 2008;586:25–34.

36. Esfandiari S, Wolsk E, Granton D, Azevedo L, Valle FH, Gustafsson F, Mak S. Pulmonary artery wedge pressure at rest and during exercise in healthy adults: a systematic review and meta-analysis. J Card Fail. 2019;25(2):114–22.

37. Pandey A, Kraus WE, Brubaker PH, Kitzman DW. Healthy aging and cardiovascular function: invasive hemodynamics during rest and exercise in 104 healthy volunteers. JACC Heart Fail. 2020;8:111–21.

38. Dawson CA. Role of pulmonary vasomotion in physiology of the lung. Physiol Rev. 1984;64:544–616.

39. Lewis GD, Bossone E, Naeije R, Grunig E, Saggar R, Lancellotti P, Ghio S, Varga J, Rajagopalan S, Oudiz

R, Rubenfire M. Pulmonary vascular hemodynamic response to exercise in cardiopulmonary diseases. Circulation. 2013;128:1470–9.

40. McLaughlin VV, Langer A, Tan M, Clements PJ, Oudiz RJ, Tapson VF, Channick RN, Rubin LJ, Pulmonary Arterial Hypertension-Quality Enhancement Research Investigators. Contemporary trends in the diagnosis and management of pulmonary arterial hypertension: an initiative to close the care gap. Chest. 2013;143:324–32.

41. Jacobs KA, Kressler J, Stoutenberg M, Roos BA, Friedlander AL. Sildenafil has little influence on cardiovascular hemodynamics or 6-km time trial performance in trained men and women at simulated high altitude. High Alt Med Biol. 2011;12:215–22.

42. La Gerche A, Heidbuchel H, Burns AT, Mooney DJ, Taylor AJ, Pfluger HB, Inder WJ, Macisaac AI, Prior DL. Disproportionate exercise load and remodeling of the athlete's right ventricle. Med Sci Sports Exerc. 2011;43:974–81.

43. La Gerche A, MacIsaac AI, Burns AT, Mooney DJ, Inder WJ, Voigt JU, Heidbuchel H, Prior DL. Pulmonary transit of agitated contrast is associated with enhanced pulmonary vascular reserve and right ventricular function during exercise. J Appl Physiol. 2010;109:1307–17.

44. Bidart CM, Abbas AE, Parish JM, Chaliki HP, Moreno CA, Lester SJ. The noninvasive evaluation of exercise-induced changes in pulmonary artery pressure and pulmonary vascular resistance. J Am Soc Echocardiogr. 2007;20:270–5.

45. Argiento P, Chesler N, Mule M, D'Alto M, Bossone E, Unger P, Naeije R. Exercise stress echocardiography for the study of the pulmonary circulation. Eur Respir J. 2010;35:1273–8.

46. Argiento P, Vanderpool RR, Mule M, Russo MG, D'Alto M, Bossone E, Chesler NC, Naeije R. Exercise stress echocardiography of the pulmonary circulation: limits of normal and sex differences. Chest. 2012;142:1158–65.

47. Kovacs G, Berghold A, Scheidl S, Olschewski H. Pulmonary arterial pressure during rest and exercise in healthy subjects: a systematic review. Eur Respir J. 2009;34:888–94.

48. Oliveira RK, Waxman AB, Agarwal M, Badr Eslam R, Systrom DM. Pulmonary haemodynamics during recovery from maximum incremental cycling exercise. Eur Respir J. 2016;48:158–67.

49. Esfandiari S, Wright SP, Goodman JM, Sasson Z, Mak S. Pulmonary artery wedge pressure relative to exercise work rate in older men and women. Med Sci Sports Exerc. 2017;49:1297–304.

50. Wright SP, Esfandiari S, Gray T, Fuchs FC, Chelvanathan A, Chan W, Sasson Z, Granton JT, Goodman JM, Mak S. The pulmonary artery wedge pressure response to sustained exercise is time-variant in healthy adults. Heart. 2016;102:438–43.

51. Wright SP, Opotowsky AR, Buchan TA, Esfandiari S, Granton JT, Goodman JM, Mak S. Flow-related right ventricular to pulmonary arterial pressure gradients during exercise. Cardiovasc Res. 2019;115:222–9.

52. van Riel A, Systrom DM, Oliveira RKF, Landzberg MJ, Mulder BJM, Bouma BJ, Maron BA, Shah AM, Waxman AB, Opotowsky AR. Hemodynamic and metabolic characteristics associated with development of a right ventricular outflow tract pressure gradient during upright exercise. PLoS One. 2017;12:e0179053.

53. Claessen G, La Gerche A, Voigt JU, Dymarkowski S, Schnell F, Petit T, Willems R, Claus P, Delcroix M, Heidbuchel H. Accuracy of echocardiography to evaluate pulmonary vascular and RV function during exercise. JACC Cardiovasc Imaging. 2016;9:532–43.

54. Buechel EV, Kaiser T, Jackson C, Schmitz A, Kellenberger CJ. Normal right and left ventricular volumes and myocardial mass in children measured by steady state free precession cardiovascular magnetic resonance. J Cardiovasc Magn Reson. 2009;11:19.

55. Faber MJ, Dalinghaus M, Lankhuizen IM, Steendijk P, Hop WC, Schoemaker RG, Duncker DJ, Lamers JM, Helbing WA. Right and left ventricular function after chronic pulmonary artery banding in rats assessed with biventricular pressure-volume loops. Am J Physiol Heart Circ Physiol. 2006;291:H1580–6.

56. Chin KM, Kim NH, Rubin LJ. The right ventricle in pulmonary hypertension. Coron Artery Dis. 2005;16:13–8.

57. MacNee W. Pathophysiology of cor pulmonale in chronic obstructive pulmonary disease. Part One. Am J Respir Crit Care Med. 1994;150:833–52.

58. Stanek V, Jebavy P, Hurych J, Widimsky J. Central haemodynamics during supine exercise and pulmonary artery occlusion in normal subjects. Bull Physiopathol Respir (Nancy). 1973;9:1203–17.

59. Gurtner HP, Walser P, Fassler B. Normal values for pulmonary haemodynamics at rest and during exercise in man. Prog Respir Res. 1975;9:1203–17.

60. Stanek V, Widimsky J, Degre S, Denolin H. The lesser circulation during exercise in healthy subjects. Prog Respir Res. 1975;9:295–315.

61. Morrison D, Sorensen S, Caldwell J, Wright AL, Ritchie J, Kennedy JW, Hamilton G. The normal right ventricular response to supine exercise. Chest. 1982;82:686–91.

62. Hirata N, Shimazaki Y, Sakakibara T, Watanabe S, Nomura F, Akamatsu H, Sasaki J, Nakano S, Matsuda H. Response of right ventricular systolic function to exercise stress: effects of pulmonary vascular resistance on right ventricular systolic function. Ann Nucl Med. 1994;8:125–31.

63. Yang HS, Mookadam F, Warsame TA, Khandheria BK, Tajik JA, Chandrasekaran K. Evaluation of right ventricular global and regional function during stress echocardiography using novel velocity vector imaging. Eur J Echocardiogr. 2010;11:157–64.

64. Lurz P, Muthurangu V, Schievano S, Nordmeyer J, Bonhoeffer P, Taylor AM, Hansen MS. Feasibility

and reproducibility of biventricular volumetric assessment of cardiac function during exercise using real-time radial k-t SENSE magnetic resonance imaging. J Magn Reson Imaging. 2009;29:1062–70.

65. Merlocco A, Olivieri L, Kellman P, Xue H, Cross R. Improved workflow for quantification of right ventricular volumes using free-breathing motion corrected cine imaging. Pediatr Cardiol. 2019;40:79–88.

66. Lewis GD, Shah RV, Pappagianopolas PP, Systrom DM, Semigran MJ. Determinants of ventilatory efficiency in heart failure: the role of right ventricular performance and pulmonary vascular tone. Circ Heart Fail. 2008;1:227–33.

67. Claeys M, Claessen G, La Gerche A, Petit T, Belge C, Meyns B, Bogaert J, Willems R, Claus P, Delcroix M. Impaired cardiac reserve and abnormal vascular load limit exercise capacity in chronic thromboembolic disease. JACC Cardiovasc Imaging. 2019;12:1444–56.

68. La Gerche A, Claessen G, Dymarkowski S, Voigt JU, De Buck F, Vanhees L, Droogne W, Van Cleemput J, Claus P, Heidbuchel H. Exercise-induced right ventricular dysfunction is associated with ventricular arrhythmias in endurance athletes. Eur Heart J. 2015;36:1998–2010.

69. Claessen G, Claus P, Delcroix M, Bogaert J, La Gerche A, Heidbuchel H. Interaction between respiration and right versus left ventricular volumes at rest and during exercise: a real-time cardiac magnetic resonance study. Am J Physiol Heart Circ Physiol. 2014;306:H816–24.

70. Neilan TG, Januzzi JL, Lee-Lewandrowski E, Ton-Nu TT, Yoerger DM, Jassal DS, Lewandrowski KB, Siegel AJ, Marshall JE, Douglas PS, Lawlor D, Picard MH, Wood MJ. Myocardial injury and ventricular dysfunction related to training levels among nonelite participants in the Boston marathon. Circulation. 2006;114:2325–33.

71. Mousavi N, Czarnecki A, Kumar K, Fallah-Rad N, Lytwyn M, Han SY, Francis A, Walker JR, Kirkpatrick ID, Neilan TG, Sharma S, Jassal DS. Relation of biomarkers and cardiac magnetic resonance imaging after marathon running. Am J Cardiol. 2009;103:1467–72.

72. Trivax JE, Franklin BA, Goldstein JA, Chinnaiyan KM, Gallagher MJ, de Jong AT, Colar JM, Haines DE, McCullough PA. Acute cardiac effects of marathon running. J Appl Physiol. 2010;108:1148–53.

73. Oxborough D, Shave R, Warburton D, Williams K, Oxborough A, Charlesworth S, Foulds H, Hoffman MD, Birch K, George K. Dilatation and dysfunction of the right ventricle immediately after ultraendurance exercise: exploratory insights from conventional two-dimensional and speckle tracking echocardiography. Circ Cardiovasc Imaging. 2011;4:253–63.

74. La Gerche A, Burns AT, Mooney DJ, Inder WJ, Taylor AJ, Bogaert J, Macisaac AI, Heidbuchel H, Prior DL. Exercise-induced right ventricular dysfunction and structural remodelling in endurance athletes. Eur Heart J. 2012;33:998–1006.

75. La Gerche A, Connelly KA, Mooney DJ, MacIsaac AI, Prior DL. Biochemical and functional abnormalities of left and right ventricular function after ultra-endurance exercise. Heart. 2008;94:860–6.

76. La Gerche A, Claessen G. Is exercise good for the right ventricle? Concepts for health and disease. Can J Cardiol. 2015;31:502–8.

77. D'Andrea A, La Gerche A, Golia E, Teske AJ, Bossone E, Russo MG, Calabro R, Baggish AL. Right heart structural and functional remodeling in athletes. Echocardiography. 2015;32(Suppl 1):S11–22.

78. Teske AJ, Prakken NH, De Boeck BW, Velthuis BK, Martens EP, Doevendans PA, Cramer MJ. Echocardiographic tissue deformation imaging of right ventricular systolic function in endurance athletes. Eur Heart J. 2009;30:969–77.

79. La Gerche A. Exercise-induced arrhythmogenic (right ventricular) cardiomyopathy is real…if you consider it. JACC Cardiovasc Imaging. 2021;14:159–61.

80. Rozenbaum Z, Ben-Gal Y, Kapusta L, Hochstadt A, Sadeh Md B, Aviram Md G, Havakuk Md O, Shimiaie Md J, Ghermezi Md M, Laufer-Perl Md M, Shacham Md Y, Keren G, Topilsky Y. Combined echocardiographic and cardiopulmonary exercise to assess determinants of exercise limitation in chronic obstructive pulmonary disease. J Am Soc Echocardiogr. 2021;34:146–55. e5

81. Oliveira RKF, Waxman AB, Hoover PJ, Dellaripa PF, Systrom DM. Pulmonary vascular and right ventricular burden during exercise in interstitial lung disease. Chest. 2020;158:350–8.

82. Claessen G, La Gerche A, Petit T, Gillijns H, Bogaert J, Claeys M, Dymarkowski S, Claus P, Delcroix M, Heidbuchel H. Right ventricular and pulmonary vascular reserve in asymptomatic BMPR2 mutation carriers. J Heart Lung Transplant. 2017;36:148–56.

83. Claessen G, La Gerche A, Wielandts JY, Bogaert J, Van Cleemput J, Wuyts W, Claus P, Delcroix M, Heidbuchel H. Exercise pathophysiology and sildenafil effects in chronic thromboembolic pulmonary hypertension. Heart. 2015;101:637–44.

84. Claessen G, La Gerche A, Dymarkowski S, Claus P, Delcroix M, Heidbuchel H. Pulmonary vascular and right ventricular reserve in patients with normalized resting hemodynamics after pulmonary endarterectomy. J Am Heart Assoc. 2015;4:e001602.

85. Plehn G, Vormbrock J, Perings S, Plehn A, Meissner A, Butz T, Trappe HJ. Comparison of right ventricular functional response to exercise in hypertrophic versus idiopathic dilated cardiomyopathy. Am J Cardiol. 2010;105:116–21.

86. Guazzi M, Cahalin LP, Arena R. Cardiopulmonary exercise testing as a diagnostic tool for the detection of left-sided pulmonary hypertension in heart failure. J Card Fail. 2013;19:461–7.

87. Guazzi M, Myers J, Peberdy MA, Bensimhon D, Chase P, Arena R. Ventilatory efficiency and dyspnea on exertion improvements are related to reduced pulmonary pressure in heart failure patients receiving Sildenafil. Int J Cardiol. 2010;144:410–2.

88. Gorter TM, Obokata M, Reddy YNV, Melenovsky V, Borlaug BA. Exercise unmasks distinct pathophysiologic features in heart failure with preserved ejection fraction and pulmonary vascular disease. Eur Heart J. 2018;39:2825–35.

89. Huang CY, Lee JK, Chen ZW, Cheng JF, Chen SY, Lin LY, Wu CK. Inhaled prostacyclin on exercise echocardiographic cardiac function in preserved ejection fraction heart failure. Med Sci Sports Exerc. 2020;52:269–77.

90. Redfield MM, Chen HH, Borlaug BA, Semigran MJ, Lee KL, Lewis G, LeWinter MM, Rouleau JL, Bull DA, Mann DL, Deswal A, Stevenson LW, Givertz MM, Ofili EO, O'Connor CM, Felker GM, Goldsmith SR, Bart BA, McNulty SE, Ibarra JC, Lin G, Oh JK, Patel MR, Kim RJ, Tracy RP, Velazquez EJ, Anstrom KJ, Hernandez AF, Mascette AM, Braunwald E, Trial RELAX. Effect of phosphodiesterase-5 inhibition on exercise capacity and clinical status in heart failure with preserved ejection fraction: a randomized clinical trial. JAMA. 2013;309:1268–77.

91. Udelson JE, Lewis GD, Shah SJ, Zile MR, Redfield MM, Burnett J Jr, Parker J, Seferovic JP, Wilson P, Mittleman RS, Profy AT, Konstam MA. Effect of praliciguat on peak rate of oxygen consumption in patients with heart failure with preserved ejection fraction: the CAPACITY HFpEF randomized clinical trial. JAMA. 2020;324:1522–31.

92. Kusunose K, Popovic ZB, Motoki H, Marwick TH. Prognostic significance of exercise-induced right ventricular dysfunction in asymptomatic degenera-tive mitral regurgitation. Circ Cardiovasc Imaging. 2013;6:167–76.

93. Helsen F, Claus P, Van De Bruaene A, Claessen G, La Gerche A, De Meester P, Claeys M, Gabriels C, Petit T, Santens B, Troost E, Voigt JU, Bogaert J, Budts W. Advanced imaging to phenotype patients with a systemic right ventricle. J Am Heart Assoc. 2018;7:e009185.

94. Vachiery JL, Gaine S. Challenges in the diagnosis and treatment of pulmonary arterial hypertension. Eur Respir Rev. 2012;21:313–20.

95. Ghofrani HA, Reichenberger F, Kohstall MG, Mrosek EH, Seeger T, Olschewski H, Seeger W, Grimminger F. Sildenafil increased exercise capacity during hypoxia at low altitudes and at Mount Everest base camp: a randomized, double-blind, placebo-controlled crossover trial. Ann Intern Med. 2004;141:169–77.

96. Faoro V, Boldingh S, Moreels M, Martinez S, Lamotte M, Unger P, Brimioulle S, Huez S, Naeije R. Bosentan decreases pulmonary vascular resistance and improves exercise capacity in acute hypoxia. Chest. 2009;135:1215–22.

97. Hsu AR, Barnholt KE, Grundmann NK, Lin JH, McCallum SW, Friedlander AL. Sildenafil improves cardiac output and exercise performance during acute hypoxia, but not normoxia. J Appl Physiol. 2006;100:2031–40.

98. Guidetti L, Emerenziani GP, Gallotta MC, Pigozzi F, Di Luigi L, Baldari C. Effect of tadalafil on anaerobic performance indices in healthy athletes. Br J Sports Med. 2008;42:130–3.

Echocardiography of the Right Heart

Bouchra Lamia and Timothee Lambert

Introduction

Echocardiography of the pulmonary circulation and the right heart is essential for the screening, differential diagnosis, and follow-up of pulmonary hypertension [1–3]. However, the screening of pulmonary hypertension using transthoracic echocardiography (TTE) is not limited to the estimation of pulmonary vascular pressures or resistances only as it has been shown that echo Doppler technic may be insufficiently accurate [4–6]. Instead the addition of different parameters of RV structure and function increases the probability of PH diagnosis. This is now being improved with better Bayesian integration of measurements in a clinical probability context [7] and understanding that measurements by adequately trained examiners and updated equipment may fail on precision rather than on accuracy [8]. Echocardiographic measurements of the pulmonary circulation at rest and at exercise have recently contributed to a better functional understanding and definition of the limits of normal of the pulmonary circulation [9]. Echocardiographic indices of right ventricular (RV) systolic and diastolic function that are of diagnostic and prognostic relevance are being developed [10, 11]. The advent of portable devices is improving the bedside diagnosis and follow-up of pulmonary hypertension and RV failure.

This chapter focuses on the functional significance of the current echocardiographic imaging of the right heart of patients with pulmonary hypertension, which is by far the most common cause of RV failure. Technical issues have been extensively reviewed in recent guidelines [10, 12].

B. Lamia (✉)
Pulmonary Department, Groupe Hospitalier du Havre, Montivilliers, France

Rouen University Hospital, Normandie University, UNIROUEN, EA3830-GRHV, Rouen, France

Institute for Research and Innovation in Biomedicine (IRIB), Rouen, France
e-mail: bouchra.lamia@chu-rouen.fr

T. Lambert
Department of Pulmonology, Alpes Leman Hospital, Contamine sur Arve, France
e-mail: tlambert@ch-alpes-leman.fr

Measurement of the Pulmonary Pressures and Cardiac Output

Pulmonary hypertension is the most common cause of RV failure. Therefore, in the presence of a patient with signs and symptoms of RV failure, it is essential to evaluate the pulmonary circulation. The definition of pulmonary hypertension relies on the recording of a mean pulmonary artery pressure (PAP) higher than 20 mmHg [1–3].

© The Author(s), under exclusive license to Springer Nature Switzerland AG 2021
S. P. Gaine et al. (eds.), *The Right Heart*, https://doi.org/10.1007/978-3-030-78255-9_7

Mean PAP (PAMP) increases with any pulmonary vascular disease causing an increased resistance (PVR) to pulmonary blood flow (CO) but also with increased left atrial pressure (LAP):

$$PVR = (PAMP - LAP)/CO$$

$$PAMP = PVR \times CO + LAP$$

Therefore, the diagnosis and estimation of the severity of pulmonary hypertension require three measurements: PAP, CO, and LAP.

Systolic PAP (PASP) can be estimated from the continuous Doppler maximum velocity of tricuspid regurgitation (TRV), in m/s, to calculate a trans-tricuspid pressure gradient, in mmHg using the simplified form of the Bernoulli equation and an estimate of right atrial pressure (RAP) [13]:

$$PASP = 4 \times TRV^2 + RAP, mmHg$$

The assumptions of this measurement are that PASP and RV peak systolic pressures are equal, and that the Bernoulli equation is applicable [14]. RAP is estimated clinically, or preferably from the diameter of the inferior vena cava and its inspiratory collapsibility [15] (Fig. 7.1).

PAMP can be calculated from PASP [16]:

$$PAMP = 0.6 \times PASP + 2mmHg$$

A limitation to estimates of PAP from TRV is that a good-quality signal cannot always be recovered, especially in the presence of hyperinflated chests and/or normal or only modestly elevated PAP [17]. However, the single use of TRV has disclosed a higher-than-normal frequency of increased pulmonary vaso-reactivity in family members of patients with pulmonary arterial hypertension (PAH), independently of identified mutations [18]. The single use of TRV to estimate exercise-induced pulmonary hypertension has been shown to be of prognostic relevance in patients with aortic or mitral valvulopathies [19, 20].

Since PAP is a flow-dependent variable, it is important to couple it with a measurement of cardiac output (CO). This can be measured from the left ventricular outflow tract (LVOT) diameter and velocity time integral (VTI) multiplied by heart rate (HR) [21]:

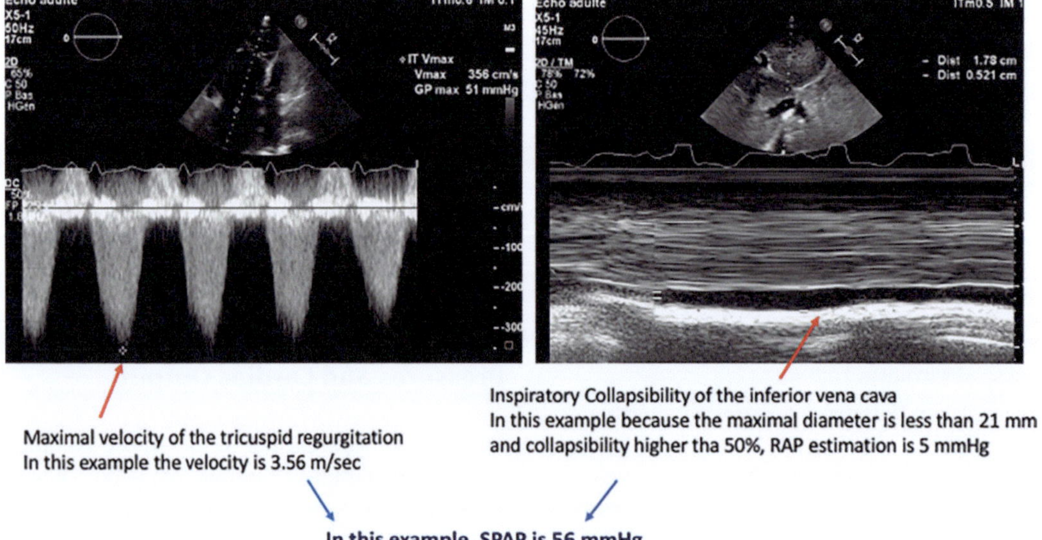

Fig. 7.1 Apical four-chamber view and continuous Doppler analysis: measurement of the maximal velocity of TR, subcostal view, and M mode: measurement of IVC inspiratory and expiratory diameters

$$CO = [0.785 \times (LVOT\ diameter)^2 \times LVOT - VTI] \times HR$$

It is also possible to record a pulmonary flow velocity sampled in the RV outflow tract (RVOT) [22]:

$$PVR = 0.1618 \times 10 \times VTI_{RVOT} / TRV$$

For the direct calculation of PVR, it is also necessary to know LAP. This can be calculated from the ratio of trans-mitral Doppler and mitral tissue Doppler E and e′ waves [23]:

$$LAP = (1.24 \times E / e') + 1$$

The echocardiographic PVR calculated from measurements of PAMP, LAP, and CO has been recently shown to be more accurate than that based on the VTI_{RVOT}/TRV ratio [24].

The simplified form of the Bernoulli equation has also been applied to pulmonary insufficiency jets to calculate mean and diastolic PAP [10].

Perhaps a more useful independent method to estimate mean PAP is based on the pulsed Doppler measurement of the acceleration time (AT) of pulmonary flow (sampled at the RVOT) [25]:

$$PAMP = 79 - (0.6 \times AT)$$

There has been less validation of PAMP calculated from the AT against invasive measurements than reported on the basis of TRV. Accurate estimates of PAMP are less reliable when AT exceeds 100 ms, the lower limit of normal, and the measurement may need a correction for ejection time at high heart rates [14]. However, there are data suggesting that AT may be more sensitive than TRV to early or latent pulmonary vasculopathy [26]. This may be due to its sensitivity to changes in pulmonary vascular impedance more than PVR [14, 17]. The advantage of the measurement of PAP on the basis of the shape of pulmonary flow is in a quasi-100% recovery of good-quality signals [17], independently on the level of PAP. In addition to AT, the shape of the flow wave is of interest, as pulmonary hypertension is associated with a deceleration of flow in late or in mid-systole (notching) [17]. A decreased time to notching has been reported to identify proximal obstruction in patients with chronic thromboembolic pulmonary hypertension (CTEPH) [27]. Notching is explained by wave reflection [28]. The impact of the first reflected wave on the forward wave may be caused either by a proximal reflection site, such as in CTEPH, or by increased wave velocity on severe pulmonary arterial stiffening caused by high PAP, such as in advanced PAH [28]. The presence of mid-systolic notching indicates a high likelihood of a PVR >5 Wood units and associated RV dysfunction [29]. An acceleration time <90 ms has been shown to be highly predictive of a PVR ≥3 WU [30].

Accuracy of Echocardiographic Measurements of the Pulmonary Circulation

Previous validation studies of Doppler echocardiographic measurements of pulmonary vascular pressures and flows have much relied on correlation calculations [4–6, 13, 21–25]. This is misleading, as correlation coefficients largely reflect the variability of the subjects being measured. If one measurement is always twice as big as the other, they are highly correlated but do not agree. Bland and Altman addressed this problem by designing difference versus average plots. This analysis has since become the gold standard to compare methods of measurements [31]. Two crucial information are provided: (1) the bias, or the difference between the means and whether it is constant over the range of measurements, and (2) the limits of agreement, or the range of possible errors. Bias informs about accuracy, and agreement informs about precision.

Two previous studies which concluded that echocardiography was insufficiently accurate when compared to catheterization for the assessment of pulmonary hypertension [4, 5] reported Bland and Altman plots showing almost no bias, and thus actually good accuracy, but large limits of agreement, rather indicating insufficient precision. More recently, D'Alto et al. compared PAP,

LAP, and CO measured by echocardiography and right-heart catheterization performed within an hour in 151 patients referred for a pulmonary hypertension [8]. The results showed nearly identical means and almost no bias, confirming the accuracy of echocardiographic measurements compared to invasive measurements. However, the limits of agreement appeared to be wide, indicating potentially insufficient precision. This may be a problem for single-number-derived decision in relation to guidelines [1, 2].

Agreed statistics are straightforward when one of the two methods of measurement is a recognized reference, or "gold standard." There is currently a consensus that right-heart catheterization provides gold standard measurements of the pulmonary circulation [1, 2].

In summary, echocardiography at rest provides accurate measurements of the pulmonary circulation, and is therefore suitable for population studies. Insufficient precision may be a problem for individual decision-making based on single numbers, such as a PAMP >20 mmHg to diagnose PH or a PAWP >15 mmHg to diagnose left-heart failure [1–3]. It may then be necessary to take the clinical context into account, and to use repetition of measurements and internal controls.

RV Systolic Function and RV-Arterial Coupling

The gold standard measurement of contractility in an intact being is maximal elastance (Emax), or the maximum value of the ratio between ventricular pressure and volume during the cardiac cycle [32–34]. Left ventricular (LV) Emax coincides with end systole, and is thus equal to the ratio between end-systolic pressure (ESP) and end-systolic volume (ESV). End-systolic elastance (Ees) of the LV is measured at the upper left corner of a square-shape pressure-volume loop [35]. Because of low pulmonary vascular impedance, the normal RV pressure-volume loop has a triangular shape and Emax occurs before the end of ejection, or end systole [36]. However, a satisfactory definition of RV Emax can be obtained by the generation of a family of pressure-volume loops at decreasing venous return [36]. Instantaneous measurements of RV volumes are difficult at the bedside, and so are manipulations of venous return. This is why single-beat methods have been developed, initially for the left ventricle [37] and then for the RV [38]. The single-beat method relies on a maximum pressure Pmax calculation from a nonlinear extrapolation of the early and late portions of a RV pressure curve, an integration of pulmonary flow, and synchronization of the signals. Emax is estimated from the slope of a tangent from Pmax to the pressure-volume curve (Fig. 7.2).

It is important to note that this graphic analysis uses relative changes in volume without assumption on absolute volumes. This is acceptable because Emax is essentially preload or end-diastolic volume (EDV) independent [34]. As contractility is homeometrically adjusted to afterload [32–34], its adequacy is best evaluated as a ratio of Emax to Ea, which defines RV-arterial coupling. The optimal mechanical coupling of Emax to Ea is equal to 1. The optimal energy transfer from the RV to the pulmonary circulation is measured at Emax/Ea ratios of 1.5–2. Patients with PAH and no clinical symptomatology of heart failure may present with a severalfold increase in Emax matching increased Ea, so that RV-arterial coupling is relatively maintained or only slightly decreased [39, 40].

There is current interest in the ratio of TAPSE (Ees surrogate) to sPAP (Ea surrogate) for the assessment of RV-PA coupling. Both are easily measured during a standard 2D Doppler echocardiography. The TAPSE/sPAP ratio has been validated against invasive measurements of the Ees/Ea ratio [41, 42] and shown to be of prognostic relevance in heart failure [41, 43], in PAH [44], in PH on chronic lung diseases [45], and even in COVID-19-induced ARDS [46].

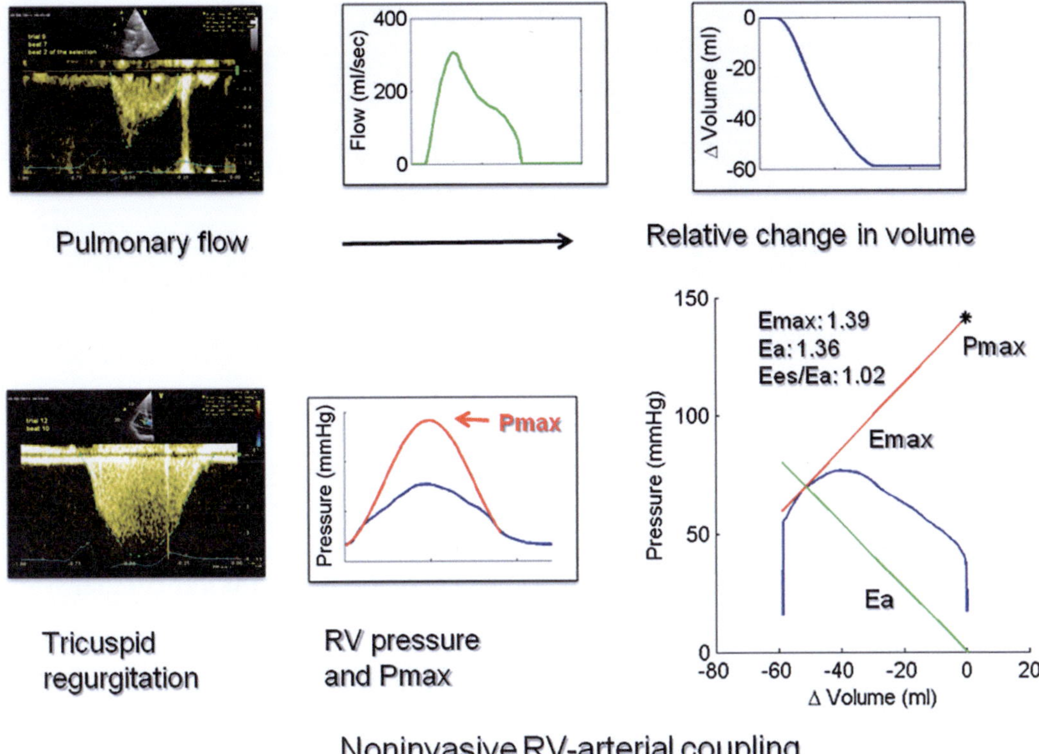

Fig. 7.2 Single-beat method applied to echocardiographic measurements of pulmonary flow and tricuspid regurgitation (TR) for the calculation of right ventricular (RV) maximum elastance (Ees) and arterial elastance (Ea) in a patient with pulmonary hypertension. A RV pressure curve is synthetized from the envelope of the TR wave. A relative change in RV volume is derived from the integration of the pulmonary flow wave

Echocardiographic Indices of RV Systolic Function

Right ventricular systolic function is usually estimated at echocardiography by the fractional area change (FAC) measured in the four-chamber view, tricuspid annual plane systolic excursion (TAPSE), tissue Doppler imaging (TDI) of the tricuspid annulus systolic velocity S wave and isovolumic contraction maximum velocity (IVV), right ventricular index of myocardial performance (defined by the ratio: isovolumic contraction time + isovolume relaxation time/ ejection time) strain or strain rate measurements, and even SV calculated from aortic flow-derived cardiac output divided by heart rate [9].

RVFAC is determined from the planimetric areas of the RV end systole and end diastole from the apical four-chamber view. RVFAC does not require geometric assumptions and correlates with RVEF, but incomplete visualization of RV cavity and suboptimal endocardial definition are causes of high inter- and intra-observer variability [9]. RVFAC was recently shown in one study to be of prognostic relevance in patients with idiopathic PAH [47].

Because of the predominantly longitudinal contraction pattern of the RV, a more suitable measure of systolic function is TAPSE, which can be derived from 2D and M-mode echocardiography, is easy to perform, and is highly reproducible. A decreased TAPSE has been shown to be associated with a decreased survival in patients with left-heart failure [47, 48] and with PH [47, 49].

A TDI measurement of the longitudinal velocity of RV contraction measured at the tricuspid

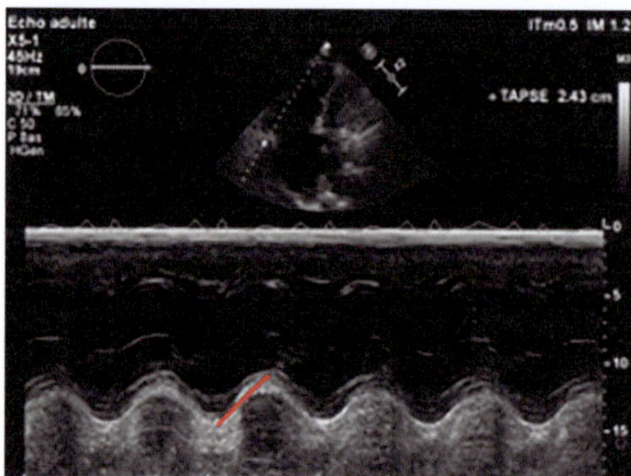
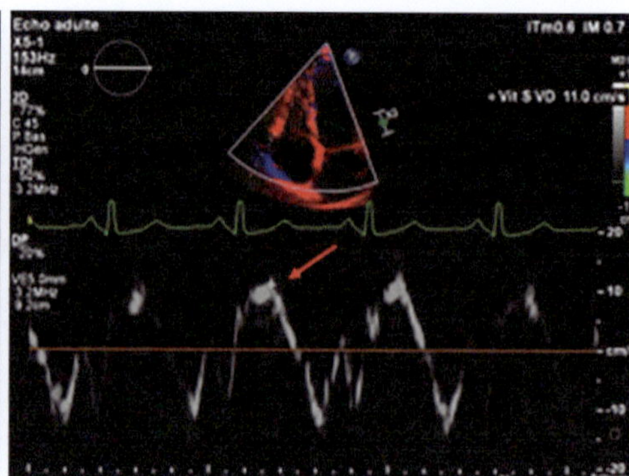

Tricuspid Annular Plane Systolic Excursion (TAPSE)
In this example TAPSE is 24.3 mm

Tissue Dopple Tricuspid Velocity, S Wave
In this example S Wave is 11 cm/sec.

Fig. 7.3 Parameters of RV systolic function: TAPSE, TDI S wave

annulus, or S wave, correlates with TAPSE and RVFAC [50, 51] and offers an additional internal control measure of systolic function.

The problem of RVFAC, TAPSE, and S wave is preload dependency. This may be less of a problem for isovolumic phase indices such as IVV [52]. IVV was recently reported to be a good predictor of survival in a series of 142 patients with PAH or CTEPH [53]. This is illustrated below (Fig. 7.3).

Strain and strain rate are also parameters of contractility. Their measurements have been shown to be closely correlated with myocardial contractility in in vitro and in vivo experimental settings, with minimal preload dependency [54]. Strain is defined as percentage change in myocardial deformation, while its derivative, strain rate, represents the rate of deformation of myocardium over time [10]. Strain and strain rate are decreased in patients with severe pulmonary hypertension [55, 56] and rapidly improve with only partial reversibility during testing with inhaled pulmonary vasodilators [57]. The addition of speckle tracking has made strain measurements less angle and operator dependent, and as such emerge as potent predictors of functional state and outcome in patients with severe pulmonary hypertension [58, 59].

RV Systolic Function Assessed by 3D Echo and 3D Right Ventricular Ejection Fraction

Because of the complexity of the RV shape and anatomy, assessment of RV volumes and thus RV ejection fraction is not possible using 2D echocardiography.

With the availability of 3D echocardiography, assessment of shape and functional changes in the right ventricle is feasible. Three-dimensional modalities allow accuracy and reproducibility in the assessment of RV shape and function. Three-dimensional echocardiography is more and more available and well validated against the gold standard MR. The most recent guideline recommends 3D echocardiography measurements of RV volumes. New generations of 3D software allow auto-segmentation and provide contour positioning and the user may still adjust images. 3D volumes are computed numerically from the dynamic surface model and used to calculate end-diastolic volume (EDV), end-systolic volume (ESV), ejection fraction (EF), and systolic volume (SV) [60–64]. As we previously discussed, RV function including RV remodeling and RV contractility plays a key role in the prognosis of pulmonary hypertension (PH) patients.

Right-heart analysis using 2D echocardiography is useful to assess RV size and surrogate of RV contractility as TAPSE. However RV ejection fraction, gold standard of systolic RV function, is missing because of RV morphology and physiology. Three-dimensional (3D) echocardiography has been recently improved to assess RV ejection fraction and volumes.

In a prospective study in our center [65], we analyzed right-heart (RH) function in PH patients using 3D echo at baseline and during follow-up. All patients prospectively underwent a right-heart catheterization (RHC), and 2D and 3D echocardiography within 1 h. We measured right-heart sizes and volumes, TAPSE, DTI S wave, RV fractional area change (FAC), global and regional longitudinal strain, and RV ejection fraction. All measurements were performed at baseline and after treatment as suggested by the guidelines. Thirty-six patients (15 women, 21 men; age 69 ± 11) were included. At baseline, mPAP was 41 ± 12 mmHg, cardiac index (CI) was 2.9 ± 0.9 L/min/m^2, pulmonary capillary wedge pressure was 11 ± 4 mmHg, right atrial pressure (RAP) was 14 ± 6 mmHg, and pulmonary vascular resistance (PVR) was 7 ± 4 WU. At baseline RVEF was decreased 40 ± 13% (normal value 58 ± 6% and abnormality threshold <45%), and RVFAC as well, 34 ± 13%, whereas TAPSE was slightly decreased and 20 ± 5% RV remodeling analysis showed dilated RV: RV/left ventricle area = 1 ± 0.6 (normal <0.6). Using univariate analysis RVEF was significantly correlated to mPAP, PVR, RV size, TAPSE (r^2 = 0.14; p = 0.0363), DTI S wave (r^2 = 0.2; p = 0.0135), and global strain (r^2 = 0.57; p = 0.0002). Using multivariate analysis RVEF was significantly correlated to TAPSE (p = 0.0243) and strain global (p = 0.0007). Ten patients (31%) had decreased RVEF while TAPSE remained normal. In patients treated with pulmonary vasodilators (n = 12) who had RHC and 2D and 3D echo analysis during follow-up RVEF increased from 32 ± 12% to 42 ± 4% while TAPSE remained stable from 20 ± 6% to 21 ± 5%. Thus in PH patients, assessment of right-heart function using 3D echocardiography was easy and reproducible. RVEF was independently correlated to TAPSE and global strain. However RVEF was altered while TAPSE remained normal and during follow-up 3D RVEF variation occurred first. 3D echo RVEF seems to be useful as an early parameter of RV systolic dysfunction and may be superior to other echo parameters of right-heart function in severe PH. This may be explained by the fact that, in spite of load dependency, EF is linked to the Ees/Ea ratio simplified for common pressure terms [66]: Ees/Ea = EF/(1 − EF).

RVEF values around 40% correspond to Ees/Ea decreased from normal values of 1.5–2 to 0.8 associated with the onset of RV dilatation [67]. A recent study reported on the negative impact on the outcome of decreased RVEF measured by MRI in spite of targeted therapy-associated decreased PVR in patients with PAH. RVEF is an independent predictor of survival in PAH [68] and correlated to risk scores [69]. Cutoff values are around 40% RVEF >54%, 37–54%, and <37% that are associated with low risk, intermediate risk, and high risk of 1-year mortality in PAH. A recent meta-analysis showed that a decrease in RVEF by 1% increases the risk of clinical deterioration by 6% at 2 years and death by 2% at 5 years (numbers rounded up) [70]. Images of 3D RV analysis and tracking are illustrated in Fig. 7.4.

RV Dimensions, Remodeling, and Diastolic Function

The heterometric adaptation of the RV inevitably results in a competition for space with the LV within the relatively non-distensible pericardium. This diastolic interaction is usually quantified by an apical four-chamber view as a ratio of RV and LV diastolic surface areas. The RV/LV ratio is normally 0.5–0.7, increasing to 0.8–1.0, 1.1–1.4, and >1.5 in mild, moderate, and severe RV dilatation [10, 12].

The dilatation of the RV compressing the LV can also be measured by an end-systolic parasternal short-axis view of a D-shape instead of circular shape of the LV, with an increased ratio of parallel to perpendicular to septum LV diameters, called eccentricity index (EI). The EI is normally

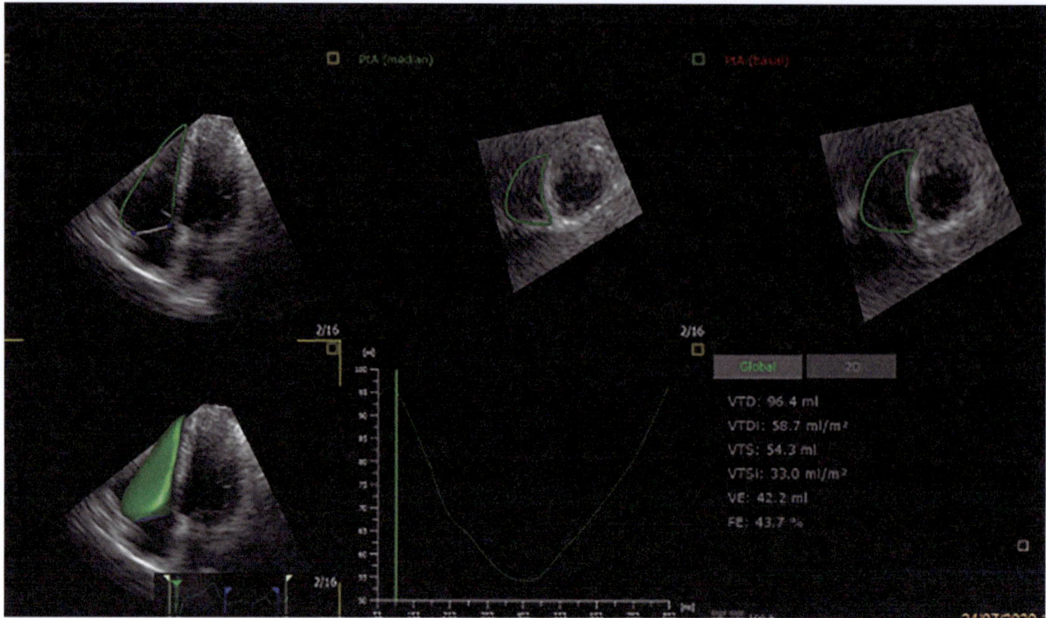

3D RV volumes : end diastolic and end systolic volumes of the RV, the RV ejection fraction is calculted. In this example RV EF is 43.7% (normal value higher than 45%).
The volume over time is also displayed in a volume-versus-time curve (at the bottom).

Fig. 7.4 3D right ventricular volumes and right ventricular ejection fraction

equal to 1, and increases to 1.1–1.4, 1.5–1.8, and >1.8 referring to mild, moderate, and severe septal bowing, respectively. However, some degree of septal flattening is invariably present in patients with pulmonary hypertension, and actually also reflects a delay in the time to peak RV contraction [71]. An increased EI enhances the prognostic impact of a given degree of RV systolic dysfunction [72].

Impaired relaxation and filling of the RV are also a consequence of altered systolic function and increased dimensions, which causes an increase in the RV isovolumic relaxation time (IVRT), with reversal of trans-tricuspid flow and tricuspid annulus velocity E and A waves. Compression of the LV by an enlarged RV alters LV diastolic compliance, with prolonged mitral E-wave deceleration, inversed E/A, and eventually an increased E/E′ indicating increased LV end-diastolic pressure (LVEDP). Altered diastolic function of the LV as a consequence of RV failure is sometimes called the "inverse Bernheim effect," after the initial report more than a century ago of altered RV function by LV failure [73].

Dilatation of the RV under pressure is inevitably associated with tricuspid insufficiency. The greatest degrees of tricuspid regurgitation are observed in dilated RV on severe PH. The combination of a marked tricuspid regurgitation and depressed TAPSE is of particularly poor prognosis in patients with severe pulmonary hypertension [47].

Right atrial enlargement is a component of right-heart failure. An increased RA area has been shown to predict decreased clinical stability and shorter survival in idiopathic PAH [74]. Whether the dilatation of the RA is more than just the mechanical consequence of RV dilatation and tricuspid insufficiency is not exactly known. Right atrial enlargement goes along with inferior vena cava dilatation and decreased inspiratory collapse.

The presence and severity of pericardial effusion are another important sign of RV failure. It is the consequence of increased central venous pressures, with increased coronary capillary filtration. It may be aggravated by coexistent inflammation in patients with PAH associated with connective tissue diseases. Pericardial effusion predicts clinical worsening and decreased survival [74].

RV Dyssynchrony

Studies using MRI imaging with myocardial tagging have shown that RV failure in patients with severe PH is characterized by prolonged systolic shortening with late peaking, and that this contributes to septal bowing, decreased LV filling, and decreased SV [71]. This interventricular asynchrony causes a typical aspect of postsystolic shortening on the TDI imaging of tricuspid annulus tissue velocity [75].

However, RV failure is also associated with regional contraction abnormalities responsible for dyssynchrony, as can be shown by speckle tracking strain measurements. This is illustrated in Fig. 7.5.

The speckle tracking analysis is used to generate regional strain from echocardiographic images [76, 77]. A region of interest is traced on the endocardial and epicardial border of the right ventricle apical four-chamber view, using a point-and-click approach. Natural acoustic markers, or speckles within the region of interest, are tracked over the cardiac cycle. The location shift of these speckles from frame to frame, which represents tissue movement, provides the spatial and temporal data. Longitudinal strain is calculated as the change in length/initial length between endocardial and epicardial trace. Accordingly, in the longitudinal view, RV myocardial shortening is represented as a negative strain and myocardial lengthening as a positive strain. The software then automatically divides the RV long-axis image into six standard segments and generates global and individual strain-time waveforms for basal septum, mid septum, apical septum, basal free wall, mid free wall, and apical free wall segments. Peak strain and time to peak strain from each of the four or six time-strain curves are

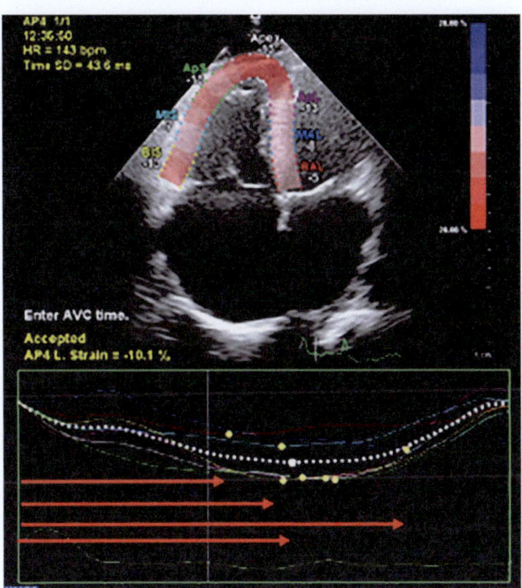

Fig. 7.5 Regional right ventricular function analyzed with speckle tracking strain of a patient with pulmonary hypertension. Global strain and individual segments are color coded: global longitudinal strain (dashed white curve); basal (yellow curve), mid (cyan curve), and apical (green curve) segments of the right ventricular septum; and basal (red curve), mid (blue curve), and apical (magenta curve) segments of the right ventricular free wall. Note that some segments shorten early and the remaining segments shorten late, similar to dyssynchrony. Hemodynamics; global, early, and late segmental contraction; and dyssynchrony are reported below each example

determined with dyssynchrony defined as the difference between earliest and latest segments as previously described [78–80]. Global longitudinal RV septal wall strain is calculated as averaged longitudinal strain from three septum segments. Global longitudinal RV free wall strain is calculated as averaged longitudinal strain from three free wall segments. Finally, global longitudinal RV strain is calculated as averaged longitudinal strain from six segments. The maximum time difference from the earliest to latest peak strain among six segments, as a measure of contraction synchrony, is increased in pulmonary hypertension patients.

Asynchrony and dyssynchrony decrease the efficiency of RV contraction, and thus depress global indices of systolic function such as FAC or TAPSE, even though this has not until now been systematically evaluated. Asynchrony also impairs LV diastolic filling. Dyssynchrony of RV contraction in advanced PAH is associated with worse functional state and decreased survival [80].

In a previous study in our center [81], we defined dyssynchrony as the R-R interval-corrected standard deviation of the times to peak systolic strain for the basal and medium segments of the RV. All the PH patients underwent a right-heart catheterization. RV dyssynchrony amounted to 69 ± 34 ms in PAH patients with mean PAP higher than 25 mmHg, 47 ± 23 ms in patients with mean PAP between 20 and 25 mmHg, and 8 ± 6 ms in controls, all different from each other ($p < 0.05$). RV dyssynchrony in patients with mean PAP between 20 and 25 mmHg was the only parameter of RV systolic dysfunction in 11 of 13 (85%) patients. RV dyssynchrony was accompanied by postsystolic shortening and correlated to RV fractional area change, not to mPAP or pulmonary vascular resistance. These results confirm that RV dyssynchrony is typical of advanced PH [80], but that it also occurs in the early stages of the disease. It has indeed also been shown that hypoxic breathing in healthy volunteers to bring mean PAP at the upper limit of normal or slightly above is already associated with a significant increase in RV dyssynchrony [82].

Conclusions

Echocardiography is essential for the diagnosis and serial assessments of RV dysfunction.

The echocardiographic approach provides accurate assessments of the pulmonary circulation and RV function. RV remodeling and RV systolic function can be analyzed with accuracy for an early diagnosis of RV dysfunction and for the follow-up. New-generation software allow sophisticated diagnosis as dyssynchrony and assessments of RV volumes to calculate RV ejection fraction. This last parameter is essential to take care of PH patients and has been for a long while available through MRI only. RV EF is now easily available using echocardiography.

Echocardiography must be understood as an extension of clinical examination.

References

1. Galiè N, Hoeper M, Humbert M, Torbicki A, Vachiéry JL, Barbera J, Beghetti M, Corris P, Gaine S, Gibbs S, Gomez-Sanchez M, Jondeau C, Klepetko W, Opitz C, Peacock A, Rubin L, Zellweger M, Simonneau G, Task force for diagnosis and treatment of pulmonary hypertension of European Society of Cardiology (ESC); European Respiratory Society (ERS); International Society of Heart and Lung Transplantation (ISHLT). Guidelines for the diagnosis and treatment of pulmonary hypertension. Eur Respir J. 2009;34:1219–63.
2. Simonneau G, Montani D, Celermajer DS, Denton CP, Gatzoulis MA, Krowka M, et al. Haemodynamic definitions and updated clinical classification of pulmonary hypertension. Eur Respir J. 2019;53(1):1801913.
3. Frost A, Badesch D, Gibbs JSR, Gopalan D, Khanna D, Manes A, et al. Diagnosis of pulmonary hypertension. Eur Respir J. 2019;53(1):1801904.
4. Fisher MR, Forfia PR, Chamera E, Housten-Harris T, Champion HC, Girgis RE, Corretti MC, Hassoun PM. Accuracy of Doppler echocardiography in the hemodynamic assessment of pulmonary hypertension. Am J Respir Crit Care Med. 2009;179:615–21.
5. Rich JD, Shah SJ, Swamy RS, Kamp A, Rich S. Inaccuracy of Doppler echocardiographic estimates of pulmonary artery pressures in patients with pulmonary hypertension. Chest. 2011;139:988–93.
6. Rich JD. Counterpoint: can Doppler echocardiography estimates of pulmonary artery systolic pressures be relied upon to accurately make the diagnosis of pulmonary hypertension? No. Chest. 2013;143:1536–9.
7. Rudski LG. Point: can Doppler echocardiography estimates of pulmonary artery systolic pressures be relied upon to accurately make the diagnosis of pulmonary hypertension? Yes. Chest. 2013;143:1533–6.
8. D'Alto M, Romeo E, Argiento P, D'Andrea A, Vanderpool R, Correra A, Bossone E, Sarubbi B, Calabrò R, Russo MG, Naeije R. Accuracy and precision of echocardiography versus right heart catheterization for the assessment of pulmonary hypertension. Int J Cardiol. 2013;168:4058–62.
9. Naeije R, Vanderpool R, Dhakal BP, Saggar R, Saggar R, Vachiery JL, Lewis GD. Exercise-induced pulmonary hypertension physiological basis and methodological concerns. Am J Respir Crit Care Med. 2013;187:576–853.
10. Rudski LG, Lai WW, Afilalo J, Hua L, Handschumacher MD, Chandrasekaran K, Solomon SD, Louie EK, Schiller NB. Guidelines for the echocardiographic assessment of the right heart in adults: a report from the American Society of Echocardiography endorsed by the European Association of Echocardiography, a registered branch of the European Society of Cardiology, and the Canadian Society of Echocardiography. J Am Soc Echocardiogr. 2010;23:685–713.

11. Bossone E, D'Andrea A, D'Alto M, Citro R, Argiento P, Ferrara F, Cittadini A, Rubenfire M, Naeije R. Echocardiography in pulmonary arterial hypertension: from diagnosis to prognosis. J Am Soc Echocardiogr. 2013;26:1–14.

12. Lang RM, Badano LP, Mor-Avi V, Afilalo J, Armstrong A, Ernande L, et al. Recommendations for cardiac chamber quantification by echocardiography in adults: an update from the American Society of Echocardiography and the European Association of Cardiovascular Imaging. Eur Heart J Cardiovasc Imaging. 2015;16(3):233–70.

13. Yock PG, Popp RL. Noninvasive estimation of right ventricular systolic pressure by Doppler ultrasound in patients with tricuspid regurgitation. Circulation. 1984;70:657–62.

14. Hatle L, Angleson B. Doppler ultrasound in cardiology: physical principles and clinical applications. 2nd ed. Philadelphia: Lea & Febiger; 1985. p. 252–63.

15. Kircher BJ, Himelman RB, Schiller NB. Noninvasive estimation of right atrial pressure from the inspiratory collapse of the inferior vena cava. Am J Cardiol. 1990;66:493–6.

16. Chemla D, Castelain V, Humbert M, Hébert JL, Simonneau G, Lecarpentier Y, Hervé P. New formula for predicting mean pulmonary artery pressure using systolic pulmonary artery pressure. Chest. 2004;126:1313–7.

17. Naeije R, Torbicki A. More on the noninvasive diagnosis of pulmonary hypertension. Doppler echocardiography revisited (editorial). Eur Respir J. 1995;8:1445–9.

18. Grünig E, Weissmann S, Ehlken N, et al. Stress-Doppler-echocardiography in relatives of patients with idiopathic and familial pulmonary arterial hypertension: results of a multicenter European analysis of pulmonary artery pressure response to exercise and hypoxia. Circulation. 2009;119:1747–57.

19. Lancellotti P, Magne J, Donal E, O'Connor K, Dulgheru R, Rosca M, Pierard LA. Determinants and prognostic significance of exercise pulmonary hypertension in asymptomatic severe aortic stenosis. Circulation. 2012;126:851–9.

20. Magne J, Lancellotti P, Piérard LA. Exercise pulmonary hypertension in asymptomatic degenerative mitral regurgitation. Circulation. 2010;122:33–41.

21. Christie J, Sheldahl LM, Tristani FE, Sagar KB, Ptacin MJ, Wann S. Determination of stroke volume and cardiac output during exercise: comparison of two-dimensional and Doppler echocardiography, Fick oximetry, and thermodilution. Circulation. 1987;76:539–47.

22. Abbas AE, Fortuin FD, Schiller NB, Appleton CP, Moreno CA, Lester SJ. A simple method for noninvasive estimation of pulmonary vascular resistance. J Am Coll Cardiol. 2003;41:1021–7.

23. Nagueh S, Middleton K, Kopelen H, Zoghbi W, Quinones M. Doppler tissue imaging: a noninvasive technique for evaluation of left ventricular relaxation and estimation of filling pressures. J Am Coll Cardiol. 1997;30:1527–33.

24. Lindqvist P, Söderberg S, Gonzalez MC, Tossavainen E, Henein MY. Echocardiography based estimation of pulmonary vascular resistance in patients with pulmonary hypertension: a simultaneous Doppler echocardiography and cardiac catheterization study. Eur J Echocardiogr. 2011;12:961–6.

25. Kitabatake A, Inoue M, Asao M, et al. Noninvasive evaluation of pulmonary hypertension by a pulsed Doppler technique. Circulation. 1983;68:302–9.

26. Huez S, Roufosse F, Vachièry JL, Pavelescu A, Derumeaux G, Wautrecht JC, Cogan E, Naeije R. Isolated right ventricular dysfunction in systemic sclerosis: latent pulmonary hypertension? Eur Respir J. 2007;30:928–36.

27. Hardziyenka M, Reesink HJ, Bouma BJ, de Bruin-Bon HA, Campian ME, Tanck MW, van den Brink RB, Kloek JJ, Tan HL, Bresser P. A novel echocardiographic predictor of in-hospital mortality and mid-term haemodynamic improvement after pulmonary endarterectomy for chronic thrombo-embolic pulmonary hypertension. Eur Heart J. 2007;28:842–9.

28. Naeije R, Huez S. Reflections on wave reflections in chronic thromboembolic pulmonary hypertension. Eur Heart J. 2007;28:785–7.

29. Arkles JS, Opotowsky AR, Ojeda J, Rogers F, Liu T, Prassana V, Marzec L, Palevsky HI, Ferrari VA, Forfia PR. Shape of the right ventricular Doppler envelope predicts hemodynamics and right heart function in pulmonary hypertension. Am J Respir Crit Care Med. 2011;183:268–76.

30. Tossavainen E, Söderberg S, Grönlund C, Gonzalez M, Henein MY, Lindqvist P. Pulmonary artery acceleration time in identifying pulmonary hypertension patients with raised pulmonary vascular resistance. Eur Heart J Cardiovasc Imaging. 2013;14:890–7.

31. Bland JM, Altman DG. Statistical methods for assessing agreement between two different methods of clinical measurement. Lancet. 1986;1:307–10.

32. Vonk-Noordegraaf A, Westerhof N. Describing right ventricular function. Eur Respir J. 2013;41:1419–23.

33. Chesler NC, Roldan A, Vanderpool RR, Naeije R. How to measure pulmonary vascular and right ventricular function. Conf Proc IEEE Eng Med Biol Soc. 2009;1:177–80.

34. Sagawa K, Maughan L, Suga H, Sunagawa K. Cardiac contraction and the pressure-volume relationship. New York: Oxford University Press; 1988.

35. Suga H, Sagawa K, Shoukas AA. Load independence of the instantaneous pressure-volume ratio of the canine left ventricle and effects of epinephrine and heart rate on the ratio. Circ Res. 1973;32:314–22.

36. Maughan WL, Shoukas AA, Sagawa K, Weisfeldt ML. Instantaneous pressure-volume relationship of the canine right ventricle. Circ Res. 1979;44:309–15.

37. Sunagawa K, Yamada A, Senda Y, Kikuchi Y, Nakamura M, Shibahara T. Estimation of the hydromotive source pressure from ejecting beats of the left ventricle. IEEE Trans Biomed Eng. 1980;57:299–305.

38. Brimioulle S, Wauthy P, Ewalenko P, Rondelet B, Vermeulen F, Kerbaul F, Naeije R. Single-beat estimation of right ventricular end-systolic pressure-volume relationship. Am J Physiol Heart Circ Physiol. 2003;284:H1625–30.

39. Kuehne T, Yilmaz S, Steendijk P, Moore P, Groenink M, Saaed M, et al. Magnetic resonance imaging analysis of right ventricular pressure-volume loops: in vivo validation and clinical application in patients with pulmonary hypertension. Circulation. 2004;110:2010–6.

40. Tedford RJ, Mudd JO, Girgis RE, Mathai SC, Zaiman AL, Housten-Harris T, et al. Right ventricular dysfunction in systemic sclerosis associated pulmonary arterial hypertension. Circ Heart Fail. 2013; 6(5):953–63.

41. Guazzi M, Dixon D, Labate V, Beussink-Nelson L, Bandera F, Cuttica MJ, Shah SJ. RV contractile function and its coupling to pulmonary circulation in heart failure with preserved ejection fraction: stratification of clinical phenotypes and outcomes. JACC Cardiovasc Imaging. 2017;10:1211–21.

42. Tello K, Wan J, Dalmer A, Vanderpool R, Ghofrani HA, Naeije R, Roller F, Mohajerani E, Seeger W, Herberg U, Sommer N, Gall H, Richter MJ. Validation of the tricuspid annular plane systolic excursion/systolic pulmonary artery pressure ratio for the assessment of right ventricular-arterial coupling in severe pulmonary hypertension. Circ Cardiovasc Imaging. 2019;12(9):e009047. https://doi.org/10.1161/CIRCIMAGING.119.00904.

43. Guazzi M, Bandera F, Pelissero G, et al. A tricuspid annular plane systolic excursion and pulmonary arterial systolic pressure relationship in heart failure: an index of right ventricular contractile function and prognosis. Am J Physiol Heart Circ Physiol. 2013;305:H1373–81.

44. Tello K, Axmann J, Ghofrani HA, Naeije R, Rieth A, Seeger W, Gall H, Richter MJ. Relevance of the TAPSE/PAPS ratio in pulmonary arterial hypertension. Int J Cardiol. 2018;266:229–3.

45. Tello K, Ghofrani HA, Heinze C, et al. A simple echocardiographic estimate of right ventricular-arterial coupling to assess severity and outcome in pulmonary hypertension on chronic lung disease. Eur Respir J. 2019;54:1802435.

46. D'Alto M, Marra AM, Severino S, Salzano A, Romeo E, De Rosa R, Stagnaro FM, Pagnano G, Verde R, Murino P, Farro A, Ciccarelli G, Vargas M, Fiorentino G, Servillo G, Gentile I, Corcione A, Cittadini A, Naeije R, Golino P. Right ventricular-arterial coupling independently predicts survival in COVID-19 ARDS. Crit Care. 2020;24(1):670.

47. Ghio S, Klersy C, Magrini G, D'Armini AM, Scelsi L, Raineri C, Pasotti M, Serio A, Campana C, Viganò M. Prognostic relevance of the echocardiographic assessment of right ventricular function in patients with idiopathic pulmonary arterial hypertension. Int J Cardiol. 2010;140:272–8.

48. Ghio S, Recusani F, Klersy C, Sebastiani R, Laudisa ML, Campana C, Gavazzi A, Tavazzi L. Prognostic usefulness of the tricuspid annular plane systolic excursion in patients with congestive heart failure secondary to idiopathic or ischemic dilated cardiomyopathy. Am J Cardiol. 2000;85:837–42.

49. Forfia PR, Fisher MR, Mathai SC, Housten-Harris T, Hemnes AR, Borlaug BA, Chamera E, Corretti MC, Champion HC, Abraham TP, Girgis RE, Hassoun PM. Tricuspid annular displacement predicts survival in pulmonary hypertension. Am J Respir Crit Care Med. 2006;174:1034–41.

50. Meluzín J, Spinarová L, Bakala J, Toman J, Krejcí J, Hude P, Kára T, Soucek M. Pulsed Doppler tissue imaging of the velocity of tricuspid annular systolic motion; a new, rapid, and non-invasive method of evaluating right ventricular systolic function. Eur Heart J. 2001;22:340–8.

51. Saxena N, Rajagopalan N, Edelman K, López-Candales A. Tricuspid annular systolic velocity: a useful measurement in determining right ventricular systolic function regardless of pulmonary artery pressures. Echocardiography. 2006;23:750–5.

52. Vogel M, Schmidt MR, Christiansen SB, et al. Validation of myocardial acceleration during isovolumic contraction as a novel non-invasive index of right ventricular contractility. Circulation. 2003;105:1693–9.

53. Ernande L, Cottin V, Leroux PY, Girerd N, Huez S, Mulliez A, Bergerot C, Ovize M, Mornex JF, Cordier JF, Naeije R, Derumeaux G. Right isovolumic contraction velocity predicts survival in pulmonary hypertension. J Am Soc Echocardiogr. 2013; 26:297–306.

54. Jamal F, Bergerot C, Argaud L, Loufouat J, Ovize M. Longitudinal strain quantitates regional right ventricular contractile function. Am J Physiol Heart Circ Physiol. 2003;285:H2842–7.

55. Dambrauskaite V, Delcroix M, Claus P, et al. Regional right ventricular dysfunction in chronic pulmonary hypertension. J Am Soc Echocardiogr. 2007;2010:1172–80.

56. Huez S, Vachiéry JL, Unger P, Brimioulle S, Naeije R. Tissue Doppler imaging evaluation of cardiac adaptation to severe pulmonary hypertension. Am J Cardiol. 2007;100:1473–8.

57. Huez S, Vachiéry JL, Naeije R. Improvement in right ventricular function during reversibility testing in pulmonary arterial hypertension: a case report. Cardiovasc Ultrasound. 2009;7:9.

58. Sachdev A, Villarraga HR, Frantz RP, McGoon MD, Hsiao JF, Maalouf JF, Ammash NM, McCully RB, Miller FA, Pellikka PA, Oh JK, Kane GC. Right ventricular strain for prediction of survival in patients with pulmonary arterial hypertension. Chest. 2011;139:1299–309.

59. Fine NM, Chen L, Bastiansen PM, Frantz RP, Pellikka PA, Oh JK, Kane GC. Outcome prediction by quantitative right ventricular function assessment in 575 subjects evaluated for pulmonary hypertension. Circ Cardiovasc Imaging. 2013;6:711–21.

60. Leary PJ, et al. Three-dimensional analysis of right ventricular shape and function in pulmonary hyper-

tension. Pulm Circ. 2012;2(1):34–40. https://doi.org/10.4103/2045-8932.94828.

61. Messner AM, Taylor GQ. Algorithm 550, solid polyhedron measures. ACM Trans Math Softw. 1980;6(1):121–30.

62. Muraru D, et al. New speckle-tracking algorithm for right ventricular volume analysis from three-dimensional echocardiographic data sets: validation with cardiac magnetic resonance and comparison with the previous analysis tool. Eur Heart J Cardiovasc Imaging. 2016;17(11):1279–89.

63. Laser KT, Karabiyik A, Korperich H, Horst JP, Barth P, Kececioglu D, Burchert W, Dalla Pozza R, Herberg U. Validation and reference values for three-dimensional echocardiographic right ventricular volumetry in children: a multicenter study. J Am Soc Echocardiogr. 2018;31(9):1050–63. https://doi.org/10.1016/j.echo.2018.03.010.

64. Medvedofsky D, et al. Novel approach to three-dimensional echocardiographic quantification of right ventricular volumes and function from focused views. J Am Soc Echocardiogr. 2015;28(10):1222–31. https://doi.org/10.1016/j.echo.2015.06.013.

65. Bouchra Lamia, Timothée Lambert, Mathilde Azzi, Fatoi Bidar, Angélique Picard, Philippe Bonnet. Right ventricular function in pulmonary hypertension: prospective 3D echocardiographic analysis of RV remodeling and contractility. American Thoracic Society Meeting, 2020.

66. Vanderpool RR, Rischard F, Naeije R, Hunter K, Simon MA. Simple functional imaging of the right ventricle in pulmonary hypertension: can right ventricular ejection fraction be improved? Int J Cardiol. 2016;223:93–4.

67. Tello K, Dalmer A, Axmann J, Vanderpool R, Ghofrani HA, Naeije R, Roller F, Seeger W, Sommer N, Wilhelm J, Gall H, Richter MJ. Reserve of right ventricular-arterial coupling in the setting of chronic overload. Circ Heart Fail. 2019;12(1):e005512.

68. Brewis MJ, Bellofiore A, Vanderpool RR, Chesler NC, Johnson MK, Naeije R, Peacock AJ. Imaging right ventricular function to predict outcome in pulmonary arterial hypertension. Int J Cardiol. 2016;218:206–11.

69. Lewis RA, Johns CS, Cogliano M, Capener D, Tubman E, Elliot CA, Charalampopoulos A, Sabroe I, Thompson AAR, Billings CG, Hamilton N, Baster K, Laud PJ, Hickey PM, Middleton J, Armstrong IJ, Hurdman JA, Lawrie A, Rothman AMK, Wild JM, Condliffe R, Swift AJ, Kiely DG. Identification of cardiac magnetic resonance imaging thresholds for risk stratification in pulmonary arterial hypertension. Am J Respir Crit Care Med. 2020;201(4):458.

70. Alabed S, Shahin Y, Garg P, Alandejani F, Johns CS, Lewis RA, Condliffe R, Wild JM, Kiely DG, Swift AJ. Cardiac-MRI predicts clinical worsening and mortality in pulmonary arterial hypertension: a systematic review and analysis. JACC Cardiovasc Imaging. 2020;14(5):931–42.

71. Marcus JT, Gan CT, Zwanenburg JJ, Boonstra A, Allaart CP, Götte MJ, Vonk-Noordegraaf A. Interventricular mechanical asynchrony in pulmonary arterial hypertension: left-to-right delay in peak shortening is related to right ventricular overload and left ventricular underfilling. J Am Coll Cardiol. 2008;51:750–7.

72. Ryan T, Petrovic O, Dillon JC, Feigenbaum H, Conley MJ, Armstrong WF. An echocardiographic index for separation of right ventricular volume and pressure overload. J Am Coll Cardiol. 1985;5:918–27.

73. Bernheim PI. De l'asystolie veineuse dans l'hypertrophie du coeur gauche par stenose concomitante du ventricule droit. Rev Med. 1910;30:785–801.

74. Raymond RJ, Hinderliter AL, Willis PW, Ralph D, Caldwell EJ, Williams W, Ettinger NA, Hill NS, Summer WR, de Boisblanc B, Schwartz T, Koch G, Clayton LM, Jöbsis MM, Crow JW, Long W. Echocardiographic predictors of adverse outcomes in primary pulmonary hypertension. J Am Coll Cardiol. 2002;39:1214–9.

75. Huez S, Faoro V, Vachiery JL, Unger P, Martinot JB, Naeije R. Images in cardiovascular medicine. High-altitude-induced right-heart failure. Circulation. 2007;115:e308–9.

76. Leitman M, Lysyansky P, Sidenko S, Shir V, Peleg E, Binenbaum M, Kaluski E, Krakover R, Vered Z. Two-dimensional strain-a novel software for real-time quantitative echocardiographic assessment of myocardial function. J Am Soc Echocardiogr. 2004;17:1021–9.

77. Reisner SA, Lysyansky P, Agmon Y, Mutlak D, Lessick J, Friedman Z. Global longitudinal strain: a novel index of left ventricular systolic function. J Am Soc Echocardiogr. 2004;17:630–3.

78. Lamia B, Tanabe M, Kim HK, Johnson L, Gorcsan J III, Pinsky MR. Quantifying the role of regional dyssynchrony on global left ventricular performance. JACC Cardiovasc Imaging. 2009;2:1350–6.

79. Tanabe M, Lamia B, Tanaka H, Schwartzman D, Pinsky MR, Gorcsan J III. Echocardiographic speckle tracking radial strain imaging to assess ventricular dyssynchrony in a pacing model of resynchronization therapy. J Am Soc Echocardiogr. 2008;21:1382–8.

80. Badagliacca R, Reali M, Poscia R, Pezzuto B, Papa S, Mezzapesa M, Nocioni M, Valli G, Giannetta E, Sciomer S, Iacoboni C, Fedele F, Vizza CD. Right intraventricular dyssynchrony in idiopathic, heritable, and anorexigen-induced pulmonary arterial hypertension: clinical impact and reversibility. JACC Cardiovasc Imaging. 2015;6:642–52.

81. Lamia B, Muir JF, Molano LC, Viacroze C, Benichou J, Bonnet P, Quieffin J, Cuvelier A, Naeije R. Altered synchrony of right ventricular contraction in borderline pulmonary hypertension. Int J Cardiovasc Imaging. 2017;33:1331–9.

82. Pezzuto B, Forton K, Badagliacca R, Motoji Y, Faoro V, Naeije R. Right ventricular dyssynchrony during hypoxic breathing but not during exercise in healthy subjects a speckle tracking echocardiography study. Exp Physiol. 2018;103:1338–46.

Causes of Right Heart Dysfunction

Volume Overload and the Right Heart

8

Javier Sanz

Introduction

Abnormalities in anatomy and function of the right ventricle (RV) can be due predominantly to a myocardial disorder or increased load. Myocardial diseases may be primary (i.e., idiopathic dilated cardiomyopathy) or secondary to other processes (such as myocarditis or toxicity). They are often accompanied by concomitant left ventricular (LV) involvement, although some may predominantly affect the RV (for example, arrhythmogenic cardiomyopathy or Uhl's anomaly). Regarding the overloaded RV, mechanisms may be divided into a predominant increase in volume (preload) or a predominant increase in pressure (afterload). This classification into three main categories (myocardial disease, pressure overload, and volume overload) is useful from a clinical perspective because clinical management and prognostic implication can vary markedly amongst these three groups [1]. Nevertheless, it must be realized that this categorization is necessarily artificial because at some point during their clinical course they may all be present simultaneously to some degree. As an example, patients with cardiomyopathies often have secondary pulmonary hypertension (PH) or may develop secondary tricuspid regurgitation (TR) as a consequence of RV dilatation (and thus superimposed RV volume overload). Similarly, patients with RV pressure overload may not only demonstrate TR by similar mechanisms or pulmonary regurgitation (PR) due to pulmonary artery dilatation, but also develop functional, metabolic, and pathologic abnormalities of the RV myocardium, either because of the chronic pressure overload (as reviewed elsewhere in the book) or because of direct myocardial involvement of the diseases causing PH (i.e., scleroderma) [2]. As we will see below, the chronically volume-overloaded RV may also develop intrinsic functional abnormalities, although to a much lesser degree than the pressure-overloaded RV. Consequently, the final adaptation of the RV to a specific pathological condition will depend on the presence and extent of abnormalities in these three intertwined facets.

While all three mechanistic groups may present with RV enlargement, in this chapter we review the group in which the main, original mechanism of RV dilatation is volume overload predominantly affecting the RV. We will not address the group with secondary RV volume overload and/or dilatation that can be seen in cardiomyopathies or advanced PH, patients with LV assist device, systemic RV, or situations where

J. Sanz (✉)
Icahn School of Medicine at Mount Sinai,
New York, NY, USA

The Zena and Michael A. Wiener Cardiovascular
Institute/Marie-Josée and Henry R. Kravis Center for
Cardiovascular Health, Mount Sinai Hospital,
New York, NY, USA

Centro Nacional de Investigaciones Cardiovasculares
Carlos III (CNIC), Madrid, Spain
e-mail: Javier.Sanz@mountsinai.org

S. P. Gaine et al. (eds.), *The Right Heart*, https://doi.org/10.1007/978-3-030-78255-9_8

volume overload affects both ventricles (high-output heart failure) [1, 3].

Overview of RV Volume Overload

Anatomic and Functional Adaptation to RV Volume Overload

From a macroscopic perspective, the anatomic hallmarks of isolated or predominant chronic RV volume overload typically include RV enlargement, normal RV wall thickness (albeit with an increase in free wall mass secondary to dilatation), and predominantly diastolic septal flattening with concomitant reduction in LV diastolic volume (Fig. 8.1) [1]. These features can be studied experimentally and/or clinically in vivo using different imaging modalities including echocardiography, cardiac magnetic resonance (CMR), computed tomography (CT), and, to a limited extent, nuclear techniques such as single-photon emission computed tomography (SPECT). Describing the role of these modalities in the evaluation of the RV in general or the volume-overloaded RV in particular is beyond the scope of this chapter and the interested reader is referred to dedicated reviews [4–6]. Suffice it to say that while echocardiography is the most widely available modality and can provide important information regarding diastolic function and hemodynamics, as detailed in other chapters of this book, CMR is considered the gold standard for quantification of biventricular size and systolic function, with CT being a good (although irradiating) alternative to both in the event they are nondiagnostic or they cannot be performed. Representative examples of volume-overloaded RVs as depicted by different modalities are displayed in Fig. 8.2.

In comparison with the LV, the RV has thinner wall and lower volume-to-wall surface area ratio, which renders the RV more compliant [7]. The RV is therefore capable of accepting varying amounts of venous return and pumping them into the low-impedance pulmonary circulation at a relatively constant stroke volume [1]. In other words, the RV is much better suited to face increases in preload than afterload. RV volume overload represents an increase of *predominantly* preload; however, according to Laplace's law (even though for spherical structures), as the RV dilates the curvature of the wall decreases and thus wall tension (afterload) increases. Therefore,

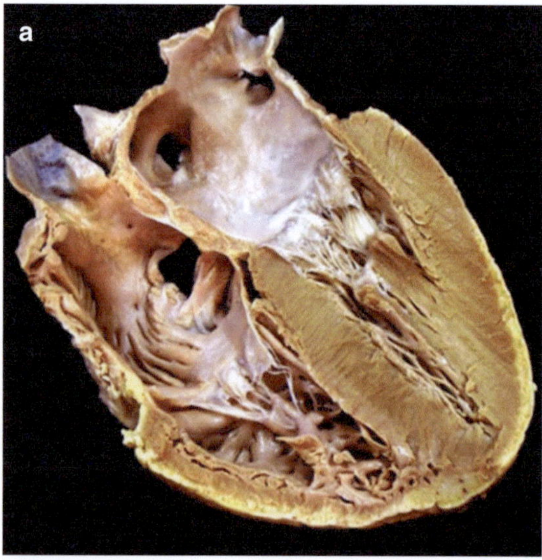
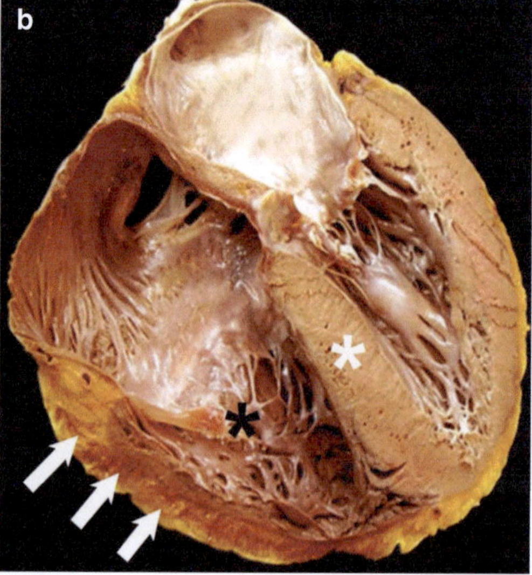

Fig. 8.1 Pathology specimens of a normal heart (**a**) and a heart with RV volume overload (**b**). Note the enlargement of the RV cavity (black asterisk), the leftward shift of the interventricular septum (white asterisk), and the mild hypertrophy of the RV free wall (arrows). (Modified from [1] with permission)

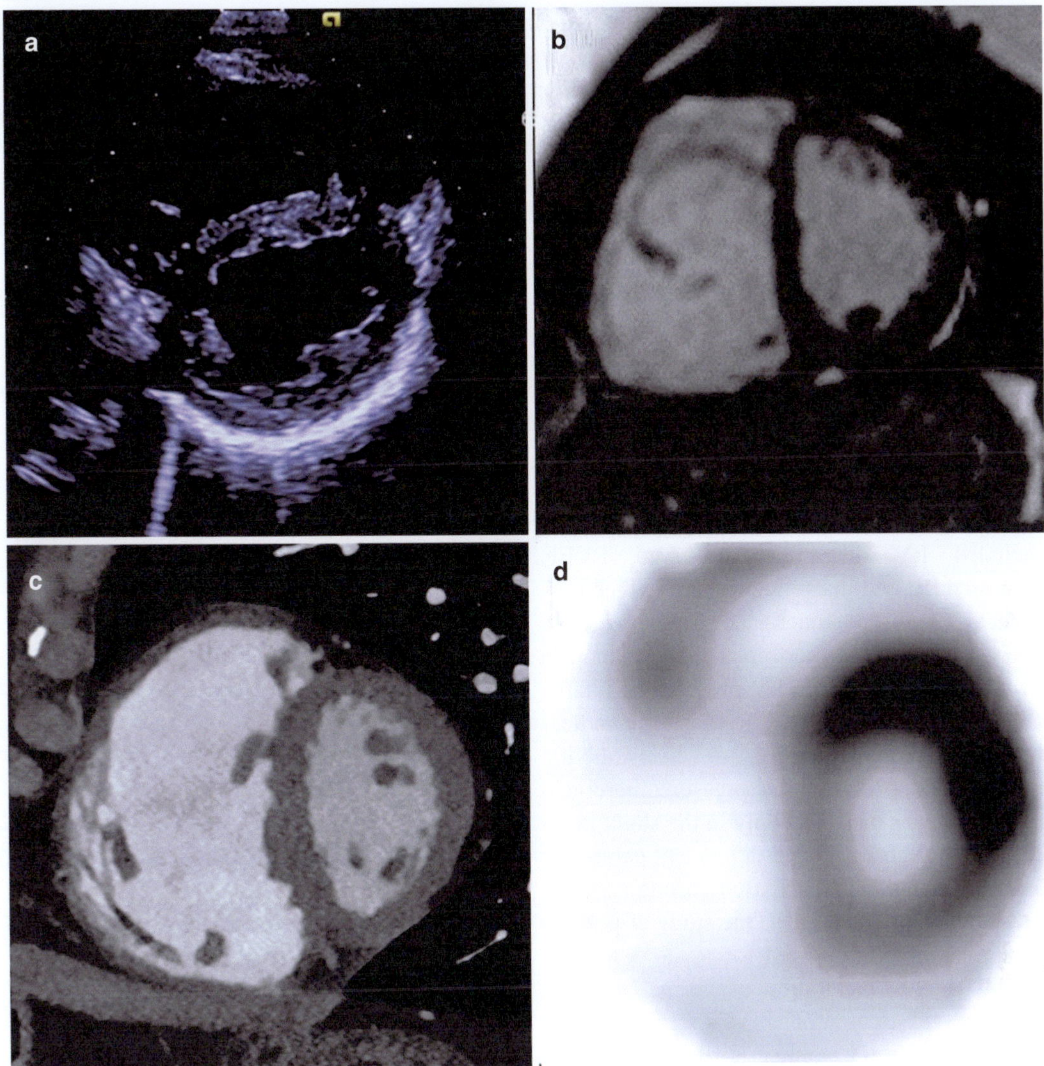

Fig. 8.2 Typical morphological features in diastole of RV volume overload (RV dilatation, septal flattening, and "D-shaped" LV with reduced volume) as demonstrated by echocardiography (**a**), CMR (**b**), CT (**c**), and SPECT (**d**)

although preload and afterload can be conceptualized separately, they are closely interrelated and cannot be fully dissociated as separate aspects.

It has been generally believed that RV volume overload courses with preserved RV systolic function, although this depends on the technique employed for quantification, underlying etiology, coexistent PH, and, importantly, disease stage. Early experimental studies in cats subjected to volume overload by surgically creating an atrial septal defect (ASD) for 4–8 weeks demonstrated normal contractility and energetics of RV myocytes studied in vitro [8, 9]. A longer follow-up of 3.5–4 years in dogs with experimentally induced TR also reported no differences in sarcomere shortening in comparison with controls [10]. Regarding in vivo investigations, a study of RV performance with both CMR and conductance catheters in pigs after 3 months of experimental PR demonstrated reduced baseline RV ejection fraction (RVEF) with no significant increase with dobutamine. End-systolic elastance was normal at rest but also failed to increase under inotropic challenge, suggesting an intrinsic alteration in contractility. In addition, RV compliance was enhanced while LV compliance was decreased [11]. A similarly diminished contractile response was noted in dogs with overload induced by femoral arterio-venous shunting and subsequently exposed to increasing afterload [12]. A systematic review of animal models of RV volume overload identified two main models: aorto-caval shunt in rodents and PR in pigs. The authors found significant heterogeneity in terms of volume load, duration of load, and surgical technique indicating that these models and species are not interchangeable and may not reflect human pathophysiology accurately. Consistent findings in both models included RV dilatation, preserved RVEF, increased RV end-diastolic pressure (which may reflect diastolic dysfunction or simply volume overload), and RV hypertrophy. The PR models demonstrated decreased RV preload recruitable stroke work and end-systolic elastance indicative of reduced contractility. Conversely, the RV maximal slope of systolic pressure increment (dP/dT_{max}) was increased only in the shunt models, although this is a load-dependent parameter and may have been increased through Frank-Starling mechanisms [13]. One study of porcine experimental PR followed for up to 3 months tested whether restoration of normal valvular function via transcatheter valve implantation would result in RV volume normalization after 1 month. The only predictor of non-recovery was the degree of RV dilatation defined as change from baseline to pre-intervention (>120 ml/m^2 for end-diastolic volume and >45 ml/m^2 for end-systolic volume; Fig. 8.3) [14], which is consistent with clinical observations described below. Regarding RV adaptation to acute volume overload, experimental studies have indicated rapid dilatation, reductions in RVEF and contractility, and increments in end-diastolic pressure without clear change in diastolic properties [15, 16].

With respect to human data, studies of RV volume overload have consistently shown the features indicated above of RV dilatation with abnormal septal motion and decreased LV dimen-

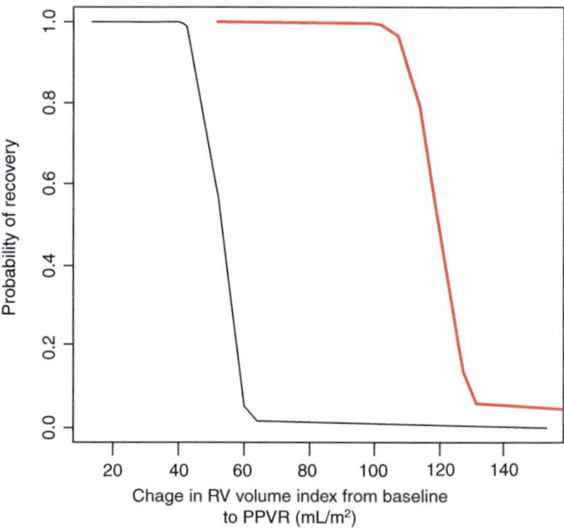

Fig. 8.3 Probability of recovery of right ventricular (RV) volumes to normal values after percutaneous pulmonary valve replacement (PPVR) in a porcine model of experimental pulmonary regurgitation (PR). The probability dropped dramatically when the increase in RV end-diastolic and end-systolic volume indices (RVEDVi and RVESVi) from PR induction to PPVR was >120 ml/m^2 and >45 ml/m^2, respectively. (Reproduced from [14] with permission)

sions [17–19]. In an early pioneer investigation evaluating RV pressure-volume relationships invasively, the shape of the loops was indistinguishable from that of the normal RV in five young patients (median age 14 years) with RV volume overload secondary to ASD [20] (graphical representations of pressure-volume loops in normal and volume-overloading conditions, and their comparison with pressure overload, are presented in Fig. 8.4). However, a study in patients with PR due to dysfunctional RV to pulmonary artery conduits who underwent percutaneous pulmonary valve implantation suggested limited contractile reserve as demonstrated by lack of improvement in cardiopulmonary exercise testing after intervention. The authors hypothesized that the volume-overloaded RV is already working at a high level at rest with limited ability to increase performance [21]. Myocardial deformation may be altered, and regional patterns appear to differ according to the underlying disease (see section "Specific Etiologies of RV Volume Overload").

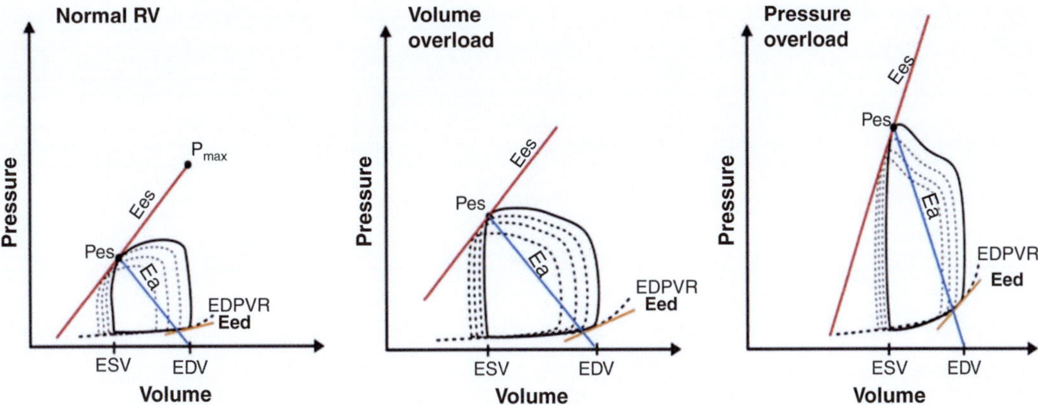

Fig. 8.4 Graphical representation of RV pressure-volume relationships in a normal RV, a volume-overloaded RV, and, for comparison, a pressure-overloaded RV. Note that in both RV volume and pressure overload there is a rightward shift of the loops reflecting RV dilatation. However, contractility (end-systolic elastance) does not differ between the normal and the volume-overloaded RV, whereas it is significantly increased in the pressure-overloaded RV to match pulmonary arterial load (arterial elastance) and maintain ventriculoarterial coupling. There is mild increase in the end-diastolic pressure-volume relationship in volume overload, but it is less prominent than in pressure overload. *Ea* arterial elastance, *Eed* end-diastolic elastance, *Ees* end-systolic elastance, *EDPVR* end-diastolic pressure-volume relationship, *EDV* end-diastolic volume, *ESV* end-systolic volume, *Pes* end-systolic RV pressure, P_{max} maximal RV pressure. (Modified from [1] with permission)

An important consequence of RV volume overload is its effects on LV geometry and performance because of ventricular interdependence. As reviewed in other chapters, the RV and LV are intimately interrelated through the interventricular septum, pericardium, and shared coronary blood flow and epicardial circumferential myocyte bundles [7, 22]. Experimental and clinical studies demonstrate that dilatation in one ventricle leads to decrease in size and an upward shift of the pressure-volume curves in the other, thus leading to higher diastolic pressures for the same volume. Therefore, RV volume overload and dilatation are associated with a reduction in LV compliance [11, 22]. In addition, it leads to a decrease in LV ejection, probably via Frank-Starling mechanisms in the setting of reduced LV size [11, 22, 23]. The primary mechanism for these changes is LV underfilling due predominantly to septal displacement and changes in LV geometry (Fig. 8.5) [3]. Septal flattening is mediated by changes in transeptal pressure gradients during diastole (likely secondary to the inability of the RV to sufficiently accommodate excess volume due to pericardial constraint), as well as septal wall tension and stiffness [7, 24]. An additional potential mechanism for impaired systolic performance was reported in pigs with experimental PR and evaluated ex vivo with diffusion tensor CMR. This study found changes in the orientations of cardiomyocyte aggregates of both ventricles compared to sham controls, which could in theory interfere with normal myocardial mechanics and ventricular interdependence [25].

Cellular and Molecular Adaptation to RV Volume Overload

RV response to pressure overload has been extensively characterized [26, 27]. One of the features is cardiomyocyte hypertrophy, which occurs through accumulation of sarcomeric proteins and is usually accompanied by the re-emergence of a fetal gene expression pattern with an increased expression of natriuretic peptides and a "proteomic switch" from α- to β-myosin heavy chain. The advantage of the β-myosin heavy chain is that it exhibits reduced energy requirements, but at the cost of decreased contractility [26]. In addition, there is experimental and some human evidence of a "metabolic switch" from

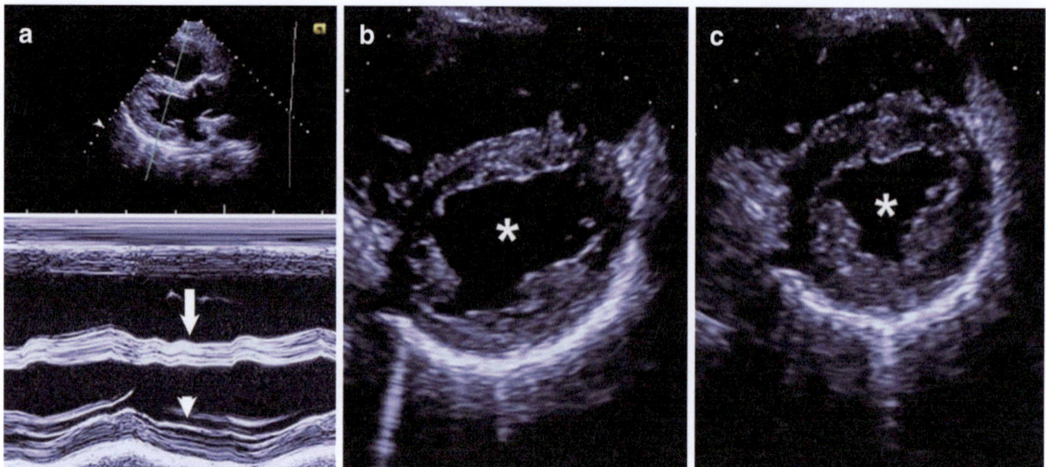

Fig. 8.5 Demonstration of diastolic septal flattening. (**a**) M-mode echocardiogram in the parasternal long-axis view demonstrating the shift of the septum towards the center of the LV during diastole (arrow) while the inferolateral wall is moving away from the LV center (arrowhead). (**b**, **c**) The images show two-dimensional echocardiograms in the parasternal short-axis view in diastole and systole, respectively. Note the flattening of the septum in diastole with a "D" shape of the LV (asterisks) with normalization to a spherical shape during systole

mitochondrial oxidation of fatty acids or glucose as the main mechanism for energy production to increased cytosolic aerobic glycolysis, which has lower oxygen requirements but also reduced energy efficiency [27].

In contrast, there is a paucity of data regarding cellular and molecular mechanisms of RV adaptation to volume overload, and the need for experimental models of pure RV volume overload has been identified as one of the current gaps in knowledge in right-heart failure [28]. In a feline model of RV volume overload induced by a surgically created ASD, the degree of RV hypertrophy at 7–10 weeks was comparable to that in animals subjected to pressure overload, with similar ultrastructural cardiomyocyte changes and capillary density. Whereas myocyte density decreased and collagen density increased in pressure overload, this was not observed in volume overload [29]. In an experimental study of aorto-caval shunting in mice, volume overload led to similar degrees of hypertrophy and gene expression of markers of fibrosis compared to pressure loading. An increase in β/α-myosin ratio and in calcineurin activity was noted in both, but it was only significant with pressure overload [30]. It should be noted though that aorto-caval

shunting may also induce PH due to increased flow through the pulmonary artery and therefore elicit different molecular responses from pure volume overload [13]. However, in another mice model of RV volume overload secondary to experimentally induced PR there were progressive increases in RV fibrosis and cardiomyocyte apoptosis [31]. Comprehensive, serial gene expression profiling suggested that early during RV volume overload β-oxidation of fatty acids remained the main energy source, but there was a late transition towards glycogenolysis. There was also a reactivation of fetal gene programs with increases in atrial natriuretic peptide and β-myosin heavy chain. Persistent downregulation of genes involved in calcium-handling genes as well as upregulation of transforming growth factor-β signaling may have contributed, respectively, to contractile dysfunction and extracellular matrix remodeling [31]. The systematic review on animal models of RV volume overload mentioned before found limited description of molecular mechanisms of RV adaptation, the most consistent ones being change in the β/α--myosin heavy chain ratio, initial activation of the renin system, and modest increase in inductors of hypertrophy such as angiotensin II or calcineurin

[13]. This review also identified, in both PR and aorto-caval shunting models, the presence of myocardial fibrosis [13], which may also be found in human hearts (Fig. 8.6).

The findings above resemble to some extent those noted in RV pressure overload; however, with the exception of fibrosis, it is uncertain if similar changes take place in humans. A small study in 11 patients with ASD evaluated with positron-emission tomography and SPECT demonstrated an increased uptake of glucose in the interventricular septum compared to the LV free wall, and a similar trend in the RV free wall that did not reach statistical significance. No differences between the septal and LV free walls were noted for the uptake of thallium as a surrogate of perfusion or β-methyl-*p*-iodophenyl-pentadecanoic acid, a fatty acid analogue. The increased glucose metabolic rate might represent metabolic switch, although other explanations such as increased septal contribution to RV ejection, relative ischemia, or technical factors cannot be excluded [32]. RV hypertrophy and increased afterload can be associated with increased oxygen requirements and relative ischemia [1, 3]. While this has been well documented in RV pressure overload with associated right-heart failure [33, 34], it is uncertain if the smaller degrees of increased wall tension expected in RV volume overload are enough to cause imbalance in oxygen supply/demand, which in turn might contribute to ischemia-related fibrosis. In the normal RV, and as opposed to the LV, there is substantial coronary blood flow during systole [35], which in theory would make systolic (pressure) overload more susceptible to ischemia than diastolic (volume) overload.

A summary of the physiopathology of RV volume overload is presented in Fig. 8.7.

Clinical Course and Management of RV Volume Overload

Because of the anatomic and physiological features discussed above, chronic volume overload is much better tolerated than pressure overload, and patients may be clinically and hemodynamically compensated for decades, particularly in the absence of PH [3, 7, 36]. However, it has become increasingly evident that chronic volume overload eventually leads to increased morbimortality, particularly in the presence of superimposed pressure overload or marked RV enlargement and/or systolic dysfunction [37–41]. Ultimately the latter ensue (and may be irreversible to some degree) together with right atrial dilatation, reaching a final symptomatic state with symptoms and signs of right-heart failure such as edema, abdominal bloating, fatigue or

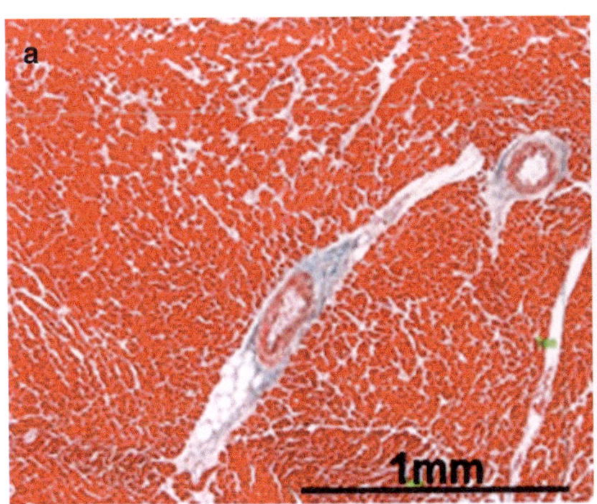
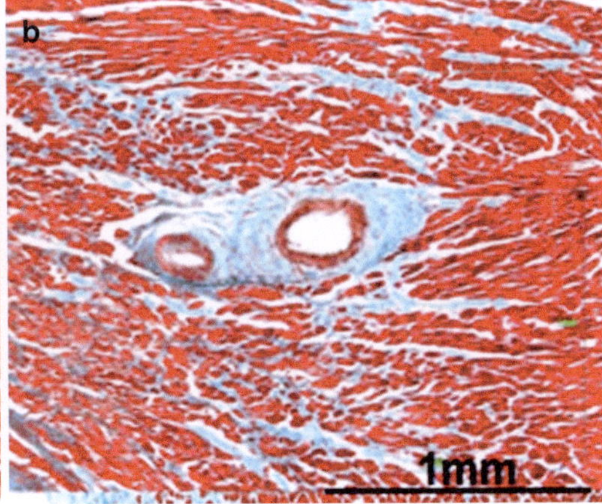

Fig. 8.6 Myocardial samples of a normal (**a**) and a volume-overloaded (**b**) human heart stained with hematoxylin and eosin and Masson's trichrome, demonstrating mildly increased interstitial fibrosis (in blue) in the volume-overloaded heart. (Reproduced from [1] with permission)

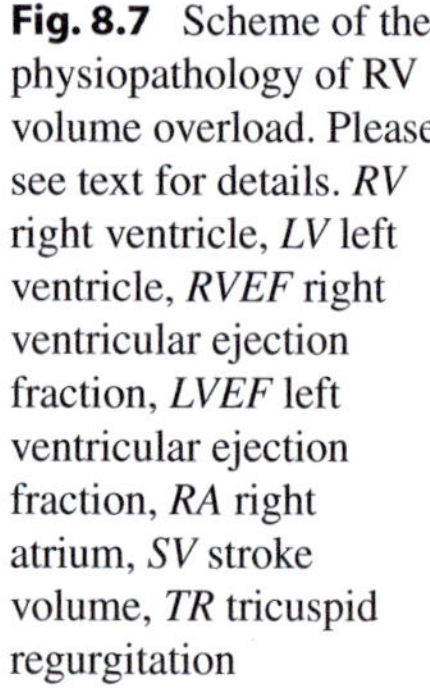

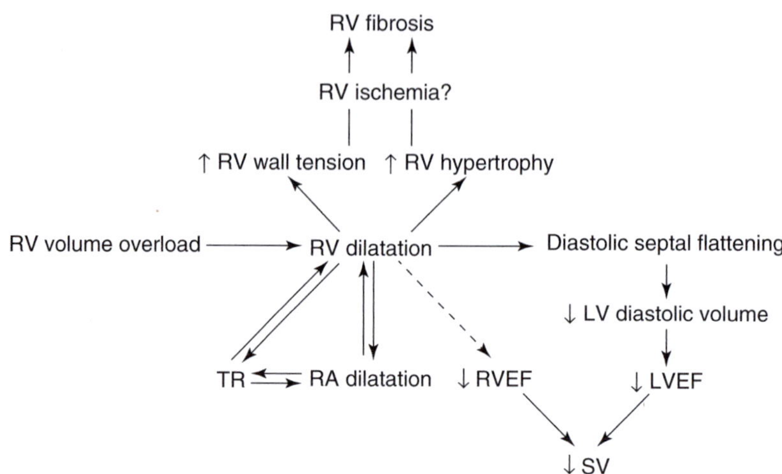

Fig. 8.7 Scheme of the physiopathology of RV volume overload. Please see text for details. *RV* right ventricle, *LV* left ventricle, *RVEF* right ventricular ejection fraction, *LVEF* left ventricular ejection fraction, *RA* right atrium, *SV* stroke volume, *TR* tricuspid regurgitation

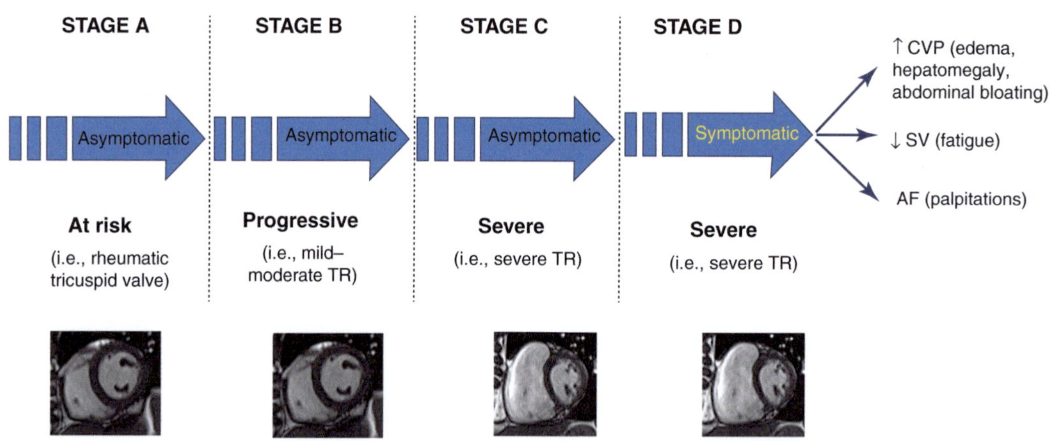

Fig. 8.8 Stages of TR as per the ACC/AHA guidelines [38], which can be conceptualized as a generalization for RV volume overload. After an initial "at-risk" phase (stage A) which may be present in some cases (for example primary or secondary valvular abnormalities) the disease progresses silently (stage B; in patients with congenital shunts the disease would start in this stage) until there is severe dilatation of the RV and often right atrium (stage C). Eventually clinical decompensation takes place (stage D). As indicated in the text, please note that in cases of associated pulmonary hypertension (PH; for example, secondary to shunt) symptoms/signs of PH may predominate. *CVP* central venous pressure, *SV* stroke volume, *AF* atrial fibrillation (or other atrial arrythmias), *TR* tricuspid regurgitation

palpitations in relation, respectively, to elevated central venous pressure, hepatic congestion, reduced output, or arrhythmia, particularly atrial fibrillation [37, 38]. Figure 8.8 represents guideline-based stages of TR [38], which can serve as a conceptual framework for the natural history of RV volume overload in general. It must be noted that if volume overload is associated with, or leads to, elevated pulmonary pressures (i.e., systemic-to-pulmonary shunts), symptoms of PH such as dyspnea, chest pain, or near syncope, rather than signs and symptoms of congestive right-heart failure, may be dominant in the clinical presentation.

Although infrequent, acute RV volume overload can occur in cases of acute right-sided valvular regurgitation secondary to endocarditis, iatrogenic or blunt trauma, or myocardial infarction. These are usually well tolerated hemodynamically in the short term, but acute decompensation has been reported [42]. As in other chronic situations, there is impaired prognosis on long-term follow-up if volume overload persists [43].

The basis of clinical management for RV volume overload is serial imaging to evaluate for progressive RV dilatation and/or systolic function that would trigger surgical or percutaneous repair of the underlying responsible lesion [37–41]. There is limited role of medical therapy with two main exceptions. In advanced, clinically manifest right-heart failure, diuretics (typically loop diuretics and/or aldosterone antagonists) may help alleviate systemic venous congestion [38]. The second situation is when PH coexists or develops during disease course, in which case PH-targeted therapy such as prostaglandins, endothelin blockers, and phosphodiesterase-5 inhibitors may also play a role [40, 41]. In addition, specific etiologies of valvular dysfunction may require dedicated medical therapy, for example antibiotics in infective endocarditis.

A comparison of main, general differences between compensated RV adaptation to chronic volume or pressure overload is summarized in Table 8.1.

Specific Etiologies of RV Volume Overload

Isolated or predominant RV volume overload can be secondary to right-sided regurgitant valve disease and pre-tricuspid systemic-to-pulmonary shunts (Table 8.2). Valvular regurgitation can be classified as primary if the abnormality leading to insufficiency resides in the valve itself, or secondary (or functional) when it develops as a result of RV or pulmonary artery dilatation in the setting of other processes such as PH. In the latter case, the valvular abnormality cannot be seen as the trigger of RV volume overload, but it can contribute to its magnification. Congenital abnormalities with sufficient pre-tricuspid systemic-to-pulmonary shunting can also cause RV volume overload. This therefore includes an ASD or partial anomalous pulmonary venous return (PAPVR). While ventricular septal defects also cause increased volume to the RV, the higher pressure component of the shunt leads to faster development of PH and thus combined pressure and volume overload [44]. PAPVR involving only one vein without an associated ASD typically does not cause enough left-to-right shunting to justify significant RV overload or therapeutic

Table 8.1 Comparison of main features in compensated, chronic RV volume versus pressure overload in humans[a]

Parameters	Volume overload	Pressure overload
RV volume	Moderate/severe increase	Preserved/mild increase
RV mass	Mild increase	Moderate/severe increase
RV ejection fraction	Preserved/mild decrease	Preserved/mild decrease
RV contractility	Preserved/mild decrease	Increased
RV compliance	Preserved/increased	Decreased
RV fibrosis	Mild	Moderate/severe
RV metabolic switch[b]	Possible	Probable
RV proteomic switch[c]	Possible	Probable
RV ischemia	Unknown	Yes
Clinical deterioration	Long term	Midterm[d]
Principles of management	Serial imaging Surgical/percutaneous repair	Treatment of underlying etiology PH-directed drug therapy

RV right ventricle, *PH* pulmonary hypertension

[a]Please note that this table represents a generalization that assumes clinical and hemodynamic compensation. Findings in a decompensated state would differ

[b]Switch from fatty acid and glucose oxidation towards glycolysis

[c]Switch from α- to β-myosin heavy chain

[d]Varies according to severity and etiology [90]

Table 8.2 Etiologies of RV volume overload

Valvular regurgitation
• Tricuspid
– Primary
– Secondary
• Pulmonary
– Primary
– Secondary
Systemic-to-pulmonary shunt
• Atrial septal defect (ASD)
– Ostium primum
– Ostium secundum
– Sinus venosus
– Unroofed coronary sinus
• Partial anomalous pulmonary vein drainage[a]
– Right upper (±middle) vein to SVC
With sinus venosus ASD
Without sinus venosus ASD
– Left upper vein to left brachiocephalic vein
– Right lower vein to IVC (scimitar syndrome)
– Other

ASD atrial septal defect, *IVC* inferior vena cava, *SVC* superior vena cava

[a]Most common variants

intervention [40]. Thus, most of the evidence regarding RV performance in simple systemic-to-pulmonary shunts derives from ASD, particularly the ostium secundum type or to a lesser extent the combination of sinus venosus ASD and PAPVR, so ASD and PAPVR will be considered together. Representative examples of the main causes of RV volume overload are shown in Fig. 8.9.

In the next sections we will review some evidence pertaining to each of the etiologic entities mentioned above, with a specific emphasis on how RV status can influence clinical course and/ or management.

Tricuspid Regurgitation

Isolated TR is usually well tolerated clinically for prolonged periods of time (Fig. 8.8) [37, 38, 45]. TR can be caused by intrinsic valvular abnormalities of various etiologies such as prolapse, radiation, endocarditis, and others. However, functional TR secondary to annular dilatation and/or distortion, most commonly in the setting of RV enlargement, represents 80% of cases of significant TR and is often associated with left-sided valvular or ventricular abnormalities and/or PH [37–39]. In these cases, TR development may contribute to additional overload and a spiral of progressive RV dilatation, systolic dysfunction, and further regurgitation [46].

It is well known that the presence of severe TR is related to poor prognosis in the long term, which has been mostly studied in the context of chronic heart failure or left-sided valvular disease [37, 38], but also in isolated TR [47]. It is generally accepted that the excess mortality associated with severe TR is independent from RV dilatation and systolic dysfunction [38] as suggested by both early echocardiographic [48] and more recent echocardiographic and CMR data [47, 49, 50]. However, not all studies have confirmed this [51], so how RV status modulates the clinical natural history of TR is not fully understood. Nonetheless, its evaluation may be helpful for the timing of intervention. In 69 patients undergoing surgical repair of severe residual TR after prior left-sided valve surgery, an RV end-systolic area <20 cm^2 as measured by echocardiography predicted reduced risk of death and cardiovascular rehospitalization [36]. Analogous data were reported in 75 patients evaluated with CMR and in whom a preoperative RVEF ≥45% (Fig. 8.10) or an RV end-systolic volume ≤75 ml/m^2 were linked to improved survival [52]. In 32 patients undergoing surgical repair of residual functional TR following previous left-sided valve surgery, a threshold of RV end-diastolic volume <164 ml/m^2 by CMR could identify those demonstrating normal postoperative RVEF, although the authors acknowledged that there was no threshold above which the RV did not show improvement [53]. Based on these and other data, and in addition to symptomatic patients or those undergoing left-sided valve surgery, clinical guidelines give consideration to the surgical repair of severe TR in patients with no or minimal symptoms if there is progressive RV dilatation and/or systolic dysfunction [38, 39], although the criteria of what constitutes meaningful progression need to be refined. The ongoing development of novel transcatheter tricuspid valve interventions [54] may

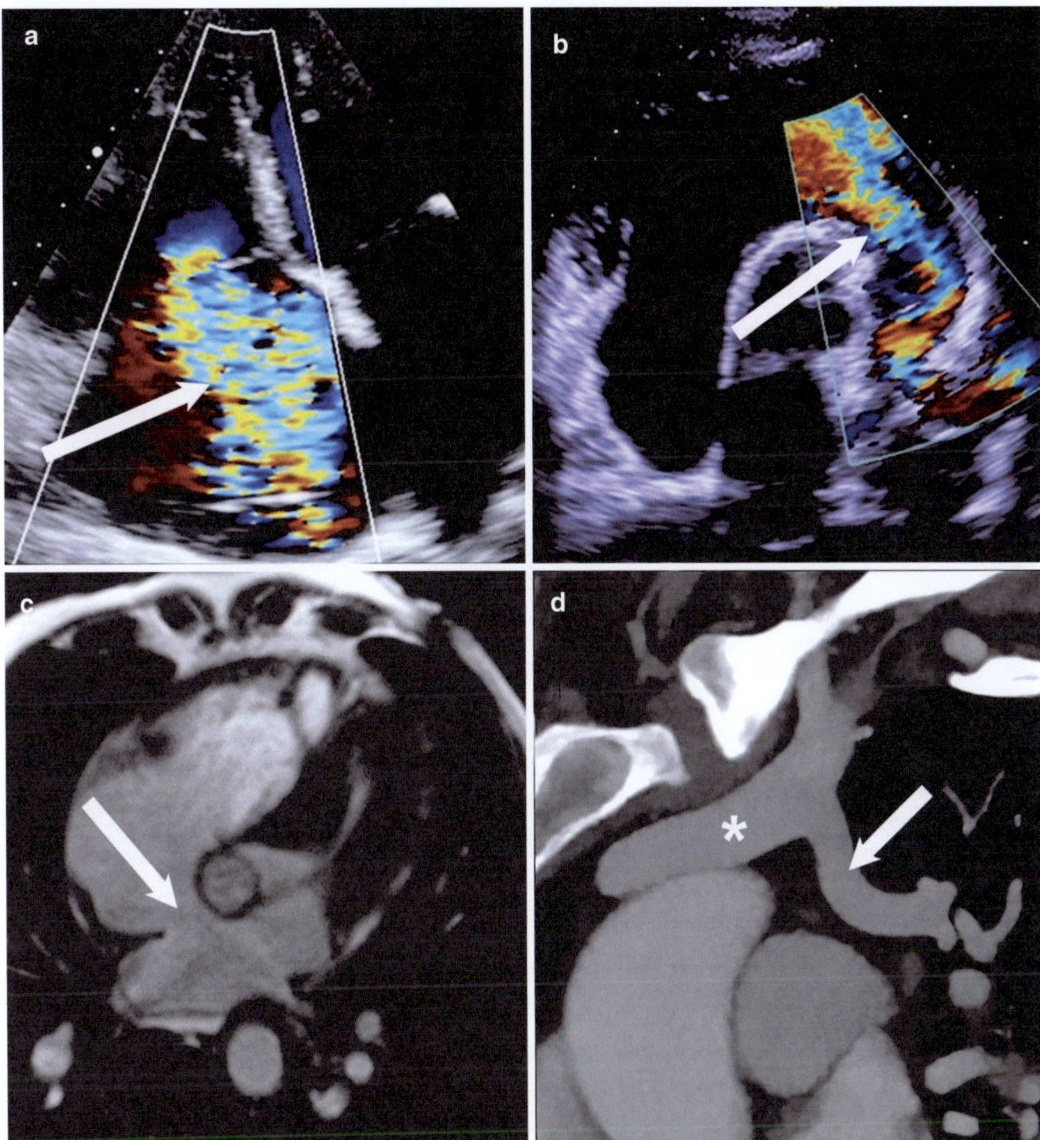

Fig. 8.9 Representative examples of different etiologies of RV volume overload. (**a**) Two-dimensional echocardiogram with color Doppler in an apical, long-axis, four-chamber view demonstrating severe tricuspid regurgitation (arrow) into the right atrium. (**b**) Two-dimensional echocardiogram with color Doppler in a parasternal short-axis view at the level of the aortic valve, displaying severe pulmonary regurgitation (arrow) into the RV outflow tract. (**c**) Cine CMR in a four-chamber orientation demonstrating an ostium secundum atrial septal defect (arrow). (**d**) Double-oblique multiplanar reformat of a CT angiogram depicting an anomalous left upper pulmonary vein (arrow) draining into the left brachiocephalic vein (asterisk)

lead to a change in the landscape of indications for repair in both primary and functional TR, as well as redefinition of the roles of RV size and function quantification in guiding the timing of therapies.

Pulmonary Regurgitation

Apart from the general considerations discussed above regarding RV adaptation to volume overload, there are regional differences in systolic

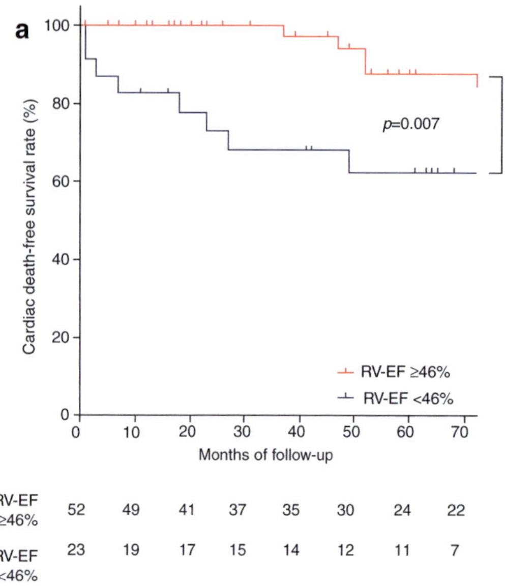

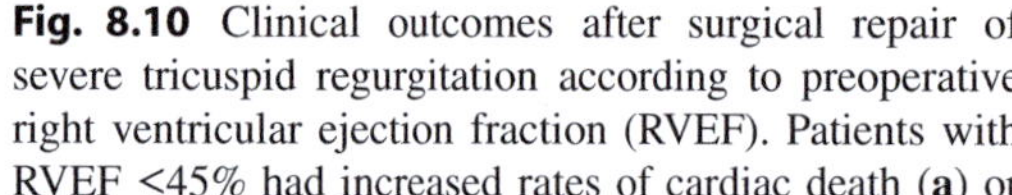

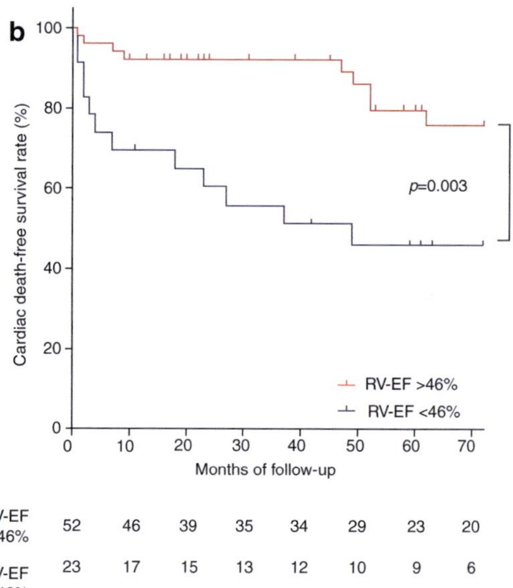

Fig. 8.10 Clinical outcomes after surgical repair of severe tricuspid regurgitation according to preoperative right ventricular ejection fraction (RVEF). Patients with RVEF ≤45% had increased rates of cardiac death (**a**) or the combination of cardiac death and unplanned cardiac related readmission (**b**). (Reproduced from [52] with permission)

function in patients with tetralogy of Fallot (TOF). One obvious reason is the presence of wall motion abnormalities in the outflow tract as sequalae of surgical infundibulotomy and/or RV outflow tract patch enlargement. Using CMR volumetric analysis of three RV components, it was shown that the contribution of the inlet to global RVEF was unchanged in patients with repaired TOF compared with controls, but it was increased for the apical trabecular portion and reduced for the outlet, suggesting that the former is assuming the additional load for maintaining ejection [55]. Preferential dilatation and a more spherical shape in the apex were also described in another series [56]. Studies using echocardiography have shown a reduction in RV free wall longitudinal strain that correlated with the severity of PR [57] and that became more severe towards the apex [58, 59]. It has been hypothesized that the apical changes in size and configuration after TOF repair may increase wall tension and result in reduced myocardial deformation in this region [58]. Unsurprisingly, given interventricular interactions described above, there is evidence also in TOF of a relation between PR-related RV dilata-

tion and systolic dysfunction with LV functional abnormalities, such as decreased torsion, increased dyssynchrony, or abnormal hemodynamic forces [59–61].

It needs to be recognized, however, that PR in TOF represents a relatively unique situation of RV volume overload that may not be directly extrapolatable to other conditions such as PR secondary to carcinoid heart disease or congenital PR. While the latter usually occur in an otherwise "normal" RV, the RV in repaired TOF demonstrates surgical sequelae with areas of scar and dyssynchrony [62, 63]. In addition, there may be residual outflow tract obstruction or pulmonary artery stenosis after surgery, with concomitant increase in afterload that can modulate the degree of PR and associated RV remodeling [64, 65]. Furthermore, the RV in TOF is exposed to persistently increased pressure overload between birth and time of repair. Indeed, the RV wall in TOF demonstrates an intermediate layer of predominantly circumferential myocyte aggregates [66], somewhat similar to the LV and in contrast to the normal RV "two-layer" structure of superficial, predominantly circumferential aggregates, and deep, predominantly longitudinal aggregates [1]. This has nonetheless been hypothesized to be part of the congenital derangement of TOF as opposed to just adaption to increased pressure load [66].

Similar to isolated TR, isolated PR is usually well tolerated and may not require intervention in patients without TOF, although a series of 72 cases with isolated congenital PR demonstrated development of symptoms and increase in mortality, particularly after age 40 [67]. If PR occurs in the setting of significant PH, there is a possible role of medical therapy with drugs aimed at decreasing pulmonary vascular resistance or treating underlying PH etiology. In a patient with normal pulmonary artery pressures and significant PR, serial noninvasive testing (particularly CMR) is advised to identify worsening RV enlargement or dysfunction, which would prompt transcatheter or surgical valve replacement [40, 45].

RV characteristics play an important role in determining prognosis in repaired TOF. Higher baseline RV size and presence of significant TR were identified as predictors of more rapid RV dilatation in 63 patients with PR secondary to surgical repair of TOF or pulmonary valve stenosis [68]. An international multicenter CMR registry of 452 patients with repaired TOF identified preoperative RVEF <40%, an RV mass-to-volume ratio $\geq$0.45 g/ml, and, in a subgroup of 230 patients with available Doppler data, an RV systolic pressure $\geq$40 mmHg as predictors of incident death or sustained ventricular tachycardia [69]. In another multicenter study of 575 patients, similar outcomes were best predicted by an RVEF <30%, an LV ejection fraction <45%, or, particularly, the combination of both [70]. Thus, in addition to symptomatic patients, clinical guidelines give consideration to valve replacement in cases of asymptomatic severe PR with significant or progressive RV dilatation and/or dysfunction [40, 41]. A number of CMR studies [71–78], summarized in Table 8.3, have also addressed the potential role of RV size quantification to determine the optimal timing for surgical intervention for PR. As can be seen, suggested preoperative thresholds have ranged between 80 and 100 ml/m² for RV end-systolic volume and 150–190 ml/m² for RV end-diastolic volume. One study [78] performed CMR very early (median 6 days) after surgery in 47 TOF patients and demonstrated immediate reductions in RV end-diastolic volume without further improvements midterm (median 3 years of follow-up). However, RV end-systolic volume, RV mass, and RVEF improved postoperatively and continued to do so midterm, suggesting that RV recovery

Table 8.3 Studies evaluating optimal preoperative values of RV volumes for RV recovery after surgical pulmonary valve replacement in PR secondary to TOF

Authors	Year	N	Age (years)	Male (%)	Median f/u (years)	Postoperative RV normalization (%)[a]	Proposed RVEDV (ml/m²)	Proposed RVESVi (ml/m²)
Therrien et al. [71]	2005	17	34 ± 12	41.2	1.8 ± 0.9	59.9	170	85
Oosterhof et al. [72]	2007	70	29 [23–37]	59.1	1.6 [0.9–5.2]	16.9	160	82
Henkens et al. [73]	2007	27	30.8 ± 8.2	63.0	0.6 (0.4–1.6)	51.8	N/R	100
Frigiola et al. [74][b]	2008	60	22 ± 11	54.9	1	60.0	150	N/R
Geva et al. [75]	1010	61	21 [11–58]	50.0	0.5	18.3	190	90
Lee et al. [76]	2012	67	16.7 (4.6–60.2)	60.1	5.9 (0.3–13.5)	50.7	163	80
Bokma et al. [77]	2016	65	29 ± 8.3	61.5	6.3 [4.9–9.5]	21.5	160	80
Heng et al. [78]	2017	47	35.8 ± 10.1	66.6	3 [1–4.1]	70.2	158	82

Continuous data expressed as mean ± standard deviation, median [interquartile range], or median (range)

RV right ventricle, *RVEDV* right ventricular end-diastolic volume, *RVESV* right ventricular end-systolic volume, *N/R* not reported

[a]Definition varied according to the study

[b]Seventy-two percent tetralogy of Fallot; remaining, other forms of outflow obstruction

evolves over time. LV volumes and ejection fraction decreased postoperatively but increased to levels above baseline at 3 years [78]. Conversely, in another series, 30 patients with predominant PR (two-thirds with TOF) underwent CMR before, within 1 month and 12 months after percutaneous valve replacement. This study also identified early reductions in RV and increments in LV volumes but no improvements in RVEF or any further late changes [79], which might be due to smaller sample size, shorter follow-up, or different repair technique. The ACC/AHA clinical guidelines have adopted thresholds of RV end-diastolic volume <160 ml/m^2 and end-systolic volume <80 ml/m^2 to recommend valve intervention [40], although recent data has challenged the prognostic significance of persistent RV dilatation after valve repair [80]. There are no specific optimal volumetric thresholds for intervention for residual PR after surgery for congenital pulmonary valve stenosis, but RV dilatation tends to be less severe than in TOF [40].

ASD/PAPVR

As opposed to the studies showing that patients with repaired TOF had reduced deformation of the RV free wall that was more severe in the apex (see above), patients with ASD had preserved global longitudinal strain with supranormal apical strain. Strain values correlated with RV dimensions, which may represent load dependency and/or suggest that RV apical contraction contributes significantly to the increased RV output [58, 81]. However, after surgical correction (even 35 years later) longitudinal strain was reduced, particularly in the apex [81, 82], and apical strain correlated with functional capacity post-repair [81]. It is uncertain if these residual abnormalities are sequelae of long-standing RV volume overload, surgical intervention, or both [82].

As expected, RV volume overload in this setting can also lead to subclinical LV abnormalities. A study comparing invasive pressure-volume relationships in patients with ostium secundum ASD versus controls reported alterations in indices of LV diastolic function (increases in the isovolumic relaxation time and diastolic time constant), and leftward and upward shifts of the pressure-volume relationships [83]. Imaging studies have also shown impairment in pump function as demonstrated by reduced LV ejection fraction [84] or septal longitudinal strain [85].

Long-term RV volume overload due to an ostium secundum ASD can lead to impaired morbidity and mortality, which can be improved with defect closure [45]. Surgical or percutaneous closure is thus the cornerstone of therapy in ASD and PAVPR except in the presence of Eisenmenger physiology or significant PH, in which case there is a role for PH-targeted medical therapy [40]. Together with the absence of significant PH and confirmed systemic-to-pulmonary shunting with a Qp/Qs ≥1.5, the presence of RV dilatation is an important factor to advocate for closure, even in the absence of symptoms [40, 41]. A small retrospective study identified a preoperative RV end-systolic volume <75 ml/m^2 as a predictor of RV size normalization after percutaneous closure [86], but further data is needed before a specific threshold can be recommended to trigger intervention. Shunt closure is associated with rapid and large improvements in biventricular size, geometry, and systolic function as well as in atrial dilatation (Fig. 8.11), although recovery may not be complete (even up to 5 years of follow-up), particularly in older individuals [45, 87–89].

Conclusions

RV volume overload is characterized by RV dilatation, diastolic septal flattening, and reductions in LV diastolic volume. Clinical course is much better than that of RV pressure overload but, although it may be well tolerated for decades, there is extensive evidence of increased morbi-mortality in the long term as a consequence of RV volume overload. In the absence of symptoms, RV dilatation and/or systolic dysfunction play an important role in triggering interventions for the repair of underlying etiologies (right-sided valvu-

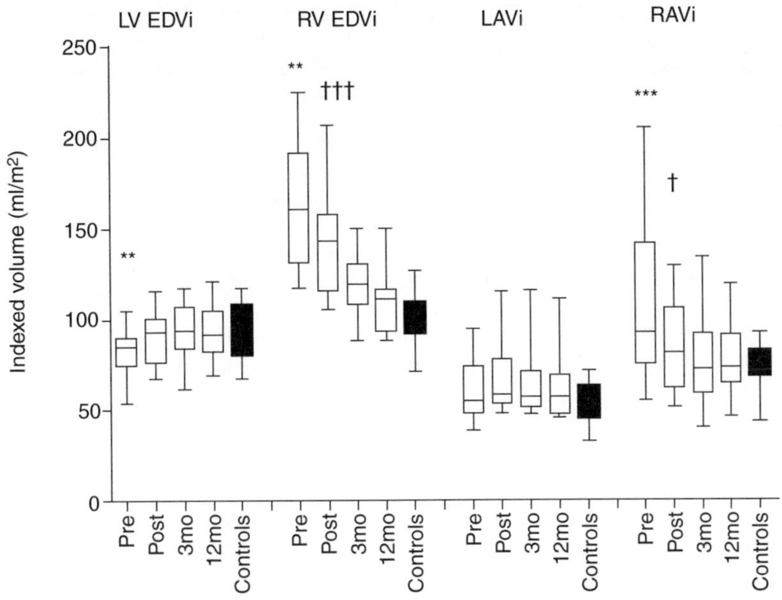

Fig. 8.11 Serial ventricular and atrial volumes measured with CMR before and up to 1 year after transcatheter closure of atrial septal defect (ASD) and compared to controls. Immediately after closure there were significant increases in left ventricular (LV) and decreases in right ventricular (RV) and right atrial volumes, with further significant reductions after 3 months for right-heart chambers. RV volume continued to decrease over a year, although changes did not reach statistical significance. Left atrial volume did not change after closure. $**P < 0.01$ pre- versus post-ASD closure; $^{†}P < 0.05$ post versus 3 months, $^{†††}P < 0.001$ post versus 3 months. *LAVi* maximal left atrial volume index, *LV EDVi* LV end-diastolic volume index, *RV EDVi* RV end-diastolic volume index, *RAVi* maximal right atrial volume index. (Reproduced from [89] with permission)

lar disease or pre-tricuspid systemic-to-pulmonary shunts). Late repair may lead to irreversible changes in RV performance and impaired outcomes. The molecular biology of RV volume overload and the mechanisms eliciting the transition from compensated to decompensated status are not well characterized, and research efforts in appropriate experimental models are needed to improve our understanding of this condition.

Disclosures None.

References

1. Sanz J, Sanchez-Quintana D, Bossone E, Bogaard HJ, Naeije R. Anatomy, function, and dysfunction of the right ventricle: JACC state-of-the-art review. J Am Coll Cardiol. 2019;73:1463–82.
2. Hsu S, Houston BA, Tampakakis E, et al. Right ventricular functional reserve in pulmonary arterial hypertension. Circulation. 2016;133:2413–22.
3. Konstam MA, Kiernan MS, Bernstein D, et al. Evaluation and management of right-sided heart failure: a scientific statement from the American Heart Association. Circulation. 2018;137:e578–622.
4. Mertens LL, Friedberg MK. Imaging the right ventricle—current state of the art. Nat Rev Cardiol. 2010;7:551–63.
5. Sanz J, Conroy J, Narula J. Imaging of the right ventricle. Cardiol Clin. 2012;30:189–203.
6. van de Veerdonk MC, Marcus JT, Bogaard HJ, Vonk Noordegraaf A. State of the art: advanced imaging of the right ventricle and pulmonary circulation in humans (2013 Grover Conference series). Pulm Circ. 2014;4:158–68.
7. Dell'Italia LJ. The right ventricle: anatomy, physiology, and clinical importance. Curr Probl Cardiol. 1991;16:653–720.
8. Cooper G, Puga FJ, Zujko KJ, Harrison CE, Coleman HN III. Normal myocardial function and energetics in volume-overload hypertrophy in the cat. Circ Res. 1973;32:140–8.
9. Carey RA, Natarajan G, Bove AA, Coulson RL, Spann JF. Myosin adenosine triphosphatase activity in the volume-overloaded hypertrophied feline right ventricle. Circ Res. 1979;45:81–7.
10. Ishibashi Y, Rembert JC, Carabello BA, et al. Normal myocardial function in severe right ventricular vol-

ume overload hypertrophy. Am J Physiol Heart Circ Physiol. 2001;280:H11–6.

11. Kuehne T, Saeed M, Gleason K, et al. Effects of pulmonary insufficiency on biventricular function in the developing heart of growing swine. Circulation. 2003;108:2007–13.

12. Szabo G, Soos P, Bahrle S, et al. Adaptation of the right ventricle to an increased afterload in the chronically volume overloaded heart. Ann Thorac Surg. 2006;82:989–95.

13. Bossers GPL, Hagdorn QAJ, Ploegstra MJ, et al. Volume load-induced right ventricular dysfunction in animal models: insights in a translational gap in congenital heart disease. Eur J Heart Fail. 2018;20:808–12.

14. Ersboell M, Vejlstrup N, Nilsson JC, et al. Percutaneous pulmonary valve replacement after different duration of free pulmonary regurgitation in a porcine model: effects on the right ventricle. Int J Cardiol. 2013;167:2944–51.

15. Bove T, Vandekerckhove K, Bouchez S, Wouters P, Somers P, Van Nooten G. Role of myocardial hypertrophy on acute and chronic right ventricular performance in relation to chronic volume overload in a porcine model: relevance for the surgical management of tetralogy of Fallot. J Thorac Cardiovasc Surg. 2014;147:1956–65.

16. Shah AS, Atkins BZ, Hata JA, et al. Early effects of right ventricular volume overload on ventricular performance and beta-adrenergic signaling. J Thorac Cardiovasc Surg. 2000;120:342–9.

17. Weyman AE, Wann S, Feigenbaum H, Dillon JC. Mechanism of abnormal septal motion in patients with right ventricular volume overload: a cross-sectional echocardiographic study. Circulation. 1976;54:179–86.

18. Feneley M, Gavaghan T. Paradoxical and pseudo-paradoxical interventricular septal motion in patients with right ventricular volume overload. Circulation. 1986;74:230–8.

19. Chalard A, Sanchez I, Gouton M, et al. Effect of pulmonary valve replacement on left ventricular function in patients with tetralogy of Fallot. Am J Cardiol. 2012;110:1828–35.

20. Redington AN, Rigby ML, Shinebourne EA, Oldershaw PJ. Changes in the pressure-volume relation of the right ventricle when its loading conditions are modified. Br Heart J. 1990;63:45–9.

21. Coats L, Khambadkone S, Derrick G, et al. Physiological consequences of percutaneous pulmonary valve implantation: the different behaviour of volume- and pressure-overloaded ventricles. Eur Heart J. 2007;28:1886–93.

22. Naeije R, Badagliacca R. The overloaded right heart and ventricular interdependence. Cardiovasc Res. 2017;113:1474–85.

23. Belenkie I, Dani R, Smith ER, Tyberg JV. Effects of volume loading during experimental acute pulmonary embolism. Circulation. 1989;80:178–88.

24. Kingma I, Tyberg JV, Smith ER. Effects of diastolic transseptal pressure gradient on ventricular septal position and motion. Circulation. 1983;68:1304–14.

25. Agger P, Ilkjaer C, Laustsen C, et al. Changes in overall ventricular myocardial architecture in the setting of a porcine animal model of right ventricular dilation. J Cardiovasc Magn Reson. 2017;19:93.

26. Bogaard HJ, Abe K, Vonk Noordegraaf A, Voelkel NF. The right ventricle under pressure: cellular and molecular mechanisms of right-heart failure in pulmonary hypertension. Chest. 2009;135:794–804.

27. Ryan JJ, Archer SL. The right ventricle in pulmonary arterial hypertension: disorders of metabolism, angiogenesis and adrenergic signaling in right ventricular failure. Circ Res. 2014;115:176–88.

28. Lahm T, Douglas IS, Archer SL, et al. Assessment of right ventricular function in the research setting: knowledge gaps and pathways forward. An official American Thoracic Society Research Statement. Am J Respir Crit Care Med. 2018;198:e15–43.

29. Marino TA, Kent RL, Uboh CE, Fernandez E, Thompson EW, Cooper G. Structural analysis of pressure versus volume overload hypertrophy of cat right ventricle. Am J Phys. 1985;249:H371–9.

30. Bartelds B, Borgdorff MA, Smit-van Oosten A, et al. Differential responses of the right ventricle to abnormal loading conditions in mice: pressure vs. volume load. Eur J Heart Fail. 2011;13:1275–82.

31. Reddy S, Zhao M, Hu DQ, et al. Physiologic and molecular characterization of a murine model of right ventricular volume overload. Am J Physiol Heart Circ Physiol. 2013;304:H1314–27.

32. Otani H, Kagaya Y, Yamane Y, et al. Long-term right ventricular volume overload increases myocardial fluorodeoxyglucose uptake in the interventricular septum in patients with atrial septal defect. Circulation. 2000;101:1686–92.

33. Gomez A, Bialostozky D, Zajarias A, et al. Right ventricular ischemia in patients with primary pulmonary hypertension. J Am Coll Cardiol. 2001;38:1137–42.

34. Vogel-Claussen J, Skrok J, Shehata ML, et al. Right and left ventricular myocardial perfusion reserves correlate with right ventricular function and pulmonary hemodynamics in patients with pulmonary arterial hypertension. Radiology. 2011;258:119–27.

35. Zong P, Tune JD, Downey HF. Mechanisms of oxygen demand/supply balance in the right ventricle. Exp Biol Med (Maywood). 2005;230:507–19.

36. Kim YJ, Kwon DA, Kim HK, et al. Determinants of surgical outcome in patients with isolated tricuspid regurgitation. Circulation. 2009;120:1672–8.

37. Pellikka PA. Tricuspid, pulmonic, and multivalvular disease. In: Zipes DP, Libby P, Bonow RO, Mann DL, Tomaselli GF, Braunwald E, editors. Braunwald's heart disease: a textbook of cardiovascular medicine. 11th ed. Philadelphia, PA: Elsevier/Saunders; 2018. p. 1445–54.

38. Nishimura RA, Otto CM, Bonow RO, et al. 2014 AHA/ACC guideline for the management of patients with valvular heart disease: a report of the American College of Cardiology/American Heart Association Task Force on Practice Guidelines. J Am Coll Cardiol. 2014;63:e57–185.

39. Baumgartner H, Falk V, Bax JJ, et al. 2017 ESC/
    EACTS guidelines for the management of valvular
    heart disease. Eur Heart J. 2017;38:2739–91.
40. Stout KK, Daniels CJ, Aboulhosn JA, et al. 2018 AHA/
    ACC guideline for the management of adults with con-
    genital heart disease: a report of the American College
    of Cardiology/American Heart Association Task
    Force on Clinical Practice Guidelines. Circulation.
    2019;139:e698–800.
41. Baumgartner H, Bonhoeffer P, De Groot NM, et al.
    ESC guidelines for the management of grown-up con-
    genital heart disease (new version 2010). Eur Heart J.
    2010;31:2915–57.
42. Harjola VP, Mebazaa A, Celutkiene J, et al.
    Contemporary management of acute right ventricular
    failure: a statement from the Heart Failure Association
    and the Working Group on Pulmonary Circulation and
    Right Ventricular Function of the European Society of
    Cardiology. Eur J Heart Fail. 2016;18:226–41.
43. Messika-Zeitoun D, Thomson H, Bellamy M, et al.
    Medical and surgical outcome of tricuspid regurgita-
    tion caused by flail leaflets. J Thorac Cardiovasc Surg.
    2004;128:296–302.
44. van der Feen DE, Bartelds B, de Boer RA, Berger
    RMF. Pulmonary arterial hypertension in congenital
    heart disease: translational opportunities to study the
    reversibility of pulmonary vascular disease. Eur Heart
    J. 2017;38:2034–41.
45. Davlouros PA, Niwa K, Webb G, Gatzoulis MA. The
    right ventricle in congenital heart disease. Heart.
    2006;92(Suppl 1):i27–38.
46. Shiran A, Sagie A. Tricuspid regurgitation in mitral
    valve disease incidence, prognostic implications,
    mechanism, and management. J Am Coll Cardiol.
    2009;53:401–8.
47. Topilsky Y, Nkomo VT, Vatury O, et al. Clinical
    outcome of isolated tricuspid regurgitation. JACC
    Cardiovasc Imaging. 2014;7:1185–94.
48. Nath J, Foster E, Heidenreich PA. Impact of tricus-
    pid regurgitation on long-term survival. J Am Coll
    Cardiol. 2004;43:405–9.
49. Bartko PE, Arfsten H, Frey MK, et al. Natural history
    of functional tricuspid regurgitation: implications of
    quantitative Doppler assessment. JACC Cardiovasc
    Imaging. 2019;12:389–97.
50. Zhan Y, Debs D, Khan MA, et al. Natural history of
    functional tricuspid regurgitation quantified by car-
    diovascular magnetic resonance. J Am Coll Cardiol.
    2020;76:1291–301.
51. Neuhold S, Huelsmann M, Pernicka E, et al. Impact
    of tricuspid regurgitation on survival in patients
    with chronic heart failure: unexpected findings
    of a long-term observational study. Eur Heart J.
    2013;34:844–52.
52. Park JB, Kim HK, Jung JH, et al. Prognostic value of
    cardiac MR imaging for preoperative assessment of
    patients with severe functional tricuspid regurgitation.
    Radiology. 2016;280:723–34.
53. Kim HK, Kim YJ, Park EA, et al. Assessment of
    haemodynamic effects of surgical correction for
    severe functional tricuspid regurgitation: cardiac
    magnetic resonance imaging study. Eur Heart J.
    2010;31:1520–8.
54. Taramasso M, Benfari G, van der Bijl P, et al.
    Transcatheter versus medical treatment of patients
    with symptomatic severe tricuspid regurgitation. J Am
    Coll Cardiol. 2019;74:2998–3008.
55. Bodhey NK, Beerbaum P, Sarikouch S, et al.
    Functional analysis of the components of the right
    ventricle in the setting of tetralogy of Fallot. Circ
    Cardiovasc Imaging. 2008;1:141–7.
56. Sheehan FH, Ge S, Vick GW III, et al. Three-
    dimensional shape analysis of right ventricular
    remodeling in repaired tetralogy of Fallot. Am J
    Cardiol. 2008;101:107–13.
57. Eyskens B, Brown SC, Claus P, et al. The influence of
    pulmonary regurgitation on regional right ventricular
    function in children after surgical repair of tetralogy
    of Fallot. Eur J Echocardiogr. 2010;11:341–5.
58. Dragulescu A, Grosse-Wortmann L, Redington A,
    Friedberg MK, Mertens L. Differential effect of
    right ventricular dilatation on myocardial defor-
    mation in patients with atrial septal defects and
    patients after tetralogy of Fallot repair. Int J Cardiol.
    2013;168:803–10.
59. Dragulescu A, Friedberg MK, Grosse-Wortmann L,
    Redington A, Mertens L. Effect of chronic right ven-
    tricular volume overload on ventricular interaction
    in patients after tetralogy of Fallot repair. J Am Soc
    Echocardiogr. 2014;27:896–902.
60. Liang XC, Cheung EW, Wong SJ, Cheung YF. Impact
    of right ventricular volume overload on three-
    dimensional global left ventricular mechanical dys-
    synchrony after surgical repair of tetralogy of Fallot.
    Am J Cardiol. 2008;102:1731–6.
61. Sjoberg P, Toger J, Hedstrom E, et al. Altered biven-
    tricular hemodynamic forces in patients with repaired
    tetralogy of Fallot and right ventricular volume
    overload because of pulmonary regurgitation. Am J
    Physiol Heart Circ Physiol. 2018;315:H1691–H702.
62. Hui W, Slorach C, Dragulescu A, Mertens L, Bijnens
    B, Friedberg MK. Mechanisms of right ventricular
    electromechanical dyssynchrony and mechanical
    inefficiency in children after repair of tetralogy of fal-
    lot. Circ Cardiovasc Imaging. 2014;7:610–8.
63. Wald RM, Haber I, Wald R, Valente AM, Powell AJ,
    Geva T. Effects of regional dysfunction and late gado-
    linium enhancement on global right ventricular func-
    tion and exercise capacity in patients with repaired
    tetralogy of Fallot. Circulation. 2009;119:1370–7.
64. Yoo BW, Kim JO, Kim YJ, et al. Impact of pressure
    load caused by right ventricular outflow tract obstruc-
    tion on right ventricular volume overload in patients
    with repaired tetralogy of Fallot. J Thorac Cardiovasc
    Surg. 2012;143:1299–304.
65. Maskatia SA, Spinner JA, Morris SA, Petit CJ,
    Krishnamurthy R, Nutting AC. Effect of branch pul-
    monary artery stenosis on right ventricular volume
    overload in patients with tetralogy of Fallot after ini-
    tial surgical repair. Am J Cardiol. 2013;111:1355–60.

66. Sanchez-Quintana D, Anderson RH, Ho SY. Ventricular myoarchitecture in tetralogy of Fallot. Heart. 1996;76:280–6.
67. Shimazaki Y, Blackstone EH, Kirklin JW. The natural history of isolated congenital pulmonary valve incompetence: surgical implications. Thorac Cardiovasc Surg. 1984;32:257–9.
68. El-Harasis MA, Connolly HM, Miranda WR, et al. Progressive right ventricular enlargement due to pulmonary regurgitation: clinical characteristics of a "low-risk" group. Am Heart J. 2018;201:136–40.
69. Geva T, Mulder B, Gauvreau K, et al. Preoperative predictors of death and sustained ventricular tachycardia after pulmonary valve replacement in patients with repaired tetralogy of Fallot enrolled in the INDICATOR cohort. Circulation. 2018;138:2106–15.
70. Bokma JP, de Wilde KC, Vliegen HW, et al. Value of cardiovascular magnetic resonance imaging in noninvasive risk stratification in tetralogy of Fallot. JAMA Cardiol. 2017;2:678–83.
71. Therrien J, Provost Y, Merchant N, Williams W, Colman J, Webb G. Optimal timing for pulmonary valve replacement in adults after tetralogy of Fallot repair. Am J Cardiol. 2005;95:779–82.
72. Oosterhof T, van Straten A, Vliegen HW, et al. Preoperative thresholds for pulmonary valve replacement in patients with corrected tetralogy of Fallot using cardiovascular magnetic resonance. Circulation. 2007;116:545–51.
73. Henkens IR, van Straten A, Schalij MJ, et al. Predicting outcome of pulmonary valve replacement in adult tetralogy of Fallot patients. Ann Thorac Surg. 2007;83:907–11.
74. Frigiola A, Tsang V, Bull C, et al. Biventricular response after pulmonary valve replacement for right ventricular outflow tract dysfunction: is age a predictor of outcome? Circulation. 2008;118:S182–90.
75. Geva T, Gauvreau K, Powell AJ, et al. Randomized trial of pulmonary valve replacement with and without right ventricular remodeling surgery. Circulation. 2010;122:S201–8.
76. Lee C, Kim YM, Lee CH, et al. Outcomes of pulmonary valve replacement in 170 patients with chronic pulmonary regurgitation after relief of right ventricular outflow tract obstruction: implications for optimal timing of pulmonary valve replacement. J Am Coll Cardiol. 2012;60:1005–14.
77. Bokma JP, Winter MM, Oosterhof T, et al. Preoperative thresholds for mid-to-late haemodynamic and clinical outcomes after pulmonary valve replacement in tetralogy of Fallot. Eur Heart J. 2016;37:829–35.
78. Heng EL, Gatzoulis MA, Uebing A, et al. Immediate and midterm cardiac remodeling after surgical pulmonary valve replacement in adults with repaired tetralogy of Fallot: a prospective cardiovascular magnetic resonance and clinical study. Circulation. 2017;136:1703–13.
79. Lurz P, Nordmeyer J, Giardini A, et al. Early versus late functional outcome after successful percutaneous pulmonary valve implantation: are the acute effects of altered right ventricular loading all we can expect? J Am Coll Cardiol. 2011;57:724–31.
80. Pastor TA, Geva T, Lu M, et al. Relation of right ventricular dilation after pulmonary valve replacement to outcomes in patients with repaired tetralogy of Fallot. Am J Cardiol. 2020;125:977–81.
81. Van De Bruaene A, Buys R, Vanhees L, Delcroix M, Voigt JU, Budts W. Regional right ventricular deformation in patients with open and closed atrial septal defect. Eur J Echocardiogr. 2011;12:206–13.
82. Menting ME, van den Bosch AE, McGhie JS, et al. Ventricular myocardial deformation in adults after early surgical repair of atrial septal defect. Eur Heart J Cardiovasc Imaging. 2015;16:549–57.
83. Satoh A, Katayama K, Hiro T, et al. Effect of right ventricular volume overload on left ventricular diastolic function in patients with atrial septal defect. Jpn Circ J. 1996;60:758–66.
84. Walker RE, Moran AM, Gauvreau K, Colan SD. Evidence of adverse ventricular interdependence in patients with atrial septal defects. Am J Cardiol. 2004;93:1374–7, A6.
85. Hiraoka A, Symons R, Bogaert JA, et al. Assessment of long-term cardiac adaptation in adult patients with type II atrial septal defect: a cardiovascular magnetic resonance (CMR) study. Eur Radiol. 2021;31(4):1905–14.
86. Umemoto S, Sakamoto I, Abe K, et al. Preoperative threshold for normalizing right ventricular volume after transcatheter closure of adult atrial septal defect. Circ J. 2020;84:1312–9.
87. Du ZD, Cao QL, Koenig P, Heitschmidt M, Hijazi ZM. Speed of normalization of right ventricular volume overload after transcatheter closure of atrial septal defect in children and adults. Am J Cardiol. 2001;88:1450–3, A9.
88. Meyer RA, Korfhagen JC, Covitz W, Kaplan S. Long-term follow-up study after closure of secundum atrial septal defect in children: an echocardiographic study. Am J Cardiol. 1982;50:143–8.
89. Stephensen SS, Ostenfeld E, Kutty S, et al. Transcatheter closure of atrial septal defect in adults: time-course of atrial and ventricular remodeling and effects on exercise capacity. Int J Cardiovasc Imaging. 2019;35:2077–84.
90. McLaughlin VV, Presberg KW, Doyle RL, et al. Prognosis of pulmonary arterial hypertension: ACCP evidence-based clinical practice guidelines. Chest. 2004;126:78S–92S.

Right Ventricular Response to Pulmonary Arterial Hypertension and Chronic Thromboembolic Pulmonary Hypertension

Daniel N. Silverman, Chakradhari Inampudi, and Ryan J. Tedford

Introduction

Progressive pulmonary vascular remodeling belies both pulmonary arterial hypertension (PAH) and chronic thromboembolic pulmonary hypertension (CTEPH), though each condition is distinguished by distinct initial insults. Whereas PAH may be idiopathic or related to several identifiable causes (e.g., connective tissue diseases such as systemic sclerosis, drug exposure, viral infections, congenital cardiac disease with left-to-right shunting, or portal hypertension), CTEPH has a more clearly delineated etiology. In the setting of hypercoagulable states including inherited coagulopathies, malignancy, antiphospholipid antibody syndrome, or chronic inflammatory disorders, thromboemboli lead to obstruction of proximal and distal pulmonary arterioles resulting in compensatory overperfusion of the remaining non-occluded vessels which further contributes to arteriopathy.

Although the differences in fundamental etiology of PAH and CTEPH have meaningful ramifications with regard to treatment options, the response of the right ventricle (RV) is largely common to each condition. Independent of specific vascular pathobiology, the net effect of pulmonary arterial remodeling is an increase in pulmonary vascular resistance (PVR). PAH as well as other forms of precapillary pulmonary hypertension are defined by a resting mean pulmonary artery pressure (mPAP) of >20 mmHg with a PVR $\geq$3 Wood units [1]. The adaptation of the RV, while related to increased afterload, is also determined by preload and contractility.

Preload, representing wall tension during diastole, is closely tied to ventricular filling. Contractility, the intrinsic ability of the cardiomyocytes to stiffen, is a characteristic that is independent of preload and afterload. RV afterload is the RV wall stress that occurs during RV ejection and is influenced by several factors including the mean resistance, vascular compliance, and arterial wave reflections resulting from pulsatile blood flow. RV response to afterload and its adaptation are dictated by the laws of Frank-Starling (heterometric) and Anrep (homeometric) [2, 3]. As afterload increases to a threshold that overwhelms RV contractility and these compensatory mechanisms, ventricular dilatation and dysfunction ensue.

The relationship between the RV and its afterload is referred to as RV-pulmonary arterial (PA) coupling. In PAH and CTEPH, as afterload increases, RV-PA coupling is a primary determinant of outcomes, and the term "uncoupling" is used to describe a maladaptive relationship

D. N. Silverman · C. Inampudi · R. J. Tedford (✉)
Division of Cardiology, Department of Medicine, Medical University of South Carolina, Charleston, SC, USA
e-mail: dns200@musc.edu; tedfordr@musc.edu

between the ventricle and pulmonary vasculature [4]. While a progressive increase in RV afterload is a primary arbiter of RV failure, uncoupling is additionally influenced by neuroendocrine signaling as well as ensuing inflammation, fibrosis, ischemia, and myocyte death directly affecting the RV [5]. Here, the specific ways in which the RV responds in PAH and CTEPH, methods to assess RV function, and mechanisms that underlie maladaptive response are discussed.

RV Responses to Load

The normally thin-walled right ventricle is designed primarily as a director of systemic venous return rather than as a muscular pump [6]. Thus, it is not well suited to acute rises in wall stress, with experimental models intended to reproduce the effect of an acute rise in RV afterload—such as with a massive pulmonary embolism—producing acute dilation and pump failure [7, 8]. However, in contrast to the right ventricle's poor response to acute rises in afterload, chronic and gradual increases in volume and/or afterload are better tolerated. Under these circumstances, the RV is capable of remodeling with hypertrophy and adaptive autoregulation [9, 10].

The right ventricular response to load—whether preload or afterload—can be described more specifically in terms of heterometric or homeometric adaptations. The beat-to-beat variation in preload or afterload may result in heterometric adaptation, characterized by a change in ventricular geometry (dilatation under increased load) governed by the Frank-Starling mechanism. While this mechanism may allow rapid adaptation to changing preload or afterload, it does not allow for prolonged compensation. Acute and subacute changes in load may also be met with an adaptation in contractility, following the observation by von Anrep in 1912, where the sustained load is met with increased force production [3].

While von Anrep noted autocrine/paracrine responses stimulated by stretch as mediators of the increased contractility, subsequent investigation has clarified that further changes underly this

adaptation. Myocyte hypertrophy, proliferation of sarcomeres, and alterations in myofilament properties all take place as part of the remodeling that facilitates increasing contractility [3, 11–13]. At the myocyte level, the response to increased load is increased sarcolemmal Ca^{2+} influx through the Na^+/Ca^{2+} exchanger [14, 15]. Ultimately, these adaptations are accompanied by RV hypertrophy, allowing for a net reduction in wall stress and increased contractility [16].

RV Remodeling in Pulmonary Arterial Hypertension of Congenital Heart Disease

RV tolerance to increased afterload may be seen in PAH associated with congenital heart disease leading to Eisenmenger syndrome (ES) [17]. In such cases, time-dependent adaptations to increased load may best be exemplified, with the more chronic PAH developed in the setting of ES better tolerated than other forms of PAH [18]. Left-to-right shunting due to a congenital defect in ES ultimately leads to pulmonary vascular remodeling, increased PVR, increased RV afterload, and shunt reversal from right to left. This process, which typically occurs over years if not decades, yields a considerably better prognosis with regard to RV function when compared with the development of PAH later in life, at least in part due to the early and persistent exposure of the right ventricle to afterload [19].

RV Remodeling in Chronic Thromboembolic Hypertension

RV afterload can be described as a combination of both resistive and capacitive loads. More specifically, left atrial pressure, pulmonary vascular compliance, and PVR are physiologic components of afterload imparted upon the RV. In CTEPH, both proximal and distal vasculopathies contribute to elevated RV afterload. As opposed to the systemic circulation, the proximal vessels in the lung vasculature account for about only 20% of the vascular compliance, or blood storage capacity of the system [20]. Therefore, proximal obstructive lesions, which do not increase PVR, also have little impact on vascular compliance and pulsatile afterload [21]. Despite this, a few recent studies have suggested that proximal obstructive lesions may impart an additional load by altering the propagation of the pressure wave during RV ejection [22, 23]. The potential impacts of these findings on RV function are yet to be fully elucidated.

Most features of RV remodeling in response to increased afterload appear to be common between PAH and CTEPH. A feature of RV remodeling unique to CTEPH, however, may include RV-LV dyssynchrony (electrical and mechanical) [21]. In a prospective MRI study of 17 CTEPH patients, improvement in RV remodeling parameters (reduction in right ventricular mass, size, and strain) following surgical pulmonary endarterectomy (PEA) was noted. Following PEA, an initial decline in RV function as diagnosed by TAPSE is noted, likely due to postoperative changes in global heart mass; it subsequently improves but is incomplete by 1 year [24]. Multiple studies performed to date evaluated the RV remodeling process by evaluating RV geometry, RV ejection fraction (EF), and RV myocardial deformation in CTEPH patients post-PEA. These studies have noted reverse remodeling of the right heart following PEA with improvement in RV and RA dimensions, RV global longitudinal strain, and RV global circumferential strain. It is important to note that RV-PA coupling also improved following PEA but did not return to normal [25–30]. Specifically, RV reserve remained impaired, driven at least in part by chronotropic incompetence [31, 32].

Assessment of RV Contractility

Echocardiography and cardiac magnetic resonance imaging are valuable noninvasive tools capable of providing a global assessment of RV systolic function. However, they are limited in their ability to assess RV contractility due to the load-dependent nature of stroke volume-based measures. The gold standard by which RV contractility is characterized is pressure-volume (PV) relations obtained through invasive hemodynamic evaluation. Such studies allow measurement of both end-systolic elastance (E_{es})—a largely load-independent measure of contractility—and RV afterload, estimated as pulmonary arterial elastance (E_a).

Echocardiography

Due to its relative ubiquity and ease of use, echocardiography is a critical diagnostic tool for the evaluation of pulmonary hypertension and RV function. It is often the first diagnostic test to identify and initiate the workup of undifferentiated pulmonary hypertension as well as a prognostic tool [33, 34]. Nonetheless, it is not without significant limitations. The use of tissue Doppler imaging to obtain tricuspid annular plane systolic excursion (TAPSE) showed promise as a prognostic marker in an early study of subjects with PAH, but subsequent evaluation has revealed less robust predictive capacity [35, 36]. In particular, TAPSE performed more poorly in predicting outcomes in those patients with more advanced symptoms and a greater degree of RV dilatation [35]. Other two-dimensional echocardiography measures of RV function include RV fractional area change (shortening), which has also been shown to predict survival [35]. Less commonly employed due to the more time-intensive nature of its derivation is the RV myocardial performance index, which is a composite measure of both systolic and diastolic function that may also predict survival [35].

More sophisticated methods of echocardiographic imaging including 3D echocardiography longitudinal strain also hold promise. 3D echocardiography is capable of better capturing the challenging RV geometry including the right ventricular outflow tract. Thus, it allows better quantitation of RV function, with established reference values validated against cardiac MRI-derived volume measurements [37]. RV longitudinal strain, applied to either 2D or 3D echocardiography, offers another method for predicting survival amongst patients with pulmonary hypertension [38].

Cardiac Magnetic Resonance Imaging

Although 3D echocardiography has made considerable gains in its ability to reproduce high-fidelity RV volumes, cardiac MRI (cMRI) remains the gold standard for noninvasive assessment of RV morphology and function. A simple assessment of chamber volumes, as well as stroke volume obtained by cMRI, possesses prognostic value [39]. RV mass has also independently been shown to prognosticate outcomes in PAH [40]. Beyond simple measurements, indices including RV stroke volume/end-systolic volume ratio and RV mass/volume ratio offer a further characterization of prognosis particularly as it relates to therapeutic response and functional impairment [41, 42]. Just as with the application of strain with echocardiography, cMRI strain offers high-fidelity measurement of RV regional myocardial deformation. Studies measuring deformation using feature tracking have been shown to correlate with increasing RV end-diastolic volume and impaired diastolic function in chronic pressure overload states [43].

cMRI offers additional capabilities, particularly with the utilization of delayed enhancement imaging and T1 mapping. Delayed enhancement imaging using gadolinium contrast has revealed novel applications to both diagnose pulmonary hypertension and predict adverse outcomes. Specifically, delayed enhancement at the insertion point of the RV strongly associates with elevated mPAP and adverse outcomes in patients with PAH [44]. T1 mapping allows diffuse characterization of myocardial tissue and may allow sensitive detection of fibrosis in conditions including PAH, along with associated other measures of interest like end-diastolic stiffness [43].

Pressure-Volume Loops

End-Systolic Elastance as a Measure of RV Contractility

Whereas echocardiography and cMRI offer detailed quantification of chamber sizes and measures of RV performance, their assessment is indirect and affected by loading conditions. The gold standard for characterizing RV function, and more specifically RV contractility, is through pressure-volume (PV) relations. Based on the observation that the LV stiffens and relaxes predictably during the cardiac cycle, it was determined that ventricular elastance was conserved and independent from the load [45]. Thus, when a family of PV loops is produced during preload reduction, a linear regression line (or "isochrone") can be fit connecting the pressure-volume points on each loop and at the same time from the onset of the cardiac cycle. The intercept of the regression line with volume at a time t represents $V_0(t)$, the slope of each regression line is the time-varying elastance $((E)t)$, and the isochrone with the greatest slope (maximum ratio of end-systolic pressure (ESP) to end-systolic volume (ESV)) represents the maximum elastance (E_{max}) [45, 46]. While this approach was first described in the left ventricle, there was subsequent adoption for the RV [47] (Fig. 9.1). This method has two significant limitations, however.

Because the time to reach end systole varies depending on load, the isochrone with maximal slope does not necessarily fit the outer boundary of the family of PV loops (where, as described above, the points on each loop were connected at the same time point from the onset of the cardiac cycle). Rather, to find the maximum elastance, the maximal ratio of pressure and volume is determined for each loop independent of cardiac cycle timing. An approach connecting the points of end systole rather than at a specific time in the cardiac cycle allows the end-systolic pressure-volume relationship (ESPVR) slope to be calculated, and this slope represents end-systolic elastance (E_{es}) [48] (Fig. 9.2). V_0, in this method independent of time, is determined based on the volume intercept of the isochrone associated with the maximum pressure/volume ratio [48]. E_{es}, then, represents a similar but different measure than E_{max}, accounting for the effects of load on the duration of systole and providing a more accurate assessment of contractility in a relatively load-independent fashion.

Though clearly the gold standard for the assessment of ventricular function, multi-beat PV relation (Fig. 9.3a) is not suitable for clinical

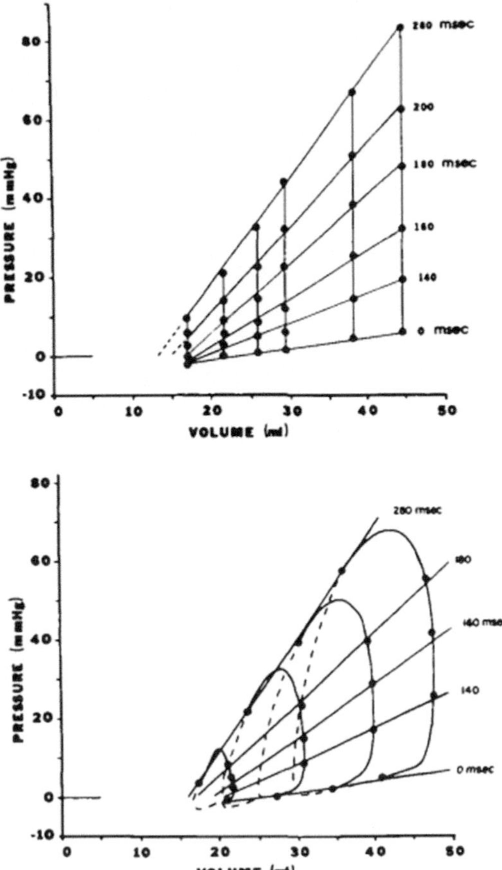

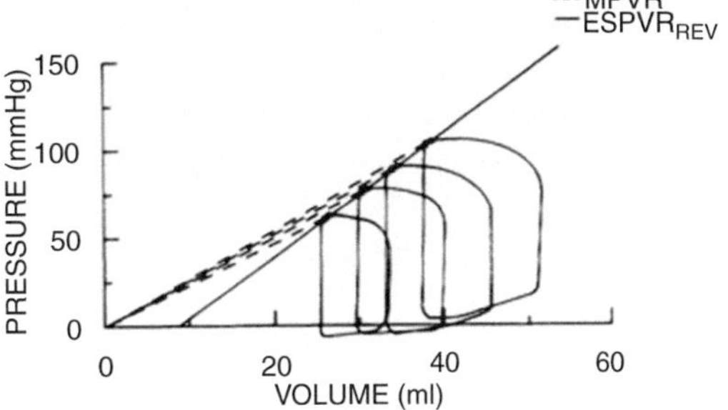

Fig. 9.2 A comparison of mean pressure-volume relationship (MPVR) ignoring V_0 (dotted lines) and the end-systolic pressure-volume relationship (ESPVR$_{REF}$) (solid line). MPVR varies with each loading condition. The four MPVR points (xs) are used to calculate the ESPVR$_{REF}$. The volume-axis intercept (V_0) derived from this first approximation is then used to determine the end-systolic P–V points (solid dots) and a new ESPVR$_{REF}$ is determined. The iterative process is repeated until V_0 does not change. (Reproduced from Kono, A., Maughan, W. L., Sunagawa, K., Hamilton, K., Sagawa, K., & Weisfeldt, M. L. (1984). The use of left ventricular end-ejection pressure and peak pressure in the estimation of the end-systolic pressure-volume relationship. Circulation, 70(6), 1057–1065. https://doi.org/10.1161/01.CIR.70.6.1057)

Fig. 9.1 Isochronal data points and the calculated regression lines for a set of isovolumetric (upper panel) and ejection (lower panel) beats. (Reproduced from Maughan, W. L., Shoukas, A. A., Sagawa, K., & Weisfeldt, M. L. (1979). Instantaneous pressure-volume relationship of the canine right ventricle. Circ Res, 44(3), 309–315. https://doi.org/10.1161/01.res.44.3.309)

practice given its complexity and requirement for specialized equipment. Consideration for simpler methods that would allow calculation of E_{es} led to the concept that a single heartbeat might be sufficient [49]. While initially tested and validated in the left ventricle [50, 51], a subsequent study revealed that E_{es} can also be estimated for the RV in a single-beat method, Brimioulle and colleagues championed a similar approach for the RV [52, 53]. By fitting a sine curve to the isovolumic portions of the RV pressure tracing, P_{max} is determined (Fig. 9.3b). P_{max} is the theoretical pressure that the RV could generate if ejecting into the infinite load. P_{max} can then be paired with

EDV, and the slope of the line through (P_{max}, EDV) and (ESP, ESV) represents E_{es}(sb) (Fig. 9.3c). In the Brimioulle study, P_{max} compared favorably to maximal RV pressure generated during acute occlusion of canine pulmonary arteries. However, the use of the single-beat estimate for diagnostic and prognostic purposes has yielded mixed results [54–58].

Inuzuka and colleagues did not find a strong correlation between E_{es}(sb) and E_{es} derived from multi-beat measures, although the correlation was better in subjects with lower E_{es} [55]. A more recent evaluation showed a good correlation with multi-beat-derived measures of contractility in a study of patients with predominant PAH (36 with PAH, 2 with CTEPH) [56]. Compared with the Inuzuka cohort, the Richter cohort had lower resting RV function. Although the Richter study also found that single-beat measures of contractility and RV-PA coupling were associated with time to clinical worsening, two prior studies had failed to illustrate similar prognostic value [57, 58].

One significant challenge of the SBE approach is the selection of the isovolumic periods on the

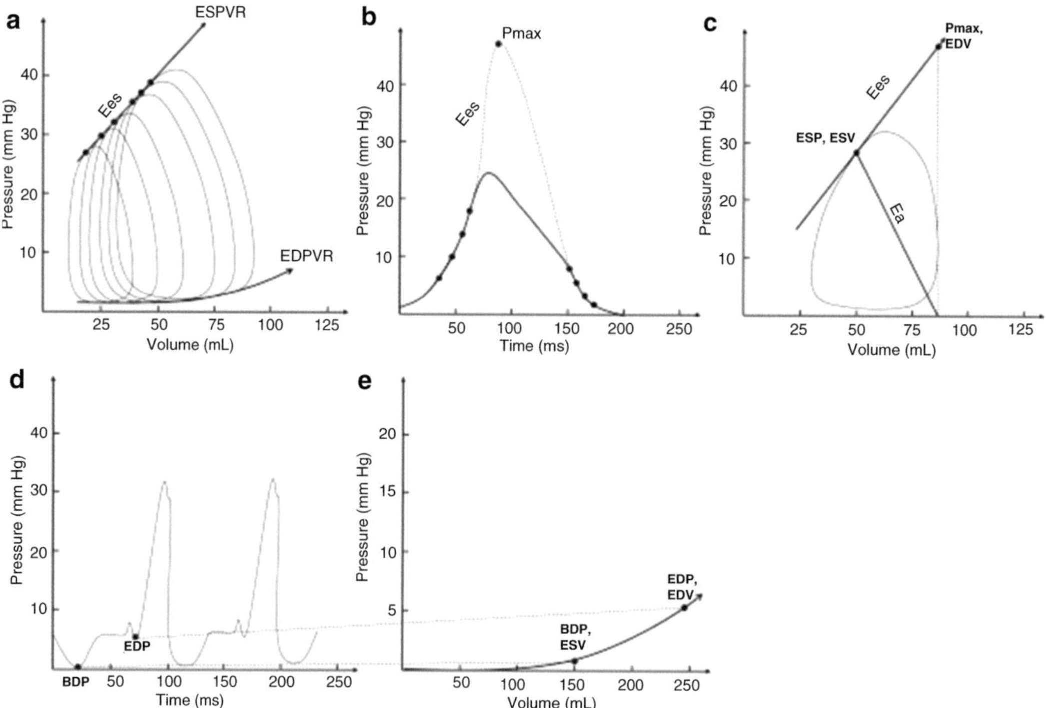

Fig. 9.3 Single-beat and multi-beat estimates of ESPVR and end-diastolic PV relationships (EDPVR). (**a**) PV loops during preload reduction. ESPVR is derived by connecting end-systolic points; its slope is the E_{es}. EDPVR, which is curvilinear, is defined by fitting end-diastolic points. (**b, c**) Single-beat estimation of ESPVR using Brimioulle and colleagues' method. Peak isovolumetric pressure (P_{max}) was extrapolated by fitting a sine curve to the isovolumetric portions of the RV pressure tracing. (**c**) A straight line is used to connect P_{max} to the RV PV diagram to form the ESPVR line; its slope is E_{es}. A line connecting the end-systolic point to end diastole is also drawn; its slope E_a. (**d, e**) Single-beat estimation of EDPVR. (**d**) End-diastolic volume (EDV) is combined with end-diastolic pressure (EDP), and end-systolic volume (ESV) is combined with beginning-diastolic pressure (BDP). (**e**) Fitting of a nonlinear expositional curve through the derived points. (Reproduced from El Hajj MC, Viray MC, Tedford RJ. Right Heart Failure: A Hemodynamic Review. Cardiol Clin. 2020;38(2):161–73)

RV pressure tracing, where inclusion or exclusion of a single time point can dramatically impact the calculated P_{max}. One study has suggested a second derivative approach to minimize interobserver variability in the estimation of isovolumic pressure [59].

Pulmonary Arterial Elastance as a Measure of Afterload

Pulmonary arterial elastance (E_a) represents a merging of the resistive and pulsatile components of afterload. While generally accepted as a reliable measure of afterload, E_a is not a direct measure of ventricular wall stress nor is it as comprehensive as pulmonary artery input imped-

ance, the latter of which requires simultaneous measures of pressure and flow [18]. Consolidation of arterial load into arterial elastance utilizing a three Windkessel model was proposed in the mid-1980s [16]. Here, E_a was a parameter that included total mean resistance, systolic and diastolic time intervals, and diastolic pressure decay time constant τ (tau) [60]. Again, these models were initially studied in the context of the LV and systemic circulation but subsequently tested and validated to evaluate RV-PA interactions [61, 62]. Kelly and Kass determined that the Windkessel E_a could be approximated by taking the ratio of end-systolic pressure to stroke volume (ESP/SV) obtained via PV loop [63]. Conveniently, ESP/

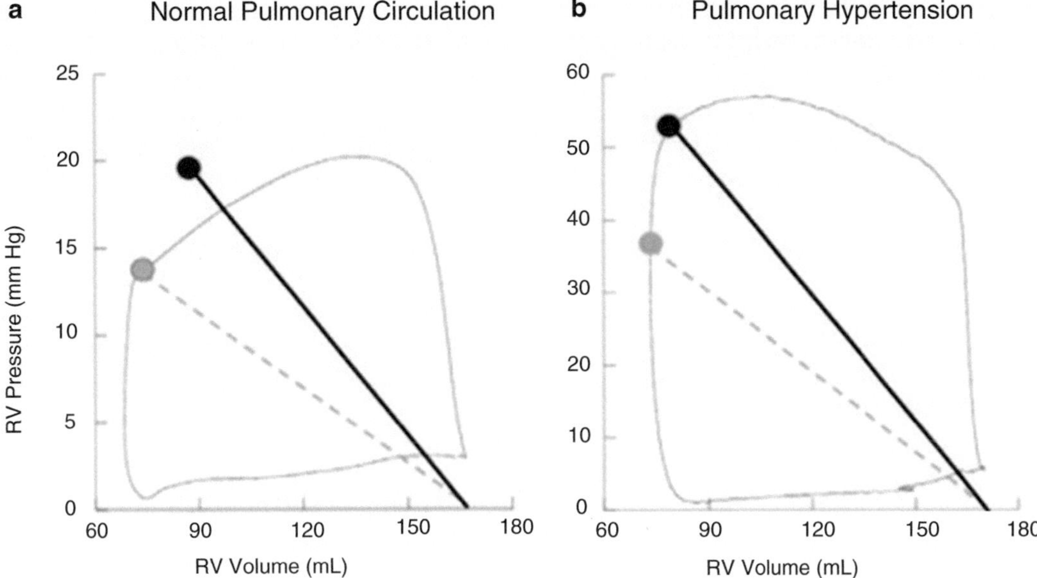

Fig. 9.4 (a) Normal pulmonary circulation-right ventricular (RV) pressure declines throughout ejection, RV systolic pressure overestimates end-systolic pressure, and end-ejection volume may be lower than end-systolic volume. Effective arterial elastance (E_a) estimated using systolic pulmonary artery pressure (solid black line) likely overestimates RV afterload. Gray dashed line represents E_a estimated using mean pulmonary artery pressure and end-ejection volume. (b) Pulmonary hypertension-RV pressure rises throughout ejection and peaks at end systole. End-ejection and end-systolic volume are similar. E_a (solid black line) is a better representation of total RV load than E_a (dashed gray line). (Reproduced from Tedford, R. J., Hsu, S., & Kass, D. A. (2020). Letter by Tedford et al Regarding Article, "Effective Arterial Elastance in the Pulmonary Arterial Circulation: Derivation, Assumptions, and Clinical Applications". Circulation. Heart failure, 13(5), e007081. https://doi.org/10.1161/circheartfailure.120.007081)

SV provides pressure as a function of volume (mmHg/ml), the same units as E_{es}, allowing comparison of a ratio of elastances, E_{es}/E_a, to characterize RV-PA coupling [18].

E_a, when estimated as ESP/SV, can be calculated noninvasively [10, 64, 65]. In the absence of pulmonary vascular pathology, the RV ejects into a low-impedance circuit and pressure falls throughout ejection (Fig. 9.4a). Therefore, ESP is best estimated as mean pulmonary artery pressure (mPAP) [66]. However, in even mild PAH, pressure rises throughout ejection and peaks near end systole (Fig. 9.4b). Therefore, RV systolic pressure or systolic pulmonary artery pressure is a better estimate of ESP than mPAP [67, 68]. Two studies have demonstrated that the use of mPAP underestimates ESP in the setting of PH [69, 70]. More importantly, the E_{es}/E_a (RV-PA coupling ratio) is significantly overestimated [68, 69].

Preload Recruitable Stroke Work as a Measure of Contractility

Another metric that describes intrinsic cardiac function is preload recruitable stroke work (PRSW). PRSW, denoted as M_{sw}, can be obtained via a ventricular function curve by plotting RV performance (stroke work) against preload (EDV). When RV contractility is increased, the stroke work versus preload relationship shifts upward, and when contractility is decreased the opposite occurs. Measuring PRSW also requires a family of PV relationships over a range of volumes just as with E_{es}. Some studies have suggested that the PRSW relationship is more linear and more load insensitive than E_{es} as a measure of RV contractility [71]. A single-beat approach has also been developed [55]. Despite the favorable characteristics of M_{sw}, the inability to couple it to afterload with similar units makes describing RV-PA coupling more difficult.

Alterations in RV Contractility and Ventricular-Arterial Coupling in PAH and CTEPH

Assessment of the interaction between the right ventricle and its afterload—described as RV-PA coupling—is critical to the characterization of RV function and prognostication in PAH and CTEPH.

Pressure-Volume Loop Evaluation of RV-Pulmonary Arterial Coupling

In PAH, homeometric adaptation, hypertrophy, and associated remodeling lead to increased contractility allowing maintenance of "coupling" early on, with E_{es} increasing as E_a also rises. The normal ratio between these values for the left (and right) ventricle is generally agreed to be between 1.5 and 2.0 [16]. A more recent evaluation of the RV in an animal model has identified that maximal RV stroke work occurs at an E_{es}/E_a ratio of around 1.0, with uncoupling occurring around 0.7 [72].

A falling E_{es}/E_a reflects this uncoupling of RV-PA interactions, with afterload outstripping the ability of the RV to adapt. Filling pressures rise and the clinical syndrome of RV failure develops. The reason for the failure of homeometric adaptation in certain individuals and not others, as well as timing, remains unclear. However, RV uncoupling may be seen earlier than clinical RV failure before the morphological changes seen in the RV manifest as ventricular dilation and reduced mass/volume ratio [43].

RV-PA Coupling Predicts Outcomes in PAH

Two recent studies are the first to show the prognostic value of multi-beat measures of RV-PA coupling. The first study found multi-beat E_{es}/E_a with an optimal cut point of 0.7 to be an independent predictor of time to clinical worsening defined as a reduction in 6-min walk test dis-

tance, worsening functional class, or clinical deterioration requiring hospital admission [56]. These findings correlated with prior data from the same group that had suggested an E_{es}/E_a cutoff of 0.805 to be associated with the onset of RV failure characterized by increased RV volumes and RV ejection fraction <35% [73]. The second study, which included subjects with more preserved RVEF (mean 49%), found a similar E_{es}/E_a ratio (0.65) to discriminate subjects with clinical worsening [74]. Traditional measures of RV function and volume were not different between groups.

Echocardiography Evaluation of RV-Arterial Coupling

Several echocardiographic approaches have been taken to develop imaging surrogates describing RV-arterial coupling. In one approach, the ratio between TAPSE/RV end-systolic area was taken to equal contractility while PASP/SV was taken to equal afterload. The ratio, then, of TAPSE/PASP was used to describe RV-arterial coupling in a study of patients with heart failure [75]. TAPSE/PASP ratio has been shown to correlate modestly with invasive measures of RV-PA coupling as well as functional class and other clinical markers [76, 77].

cMRI Evaluation of RV-PA Coupling

Methods attempting to avoid any (invasive) catheter-derived measurements to assess RV-PA coupling have been attempted. If E_{es} = (ESP, ESV − V_0), and E_a = (ESP/SV), E_{es}/E_a simplifies to (SV/ESV − V_0). If one can assume that V_0 is negligible, then E_{es}/E_a would equal SV/ESV [78]. Although this method is appealing and has prognostic value, the assumption that the volume of an unloaded right ventricle (V_0) is minimal is incorrect [79]. Indeed, several studies have shown that this approach underestimates E_{es} [80–82]. One more recent study has suggested that V_0 may be estimated as $-50.01 + 0.7 \times$ ESV, though this requires addi-

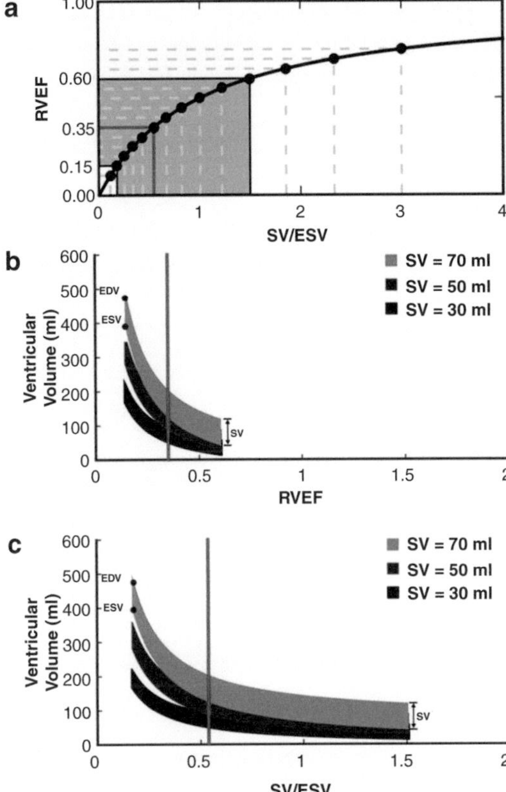

Fig. 9.5 (**a**) Nonlinear relationship between right ventricular ejection fraction (RVEF) and stroke volume (SV) to end-systolic volume (ESV). The gray region shows the pulmonary hypertension RVEF range (0.15–0.60) and the red line shows the RVEF and corresponding SV/ESV cutoff value that is predictive of outcomes. (**b, c**) Nonlinear relationship between ventricular volumes (end-diastolic volume (EDV) and ESV) and RVEF and SV/ESV at a given SV. As RVEF and SV/ESV decrease, to maintain stroke volume ventricular volumes have to increase or there needs to be changes in contractility. The red line shows the RVEF and corresponding SV/ESV cutoff value that has been shown to be predictive of outcomes. (Reproduced from Vanderpool RR, Rischard F, Naeije R, Hunter K, Simon MA. Simple functional imaging of the right ventricle in pulmonary hypertension: Can right ventricular ejection fraction be improved? Int J Cardiol. 2016;223:93–4)

tional validation [56]. It is also important to realize that SV/ESV is mathematically related to RVEF [79]. However, because of the larger physiological range and greater sensitivity to change resulting from its nonlinear relationship to RVEF (Fig. 9.5), SV/ESV may be a better predictor of outcome [79].

RV-PA Coupling and Disease

The specific circumstances leading to uncoupling in some individuals but not others with similar comorbidities remain an area of active investigation. Nonetheless, several studies have attempted to characterize RV-PA coupling in specific disease states or syndromes.

RV-PA Coupling in Idiopathic PAH and Systemic Sclerosis-Associated PAH

Patients with systemic sclerosis (SSc)-associated PAH are known to have worse survival than individuals with idiopathic PAH. Several studies have now shown impairments in RV contractility (Fig. 9.6), RV-PA coupling, and RV reserve in SSc-PAH compared with IPAH [81, 82]. Although some have suggested reduced hypertrophy for a given level of afterload [83], larger studies have not supported this observation [84]. Global RV contractile deficits have been attributed to a myofilament abnormality in the SSc-PAH group [12]. Maximal force generation from isolated, skinned myocytes (obtained from RV septal biopsies) has confirmed a deficit in the myocyte contractile apparatus (Fig. 9.7). Importantly force-calcium measures from these single myocytes obtained from the RV septum correlated well with global measures of RV contractility.

Perhaps just as interesting, IPAH subjects had supercontractile force generation compared with controls, which correlates with increased global E_{es}. This increase in E_{es} and myocyte contractility seems to be preserved even in end-stage disease [85]. This would suggest afterload as the primary culprit in RV-PA uncoupling.

RV-PA Coupling in Congenital Heart Disease

Under the umbrella of PAH related to congenital heart disease are a wide range of underlying pathology, anatomical insults, and surgical inter-

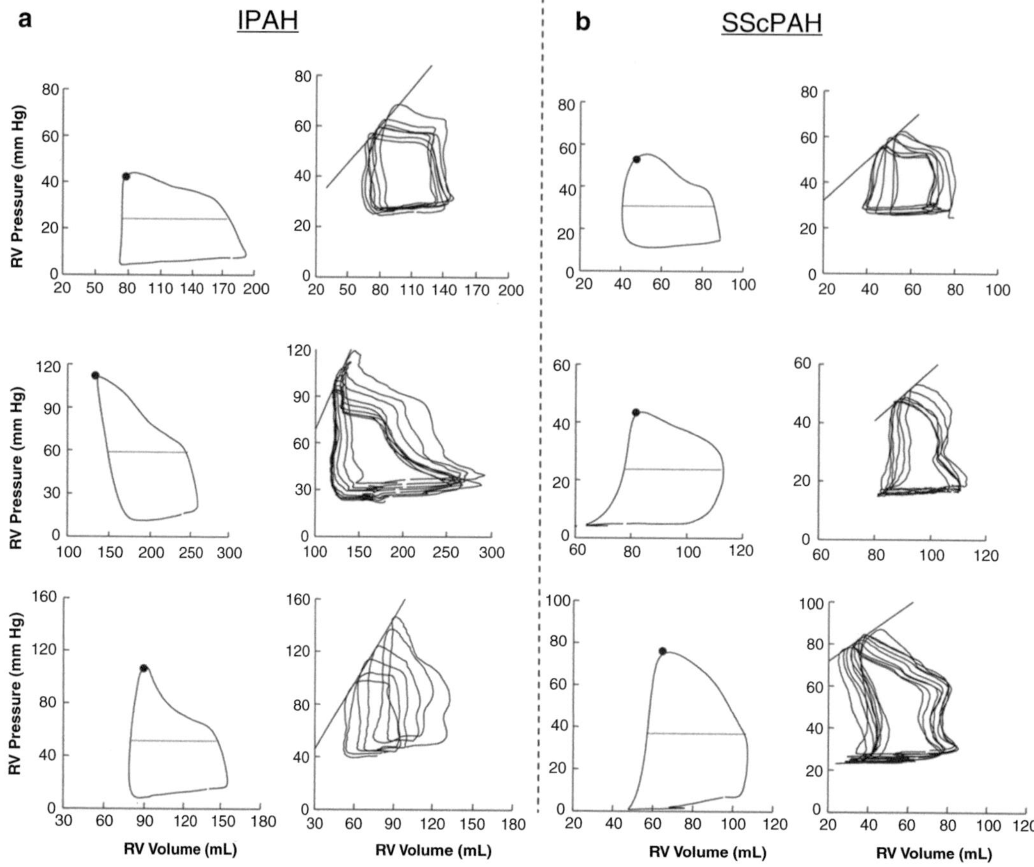

Fig. 9.6 Right ventricular (RV) pressure-volume loops in six patients, three with (**a**) idiopathic pulmonary arterial hypertension (IPAH) and three with (**b**) systemic sclerosis-associated pulmonary artery hypertension (SSc-PAH). Steady-state loops (left) in both cohorts show RV pressure rising throughout ejection and peaking at end systole, consistent with increased RV afterload from PAH. The black dot identifies the end-systolic pressure-volume point, and the dashed line mean loop width (stroke volume). E_a was determined by the ratio of end-systolic pressure to SV. In the loops generated during Valsalva maneuver (right), the data are all shifted upward because of the rise in intrathoracic pressure, but while this is held, phase 2 of the Valsalva maneuver results in a beat-to-beat decline in filling volume and various PV relations including the end-systolic pressure-volume relationship (black line). The slope is end-systolic elastance (E_{es}). (Reproduced from Tedford RJ, Mudd JO, Girgis RE, et al. Right ventricular dysfunction in systemic sclerosis associated pulmonary arterial hypertension. Circulation Heart Fail 2013; 6: 953–963)

ventions. Nonetheless, specific conditions have provided unique insights into the ways that the RV may adapt in the setting of increased load. A study of subjects who had undergone surgical repair of tetralogy of Fallot (TOF) and who had developed subsequent RV dilatation was undertaken using pressure-volume loops at baseline and with inotrope (dobutamine) infusion. While there was an increase in E_{es} with inotrope infusion, RV-PA coupling remained significantly impaired. Interestingly, uncoupling appeared to be related to the type of repair that subjects had

undergone, with transannular patch repair associated with greater uncoupling in response to dobutamine compared with a transatrial approach [86]. In a separate retrospective study, adults with TOF with at least moderate pulmonary regurgitation and preserved RV ejection fraction were compared to propensity-matched adults with normal RVEF. RV-PA coupling was assessed using the echo-derived method outlined by Guazzi et al. RV-PA coupling was significantly lower in the group with TOF despite both groups having normal RVEF [87].

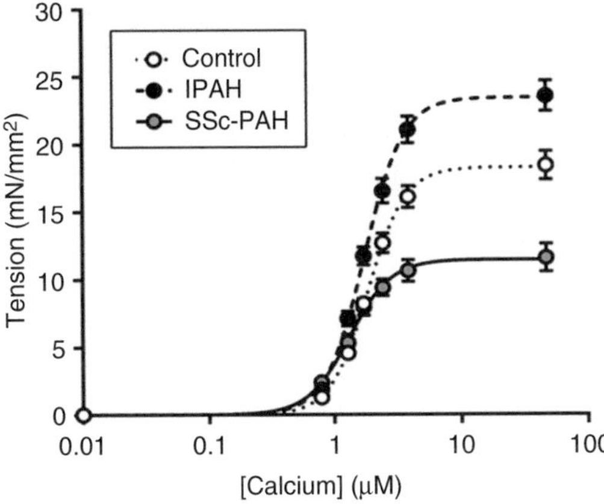

Fig. 9.7 Force-calcium data were obtained in nonfailing control, IPAH, and SSc-associated pulmonary arterial hypertension (PAH) myocytes to obtain maximal calcium-activated tension (F_{max}) and calcium sensitivity (EC_{50}) ($n = 7$ subjects per group). (Reproduced from Hsu S, Kokkonen-Simon KM, Kirk JA, Kolb TM, Damico RL, Mathai SC, et al. Right Ventricular Myofilament Functional Differences in Humans with Systemic Sclerosis-Associated Versus Idiopathic Pulmonary Arterial Hypertension. Circulation. 2018;137(22):2360–70)

RV-PA Coupling in CTEPH

In chronic thromboembolic disease (CTED), RV-PA coupling has been compared amongst individuals with and without associated pulmonary hypertension. In a study employing MRI-validated volumes and conductance catheter-derived PV loops, both E_{es} and E_a were noted to be lower in the CTED group compared with CTEPH. However, RV-PA coupling was reduced only in those with CTEPH [88]. Subsequent confirmed similar findings, though with a small proportion of patients with CTED, were also found to have impaired RV-PA coupling consistent with occult RV dysfunction [72].

Sex Differences in RV-PA Coupling

Amongst patients with IPAH, women tend to have comparatively higher RV ejection fractions than men, suggesting the possibility that sex-dependent differences in RV contractility and RV-PA coupling might exist [89]. In a prospective study of subjects with PAH or CTEPH which assessed RV function by multi-beat RV-PA coupling [90], female subjects had significantly higher E_{es} and E_{es}/E_a than male patients. Measures of diastolic function and RV mass index were also lower in female subjects. The mass/volume ratio in female subjects, however, did not differ from males, which has previously been associated with clinical worsening in PAH [41]. Collectively, these findings suggest that female patients with PAH may have higher contractility and more preserved RV-PA coupling than males, which might explain the superior survival seen in female patients with PAH [89].

RV Reserve

The capability of the ventricle to augment contractility for a given degree of loading can be determined using exercise or pharmacologic stress testing (such as with dobutamine infusion) and is referred to as RV contractile reserve [91]. RV contractile reserve may also be associated with resting RV-PA coupling, offering a less invasive surrogate [92]. A more recent study comparing patients with IPAH with SSc-PAH showed that patients with SSC-PAH were unable to augment contractility during submaximal exercise. To maintain stroke volume, the RV dilated (heterometric adaptation) resulting in increasing RV EDV (and as a result, a decline in RVEF) compared with IPAH subjects [82] (Fig. 9.8). Beyond its use to evaluate the severity of RV dysfunction, RV reserve may be useful in detecting subclinical RV failure in PAH even when resting measures of RV function appear normal [93, 94]. Finally, RV contractile reserve may provide prognostic value, having been shown to correlate well with clinical measures (6-min walk distance, peak VO_2) as well as survival [95].

Mechanisms Underlying Maladaptive RV Adaptation in PAH

Despite pulmonary vascular disease providing the stimulus, it is the adaptation and then decline of RV function with concomitant decoupling

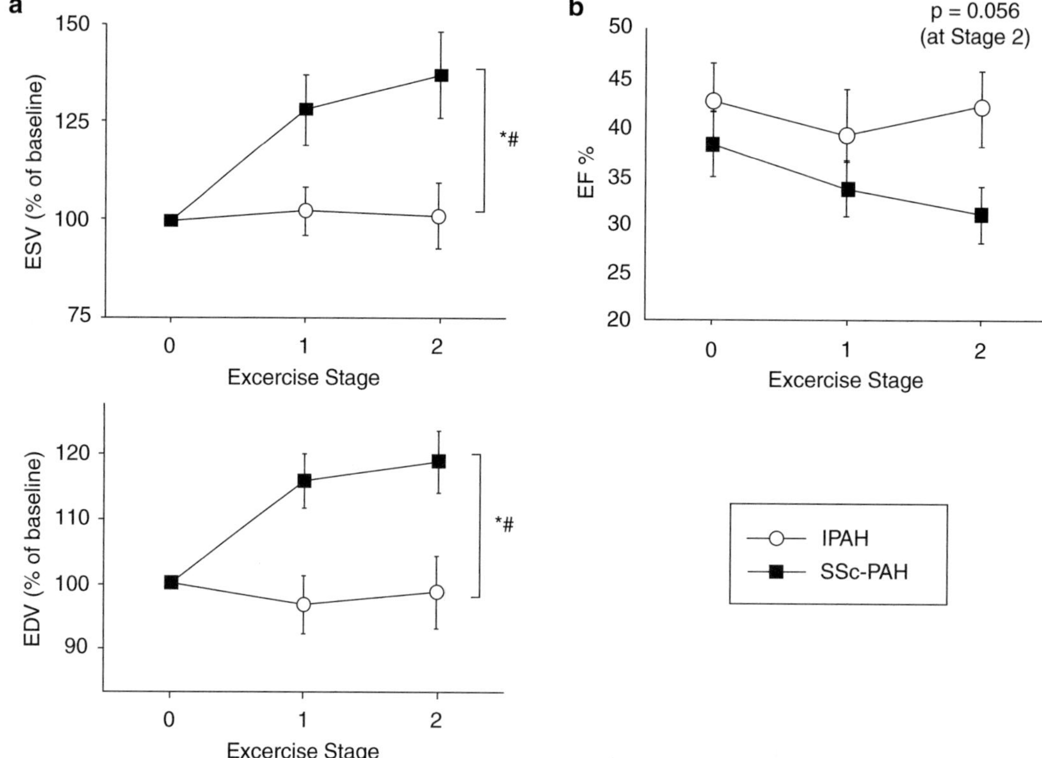

Fig. 9.8 Exercise changes in RV end-systolic volume (ESV) and end-diastolic volume (EDV): (**a**) Percent change in ESV and EDV plotted for each group from exercise stage 0–2. SSc-PAH subjects had acutely increased ESV and EDV, whereas IPAH subjects maintained stable RV volumes with increasing workload because of increase in contractility (**b**) Even though stroke volume is concerned due to Frank-Starling mechanism, RVEF declined in SSc-PAH vs. IPAH with increasing exercise, with a trend towards a decrease during submaximal exercise (25 W, stage 2). (Reproduced from Hsu, S., Houston, B. A., Tampakakis, E., Bacher, A. C., Rhodes, P. S., Mathai, S. C., et al. (2016). Right Ventricular Functional Reserve in Pulmonary Arterial Hypertension. Circulation, 133(24), 2413–2422. https://doi.org/10.1161/CIRCULATIONAHA.116.022082)

that determines prognosis in PAH. As described previously, different subtypes of PAH have varying risks for the development of RV failure [96]. The response of RV hypertrophy in PAH can vary significantly despite similar degrees of hemodynamic stress, with progression to RV failure difficult to predict [13]. Nonetheless, certain discrete characteristics identify maladaptive RV hypertrophy: fibrosis, eccentric hypertrophy, and dilatation as morphologic findings. To date, identification of metabolic and energetic changes in the failing RV has provided insights into disease progression that go beyond quantifying the degree of RV hypertrophy and aim to pinpoint the molecular underpinnings of maladaptive remodeling.

Macro- and Microvascular RV Ischemia

RV hypertrophy as an adaptation to increased afterload will lead to the generation of elevated right ventricular systolic pressures (RVSP). As RVSP approaches systemic pressure, there may be decreased systolic perfusion of the right coronary artery (RCA). In patients with severe RV hypertrophy, the total mean coronary blood flow is reduced [97]. In animal models, however, RV dysfunction only manifests when perfusion pressure drops below 50 mmHg, suggesting an alternative mechanism for ischemia. One explanation may be the reduced microvascular coronary circulation, referred to as capillary rarefaction [98].

Such a mechanism might complement the more recent findings of Hsu et al. in explaining RV myocyte dysfunction in SSc-PAH [12, 96, 99]. Increased reactive oxygen species in the setting of decompensated RV hypertrophy may also inhibit angiogenesis-promoting factors such as hypoxia inducible factor-1α, further impairing blood flow and facilitating ischemia [13].

Metabolic Shifts in the RV Myocardium

Whereas typical cardiac metabolism preferentially utilizes fatty acid oxidation as a primary source of energy, RV hypertrophy is associated with a reliance on glucose metabolism, and in general, RV failure is associated with a shift from oxidative phosphorylation to aerobic glycolysis [100]. Along with increased glycolysis comes increased pyruvate, which requires pyruvate dehydrogenase (PDH) to funnel towards the far more energy (ATP)-productive oxidative phosphorylation. With RV hypertrophy, however, there is increased pyruvate dehydrogenase kinase (PDK) expression and activity. PDK inhibits PDH and inhibits the formation of acetyl CoA, slowing the citric acid cycle and reducing energy production (as well as reducing O_2 consumption) [101]. This metabolic switch to less efficient energy production is associated with impaired RV contractility as well as impaired cardiac output and electrical abnormalities [102].

Accompanying the transition to glycolysis is an increase in the metabolism of glutamine, called glutaminolysis [103]. This metabolic pathway is also harnessed by cancer cells to facilitate rapid cell growth without apoptosis and, in the setting of RVH, appears to be caused by capillary rarefaction and RV ischemia. The downstream effects of glutaminolysis include increased pyruvate production and conversion by lactate dehydrogenase into lactate. Simultaneously, glucose oxidation is inhibited [103]. Further exacerbating the attenuated oxidative capacity described, mitochondria in RV myocytes appear to be reduced in number, and those that remain are

dysfunctional [104]. Whether this is a cause of RV dysfunction or effect is less clear.

Loss-of-function mutation in the bone morphogenetic protein receptor type 2 (BMPR2) gene is the most commonly known genetic cause of PAH, and it has been observed that the BMPR2 mutation confers more severe RV dysfunction compared with individuals with PAH but without BMPR2 mutation [105, 106]. BMPR2, a member of the transforming growth factor-beta (TGF-β) family, is expressed by cardiomyocytes as well as ventricular endothelium [107]. It is generally hypothesized that the balance of TGF-beta/BMP influences RV adaptation in response to chronic load, and in experimental models, BMPR2 mutation can result in an altered hypertrophic response to chronic pressure overload [108]. Specifically, the mutation was associated with impaired fatty acid oxidation and glycolysis with ensuing lipid accumulation and lipotoxicity involving the RV [108–110]. Further study by other groups has identified the presence of increased mRNA expression signaling glycolysis and fatty acid oxidation pathways in patients with PAH without BMPR2 mutation, suggesting impaired compensation in those with BMPR2 mutation, where the RV's metabolic programming is unable to properly adapt energy production to stress [111].

Neurohormonal Activation

Just as in left-heart failure, PAH patients with RV failure have high levels of circulating catecholamines and are unable to augment levels with exercise [112]. In addition to decreased inotropic response, reduced chronotropic response to exercise along with delayed heart rate recovery has also been shown in the failing RV [113]. Likewise, the failing RV's response to inotropic agents targeting beta-adrenergic receptor agonism is attenuated, likely due to downregulation of α1, β1, and dopamine receptors [112]. It may be that the adrenergic response is fully activated in RV failure, so that infusion of catecholaminergic agents may be nearly futile [114]. Such reduction in inotropic reserve is also prognostic, associated with poor survival [115]. Further, reduced protein kinase A (PKA) activation by catecholamine binding to the β1-adrenoreceptor leads to reduced PKA-mediated phosphorylation of proteins related to calcium handling and myofilament function. This means that in addition to impaired systolic function and inotropic reserve, the RV in PAH maintains higher diastolic stiffness with hypophosphorylation of titin along with increased fibrosis [85, 116].

Impaired RV function and alterations in kidney perfusion lead to renin release and resultant activation of the renin-angiotensin-aldosterone (RAAS) axis. This compensatory response becomes persistently activated and is associated with both progressive impairment of RV function and worse prognosis [117, 118]. These observations have already been applied in the study of pharmacologic neurohormonal blockade and renal denervation as potential therapies with promising results [119–121]. Specifically, pharmacologic parasympathetic stimulation with the acetylcholinesterase inhibitor pyridostigmine has been shown to improve RV function, reduce pulmonary vascular remodeling, and improve survival in an animal model of experimental PH [122].

Metabolic Syndrome and RV Remodeling

An emerging area of study is in the relationship between insulin resistance and PAH as it pertains to RV function. Building on animal studies suggest that metabolic syndrome (hypertension, elevated triglyceride levels, low high-density lipoproteins, obesity, and hyperglycemia) may be linked with pulmonary vascular disease. Apolipoprotein E (ApoE), for example, is thought to be protective in vascular disease as it reduces oxidized low-density lipoproteins in the blood but has reduced expression in lung tissue from patients with PAH. In mice deficient in ApoE, a high-fat diet can lead to the development of pulmonary hypertension. Just as reduced ApoE expression appears to facilitate pulmonary hypertension, other mediators such as peroxisome proliferator-activated receptor γ (PPARγ, the

target of glitazone agents for diabetes mellitus) are regulators of glucose metabolism and adipogenesis that has reduced expression in PAH [123, 124]. These findings have prompted animal studies that showed mice fed a Western diet (high-fat content) developed insulin resistance and RV hypertrophy, elevated RVSP, and increased myocardial lipid accumulation that disproportionally got deposited in the RV. In a subset of mice who also underwent pulmonary artery banding to simulate RV pressure overload, those mice with banding plus a Western diet developed more RV hypertrophy, increased lipid deposition, lower RV ejection fraction, and RV diastolic dysfunction [125, 126]. A recent single-center study of metformin in patients with PAH was completed, evaluating RV function by echo, metabolomic analysis, and MR spectroscopy for RV triglyceride content, and clinical endpoints including 6-min walk distance. Although metformin did not impact 6-min walk distance, RV fractional area change was significantly improved and, in a subset of patients who were specifically evaluated, RV triglyceride content was reduced [126]. This study opens the door to further investigation of metformin and other pharmacologic agents for the alteration of metabolic derangements and their role in RV functional impairment.

RV Diastolic Dysfunction in PAH and CTEPH

Although the focus has primarily centered on systolic function as it relates to RV failure in PAH, RV diastolic dysfunction is evident and contributes to RV dysfunction and poor outcomes [9]. Diastolic stiffness is a product of intrinsic chamber stiffness, changing volumes, and alterations in myocyte contractile machinery. RV remodeling in an animal model exposed to sustained pressure overload induced by PA banding, for example, led to increased RV free wall stiffness, reorientation of collagen fibers and myofibrils, and intrinsic stiffness of the fibers [127]. Those same changes translated to increased measures of RV diastolic stiffness during hemodynamic measurement using a conductance catheter, characterized as end-diastolic elastance (E_{ed}) [128]. Changes in phosphorylation patterns in the myocyte contractile apparatus also contribute to titin hypophosphorylation, an increase in calcium sensitivity due to hypophosphorylation of troponin I, and reduced clearance of diastolic Ca^{2+} due to hypophosphorylation of the sarcoplasmic reticulum Ca^{2+} ATPase (SERCA) and phospholamban [85, 116, 129]. In these instances, myocyte stiffness—rather than interstitial fibrosis—was the primary driver of diastolic dysfunction [129]. Similarly, even with increased interstitial fibrosis in subjects with SSc-PAH compared with IPAH, there does not appear to be significant differences in diastolic function between groups [12].

The assessment of RV diastolic function is an area of active investigation, with several methods examined in recent years. Just as for assessment of systolic function, the gold standard for assessment is via multi-beat pressure-volume relations with the construction of an end-diastolic pressure-volume relationship (EDPVR). Alternative methods utilizing a single-beat method have also been employed (Fig. 9.3d, e), utilizing beginning and end-diastolic pressure and cMRI volumetric assessment. Noninvasive techniques for the specific evaluation of RV diastolic stiffness have also been developed using cMRI strain. Using feature tracking and a ratio of RV longitudinal strain to RV end-diastolic volume indexed to body surface area, E_{ed} could be estimated in a model of chronic pressure overload [43].

Conclusion

The study of the RV and its response to PAH and CTEPH is moving from a broad characterization of the remodeling process to understanding the circumstances and risk factors that contribute to maladaptive remodeling and RV failure. Improving diagnostic techniques and evolving understanding of distinct pathophysiologic processes underlying RV responses to PAH and CTEPH will continue to foster the targeted study of the characteristics that define a transition from adaptive to maladaptive adaptations in distinct disease states. With the discovery of such pathomechanisms, so too will come new therapeutic targets.

References

1. Simonneau G, Montani D, Celermajer DS, Denton CP, Gatzoulis MA, Krowka M, et al. Haemodynamic definitions and updated clinical classification of pulmonary hypertension. Eur Respir J. 2019;53(1):1801913.
2. Ross J Jr. Afterload mismatch and preload reserve: a conceptual framework for the analysis of ventricular function. Prog Cardiovasc Dis. 1976;18(4):255–64.
3. von Anrep G. On the part played by the suprarenals in the normal vascular reactions of the body. J Physiol. 1912;45(5):307–17.
4. Vanderpool RR, Desai AA, Knapp SM, Simon MA, Abidov A, Yuan JX, et al. How prostacyclin therapy improves right ventricular function in pulmonary arterial hypertension. Eur Respir J. 2017;50(2):1700764.
5. Gomez-Arroyo J, Sandoval J, Simon MA, Dominguez-Cano E, Voelkel NF, Bogaard HJ. Treatment for pulmonary arterial hypertension-associated right ventricular dysfunction. Ann Am Thorac Soc. 2014;11(7):1101–15.
6. Haddad F, Hunt SA, Rosenthal DN, Murphy DJ. Right ventricular function in cardiovascular disease, Part I: Anatomy, physiology, aging, and functional assessment of the right ventricle. Circulation. 2008;117(11):1436–48.
7. Abel FL, Waldhausen JA. Effects of alterations in pulmonary vascular resistance on right ventricular function. J Thorac Cardiovasc Surg. 1967;54(6):886–94.
8. Guyton AC, Lindsey AW, Gilluly JJ. The limits of right ventricular compensation following acute increase in pulmonary circulatory resistance. Circ Res. 1954;2(4):326–32.
9. Trip P, Rain S, Handoko ML, van der Bruggen C, Bogaard HJ, Marcus JT, et al. Clinical relevance of right ventricular diastolic stiffness in pulmonary hypertension. Eur Respir J. 2015;45(6):1603–12.
10. Vonk Noordegraaf A, Westerhof BE, Westerhof N. The relationship between the right ventricle and its load in pulmonary hypertension. J Am Coll Cardiol. 2017;69(2):236–43.
11. Minami S, Onodera T, Okazaki F, Miyazaki H, Ohsawa S, Mochizuki S. Myocyte morphological characteristics differ between the phases of pulmonary hypertension-induced ventricular hypertrophy and failure. Int Heart J. 2006;47(4):629–37.
12. Hsu S, Kokkonen-Simon KM, Kirk JA, Kolb TM, Damico RL, Mathai SC, et al. Right ventricular myofilament functional differences in humans with systemic sclerosis-associated versus idiopathic

pulmonary arterial hypertension. Circulation. 2018;137(22):2360–70.

13. Bogaard HJ, Abe K, Vonk Noordegraaf A, Voelkel NF. The right ventricle under pressure: cellular and molecular mechanisms of right-heart failure in pulmonary hypertension. Chest. 2009;135(3):794–804.

14. Monroe RG, Gamble WJ, LaFarge CG, Kumar AE, Stark J, Sanders GL, et al. The Anrep effect reconsidered. J Clin Invest. 1972;51(10):2573–83.

15. Alvarez BV, Pérez NG, Ennis IL, Camilión de Hurtado MC, Cingolani HE. Mechanisms underlying the increase in force and Ca(2+) transient that follow stretch of cardiac muscle: a possible explanation of the Anrep effect. Circ Res. 1999;85(8):716–22.

16. Sunagawa K, Maughan WL, Burkhoff D, Sagawa K. Left ventricular interaction with arterial load studied in isolated canine ventricle. Am J Phys. 1983;245(5 Pt 1):H773–80.

17. Hopkins WE, Ochoa LL, Richardson GW, Trulock EP. Comparison of the hemodynamics and survival of adults with severe primary pulmonary hypertension or Eisenmenger syndrome. J Heart Lung Transplant. 1996;15(1 Pt 1):100–5.

18. Vonk-Noordegraaf A, Haddad F, Chin KM, Forfia PR, Kawut SM, Lumens J, et al. Right heart adaptation to pulmonary arterial hypertension: physiology and pathobiology. J Am Coll Cardiol. 2013;62(25 Suppl):D22–33.

19. Beghetti M, Galiè N. Eisenmenger syndrome a clinical perspective in a new therapeutic era of pulmonary arterial hypertension. J Am Coll Cardiol. 2009;53(9):733–40.

20. Saouti N, Westerhof N, Postmus PE, Vonk-Noordegraaf A. The arterial load in pulmonary hypertension. Eur Respir Rev. 2010;19(117):197–203.

21. Delcroix M, Vonk Noordegraaf A, Fadel E, Lang I, Simonneau G, Naeije R. Vascular and right ventricular remodelling in chronic thromboembolic pulmonary hypertension. Eur Respir J. 2013;41(1):224–32.

22. Ruigrok D, Meijboom LJ, Westerhof BE, Veld AH, van der Bruggen CEE, Marcus JT, et al. Right ventricular load and function in chronic thromboembolic pulmonary hypertension: differences between proximal and distal chronic thromboembolic pulmonary hypertension. Am J Respir Crit Care Med. 2019;199(9):1163–6.

23. Fukumitsu M, Westerhof BE, Ruigrok D, Braams NJ, Groeneveldt JA, Bayoumy AA, et al. Early return of reflected waves increases right ventricular wall stress in chronic thromboembolic pulmonary hypertension. Am J Physiol Heart Circ Physiol. 2020;19(6):H1438–50.

24. Mauritz GJ, Vonk-Noordegraaf A, Kind T, Surie S, Kloek JJ, Bresser P, et al. Pulmonary endarterectomy normalizes interventricular dyssynchrony and right ventricular systolic wall stress. J Cardiovasc Magn Reson. 2012;14:5.

25. Casaclang-Verzosa G, McCully RB, Oh JK, Miller FA Jr, McGregor CG. Effects of pulmonary thromboendarterectomy on right-sided echocardiographic parameters in patients with chronic thromboembolic pulmonary hypertension. Mayo Clin Proc. 2006;81(6):777–82.

26. Berman M, Gopalan D, Sharples L, Screaton N, Maccan C, Sheares K, et al. Right ventricular reverse remodeling after pulmonary endarterectomy: magnetic resonance imaging and clinical and right heart catheterization assessment. Pulm Circ. 2014;4(1):36–44.

27. Reesink HJ, Marcus JT, Tulevski II, Jamieson S, Kloek JJ, Vonk Noordegraaf A, et al. Reverse right ventricular remodeling after pulmonary endarterectomy in patients with chronic thromboembolic pulmonary hypertension: utility of magnetic resonance imaging to demonstrate restoration of the right ventricle. J Thorac Cardiovasc Surg. 2007;133(1):58–64.

28. Menzel T, Wagner S, Kramm T, Mohr-Kahaly S, Mayer E, Braeuninger S, et al. Pathophysiology of impaired right and left ventricular function in chronic embolic pulmonary hypertension: changes after pulmonary thromboendarterectomy. Chest. 2000;118(4):897–903.

29. Rolf A, Rixe J, Kim WK, Borgel J, Mollmann H, Nef HM, et al. Right ventricular adaptation to pulmonary pressure load in patients with chronic thrombo-embolic pulmonary hypertension before and after successful pulmonary endarterectomy—a cardiovascular magnetic resonance study. J Cardiovasc Magn Reson. 2014;16:96.

30. Waziri F, Ringgaard S, Mellemkjaer S, Bogh N, Kim WY, Clemmensen TS, et al. Long-term changes of right ventricular myocardial deformation and remodeling studied by cardiac magnetic resonance imaging in patients with chronic thromboembolic pulmonary hypertension following pulmonary thromboendarterectomy. Int J Cardiol. 2020;300:282–8.

31. Houston BA, Tedford RJ. Putting "at-rest" evaluations of the right ventricle to rest: insights gained from evaluation of the right ventricle during exercise in CTEPH patients with and without pulmonary endarterectomy. J Am Heart Assoc. 2015;4(3):e001895.

32. Claessen G, La Gerche A, Dymarkowski S, Claus P, Delcroix M, Heidbuchel H. Pulmonary vascular and right ventricular reserve in patients with normalized resting hemodynamics after pulmonary endarterectomy. J Am Heart Assoc. 2015;4(3):e001602.

33. Galiè N, Humbert M, Vachiery JL, Gibbs S, Lang I, Torbicki A, et al. 2015 ESC/ERS guidelines for the diagnosis and treatment of pulmonary hypertension: the joint task force for the diagnosis and treatment of pulmonary hypertension of the European Society of Cardiology (ESC) and the European Respiratory Society (ERS): endorsed by: Association for European Paediatric and Congenital Cardiology (AEPC), International Society for Heart and Lung Transplantation (ISHLT). Eur Heart J. 2016;37(1):67–119.

34. Grapsa J, Gibbs JS, Cabrita IZ, Watson GF, Pavlopoulos H, Dawson D, et al. The association of clinical outcome with right atrial and ventricular remodelling in patients with pulmonary arterial

hypertension: study with real-time three-dimensional echocardiography. Eur Heart J Cardiovasc Imaging. 2012;13(8):666–72.

35. Grapsa J, Pereira Nunes MC, Tan TC, Cabrita IZ, Coulter T, Smith BC, et al. Echocardiographic and hemodynamic predictors of survival in precapillary pulmonary hypertension: seven-year follow-up. Circ Cardiovasc Imaging. 2015;8(6):e002107.

36. Forfia PR, Fisher MR, Mathai SC, Housten-Harris T, Hemnes AR, Borlaug BA, et al. Tricuspid annular displacement predicts survival in pulmonary hypertension. Am J Respir Crit Care Med. 2006;174(9):1034–41.

37. Maffessanti F, Muraru D, Esposito R, Gripari P, Ermacora D, Santoro C, et al. Age-, body size-, and sex-specific reference values for right ventricular volumes and ejection fraction by three-dimensional echocardiography: a multicenter echocardiographic study in 507 healthy volunteers. Circ Cardiovasc Imaging. 2013;6(5):700–10.

38. Hulshof HG, Eijsvogels TMH, Kleinnibbelink G, van Dijk AP, George KP, Oxborough DL, et al. Prognostic value of right ventricular longitudinal strain in patients with pulmonary hypertension: a systematic review and meta-analysis. Eur Heart J Cardiovasc Imaging. 2019;20(4):475–84.

39. Swift AJ, Rajaram S, Campbell MJ, Hurdman J, Thomas S, Capener D, et al. Prognostic value of cardiovascular magnetic resonance imaging measurements corrected for age and sex in idiopathic pulmonary arterial hypertension. Circ Cardiovasc Imaging. 2014;7(1):100–6.

40. Simpson CE, Damico RL, Kolb TM, Mathai SC, Khair RM, Sato T, et al. Ventricular mass as a prognostic imaging biomarker in incident pulmonary arterial hypertension. Eur Respir J. 2019;53(4):1802067.

41. Badagliacca R, Poscia R, Pezzuto B, Papa S, Pesce F, Manzi G, et al. Right ventricular concentric hypertrophy and clinical worsening in idiopathic pulmonary arterial hypertension. J Heart Lung Transplant. 2016;35(11):1321–9.

42. van Wolferen SA, Marcus JT, Boonstra A, Marques KM, Bronzwaer JG, Spreeuwenberg MD, et al. Prognostic value of right ventricular mass, volume, and function in idiopathic pulmonary arterial hypertension. Eur Heart J. 2007;28(10):1250–7.

43. Tello K, Dalmer A, Vanderpool R, Ghofrani HA, Naeije R, Roller F, et al. Cardiac magnetic resonance imaging-based right ventricular strain analysis for assessment of coupling and diastolic function in pulmonary hypertension. JACC Cardiovasc Imaging. 2019;12(11 Pt 1):2155–64.

44. Freed BH, Gomberg-Maitland M, Chandra S, Mor-Avi V, Rich S, Archer SL, et al. Late gadolinium enhancement cardiovascular magnetic resonance predicts clinical worsening in patients with pulmonary hypertension. J Cardiovasc Magn Reson. 2012;14(1):11.

45. Suga H, Sagawa K, Shoukas AA. Load independence of the instantaneous pressure-volume ratio of the canine left ventricle and effects of epinephrine and heart rate on the ratio. Circ Res. 1973;32(3):314–22.

46. Maughan WL, Shoukas AA, Sagawa K, Weisfeldt ML. Instantaneous pressure-volume relationship of the canine right ventricle. Circ Res. 1979;44(3):309–15.

47. Redington AN, Gray HH, Hodson ME, Rigby ML, Oldershaw PJ. Characterisation of the normal right ventricular pressure-volume relation by biplane angiography and simultaneous micromanometer pressure measurements. Br Heart J. 1988;59(1):23–30.

48. Kono A, Maughan WL, Sunagawa K, Hamilton K, Sagawa K, Weisfeldt ML. The use of left ventricular end-ejection pressure and peak pressure in the estimation of the end-systolic pressure-volume relationship. Circulation. 1984;70(6):1057–65.

49. Sunagawa K, Yamada A, Senda Y, Kikuchi Y, Nakamura M, Shibahara T, et al. Estimation of the hydromotive source pressure from ejecting beats of the left ventricle. IEEE Trans Biomed Eng. 1980;27(6):299–305.

50. Takeuchi M, Igarashi Y, Tomimoto S, Odake M, Hayashi T, Tsukamoto T, et al. Single-beat estimation of the slope of the end-systolic pressure-volume relation in the human left ventricle. Circulation. 1991;83(1):202–12.

51. Senzaki H, Chen CH, Kass DA. Single-beat estimation of end-systolic pressure-volume relation in humans. A new method with the potential for noninvasive application. Circulation. 1996;94(10):2497–506.

52. Brimioulle S, Wauthy P, Ewalenko P, Rondelet B, Vermeulen F, Kerbaul F, et al. Single-beat estimation of right ventricular end-systolic pressure-volume relationship. Am J Phys Heart Circ Phys. 2003;284(5):H1625–H30.

53. Brimioulle S, Wauthy P, Naeije R. Single-beat evaluation of right ventricular contractility. Crit Care Med. 2005;33(4):917–8; author reply 8.

54. Lambermont B, Segers P, Ghuysen A, Tchana-Sato V, Morimont P, Dogne JM, et al. Comparison between single-beat and multiple-beat methods for estimation of right ventricular contractility. Crit Care Med. 2004;32(9):1886–90.

55. Inuzuka R, Hsu S, Tedford RJ, Senzaki H. Single-beat estimation of right ventricular contractility and its coupling to pulmonary arterial load in patients with pulmonary hypertension. J Am Heart Assoc. 2018;7(10):e007929.

56. Richter MJ, Peters D, Ghofrani HA, Naeije R, Roller F, Sommer N, et al. Evaluation and prognostic relevance of right ventricular-arterial coupling in pulmonary hypertension. Am J Respir Crit Care Med. 2020;201(1):116–9.

57. Brewis MJ, Bellofiore A, Vanderpool RR, Chesler NC, Johnson MK, Naeije R, et al. Imaging right ventricular function to predict outcome in pulmonary arterial hypertension. Int J Cardiol. 2016;218:206–11.

58. Vanderpool RR, Pinsky MR, Naeije R, Deible C, Kosaraju V, Bunner C, et al. RV-pulmonary arterial

coupling predicts outcome in patients referred for pulmonary hypertension. Heart. 2015;101(1):37–43.

59. Bellofiore A, Vanderpool R, Brewis MJ, Peacock AJ, Chesler NC. A novel single-beat approach to assess right ventricular systolic function. J Appl Physiol (1985). 2018;124(2):283–90.

60. Sunagawa K, Maughan WL, Sagawa K. Optimal arterial resistance for the maximal stroke work studied in isolated canine left ventricle. Circ Res. 1985;56(4):586–95.

61. Ghuysen A, Lambermont B, Kolh P, Tchana-Sato V, Magis D, Gerard P, et al. Alteration of right ventricular-pulmonary vascular coupling in a porcine model of progressive pressure overloading. Shock. 2008;29(2):197–204.

62. Morimont P, Lambermont B, Ghuysen A, Gerard P, Kolh P, Lancellotti P, et al. Effective arterial elastance as an index of pulmonary vascular load. Am J Physiol Heart Circ Physiol. 2008;294(6):H2736–42.

63. Kelly RP, Ting CT, Yang TM, Liu CP, Maughan WL, Chang MS, et al. Effective arterial elastance as index of arterial vascular load in humans. Circulation. 1992;86(2):513–21.

64. Tabima DM, Philip JL, Chesler NC. Right ventricular-pulmonary vascular interactions. Physiology (Bethesda). 2017;32(5):346–56.

65. Brener MI, Burkhoff D, Sunagawa K. Effective arterial elastance in the pulmonary arterial circulation. Circ Heart Fail. 2020;13(3):e006591.

66. Chemla D, Hébert JL, Coirault C, Salmeron S, Zamani K, Lecarpentier Y. Matching dicrotic notch and mean pulmonary artery pressures: implications for effective arterial elastance. Am J Phys. 1996;271(4 Pt 2):H1287–95.

67. Redington AN, Rigby ML, Shinebourne EA, Oldershaw PJ. Changes in the pressure-volume relation of the right ventricle when its loading conditions are modified. Br Heart J. 1990;63(1):45–9.

68. Tedford RJ, Hsu S, Kass DA. Letter by Tedford et al. Regarding Article, "Effective arterial elastance in the pulmonary arterial circulation: derivation, assumptions, and clinical applications". Circ Heart Fail. 2020;13(5):e007081.

69. Tello K, Richter MJ, Axmann J, Buhmann M, Seeger W, Naeije R, et al. More on single-beat estimation of right ventriculoarterial coupling in pulmonary arterial hypertension. Am J Respir Crit Care Med. 2018;198(6):816–8.

70. Metkus TS, Mullin CJ, Grandin EW, Rame JE, Tampakakis E, Hsu S, et al. Heart rate dependence of the pulmonary resistance × compliance (RC) time and impact on right ventricular load. PLoS One. 2016;11(11):e0166463.

71. Glower DD, Spratt JA, Snow ND, Kabas JS, Davis JW, Olsen CO, et al. Linearity of the Frank-Starling relationship in the intact heart: the concept of preload recruitable stroke work. Circulation. 1985;71(5):994–1009.

72. Axell RG, Messer SJ, White PA, McCabe C, Priest A, Statopoulou T, et al. Ventriculo-arterial coupling detects occult RV dysfunction in chronic thromboembolic pulmonary vascular disease. Physiol Rep. 2017;5(7):e13227.

73. Tello K, Dalmer A, Axmann J, Vanderpool R, Ghofrani HA, Naeije R, et al. Reserve of right ventricular-arterial coupling in the setting of chronic overload. Circ Heart Fail. 2019;12(1):e005512.

74. Hsu S, Simpson CE, Houston BA, Wand A, Sato T, Kolb TM, et al. Multi-beat right ventricular-arterial coupling predicts clinical worsening in pulmonary arterial hypertension. J Am Heart Assoc. 2020;9(10):e016031.

75. Guazzi M, Dixon D, Labate V, Beussink-Nelson L, Bandera F, Cuttica MJ, et al. RV contractile function and its coupling to pulmonary circulation in heart failure with preserved ejection fraction: stratification of clinical phenotypes and outcomes. JACC Cardiovasc Imaging. 2017;10(10 Pt B):1211–21.

76. Tello K, Axmann J, Ghofrani HA, Naeije R, Narcin N, Rieth A, et al. Relevance of the TAPSE/PASP ratio in pulmonary arterial hypertension. Int J Cardiol. 2018;266:229–35.

77. Tello K, Wan J, Dalmer A, Vanderpool R, Ghofrani HA, Naeije R, et al. Validation of the tricuspid annular plane systolic excursion/systolic pulmonary artery pressure ratio for the assessment of right ventricular-arterial coupling in severe pulmonary hypertension. Circ Cardiovasc Imaging. 2019;12(9):e009047.

78. Sanz J, García-Alvarez A, Fernández-Friera L, Nair A, Mirelis JG, Sawit ST, et al. Right ventriculo-arterial coupling in pulmonary hypertension: a magnetic resonance study. Heart. 2012;98(3):238–43.

79. Vanderpool RR, Rischard F, Naeije R, Hunter K, Simon MA. Simple functional imaging of the right ventricle in pulmonary hypertension: can right ventricular ejection fraction be improved? Int J Cardiol. 2016;223:93–4.

80. Trip P, Kind T, van de Veerdonk MC, Marcus JT, de Man FS, Westerhof N, et al. Accurate assessment of load-independent right ventricular systolic function in patients with pulmonary hypertension. J Heart Lung Transplant. 2013;32(1):50–5.

81. Tedford RJ, Mudd JO, Girgis RE, Mathai SC, Zaiman AL, Housten-Harris T, et al. Right ventricular dysfunction in systemic sclerosis-associated pulmonary arterial hypertension. Circ Heart Fail. 2013;6(5):953–63.

82. Hsu S, Houston BA, Tampakakis E, Bacher AC, Rhodes PS, Mathai SC, et al. Right ventricular functional reserve in pulmonary arterial hypertension. Circulation. 2016;133(24):2413–22.

83. Kelemen BW, Mathai SC, Tedford RJ, Damico RL, Corona-Villalobos C, Kolb TM, et al. Right ventricular remodeling in idiopathic and scleroderma-associated pulmonary arterial hypertension: two distinct phenotypes. Pulm Circ. 2015;5(2):327–34. https://doi.org/10.1086/680356. PMID: 26064458; PMCID: PMC4449244.

84. Ramjug S, Hussain N, Hurdman J, Billings C, Charalampopoulos A, Elliot CA, et al. Idiopathic and Systemic Sclerosis-Associated Pulmonary Arterial Hypertension: A Comparison of Demographic, Hemodynamic, and MRI Characteristics and Outcomes. Chest. 2017;152(1):92–102. https://doi.org/10.1016/j.chest.2017.02.010. Epub 2017 Feb 20. PMID: 28223154.

85. Rain S, Handoko ML, Trip P, Gan CT, Westerhof N, Stienen GJ, et al. Right ventricular diastolic impairment in patients with pulmonary arterial hypertension. Circulation. 2013;128(18):2016–25, 1–10.

86. Latus H, Binder W, Kerst G, Hofbeck M, Sieverding L, Apitz C. Right ventricular-pulmonary arterial coupling in patients after repair of tetralogy of Fallot. J Thorac Cardiovasc Surg. 2013;146(6):1366–72.

87. Egbe AC, Kothapalli S, Miranda WR, Pislaru S, Ammash NM, Borlaug BA, et al. Assessment of right ventricular-pulmonary arterial coupling in chronic pulmonary regurgitation. Can J Cardiol. 2019;35(7):914–22.

88. McCabe C, White PA, Hoole SP, Axell RG, Priest AN, Gopalan D, et al. Right ventricular dysfunction in chronic thromboembolic obstruction of the pulmonary artery: a pressure-volume study using the conductance catheter. J Appl Physiol (1985). 2014;116(4):355–63.

89. Jacobs W, van de Veerdonk MC, Trip P, de Man F, Heymans MW, Marcus JT, et al. The right ventricle explains sex differences in survival in idiopathic pulmonary arterial hypertension. Chest. 2014;145(6):1230–6.

90. Tello K, Richter MJ, Yogeswaran A, Ghofrani HA, Naeije R, Vanderpool R, et al. Sex differences in right ventricular–pulmonary arterial coupling in pulmonary arterial hypertension. Am J Respir Crit Care Med. 2020;202(7):1042–6.

91. Haddad F, Kudelko K, Mercier O, Vrtovec B, Zamanian RT, de Jesus Perez V. Pulmonary hypertension associated with left heart disease: characteristics, emerging concepts, and treatment strategies. Prog Cardiovasc Dis. 2011;54(2):154–67.

92. Guihaire J, Haddad F, Noly PE, Boulate D, Decante B, Dartevelle P, et al. Right ventricular reserve in a piglet model of chronic pulmonary hypertension. Eur Respir J. 2015;45(3):709–17.

93. Sharma T, Lau EM, Choudhary P, Torzillo PJ, Munoz PA, Simmons LR, et al. Dobutamine stress for evaluation of right ventricular reserve in pulmonary arterial hypertension. Eur Respir J. 2015;45(3):700–8.

94. Ireland CG, Damico RL, Kolb TM, Mathai SC, Mukherjee M, Zimmerman SL, et al. Exercise right ventricular ejection fraction predicts right ventricular contractile reserve. J Heart Lung Transplant. 2021;40(6):504-512. https://doi.org/10.1016/j.healun.2021.02.005. Epub 2021 Feb 17. PMID: 33752973; PMCID: PMC8169559.

95. Grünig E, Tiede H, Enyimayew EO, Ehlken N, Seyfarth HJ, Bossone E, et al. Assessment and prognostic relevance of right ventricular contractile reserve in patients with severe pulmonary hypertension. Circulation. 2013;128(18):2005–15.

96. Kawut SM, Taichman DB, Archer-Chicko CL, Palevsky HI, Kimmel SE. Hemodynamics and survival in patients with pulmonary arterial hypertension related to systemic sclerosis. Chest. 2003;123(2):344–50.

97. van Wolferen SA, Marcus JT, Westerhof N, Spreeuwenberg MD, Marques KM, Bronzwaer JG, et al. Right coronary artery flow impairment in patients with pulmonary hypertension. Eur Heart J. 2008;29(1):120–7.

98. Bogaard HJ, Natarajan R, Henderson SC, Long CS, Kraskauskas D, Smithson L, et al. Chronic pulmonary artery pressure elevation is insufficient to explain right heart failure. Circulation. 2009;120(20):1951–60.

99. Overbeek MJ, Lankhaar JW, Westerhof N, Voskuyl AE, Boonstra A, Bronzwaer JG, et al. Right ventricular contractility in systemic sclerosis-associated and idiopathic pulmonary arterial hypertension. Eur Respir J. 2008;31(6):1160–6.

100. Oikawa M, Kagaya Y, Otani H, Sakuma M, Demachi J, Suzuki J, et al. Increased [18F] Fluorodeoxyglucose accumulation in right ventricular free wall in patients with pulmonary hypertension and the effect of Epoprostenol. J Am Coll Cardiol. 2005;45(11):1849–55.

101. Sugden MC, Langdown ML, Harris RA, Holness MJ. Expression and regulation of pyruvate dehydrogenase kinase isoforms in the developing rat heart and in adulthood: role of thyroid hormone status and lipid supply. Biochem J. 2000;352(Pt 3): 731–8.

102. Piao L, Fang YH, Cadete VJ, Wietholt C, Urboniene D, Toth PT, et al. The inhibition of pyruvate dehydrogenase kinase improves impaired cardiac function and electrical remodeling in two models of right ventricular hypertrophy: resuscitating the hibernating right ventricle. J Mol Med (Berl). 2010;88(1):47–60.

103. Piao L, Fang YH, Parikh K, Ryan JJ, Toth PT, Archer SL. Cardiac glutaminolysis: a maladaptive cancer metabolism pathway in the right ventricle in pulmonary hypertension. J Mol Med (Berl). 2013;91(10):1185–97.

104. Gomez-Arroyo J, Mizuno S, Szczepanek K, Van Tassell B, Natarajan R, dos Remedios CG, et al. Metabolic gene remodeling and mitochondrial dysfunction in failing right ventricular hypertrophy secondary to pulmonary arterial hypertension. Circ Heart Fail. 2013;6(1):136–44.

105. Sztrymf B, Coulet F, Girerd B, Yaici A, Jais X, Sitbon O, et al. Clinical outcomes of pulmonary arterial hypertension in carriers of BMPR2 mutation. Am J Respir Crit Care Med. 2008;177(12):1377–83.

106. Evans JD, Girerd B, Montani D, Wang XJ, Galiè N, Austin ED, et al. BMPR2 mutations and survival in pulmonary arterial hypertension: an individual participant data meta-analysis. Lancet Respir Med. 2016;4(2):129–37.

107. Morrell NW, Aldred MA, Chung WK, Elliott CG, Nichols WC, Soubrier F, et al. Genetics and genomics of pulmonary arterial hypertension. Eur Respir J. 2019;53(1):1801899.

108. Hemnes AR, Brittain EL, Trammell AW, Fessel JP, Austin ED, Penner N, et al. Evidence for right ventricular lipotoxicity in heritable pulmonary arterial hypertension. Am J Respir Crit Care Med. 2014;189(3):325–34.

109. Brittain EL, Talati M, Fessel JP, Zhu H, Penner N, Calcutt MW, et al. Fatty acid metabolic defects and right ventricular lipotoxicity in human pulmonary arterial hypertension. Circulation. 2016;133(20):1936–44.

110. Hemnes AR, Luther JM, Rhodes CJ, Burgess JP, Carlson J, Fan R, et al. Human PAH is characterized by a pattern of lipid-related insulin resistance. JCI Insight. 2019;4(1):e123611.

111. van der Bruggen CE, Happé CM, Dorfmüller P, Trip P, Spruijt OA, Rol N, et al. Bone morphogenetic protein receptor type 2 mutation in pulmonary arterial hypertension: a view on the right ventricle. Circulation. 2016;133(18):1747–60.

112. Nootens M, Kaufmann E, Rector T, Toher C, Judd D, Francis GS, et al. Neurohormonal activation in patients with right ventricular failure from pulmonary hypertension: relation to hemodynamic variables and endothelin levels. J Am Coll Cardiol. 1995;26(7):1581–5.

113. Ciarka A, Doan V, Velez-Roa S, Naeije R, van de Borne P. Prognostic significance of sympathetic nervous system activation in pulmonary arterial hypertension. Am J Respir Crit Care Med. 2010;181(11):1269–75.

114. Piao L, Fang YH, Parikh KS, Ryan JJ, D'Souza KM, Theccanat T, et al. GRK2-mediated inhibition of adrenergic and dopaminergic signaling in right ventricular hypertrophy: therapeutic implications in pulmonary hypertension. Circulation. 2012;126(24):2859–69.

115. Campo A, Mathai SC, Le Pavec J, Zaiman AL, Hummers LK, Boyce D, et al. Outcomes of hospitalisation for right heart failure in pulmonary arterial hypertension. Eur Respir J. 2011;38(2):359–67.

116. Rain S, Bos Dda S, Handoko ML, Westerhof N, Stienen G, Ottenheijm C, et al. Protein changes contributing to right ventricular cardiomyocyte diastolic dysfunction in pulmonary arterial hypertension. J Am Heart Assoc. 2014;3(3):e000716.

117. de Man FS, Handoko ML, Guignabert C, Bogaard HJ, Vonk-Noordegraaf A. Neurohormonal axis in patients with pulmonary arterial hypertension: friend or foe? Am J Respir Crit Care Med. 2013;187(1):14–9.

118. de Man FS, Tu L, Handoko ML, Rain S, Ruiter G, François C, et al. Dysregulated renin-angiotensin-aldosterone system contributes to pulmonary arterial hypertension. Am J Respir Crit Care Med. 2012;186(8):780–9.

119. Maron BA, Waxman AB, Opotowsky AR, Gillies H, Blair C, Aghamohammadzadeh R, et al. Effectiveness of spironolactone plus ambrisentan for treatment of pulmonary arterial hypertension (from the [ARIES] study 1 and 2 trials). Am J Cardiol. 2013;112(5):720–5.

120. Maron BA, Leopold JA. The role of the renin-angiotensin-aldosterone system in the pathobiology of pulmonary arterial hypertension (2013 Grover Conference series). Pulm Circ. 2014;4(2):200–10.

121. da Silva Gonçalves Bos D, Happé C, Schalij I, Pijacka W, Paton JFR, Guignabert C, et al. Renal denervation reduces pulmonary vascular remodeling and right ventricular diastolic stiffness in experimental pulmonary hypertension. JACC Basic Transl Sci. 2017;2(1):22–35.

122. da Silva Gonçalves Bós D, Van Der Bruggen CEE, Kurakula K, Sun XQ, Casali KR, Casali AG, et al. Contribution of impaired parasympathetic activity to right ventricular dysfunction and pulmonary vascular remodeling in pulmonary arterial hypertension. Circulation. 2018;137(9):910–24.

123. Hansmann G, Wagner RA, Schellong S, Perez VA, Urashima T, Wang L, et al. Pulmonary arterial hypertension is linked to insulin resistance and reversed by peroxisome proliferator-activated receptor-gamma activation. Circulation. 2007;115(10):1275–84.

124. Zamanian RT, Hansmann G, Snook S, Lilienfeld D, Rappaport KM, Reaven GM, et al. Insulin resistance in pulmonary arterial hypertension. Eur Respir J. 2009;33(2):318–24.

125. Brittain EL, Talati M, Fortune N, Agrawal V, Meoli DF, West J, et al. Adverse physiologic effects of Western diet on right ventricular structure and function: role of lipid accumulation and metabolic therapy. Pulm Circ. 2019;9(1):2045894018817741.

126. Brittain EL, Niswender K, Agrawal V, Chen X, Fan R, Pugh ME, et al. Mechanistic phase II clinical trial of metformin in pulmonary arterial hypertension. J Am Heart Assoc. 2020;2020:e018349.

127. Hill MR, Simon MA, Valdez-Jasso D, Zhang W, Champion HC, Sacks MS. Structural and mechanical adaptations of right ventricle free wall myocardium to pressure overload. Ann Biomed Eng. 2014;42(12):2451–65.

128. Jang S, Vanderpool RR, Avazmohammadi R, Lapshin E, Bachman TN, Sacks M, et al. Biomechanical and hemodynamic measures of right ventricular diastolic function: translating tissue biomechanics to clinical relevance. J Am Heart Assoc. 2017;6(9):e006084.

129. Rain S, Andersen S, Najafi A, Gammelgaard Schultz J, da Silva Gonçalves Bós D, Handoko ML, et al. Right ventricular myocardial stiffness in experimental pulmonary arterial hypertension: relative contribution of fibrosis and myofibril stiffness. Circ Heart Fail. 2016;9(7):e002636.

Left-Heart Failure and Its Effects on the Right Heart

10

Stefano Ghio

Introduction

The neglected role of the right ventricle in left-heart failure is a never-ending story. For decades, cardiologists have largely underestimated the role of the right ventricle in heart failure (HF), based on the misconception that this heart chamber simply plays a passive role in maintaining cardiac output. It goes without saying that this view was completely wrong. However, now that clinicians agree that right ventricular (RV) systolic dysfunction is a robust marker of poor prognosis in patients with chronic heart failure, there is yet another overlooked topic, namely the causes of right-heart dysfunction.

Understanding the determinants of RV dysfunction in left-heart failure patients is extremely important both from a clinical and a research point of view. RV dysfunction, in particular when it is combined with pulmonary hypertension (PH), is a challenge for clinical cardiologists, since it is associated with dismal prognosis and limited efficacy of conventional medical treatments. This is one of the reasons why off-label use of specific drugs for pulmonary arterial hypertension is quite widespread in clinical practice in such patients, despite the fact that randomized clinical trials provide no evidence of their efficacy. Ultimately, mechanistic research that uncovers the pathophysiology and causes of right-sided heart failure is critical to better stratify prognosis, to target unique and specific mediators of RV dysfunction, and, therefore, possibly to develop more effective therapeutic strategies in patients with left-heart failure.

To this aim, there is no doubt that we have to address heart failure with reduced ejection fraction (HFrEF) and heart failure with preserved ejection fraction (HFpEF) separately. This is because HFrEF and HFpEF may exhibit a similar pulmonary hemodynamic profile and similar outcomes but are characterized by important differences in the underlying clinical causes, in comorbidities, in triggers and in molecular pathways for pulmonary vascular injury, and, finally, also in type and extent of remodeling of the left and the right ventricular chambers.

Causes of Right-Heart Dysfunction in HFrEF Patients

The commonly held concept is that RV dysfunction in left-heart failure is associated with elevated pressures in the pulmonary circulation. This hypothesis has a sound pathophysiological background since, due to its peculiar anatomic characteristics, the RV cannot easily tolerate pressure overload [1, 2]. In fact, since the year 1980s, sev-

S. Ghio (✉)
Divisione di Cardiologia, Fondazione IRCCS
Policlinico S Matteo, Pavia, Italy
e-mail: s.ghio@smatteo.pv.it

eral clinical studies have shown that the increase in pulmonary pressure is inversely related with RV function and global cardiac performance [3–6]. Molecular biology also supports the hypothesis that PH is a primary cause for myocardial contractile failure of the right ventricle: the integrity of the amino (N)-terminus of dystrophin (a protein which plays a key role in the transduction of physical forces in the striated muscle) is disrupted both in the left and in the right ventricle of end-stage HF patients and unloading the left ventricle via a LV assist device ameliorates the cardiac structure both in the left and in the right ventricle [7]. However, in addition to pulmonary hypertension, there are several other mechanisms which may contribute to determining the development of RV dysfunction in patients with HFrEF, and more than one mechanism can obviously contribute in individual patients. Myocardial ischemia or infarction may frequently involve both ventricles. In patients without ischemic heart disease, the same cardiomyopathic process may simultaneously affect both the left and the right ventricles. As a matter of fact, whether the genetic background influences the right ventricular phenotype in patients with dilated cardiomyopathy is not yet known, but it has been observed that desmosomal protein gene mutations, currently regarded as synonymous with another disorder, arrhythmogenic right ventricular cardiomyopathy, are also quite common in patients with HFrEF [8]. Finally, the absence of active atrial contraction in patients with atrial fibrillation (as well as in patients overtreated with diuretic drugs) might determine an excessive reduction in right ventricular preload and may be a possible cause of RV dysfunction.

To our knowledge, a single large multicenter study was specifically designed to evaluate the clinical and echocardiographic correlates of RV dysfunction and whether they differ among patients having HFrEF, or HFmrEF, or HFpEF [9]. This study had two main limitations: first, RV function was evaluated by means of the simple echocardiographic measure of TAPSE, and second, PH was defined on the basis of a Doppler echocardiographic estimate of pulmonary artery systolic pressure (PASP) rather than on the invasive evaluation of mean pulmonary pressure as recommended by international guidelines [10]. However, within these limits, the results are interesting to discuss. In this study the first parameter correlating with RV dysfunction was left ventricular systolic function itself: HFrEF patients had a more than threefold increased risk of having a reduced TAPSE. This may be explained considering that the right and the left ventricles share the same visceral cavity (the pericardium), have common myofibers, and strong ventriculo–ventricular interactions that have been well demonstrated in isolated ventricles; therefore, the mere presence of LV dysfunction may be associated with some degree of RV dysfunction [11, 12]. In addition, ischemic etiology was associated with a greater risk of RV dysfunction in HFrEF patients. Previous smaller, single-center studies yielded discrepant results on this topic; however, it is clinically common to observe large myocardial infarctions causing heart failure which involve the left and the right ventricles [13–15]. The role of pulmonary hypertension as a determinant of RV dysfunction in HFrEF did not emerge clearly in this study. An elevated PASP at Doppler echocardiography was not independently associated with a greater risk of RV dysfunction. A substantial proportion of HFrEF patients had a reduced TAPSE even in the absence of high pulmonary pressures. This observation might be explained considering the limitations of the noninvasive echocardiographic definition of PH used in the study. In contrast, a restrictive LV filling pattern (which is a robust echocardiographic indicator of elevated pulmonary artery wedge pressure in HFrEF patients) was significantly associated with RV dysfunction, thus highlighting the importance of retrograde transmission of elevated diastolic left ventricular pressure to the pulmonary circulation as a mechanism of RV dysfunction. Atrial fibrillation and permanent RV pacing were strongly related to RV dysfunction in HFrEF, in agreement with previous suggestions that the mechanical function of the atria and ventricles is closely coupled on the right side of the heart and with the results of a large study in heart failure outpatients [16–18].

Causes of Right-Heart Dysfunction in HFpEF Patients

Although it is now agreed that RV dysfunction is highly prevalent in patients with HFpEF, the underlying pathways that lead to RV dysfunction in HFpEF are far less clear than in HFrEF [19–25]. There are several reasons to hypothesize that the determinants of RV dysfunction in HFpEF may be different from those in HFrEF. HFpEF and HFrEF are characterized by important differences in the underlying clinical causes. In HFpEF, most cases are associated with common cardiac risk factors such as hypertension, diabetes, renal disease, obesity, and aging, whereas a few cases are due to specific infiltrative disorders wherein the myocardial architecture and function are altered by excess accumulation of either abnormal proteins, glycosphingolipids, glycogen, or other substances [26].

It is essential to identify these specific forms of HFpEF since they may possibly benefit of disease-specific therapies. In younger individuals (<30 years of age), HFpEF is most frequently due to genetic disorders that cause increased fibrosis and/or abnormal deposition of iron, proteins, or glycogen. In older adults, the most common cause is cardiac amyloidosis, which was previously considered a rare disease, but it is recently considered an underestimated condition, deserving full attention as an important differential diagnosis in patients with HFpEF [27].

Triggers and molecular pathways for pulmonary vascular injury are also substantially different between HFrEF and HFpEF, despite the fact that the hemodynamic definition of PH is the same in both conditions [28]. The hemodynamic drivers for PH-HFrEF are LV dilatation, secondary mitral regurgitation, and left atrial enlargement. Predominant mechanisms in PH HFpEF are diastolic stiffness, atrial myopathy (making patients more susceptible to evolve to AF), and LA functional MR. Vascular stress failure and remodeling similarly affect veins, capillaries, and small arteries, in HFrEF and HFpEF patients, but a main differential trait is the metabolic injury superimposed to the pressure-induced one, typical of HFpEF with metabolic syndrome [29].

Concerning the causes of right-heart dysfunction in HFpEF, most studies have observed a strong, significant association between pulmonary hypertension and an increased risk of reduced RV function in HFmrEF and HFpEF patients [9, 20–24]. In HFmrEF and HFpEF patients the prevalence of a reduced TAPSE was negligible when PASP was normal, in contrast to HFrEF patients in whom a reduced TAPSE could be observed even in the absence of high pulmonary pressures. If confirmed, this observation could be extremely relevant for researchers, as it would indicate that PH-HFpEF patients could be the ideal candidates to be included in trials testing the efficacy of specific pulmonary vasodilator therapy in PH due to left-heart failure [30].

Atrial fibrillation is strongly related to RV dysfunction in HFpEF. This association is also observed in HFrEF, but there is a peculiar difference between HFpEF and HFrEF. In HFpEF patients, long-standing AF may determine marked right atrial dilatation and increase in diameter of the tricuspid annulus, thus leading to severe functional tricuspid regurgitation [31, 32]. The RV volume overload caused by tricuspid regurgitation may in turn favor the onset or the worsening of right-heart failure [33, 34].

Gaps in Evidence and Perspectives

The prevalence and the prognostic significance of RV dysfunction in different types of left-heart failure are quite variable in the literature, possibly because the inclusion criteria were different among studies and not always a precise differentiation between HFrEF, HFmrEF, and HFpEF was applied.

There is no agreement on which imaging technique should be used to evaluate RV function in such patients. Cardiac magnetic resonance is the gold standard to evaluate RV structure and function; however we should agree that the simpler, more widespread, and less expensive echocardiographic examination could be routinely used in the follow-up of heart failure patients. As a matter of fact, repeated Doppler echocardiographic examinations, despite the limitations of the technique, allow to obtain relevant clinical and prognostic information in the follow-up of HFrEF patients [35]. If we decide to use echocardiography, we are left with the fact that there is no agreement on which are the best echocardiographic parameters to evaluate the function of the right ventricle. If we privilege simplicity, tricuspid annular plane systolic excursion (TAPSE) and its normalization for pulmonary artery systolic pressure (TAPSE/PASP) should be preferred. However, there are several suggestions in the literature in favor of the use of other echocardiographic modalities to assess RV structure and function. It is unfortunate that we still do not know whether and in which cases the measure of global RV strain or of three-dimensional echocardiography should be used to allow a better risk stratification or a better understanding of RV pathophysiology in left-heart failure patients.

Most importantly, rather than focusing on the search of the best echocardiographic indicator, we should realize that the assessment of ventricular function using imaging is limited by the load dependency of all parameters assessing cardiac motion, whether they are volume based as ejection fraction, or area based as fractional area change, or single plane based such as TAPSE; in all cases the presence of significant atrioventricular valve regurgitation leads to an overestimation of the systolic function of the ventricular chamber. Therefore, the degree of tricuspid regurgitation must always be taken into account when evaluating RV function. Unfortunately, current parameters used to identify the pathophysiology and describe the severity of tricuspid regurgitation lack accuracy and need to be redefined [36]. And yet, these simple parameters are already capable to improve prognostic stratification both in heart failure and in pulmonary arterial hypertension [37, 38]. A prospective, multicenter study enrolling a large number of heart failure patients in Europe and in other continents, standardizing imaging techniques and inclusion criteria, may be considered an ambitious project, but for sure it would be worthwhile.

Most importantly for clinicians, therapeutic options for RV dysfunction and failure are strongly limited and even less addressed in the context of left-heart failure than in the context of pulmonary arterial hypertension. However, a number of experimental studies employing different animal models for RV dysfunction or failure and preclinical data have identified beneficial effects of novel pharmacological agents, with most promising results obtained with modulators of metabolism and reactive oxygen species or inflammation [39].

Conclusions

Knowledge about the role of the right ventricle in heart failure patients has historically lagged behind that of the left ventricle. Nevertheless, even the proportionately limited information on the methods to evaluate right ventricular structure, on its pathophysiologic determinants, and on its impact on the outcome in the different types of heart failure suggests that the right ventricle is a crucial contributor of these diseases and that further understanding of these issues is of pivotal importance to improve our possibility to treat these patients.

References

1. Voelkel NF, Quaife RA, Leinwand LA, Barst RJ, McGoon MD, Meldrum DR, Dupuis J, Long CS, Rubin LJ, Smart FW, Suzuki YJ, Gladwin M, Denholm EM, Gail DB. Right ventricular function and failure: report of a National Heart, Lung, and Blood Institute Working Group on Cellular and Molecular Mechanisms of Right Heart Failure. Circulation. 2006;114:1883–91.
2. Haddad F, Hunt SA, Rosenthal DN, Murphy DJ. Right ventricular function in cardiovascular disease, Part I: Anatomy, physiology, aging, and functional assessment of the right ventricle. Circulation. 2008;117:1436–48.
3. Morrison D, Goldman S, Wright AL, Henry R, Sorenson S, Caldwell J, Ritchie J. The effect of pulmonary hypertension on systolic function of the right ventricle. Chest. 1983;84:250–7.

4. Drazner MH, Hamilton MA, Fonarow G, Creaser J, Flavell C, Stevenson LW. Relationship between right and left-sided filling pressures in 1000 patients with advanced heart failure. J Heart Lung Transplant. 1999;18:1126–32.

5. Ghio S, Gavazzi A, Campana C, Inserra C, Klersy C, Sebastiani R, Arbustini E, Recusani F, Tavazzi L. Independent and additive prognostic value of right ventricular systolic function and pulmonary artery pressure in patients with chronic heart failure. J Am Coll Cardiol. 2001;37:183–8.

6. Friedberg MK, Redington AN. Right versus left ventricular failure: differences, similarities, and interactions. Circulation. 2014;129:1033–44.

7. Vatta M, Stetson SJ, Jimenez S, Entman ML, Noon GP, Bowles NE, Towbin JA, Torre-Amione G. Molecular normalization of dystrophin in the failing left and right ventricle of patients treated with either pulsatile or continuous flow-type ventricular assist devices. J Am Coll Cardiol. 2004;43:811–7.

8. Elliott P, O'Mahony C, Syrris P, Evans A, Rivera Sorensen C, Sheppard MN, Carr-White G, Pantazis A, McKenna WJ. Prevalence of desmosomal protein gene mutations in patients with dilated cardiomyopathy. Circ Cardiovasc Genet. 2010;3:314–22.

9. Ghio S, Guazzi M, Scardovi AB, Klersy C, Clemenza F, Carluccio E, Temporelli PL, Rossi A, Faggiano P, Traversi E, Vriz O, Dini FL, all investigators. Different correlates but similar prognostic implications for right ventricular dysfunction in heart failure patients with reduced or preserved ejection fraction. Eur J Heart Fail. 2017;19:873–9.

10. Galiè N, Humbert M, Vachiery JL, Gibbs S, Lang I, Torbicki A, Simonneau G, Peacock A, Vonk Noordegraaf A, Beghetti M, Ghofrani A, Gomez Sanchez MA, Hansmann G, Klepetko W, Lancellotti P, Matucci M, McDonagh T, Pierard LA, Trindade PT, Zompatori M, Hoeper M, ESC Scientific Document Group. 2015 ESC/ERS guidelines for the diagnosis and treatment of pulmonary hypertension: the joint task force for the diagnosis and treatment of pulmonary hypertension of the European Society of Cardiology (ESC) and the European Respiratory Society (ERS): endorsed by: Association for European Paediatric and Congenital Cardiology (AEPC), International Society for Heart and Lung Transplantation (ISHLT). Eur Heart J. 2016;37:67–119.

11. Damiano RJ Jr, La Follette P Jr, Cox JL, Lowe JE, Santamore WP. Significant left ventricular contribution to right ventricular systolic function. Am J Phys. 1991;261:H1514–24.

12. Santamore WP, Dell'Italia LJ. Ventricular interdependence: significant left ventricular contributions to right ventricular systolic function. Prog Cardiovasc Dis. 1998;40:289–308.

13. Kjaergaard J, Iversen KK, Akkan D, Møller JE, Køber LV, Torp-Pedersen C, Hassager C. Predictors of right ventricular function as measured by tricuspid annular plane systolic excursion in heart failure. Cardiovasc Ultrasound. 2009;7:51.

14. La Vecchia L, Zanolla L, Varotto L, Bonanno C, Spadaro GL, Ometto R, Fontanelli A. Reduced right ventricular ejection fraction as a marker for idiopathic dilated cardiomyopathy compared with ischemic left ventricular dysfunction. Am Heart J. 2001;142:181–9.

15. Hirose K, Shu NH, Reed JE, Rumberger JA. Right ventricular dilatation and remodelling the first year after an initial transmural wall left ventricular myocardial infarction. Am J Cardiol. 1993;72:1126–30.

16. Bazaz R, Edelman K, Gulyasy B, Lopez-Candales A. Evidence of robust coupling of atrioventricular mechanical function of the right side of the heart: insights from M-mode analysis of annular motion. Echocardiography. 2008;25:557–61.

17. Alam M, Samad BA, Hedman A, Frick M, Nordlander R. Cardioversion of atrial fibrillation and its effect on right ventricular function as assessed by tricuspid annular motion. Am J Cardiol. 1999;84:1256–8.

18. Damy T, Kallvikbacka-Bennett A, Goode K, Khaleva O, Lewinter C, Hobkirk J, Nikitin NP, Dubois-Randé JL, Hittinger L, Clark AL, Cleland JG. Prevalence of, associations with, and prognostic value of tricuspid annular plane systolic excursion (TAPSE) among outpatients referred for the evaluation of heart failure. J Card Fail. 2012;18:216–25.

19. Puwanant S, Priester TC, Mookadam F, Bruce CJ, Redfield MM, Chandrasekaran K. Right ventricular function in patients with preserved and reduced ejection fraction heart failure. Eur J Echocardiogr. 2009;10:733–7.

20. Melenovsky V, Hwang SJ, Lin G, Redfield MM, Borlaug BA. Right heart dysfunction in heart failure with preserved ejection fraction. Eur Heart J. 2014;35:3452–62.

21. Mohammed SF, Hussain I, Abou Ezzeddine OF, Takahama H, Kwon SH, Forfia P, Roger VL, Redfield MM. Right ventricular function in heart failure with preserved ejection fraction: a community-based study. Circulation. 2014;130:2310–20.

22. Gorter TM, Hoendermis ES, van Veldhuisen DJ, Voors AA, Lam CS, Geelhoed B, Willems TP, van Melle JP. Right ventricular dysfunction in heart failure with preserved ejection fraction: a systematic review and meta-analysis. Eur J Heart Fail. 2016;18:1472–87.

23. Aschauer S, Kammerlander AA, Zotter-Tufaro C, Ristl R, Pfaffenberger S, Bachmann A, Duca F, Marzluf BA, Bonderman D, Mascherbauer J. The right heart in heart failure with preserved ejection fraction: insights from cardiac magnetic resonance imaging and invasive haemodynamics. Eur J Heart Fail. 2016;18:71–80.

24. Bosch L, Lam CSP, Gong L, Chan SP, Sim D, Yeo D, Jaufeerally F, Leong KTG, Ong HY, Ng TP, Richards AM, Arslan F, Ling LH. Right ventricular dysfunction in left-sided heart failure with preserved versus reduced ejection fraction. Eur J Heart Fail. 2017;19:1664–71.

25. Gorter TM, van Veldhuisen DJ, Bauersachs J, Borlaug BA, Celutkiene J, Coats AJS, Crespo-Leiro MG, Guazzi M, Harjola VP, Heymans S, Hill L,

Lainscak M, Lam CSP, Lund LH, Lyon AR, Mebazaa A, Mueller C, Paulus WJ, Pieske B, Piepoli MF, Ruschitzka F, Rutten FH, Seferovic PM, Solomon SD, Shah SJ, Triposkiadis F, Wachter R, Tschöpe C, de Boer RA. Right heart dysfunction and failure in heart failure with preserved ejection fraction: mechanisms and management. Position statement on behalf of the Heart Failure Association of the European Society of Cardiology. Eur J Heart Fail. 2018;20:16–37.

26. Madan N, Kalra D. Clinical evaluation of infiltrative cardiomyopathies resulting in heart failure with preserved ejection fraction. Rev Cardiovasc Med. 2020;21:181–90.

27. Ihne S, Morbach C, Obici L, Palladini G, Störk S. Amyloidosis in heart failure. Curr Heart Fail Rep. 2019;16:285–303.

28. Guazzi M, Ghio S, Adir Y. Pulmonary hypertension in HFpEF and HFrEF: JACC review topic of the week. J Am Coll Cardiol. 2020;76:1102–11.

29. Adir Y, Guazzi M, Offer A, Temporelli PL, Cannito A, Ghio S. Pulmonary hemodynamics in heart failure patients with reduced or preserved ejection fraction and pulmonary hypertension: similarities and disparities. Am Heart J. 2017;192:120–7.

30. Ghio S, D'Alto M, Badagliacca R, Vizza CD. Pulmonary hypertension in left heart disease: the need to continue to explore. Int J Cardiol. 2019;288:132–4.

31. Yamasaki N, Kondo F, Kubo T, Okawa M, Matsumura Y, Kitaoka H, et al. Severe tricuspid regurgitation in the aged: atrial remodeling associated with long-standing atrial fibrillation. J Cardiol. 2006;48:315–23.

32. Utsunomiya H, Itabashi Y, Mihara H, Berdejo J, Kobayashi S, Siegel RJ, et al. Functional tricuspid regurgitation caused by chronic atrial fibrillation: a real-time 3-dimensional transesophageal echocardiography study. Circ Cardiovasc Imaging. 2017;10(1):e004897.

33. Batchelor W, Emaminia A. Tricuspid regurgitation and right heart failure: "it all begins and ends with the RV". JACC Heart Fail. 2020;8(8):637–9.

34. DeFilippis EM, Guazzi M, Colombo PC, Yuzefpolskaya M. A right ventricular state of mind in the progression of heart failure with reduced ejection fraction: implications for left ventricular assist device therapy. Heart Fail Rev. 2020; https://doi.org/10.1007/s10741-020-09935-x.

35. Ghio S, Carluccio E, Scardovi AB, Dini FL, Rossi A, Falletta C, Scelsi L, Greco A, Temporelli PL. Prognostic relevance of Doppler echocardiographic re-assessment in HFrEF patients. Int J Cardiol. 2020;327:111–6.

36. Badano LP, Hahn R, Rodríguez-Zanella H, Araiza Garaygordobil D, Ochoa-Jimenez RC, Muraru D. Morphological assessment of the tricuspid apparatus and grading regurgitation severity in patients with functional tricuspid regurgitation: thinking outside the box. JACC Cardiovasc Imaging. 2019;12(4):652–64.

37. Benfari G, Antoine C, Miller WL, Thapa P, Topilsky Y, Rossi A, Michelena HI, Pislaru S, Enriquez-Sarano M. Excess mortality associated with functional tricuspid regurgitation complicating heart failure with reduced ejection fraction. Circulation. 2019;140(3):196–206.

38. Ghio S, Mercurio V, Fortuni F, Forfia PR, Gall H, Ghofrani A, Mathai SC, Mazurek JA, Mukherjee M, Richter M, Scelsi L, Hassoun PM, Tello K, TAPSE in PAH investigators. A comprehensive echocardiographic method for risk stratification in pulmonary arterial hypertension. Eur Respir J. 2020;56(3):2000513.

39. Klinke A, Schubert T, Müller M, Legchenko E, Zelt JGE, Shimauchi T, Napp LC, Rothman AMK, Bonnet S, Stewart DJ, Hansmann G, Rudolph V. Emerging therapies for right ventricular dysfunction and failure. Cardiovasc Diagn Ther. 2020;10(5):1735–67.

Cor Pulmonale

11

Cyril Charron, Guillaume Geri, Xavier Repessé,
and Antoine Vieillard-Baron

Abbreviations

ARDS   Acute respiratory distress syndrome
CVP   Central venous pressure
LV   Left ventricle
MRI   Magnetic resonance imaging
PAC   Pulmonary artery catheter
PAOP   Pulmonary artery occlusion pressure
PAP   Pulmonary artery pressure

Introduction

Right ventricular (RV) failure is frequent and key to be detected in the management of critically ill patients [1]. At the opposite of the left side, its definition was not so clear until recently explaining that few consensus of experts were needed to better characterize it [1–3]. Briefly, RV failure is now defined as a state in which the right ventricle is unable to meet the demands for blood flow without excessive use of the Frank-Starling mechanisms, which is "excessive" RV dilatation [1]. RV failure is always associated with systemic congestion, which is part of the definition and reflected by an increase in central venous pressure (CVP) leading to renal congestion and injury [2]. To detect RV failure, it was recently proposed in patients with septic shock to combine echocardiography, allowing RV size evaluation, with CVP measurement [4].

Cor pulmonale, when acute or decompensated, is one phenotype of RV failure, which means that RV failure is caused by a pressure overload in this case. Cor pulmonale is a frequent complication of pulmonary diseases and is associated with a poor prognosis in many different clinical settings. This is obviously true in primary pulmonary hypertension [5], but also in acute respiratory distress syndrome (ARDS) [6]. This means that routine evaluation of right ventricular (RV) function is crucial in detecting cor pulmonale.

Cor pulmonale was first described clinically in 1831 by Testa, as a chronic process, to illustrate heart-lung interactions [7]. In 1960, Harvey and Ferrer during a symposium on congestive heart failure defined it as "a complication of certain forms of lung disease" [8]. They especially focused on chronic pulmonary emphysema, leading to RV dysfunction either by alveolar hypoventilation or by destruction of the pulmonary circulation [8]. Also called pulmonary heart disease, it is often just the clinical translation of an increased pulmonary artery pressure (PAP). Later, cor pulmonale was also reported as an acute phe-

C. Charron · G. Geri · X. Repessé
A. Vieillard-Baron (✉)
Intensive Care Unit, Assistance Publique-Hôpitaux de Paris, University Hospital Ambroise Paré,
Boulogne Billancourt, France
e-mail: cyril.charron@aphp.fr; guillaume.geri@aphp.fr; xavier.repesse@aphp.fr; antoine.vieillard-baron@aphp.fr

© The Author(s), under exclusive license to Springer Nature Switzerland AG 2021
S. P. Gaine et al. (eds.), *The Right Heart*, https://doi.org/10.1007/978-3-030-78255-9_11

nomenon in pulmonary embolism, and then called acute cor pulmonale [9]. In the ICU, many situations may be responsible for such a pattern, especially in mechanically ventilated patients [10]. The reasons are briefly explained below.

Physiological Reminders

In normal conditions, the right ventricle acts as a "passive conduit." The isovolumetric contraction pressure is negligible and there is nearly no isovolumetric relaxation time because the right ventricle continues to eject blood long after the beginning of the relaxation [11]. This is only possible because the pressure in the pulmonary circulation is low. Then, for the right ventricle, ventricular-arterial coupling is the key, even though it is unfortunately difficult to assess at the bedside because it requires generation of pressure/volume loops [12]. It can be evaluated as the ratio between end-systolic elastance of the right ventricle and elastance of the pulmonary artery (Ees/Ea) [12]. The right ventricle maintains optimal coupling by adjusting its contraction to its afterload changes [12]. However, this adaptation is limited, especially in acute conditions when an abrupt increase in afterload occurs or after a long process of severe pulmonary hypertension [13]. This is also limited when hypotension, whatever the cause, occurs. Any situations leading to uncoupling between the right ventricle and the pulmonary circulation may induce a pattern of cor pulmonale. This is obvious in cases of chronic or acute pulmonary hypertension where pulmonary artery elastance is significantly increased and the right ventricle has difficulty adapting. In acute pulmonary hypertension, this has been reported to be due to either proximal obstruction of the pulmonary circulation, as in pulmonary embolism [9], or distal obstruction (at the level of the pulmonary capillaries), as in ARDS [14, 15]. But uncoupling may also occur when RV Ees is decreased compared with only a slight increase in pulmonary artery Ea. This is especially apparent in mechanically ventilated patients with depressed RV contraction related to ischemia (RV myocardial infarction) or to inflammatory cytokines (sepsis). Both situations are illustrated in Fig. 11.1. It has long been known that positive-

pressure ventilation may induce increased afterload by collapse of pulmonary capillaries [16, 17]. This is related to the tidal volume or the related transpulmonary pressure [18].

Diagnosis of Cor Pulmonale

As emphasized above, cor pulmonale was initially mainly a clinical diagnosis supported by a suggestive clinical context [1, 7, 8]. Since then, hemodynamic evaluation has been easily available at the bedside using the pulmonary artery catheter (PAC) and cor pulmonale was often defined as a central venous pressure (CVP) higher than the pulmonary artery occlusion pressure (PAOP) (Fig. 11.2) [19, 20]. But this definition is not very sensitive and is more a reflection of severe RV failure than of cor pulmonale per se. With the development of echocardiography, the recognized definition is mainly now an echocardiographic one [21, 22]. It is the association of RV dilatation in diastole with a paradoxical septal motion in end systole (Fig. 11.3). The paradoxical septal motion is the surrogate of the inverted transseptal pressure gradient between the right and the left ventricles (Fig. 11.4). Some studies have also recently reported the accuracy of CT scan in detecting RV dilatation in a clinical context of cor pulmonale [23]. Moreover, cardiac magnetic resonance imaging (MRI) has become an interesting noninvasive approach to assessment not only of chronic changes, long after embolism for example, but also of acute changes in pulmonary vascular resistance [24]. Cardiac MRI could become a key exam in the follow-up of patients suffering from pulmonary hypertension [25].

Differences between acute, chronic, and acute-on-chronic cor pulmonale are not always obvious and the diagnosis is sometimes difficult. Briefly, the clinical context is crucial. Otherwise, chronic cor pulmonale is associated with major thickening of the RV free wall (10–12 mm for a normal value of 3 mm). However, a slight thickening (5–6 mm) has been reported in patients with acute cor pulmonale related to ARDS after only 3 days on mechanical ventilation [22]. In rats, hypoxia is also able to induce some RV hypertrophy in only 3 days [26]. In chronic pulmonary hypertension, thickening is a sign of adaptation and the cardiac

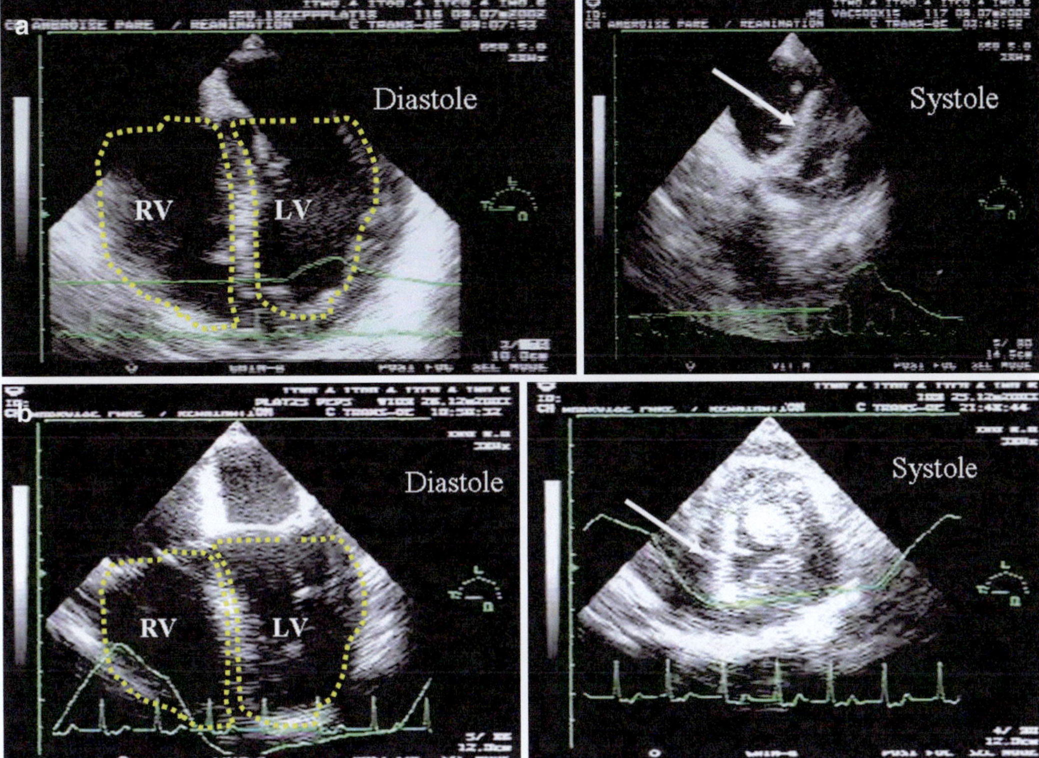

Fig. 11.1 Illustration in two mechanically ventilated patients, using transesophageal echocardiography, of uncoupling between the right ventricle and the pulmonary circulation, leading to a pattern of acute cor pulmonale. Panel (**a**): Patient with septic shock at admission. Note the severe dilatation of the right ventricle in diastole on a four-chamber view, associated with paradoxical septal motion in systole on a short-axis view (*arrow*). Panel (**b**): Patient with myocardial infarction and moderate dilatation of the right ventricle with paradoxical septal motion (D-shape of the left ventricle, *arrow*). *RV* right ventricle, *LV* left ventricle

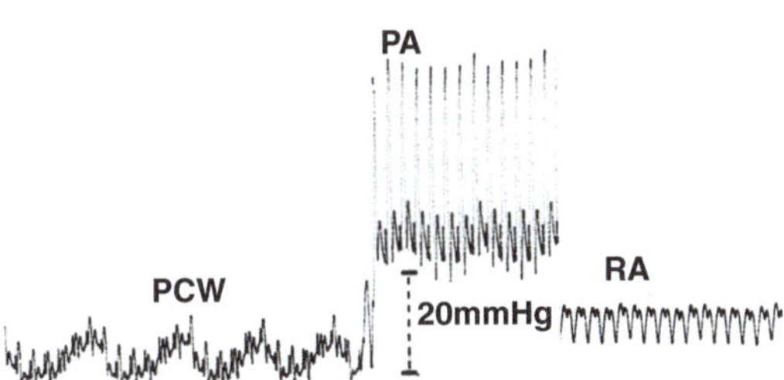

Fig. 11.2 Demonstration in a patient with massive pulmonary embolism, with right atrial pressure (*RA*) higher than pulmonary capillary wedge pressure (*PCW*), illustrating marked right ventricular failure. *PA* pulmonary artery

output is still preserved, whereas dilatation, especially when significant, is a sign of failure with a decreased cardiac output [13]. Another difference between acute and chronic is the level of pulmonary hypertension: it is usually moderate (systolic pressure ≤60 mmHg) in acute and more severe in chronic.

Treatment of Cor Pulmonale

Here we will not consider etiologic treatments, as pulmonary vasodilation, fibrinolysis, coronary reperfusion, etc. But whatever the disease, general support is needed in certain situations, including the use of vasoactive drugs and changes in respiratory settings, and some support has to be limited or even avoided, as fluid expansion.

Whereas it is clear that supporting the right ventricle is required in the case of cor pulmonale related to RV failure, the question is still debatable in the case of RV systolic dysfunction only. In the first situation, cardiac output is not always adequate, whereas in the second situation, it is always preserved. In general, moderate acute cor pulmonale

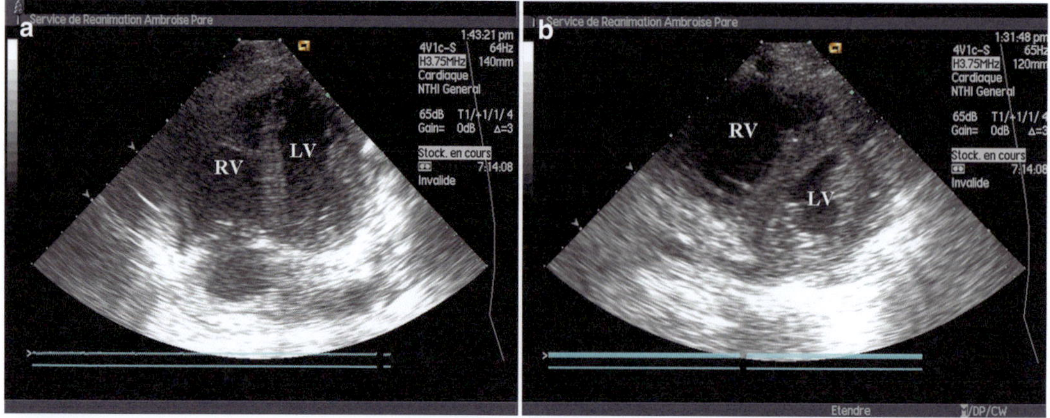

Fig. 11.3 Typical pattern of acute cor pulmonale by a transthoracic approach in a mechanically ventilated young woman with severe pneumonia related to influenza. Panel (**a**): Apical four-chamber view showing major right ventricular dilatation (the right ventricle is bigger than the left) in diastole. Panel (**b**): Parasternal short-axis view of paradoxical septal motion in systole leading to a "D-shape" of the left ventricle and reflecting right ventricular systolic overload. *RV* right ventricle, *LV* left ventricle

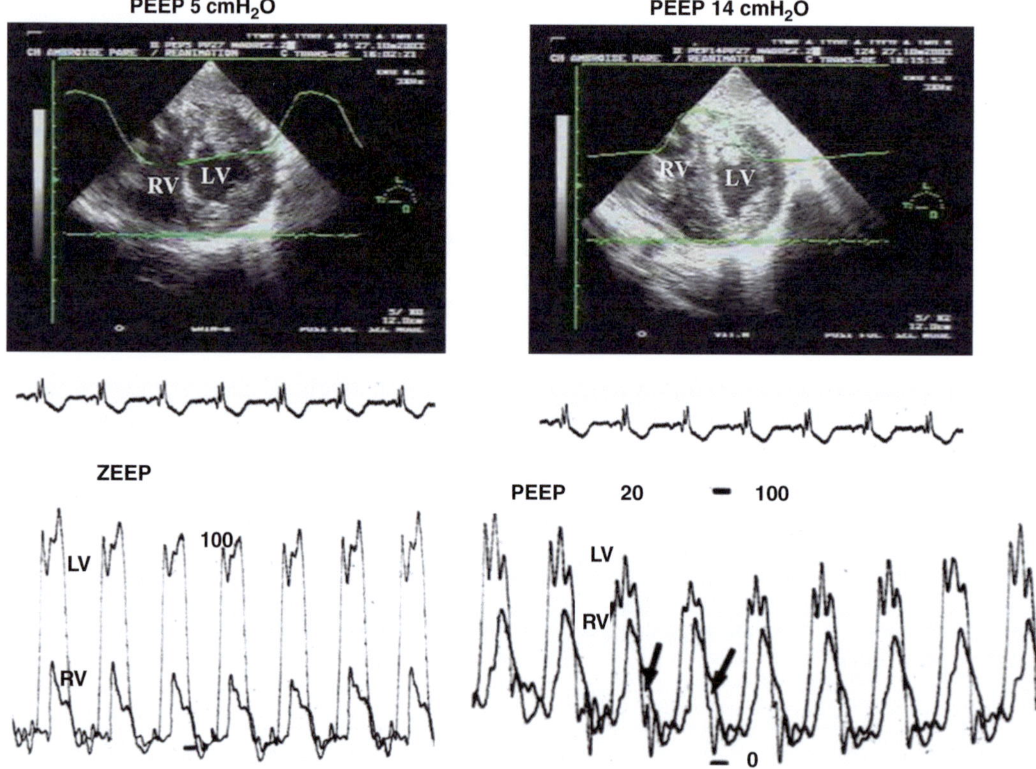

Fig. 11.4 Illustration of the mechanism of paradoxical septal motion. *Above*: Parasternal short-axis view of the left ventricle in a patient ventilated for severe ARDS with PEEP of 5 cmH₂O (no paradoxical septal motion) and after applying PEEP of 14 cmH₂O (paradoxical septal motion). *Below*: Recording of left and right ventricular pressures in a mechanically ventilated patient with ARDS. Note for PEEP of 20 cmH₂O the inverted pressure gradient between both ventricles at end systole, not occurring at PEEP 0 (ZEEP). *RV* right ventricle, *LV* left ventricle, *PEEP* positive end-expiratory pressure

(RV < LV) is associated with a preserved cardiac output, whereas severe acute cor pulmonale (RV > LV) is associated with decreased cardiac output [22]. In the former situation, it is very likely that RV failure is "in progress," while in the latter situation RV failure is already there. Some data recently published in ARDS show that acute cor pulmonale, whatever the cardiac output, is associated with a poor prognosis [6], suggesting that something has also to be adapted in these patients. But this is a special situation where a direct relationship between lung disease, effect of mechanical ventilation, and RV function is well described. This led some intensivists to call in these patients for an RV-protective approach, based on (1) a systematic decrease in tidal volume and plateau pressure, (2) a limitation of hypercapnia, and (3) the use of prone position in the most severely ill patients [27].

Most data regarding the use of vasoactive drugs come from experimental studies. They are based on the concept that a vicious circle is occurring: cor pulmonale leads to RV failure and severe RV dilatation, which results in decreased blood pressure, which leads to decreased coronary perfusion pressure and RV functional coronary ischemia, which worsens RV failure, etc. This supports the use of a vasoconstrictor as norepinephrine to restore a normal blood pressure and then coronary perfusion, helping the right ventricle to adapt to the stress. This was demonstrated by Guyton et al. [28] in animals and also confirmed by Vlahakes et al. [29]. In an experimental model of major pulmonary embolism in dogs, Molloy et al. reported that norepinephrine was much more effective in terms of hemodynamic improvement and survival than isoproterenol [30]. The same results were also reported by Rosenberg et al. [31]. An example is given in Fig. 11.5 in a patient ventilated for ARDS.

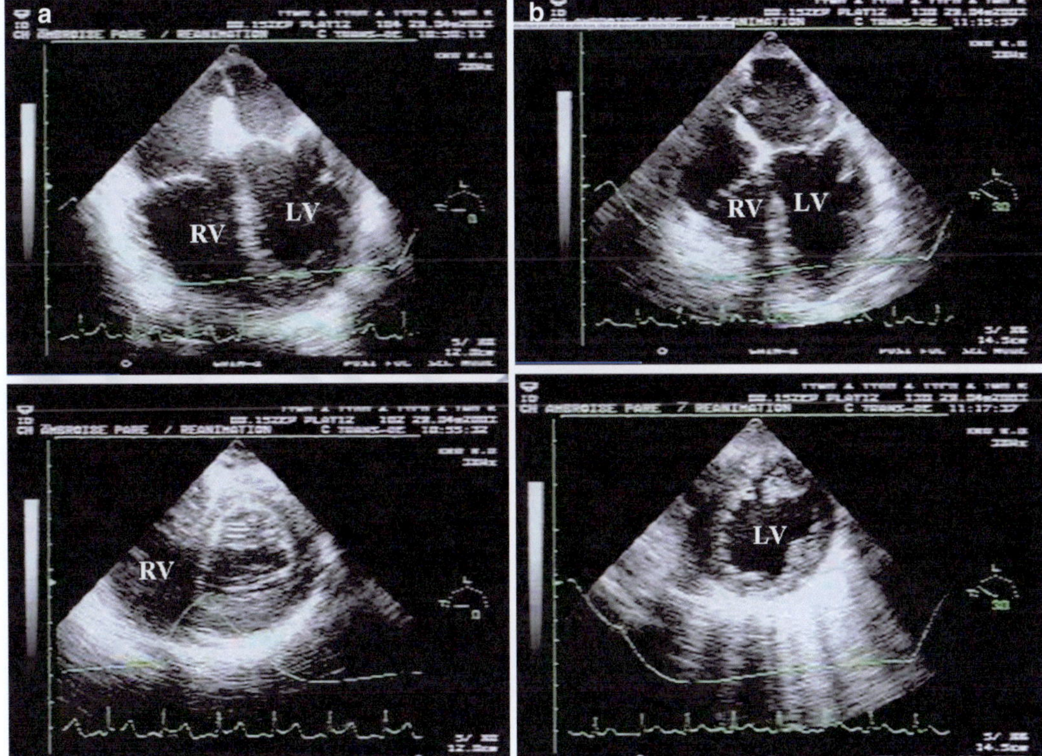

Fig. 11.5 Demonstration of the beneficial effect of norepinephrine infusion on right ventricular function. Panel (**a**): Patient with acute cor pulmonale (right ventricular dilatation above and paradoxical septal motion below) and severe hypotension. Panel (**b**): After norepinephrine infusion, leading to restoration of blood pressure, right ventricular function was normalized (the right ventricle was now non-dilated and paradoxical motion disappeared). *RV* right ventricle, *LV* left ventricle

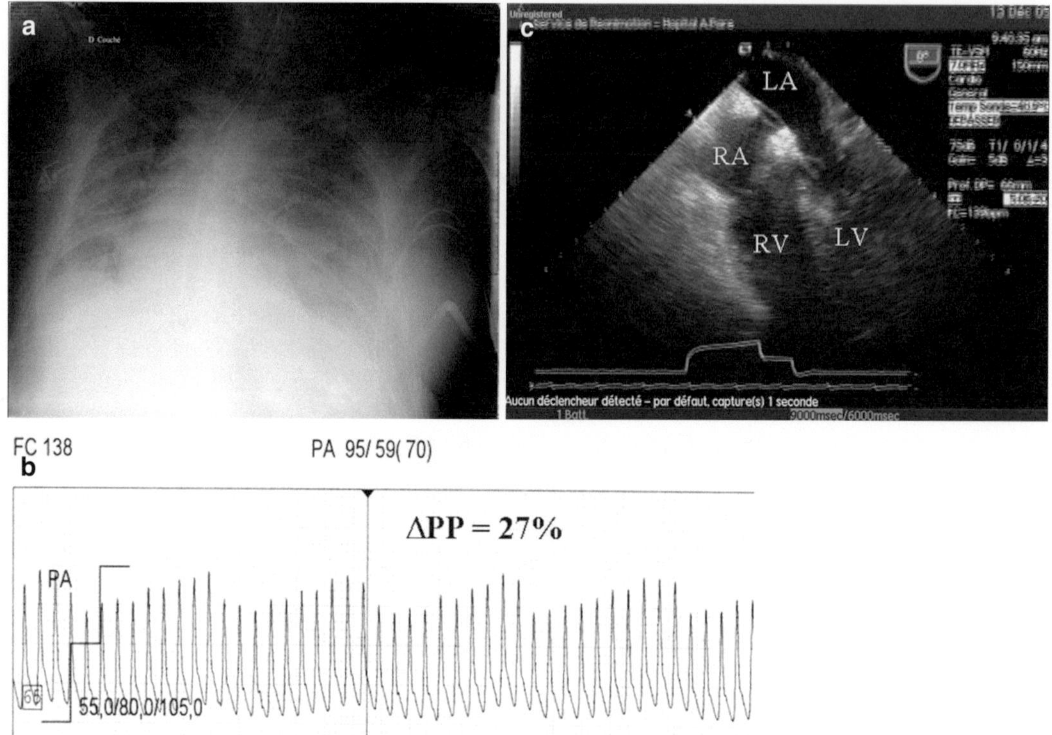

Fig. 11.6 Mechanically ventilated patient with severe ARDS, as shown by the chest X-ray (panel **a**). He exhibited significant pulse pressure variations (panel **b**, invasive blood pressure recording) due to severe acute cor pulmonale, as shown by transesophageal echocardiography, with major right ventricular dilatation (panel **c**). Cardiac output did not increase after fluid expansion. *RV* right ventricle, *LV* left ventricle, *RA* right atrium, *LA* left atrium, *ΔPP* pulse pressure variation, *FC* heart rate, *PA* systolic blood pressure

Fluid management in this situation is not obvious. Clearly, RV function is known to be the main limiting factor for the effectiveness of fluid expansion [28–32]. In mechanically ventilated ARDS patients, Mahjoub et al. showed that false-positive pulse pressure variation (i.e., patients who seemed fluid responsive but in whom cardiac output actually did not increase after fluids) had echocardiographic parameters suggesting RV systolic dysfunction [33] (Fig. 11.6). Mercat et al. demonstrated 15 years ago in patients with pulmonary embolism that changes in cardiac index related to fluids were strongly associated with baseline RV size [34]. We recently reported in 282 patients with septic shock, all mechanically ventilated, that fluid expansion is useless in case of moderate-to-severe RV dilatation even with significant pulse pressure variations [4]. Fluids may be not only useless, but also deleterious in this situation by aggravating RV dilatation and then LV constriction and finally hemodynamic failure [35]. This was also nicely demonstrated in dogs in a model of massive pulmonary embolism [36].

In conclusion, cor pulmonale may be due to many different diseases or injuries, most of them leading to uncoupling between the right ventricle and the pulmonary circulation. The most efficient tool for bedside evaluation of RV function is currently echocardiography. To support the right ventricle it is necessary to evaluate how dilated it is and to be familiar with its physiology and pathophysiology.

References

1. Vieillard-Baron A, Naeije R, Haddad F, Bogaard HJ, Bull TM, Fletcher N, et al. Diagnostic workup, etiologies and management of acute right ventricle failure. A state-of-the-art paper. Intensive Care Med. 2018;44:774–90.
2. Harjola VP, Mebazaa A, Celutkiene J, Bettex D, Bueno H, Chioncel O, et al. Contemporary management of acute right ventricular failure: a statement from the heart failure association and the working group on pulmonary circulation and right ventricular function of the European Society of Cardiology. Eur J Heart Fail. 2016;18:226–41.
3. Lahm T, Douglas I, Archer S, Bogaard H, Chesler N, Haddad F, et al. Assessment of right ventricular function in the research setting: knowledge gaps and pathway forwards. An official American Thoracic Society research statement. Am J Respir Crit Care Med. 2018;198:e15–43.
4. Vieillard-Baron A, Prigent A, Repessé X, Goudelin M, Prat G, Evrard B, et al. Right ventricular failure in septic shock: characterization, incidence and impact on fluid responsiveness. Crit Care. 2020;24:630.
5. D'Alonzo GE, Barst RJ, Ayres SM, Bergofsky EH, Brundage BH, Detre KM, et al. Survival in patients with primary pulmonary hypertension. Results from a national prospective registry. Ann Intern Med. 1991;115:343–9.
6. Boissier F, Katsahian S, Razazi K, Thille AW, Roche-Campo F, Leon R, et al. Prevalence and prognosis of cor pulmonale during protective ventilation for acute respiratory distress syndrome. Intensive Care Med. 2013;39:1725–33.
7. Testa AG. Delle malattie del cuore. Schiepatti: Milano; 1831.
8. Harvey RM, Ferrer MI. A clinical consideration of cor pulmonale. Circulation. 1960;21:236–55.
9. McGinn S, White PD. Acute cor pulmonale resulting from pulmonary embolism. JAMA. 1935;104:1473–8.
10. Piazza G, Goldhaber SZ. The acutely decompensated right ventricle: pathways for diagnosis and management. Chest. 2005;128:1836–52.
11. Redington AN, Rigby ML, Shinebourne EA, Oldershaw PJ. Changes in the pressure-volume relation of the right ventricle when its loading conditions are modified. Br Heart J. 1990;63:45–9.
12. Brimioulle S, Wauthy P, Ewalenko P, Rondelet B, Vermeulen F, Kerbaul F, et al. Single-beat estimation of right ventricular end-systolic pressure-volume relationship. Am J Physiol Heart Circ Physiol. 2003;284:1625–30.
13. Champion HC, Michelakis ED, Hassoun PM. Comprehensive invasive and noninvasive approach to the right ventricle-pulmonary circulation unit: state of the art and clinical and research implications. Circulation. 2009;120:992–1007.
14. Zapol WM, Kobayashi K, Snider MT, Greene R, Laver MB. Vascular obstruction causes pulmonary hypertension in severe acute respiratory failure. Chest. 1977;71:306–7.
15. Vieillard-Baron A, Schmitt JM, Augarde R, Fellahi JL, Prin S, Page B, et al. Acute cor pulmonale in acute respiratory distress syndrome submitted to protective ventilation: incidence, clinical implications, and prognosis. Crit Care Med. 2001;29:1551–5.
16. West JB, Dollery CT, Naimark A. Distribution of blood flow in isolated lung; relation to vascular and alveolar pressures. J Appl Physiol. 1964;19:713–24.
17. Whittenberger JL, Mc GM, Berglund E, Borst HG. Influence of state of inflation of the lung on pulmonary vascular resistance. J Appl Physiol. 1960;15:878–82.
18. Vieillard-Baron A, Loubieres Y, Schmitt JM, Page B, Dubourg O, Jardin F. Cyclic changes in right ventricular output impedance during mechanical ventilation. J Appl Physiol. 1999;87:1644–50.
19. Monchi M, Bellenfant F, Cariou A, Joly LM, Thebert D, Laurent I, et al. Early predictive factors of survival in the acute respiratory distress syndrome. A multivariate analysis. Am J Respir Crit Care Med. 1998;158:1076–81.
20. Osman D, Monnet X, Castelain V, Anguel N, Warszawski J, Teboul JL, et al. Incidence and prognostic value of right ventricular failure in acute respiratory distress syndrome. Intensive Care Med. 2009;35:69–76.
21. Jardin F, Dubourg O, Bourdarias JP. Echocardiographic pattern of acute cor pulmonale. Chest. 1997;111:209–17.
22. Vieillard-Baron A, Prin S, Chergui K, Dubourg O, Jardin F. Echo-Doppler demonstration of acute cor pulmonale at the bedside in the medical intensive care unit. Am J Respir Crit Care Med. 2002;166:1310–9.
23. Quiroz R, Kucher N, Schoepf UJ, Kipfmueller F, Solomon SD, Costello P, et al. Right ventricular enlargement on chest computed tomography: prognostic role in acute pulmonary embolism. Circulation. 2004;109:2401–4.
24. Garcia-Alvarez A, Fernandez-Friera L, Garcia-Ruiz JM, Nuno-Ayala M, Pereda D, Fernandez-Jimenez R, et al. Noninvasive monitoring of serial changes in pulmonary vascular resistance and acute vasodilator testing using cardiac magnetic resonance. J Am Coll Cardiol. 2013;62:1621–31.
25. Kreitner KF, Wirth GM, Krummenauer F, Weber S, Pitton MB, Schneider J, et al. Non-invasive assessment of pulmonary hemodynamics in patients with chronic thromboembolic pulmonary hypertension (CTEPH) by high temporal resolution phase-contrast MR imaging: correlation with simultaneous invasive pressure recordings. Circ Cardiovasc Imaging. 2013;6:722–9.
26. Rabinovitch M, Fisher K, Gamble W, Reid L, Treves S. Thallium-201: quantitation of right ventricular hypertrophy in chronically hypoxic rats. Radiology. 1979;130(1):223–5.
27. Vieillard-Baron A, Price LC, Matthay MA. Acute cor pulmonale in ARDS. Intensive Care Med. 2013;39:1836–8.
28. Guyton AC, Lindsey AW, Gilluly JJ. The limits of right ventricular compensation following acute

increase in pulmonary circulatory resistance. Circ Res. 1954;2(4):326–32.

29. Vlahakes GJ, Turley K, Hoffman JI. The pathophysiology of failure in acute right ventricular hypertension: hemodynamic and biochemical correlations. Circulation. 1981;63:87–95.

30. Molloy WD, Lee KY, Girling L, Schick U, Prewitt RM. Treatment of shock in a canine model of pulmonary embolism. Am Rev Respir Dis. 1984;130:870–4.

31. Rosenberg JC, Hussain R, Lenaghan R. Isoproterenol and norepinephrine therapy for pulmonary embolism shock. J Thorac Cardiovasc Surg. 1971;62:144–50.

32. Schneider AJ, Teule GJ, Groeneveld AB, Nauta J, Heidendal GA, Thijs LG. Biventricular performance during volume loading in patients with early septic shock, with emphasis on the right ventricle: a combined hemodynamic and radionuclide study. Am Heart J. 1988;116:103–12.

33. Mahjoub Y, Pila C, Friggeri A, Zogheib E, Lobjoie E, Tinturier F, et al. Assessing fluid responsiveness in critically ill patients: false-positive pulse pressure variation is detected by Doppler echocardiographic evaluation of the right ventricle. Crit Care Med. 2009;37:2570–5.

34. Mercat A, Diehl JL, Meyer G, Teboul JL, Sors H. Hemodynamic effects of fluid loading in acute massive pulmonary embolism. Crit Care Med. 1999;27:540–4.

35. Piazza G, Goldhaber SZ. Acute pulmonary embolism: part II: treatment and prophylaxis. Circulation. 2006;114:42–7.

36. Ghignone M, Girling L, Prewitt RM. Volume expansion versus norepinephrine in treatment of a low cardiac output complicating an acute increase in right ventricular afterload in dogs. Anesthesiology. 1984;60:132–5.

High Altitude and the Right Ventricle

12

Robert Naeije

Introduction

High-altitude exposure has long been recognized as a cause of "cardiac fatigue" [1]. Heart failure syndromes have been reported as "brisket disease" in cattle brought to high-altitude pastures [2], chronic mountain sickness or subacute mountain sickness in the Andes or the Himalayas [3–6], and occasionally high-altitude right-heart failure (HARHF) in healthy lowlander sojourners [7]. On the other hand, there is the notion that the myocardium has a good tolerance to hypoxia and that the prevalence of cardiovascular diseases is lower in high-altitude dwellers than in sea-level inhabitants [8]. Hypoxia induces an increase in pulmonary vascular resistance (PVR), but resulting pulmonary hypertension (PH) is most often mild to moderate [9]. There has been no report of hypobaric hypoxia-induced RHF in the intensive care setting. This may be due to the fact that severe environmental hypoxic stress is mainly observed in remote high-altitude areas with little access to hospital equipment. Another difficulty in the assessment of HARHF is in the use of different definitions of PH, pulmonary hypertension, and RHF by high-altitude communities and PH experts [10–13]. This pheno-type uncertainty makes epidemiological studies and drug trials difficult.

Definitions

Pulmonary hypertension used to be defined by a mean pulmonary artery pressure (mPAP) $\geq$25 mmHg, and pulmonary vascular disease by a PVR $\geq$3 Wood units (WU) [10]. The mPAP threshold for the diagnosis of PH was recently decreased to 20 mmHg at an international expert consensus conference [11]. Pre- vs. postcapillary PH is still separated on the basis of a wedged PAP (PAWP) below or above 15 mmHg, respectively [10, 11].

High-altitude experts define PH by a mPAP >30 mmHg "in the absence of excessive erythrocytosis" [12]. How to correct pulmonary hemodynamic measurements for the blood viscosity of excessive erythrocytosis has been recently remodeled with the proposal of a practical diagram [13]. This is not yet incorporated in consensus documents or recommendations.

Chronic mountain sickness (CMS) is defined by an excessive erythrocytosis and severe hypoxemia associated with neurological symptoms such as headache, somnolence, fatigue, and depression, occurring in natives or long-term residents above 2500 m [12]. The condition is reversible at lower altitudes. Diagnostic cutoff values are hemoglobin $\geq$21 g/dL in men and $\geq$19 g/dL in women.

R. Naeije (✉)
Free University of Brussels, Brussels, Belgium

While it is recognized that PH and eventual heart failure may complicate CMS, these are *not* sine qua non diagnostic criteria. In fact systemic congestion suggestive of RHF in advanced CMS may be related to carbon dioxide, salt, and water retention in the context of relative hypoventilation [14]. The same characteristics were historically called about "cor pulmonale" (right ventricular, RV hypertrophy/dilatation) in patients with chronic obstructive pulmonary disease [15].

Right-heart failure can be defined as a dyspnea-fatigue syndrome with systemic congestion caused by a failure of right ventricular (RV) systolic function adaptation to afterload resulting in insufficient flow output in response to peripheral demand without increased dimensions [16]. This definition does not propose cutoff values of measurements of systolic function, diastolic function, or dimensions, because of insufficient evidence about the optimal combination of these measurements and uncertainty about limits of normal. There is no definition of RHF in high-altitude expert consensus documents.

Altitude as a Cause of Increased RV Afterload

Hypoxic exposure induces pulmonary vasoconstriction followed by arteriolar remodeling [17, 18]. Hypoxic pulmonary vasoconstriction (HPV) may therefore be a cause of PH secondary to the hypobaric hypoxia environmental stress at high altitude [8]. It has long been known that HPV—and subsequent hypoxic PH—is characterized by marked interspecies variability: as it is intense in pig, horse, and cow; moderate in most rodents; and mild to nonexistent in dog, guinea pig, yak, and llama [17]. Human HPV is generally mild, at the low end of this spectrum, and varies considerably as well [19].

In the first report of human HPV, by Motley et al. in 1947, an acute challenge with a fraction of inspired oxygen (FIO_2) of 0.1 in five healthy subjects increased mPAP on average from 13 to 23 mmHg [20]. In later invasive studies on normal subjects challenged with a FIO_2 of 0.1–0.125 (PaO_2, 40 mmHg, corresponding to an altitude of 4000–4500 m), hypoxia-induced increases in mPAP ranged from 0 to 20 mmHg [21–24]. In these studies, 20% of the subjects had no increase in PVR with hypoxic breathing.

The time course of pulmonary vascular remodeling and its reversal after initial HPV and persistent hypoxic exposure are not exactly known. However, loss of immediate reversibility of increased PVR on reoxygenation occurs within the first 24 h of hypoxic exposure [23–26]. In high-altitude dwellers brought to stay at sea-level altitudes, PVR returns to normal but this reverse remodeling takes several weeks [27].

Chronic hypoxic exposure in high-altitude dwellers is characterized by a variable increase in mPAP. Penaloza and Arias-Stella plotted mPAP reported in high altitude studies as a function of arterial O_2 saturation and found a hyperbolic relationship [28]. When they plotted mPAP as a function of altitude of residence, they found that there were disproportionally high mPAP in Denver, and low mPAP in Lhasa. This fueled the speculation of a Darwinian selection of a lower hypoxic pulmonary pressure response for improved survival in Himalayan populations, which have been living at high altitudes for thousand years compared with more recent North American immigration. However, subsequent studies do not confirm these differences [29], which probably emerged due to selection biases, small-size study populations, and huge variability of human HPV.

A meta-analysis of echocardiographic studies of the pulmonary circulation in healthy subjects showed a mPAP of 13 mmHg in 710 sea-level residents (18 studies) and 20 mmHg in 834 high-altitude residents (12 studies) [9]. The estimates of PAP rested on the measurement of a maximum velocity of tricuspid regurgitation, and mPAP is here recalculated as $0.6 \times$ systolic PAP $+ 2$ mmHg. This method has been shown to be accurate but with limited precision and thus valid for population studies [30]. Thus most high-altitude dwellers have no PH according to high-altitude expert consensus definition [12] or traditional definition of PH by a mPAP ≥ 25 mmHg [10] but a significant proportion would have PH as recently redefined by a mPAP >20 mmHg [11]. The proportion of high-altitude dwellers with pulmonary vascular disease defined by a combination of mPAP >20 mmHg and a PVR ≥3 WU is probably very low if one considers that most of these patients have a normal cardiac output and a PAWP <15 mmHg. More simply stated, mPAP in healthy high-altitude dwellers is generally at the upper limit of sea-level normal or slightly above, and PH with underlying pulmonary vascular disease is very rare.

The same authors hypothesized that CMS would be associated with more important increase in PAP [31]. Accordingly, they performed a meta-analysis of 9 echocardiographic studies in a total of 287 CMS patients. The results showed a mPAP on average of 18 mmHg (95% confidence interval of 16–20 mmHg) at rest and 31 mmHg (95% CI of 29–33 mmHg) during exercise, suggesting that CMS would not be a cause of PH.

A review of invasive and noninvasive pulmonary hemodynamic measurements in healthy lowlander subjects at sea level [23, 32–36] and at high altitude [23, 32–37], healthy high-altitude dwellers [32, 36–40], and CMS patients [36, 40,

41] shows that patients with CMS have a higher mPAP than high-altitude healthy controls, and high-altitude dwellers have steeper mPAP-cardiac output relationships, i.e., a higher PVR during exercise [36]. This is largely explained by increased viscosity of the blood because of erythrocytosis. Hematocrit-corrected PVR smoothens out difference in PVR between high-altitude dwellers with or without CMS or high-altitude sojourners as compared to sea-level controls [14]. For example it is generally assumed that high-altitude inhabitants of the Himalayas have no hypoxic PH as compared to the inhabitants of the high-altitude Andean plateaus [37]. However, these differences smoothen out after correcting PVR for hematocrit [14, 29] (Fig. 12.1).

Hypoxic vasoconstriction is particularly intense in very few normal human subjects [24, 42]. Because hypoxia does not affect the longitudinal distribution of resistances, these subjects present with increased pulmonary capillary pressure and, accordingly, are predisposed to high-altitude pul-

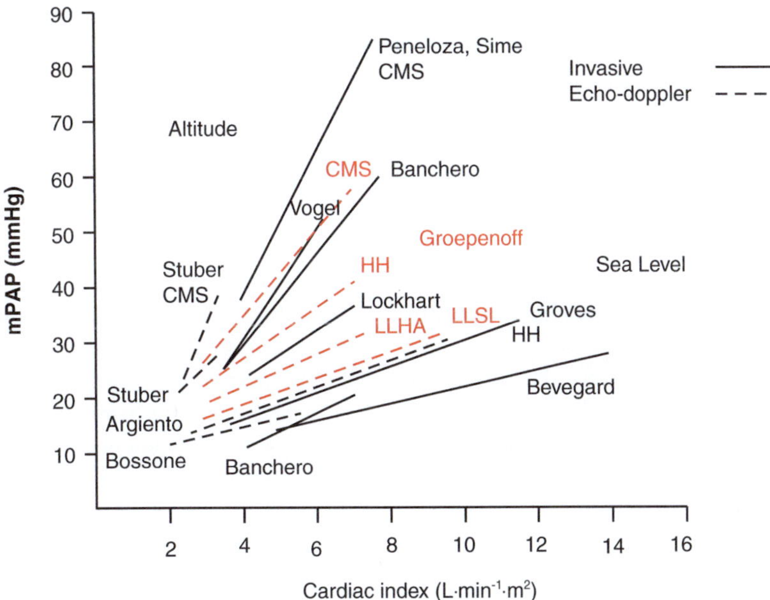

Fig. 12.1 Range of mean pulmonary artery pressures (mPAP) expressed as a function of cardiac index (CI) at exercise in high-altitude (HA) and sea-level (SL) inhabitants. Source studies are indicated by names of first authors [23, 31–41]. Highlanders present with higher resting mPAP and increased slopes of mPAP-CI. The steepest slopes of mPAP-CI occur in highlanders with chronic mountain sickness (CMS). Tibetan highlanders have mPAP-CI relationships with limits of normal measured at sea level. Invasive and noninvasive measurements generated similar averaged mPAP-CI curves. (Adapted from Groepenhoff et al. [36] with permission)

monary edema (HAPE) [43]. Brisk responders to hypoxia are also at risk of HARHF [7]. The occurrence of HARHF in the human species seems very low, but prevalence is not exactly known.

Does Hypoxic Exposure Exert Negative Inotropic Effects?

It has long been thought that the myocardium may self-limit its pump function because of decreased oxygen availability, thereby preventing potentially fatal hypoxia-induced arrhythmia or failure [44, 45]. Hypoxia has been reported to exert negative inotropic effects in intact animal preparations [46] and in isolated myocardial fibers [44]. However, stroke volume (SV) as a function of right- or left-heart filling pressures has been reported to be well maintained at extremely high simulated altitudes, indicating preserved contractility [47]. This has been confirmed by measurements of left ventricular (LV) peak systolic versus end-systolic volume relationships [48]. Yet borderline PH in association with hypoxia and inflammatory conditions such as chronic obstructive pulmonary disease and systemic sclerosis [49] or hypoxic breathing only [50] has been reported in speckle tracking echocardiography studies to be a cause of regional inhomogeneity of RV contraction and occasional postsystolic shortening. The functional relevance of these observations remains incompletely understood.

Acute hypoxic breathing at sea level in healthy adult volunteers has been reported to increase systolic PAP (estimated from the maximum velocity of tricuspid regurgitation) to 41 mmHg and not to affect echocardiographic indices of RV systolic function such as fractional area change (FAC), tricuspid annular plane systolic excursion (TAPSE), tissue Doppler tricuspid annulus S wave, or RV free wall strain, but with suggestion of altered diastolic function by decreased tricuspid inflow and annulus ratio of E and A waves [51]. However, this last effect was also obtained by an infusion of low-dose dobutamine. The authors thought that maintained systolic function in the presence of moderate increase in PAP and changes in diastolic filling patterns would be essentially explained by acute hypoxia-induced activation of the sympathetic nervous system.

This observation was confirmed by a study on children and adolescents rapidly taken to the altitude of 3450 m. Echocardiographic examinations showed a mild increase in PAP to the upper limit of normal normobaric values, inversely correlated to age, with preserved or slightly enhanced indices of both RV and LV systolic function [52]. A frequency analysis of heart rate showed an increase in low-frequency-to-high-frequency mode ratio (LF/HF) suggesting sympathetic nervous system activation [52].

The effects of chronic hypoxic exposure were assessed by a study on healthy Aymara living permanently on the Bolivian altiplano, at approximately 4000 m, compared to recently acclimatized healthy sojourners [53]. Acute exposure to high altitude caused an increase in mPAP to 20–25 mmHg, decreased RV and LV E/A with a prolonged isovolumic relaxation time of the RV, and maintained RV systolic function as estimated by TAPSE and tricuspid annulus S wave. The high-altitude natives presented with relatively lower mPAP, higher oxygen saturation, more pronounced alteration in indices of diastolic function, and a slight decrease in TAPSE and tricuspid annulus S wave. The estimated LV filling pressure was lower in native high-altitude natives. The (slight) deterioration of indices of both systolic and diastolic functions in high-altitude natives, in spite of less marked PH and better oxygenation, was explained by the authors by combined effects of a lesser degree of sympathetic nervous system activation, relative hypovolemia, and possibly some negative inotropic effects of a long-lasting hypoxic exposure [53].

A speckle tracking echocardiography study on the Peruvian altiplano showed a slight decrease in LV strain and deformation in recently acclimatized sojourners, but normal LV systolic function in Quechua natives with or without CMS [54]. Interestingly, the E/A ratio was decreased in patients with CMS. A frequency analysis of heart rate showed an increased LF/HF ratio in high-altitude sojourners and dwellers, but a decreased LF/HF ratio in CMS patients in whom therefore sympathetic nervous system activation could not explain altered indices of LV diastolic function.

A similar study performed at the altitude of 5000 m in Nepal showed a slight increase in sPAP in Sherpa (who are of Tibetan ancestry) and acclimatized lowlanders [55]. The Sherpa had smaller RV and LV volumes but similar LV systolic mechanics compared to the sojourners. In contrast to LV systolic mechanics, LV diastolic, untwisting velocity was significantly lower in Sherpa compared with lowlanders at both sea level and high altitude. After partial acclimatization, lowlanders demonstrated no change in the RV end-diastolic area; however, both RV strain and LV end-diastolic volume were reduced. The authors concluded that short-term hypoxia induced a reduction in RV systolic function that was also evident in Sherpa following chronic exposure. However, the LV appeared well adapted in spite of some alteration in diastolic relaxation.

In summary, imaging studies have shown that acute acclimatization or chronic exposure to high-altitude hypobaric hypoxia is associated with unchanged, increased, or slightly decreased systolic function and unchanged or increased dimensions of the RV, unchanged or slightly decreased systolic function and decreased dimensions of the LV, and altered indices of diastolic function of both ventricles. Most of these changes can be explained by changes in blood volume, ventricular dimensions, and sympathetic nervous system activation, but some negative inotropic effects of chronic hypoxia cannot be excluded. Similar changes are to be found in CMS, but without sympathetic nervous system activation, and possible remodeling effects of lifelong hypoxia.

The Right Ventricle During Hypoxic Exercise

There have been reports that exercise capacity in hypoxia can be improved by pharmacological interventions to decrease PVR. The phosphodiesterase-5 inhibitor sildenafil decreased PAP and increased maximum workload in healthy low-landers who hiked to Mount Everest base camp [56]. Sildenafil decreased PVR in healthy volunteers and improved their maximum oxygen uptake (VO_2max) in acute normobaric hypoxia but this was less prominent in more chronic hypoxia at the altitude of 5000 m on the Chimborazo, in Ecuador [57]. Concomitant decreases in PVR and improved VO_2max were also reported in HAPE-susceptible subjects exposed to high altitude after preventive administration of dexamethasone [58]. In these studies, improved systemic oxygenation by the intake of vasodilating interventions was a confounding factor [56–58]. Decreasing PVR by the intake of the endothelin receptor antagonists bosentan or sitaxsentan in acute or chronic hypoxia in healthy volunteers did not affect arterial O_2 content, but even so VO_2max improved by 10–25% [59, 60]. A review of exercise studies in healthy subjects with or without intake of pulmonary vasodilators reveals inverse relationships between PVR and VO_2max along with higher lung-diffusing capacity and lower ventilatory equivalents for carbon dioxide in those with the lowest PVR, in hypoxia [61]. However, hypoxia also limits maximum cardiac output and VO2max by altered coupling between peripheral convective and diffusional O_2 transport mechanisms [62], so that increased RV afterload and decreased exercise capacity may not be causally related [63]. In fact, the answer to the question whether increased afterload in hypoxia impairs the coupling of RV function to the pulmonary circulation, limits maximum cardiac output, and eventually decreases VO_2max would require measurements of RV structure and function. Such studies are few.

In perhaps the only study until now looking into RV function reserve during hypoxic exercise, pulmonary vascular pressures, cardiac output, and indices of ventricular function and dimensions were measured using Doppler echocardiography at rest and at exercise in 46 patients with CMS and 41 healthy controls all living permanently at the altitude of 3600–4000 m, in La Paz, Bolivia [64]. Pulmonary artery pressures at rest were on average at the upper limit of sea-level normal in both groups, but increased markedly at exercise, as expected. PVR increased

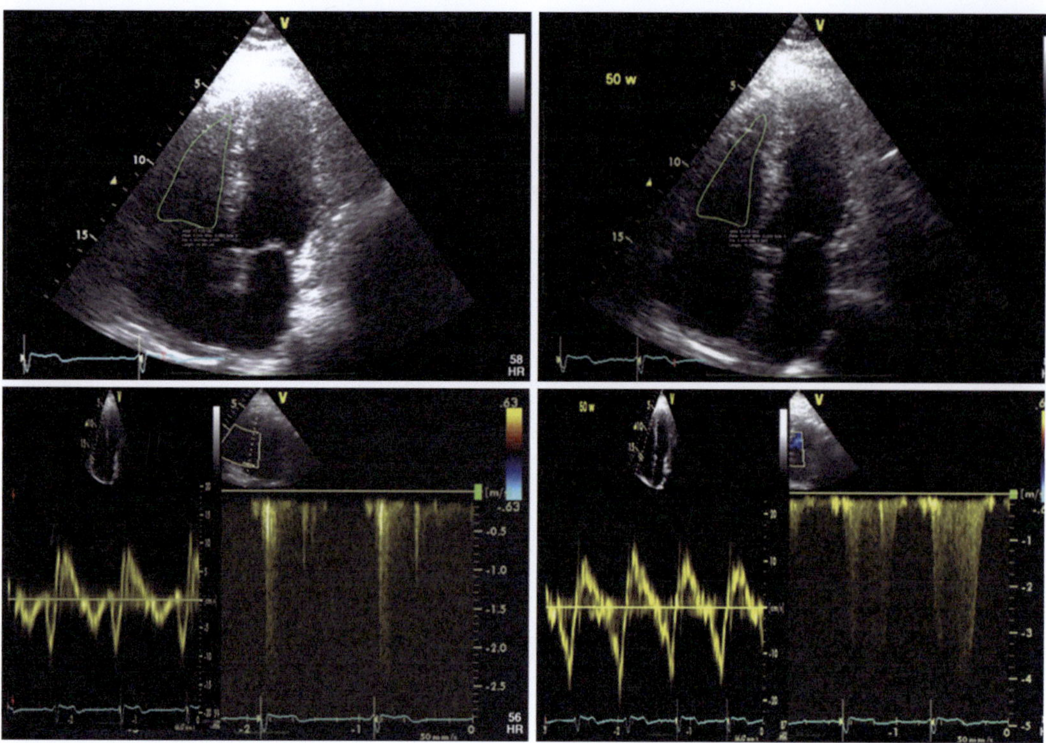

Fig. 12.2 Apical four-chamber views showing end-systolic areas (ESA) of the right ventricle (RV) at rest (left panels) and during exercise (right panels) with tissue Doppler tricuspid annulus S′ wave and tricuspid regurgitant jets in a patient with chronic mountain sickness. Exercise was associated with a maximum velocity of tricuspid regurgitation of 4 m/s, corresponding to a systolic RV pressure of 69 mmHg, an unchanged S′, and a decreased RV ESA, all compatible with preserved coupling of RV function to the hypertensive pulmonary circulation. (From Ref. [64])

in CMS patients and remained unchanged in controls, in contrast to the decrease in PVR normally seen in healthy subjects at sea level. Indices of RV or LV function at rest did not differ between CMS patients and controls, with the exception of some increase in RV dimensions and decreased FAC in CMS patients. Both healthy subjects and CMS patients had a few slight alterations in the indices of LV and RV diastolic and systolic functions, in agreement with previous studies. However, RV contractility assessed by peak systolic pressure versus end-systolic area increased in an adapted fashion in response to increased loading conditions, indicating preserved contractile reserve. This result illustrated in Fig. 12.2 is in keeping with recent report of preserved aerobic exercise capacity in CMS patients as compared to healthy high-altitude dwellers or recently acclimatized lowlanders [36].

These observations are in keeping with animal experiments showing in dogs, pigs, goats, and sheep that hypoxic breathing induces an acute increase in PAP of variable magnitudes but matched by a proportional increase in RV end-systolic elastance as the gold standard estimate of contractility, thereby preserving RV-PA coupling [65–67].

High Altitude-Induced Right-Heart Failure

Sometimes high-altitude exposure is associated with a brisk increase in PAP. How often this occurs is not known. It has been observed in a small number of mountaineers, but may be less common during high-altitude travels without strenuous exercise [43]. However, PH at high

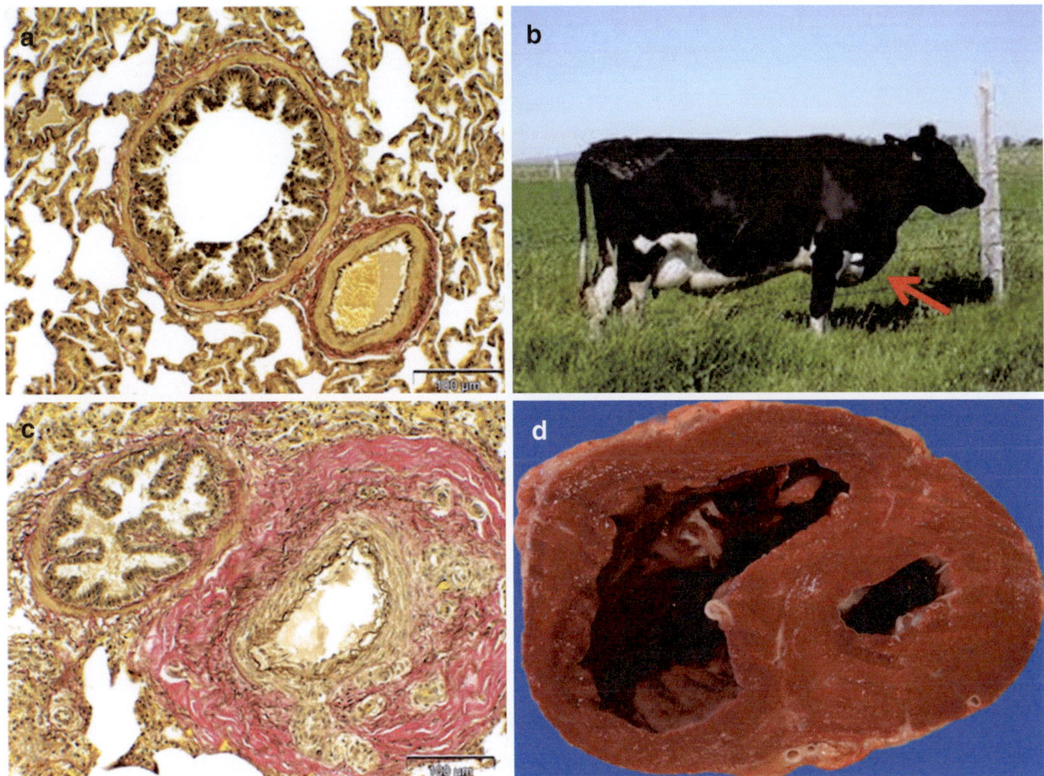

Fig. 12.3 Pulmonary arterial remodeling with medial hypertrophy and adventitial thickening (**c**) compared to normally thin medial and adventitial layers in a normal pulmonary arteriole (**a**), right ventricular hypertrophy (**d**), and cow with right clinical heart failure ("brisket disease") (**b**). The red arrow shows the typical swelling of the brisket. (From Ref. [69])

altitudes is a cause of HAPE [43] but also HARHF [68]. Severe and rapidly evolving hypoxic PH as a cause of HARHF has been documented by hemodynamic measurements in cattle, chickens, and humans [2, 3] with pathological examination showing remodeling of pulmonary arterioles and a dilated/hypertrophied RV [6]. A case of right-heart failure in cow, or "brisket disease," is illustrated in Fig. 12.3 [69].

The most detailed and actually only invasive hemodynamic study in patients with the so-called adult subacute mountain sickness or HARHF was reported in 21 Indian soldiers posted for weeks at altitudes of 5800–6700 m, and who developed a predominantly right-sided congestive heart failure syndrome, with echocardiography showing dilatation of the right heart and a normal LV EF [3]. A right-heart catheterization performed after they were returned in 3 days to the altitude of 300 m showed a mPAP of 26 ± 4 mmHg, a PAWP of 11 ± 4 mmHg, a right atrial pressure of 8 ± 4 mmHg, and a cardiac index of 3.5 L/min/m^2. Exercise was associated with a steep increase in mPAP but no change in PVR. The authors thought that this hemodynamic profile reflected RVF in response to severe hypoxic PH that developed during the high-altitude stay and had already much resolved, but did not exclude a significant contribution of left-heart failure due to strenuous exercise in extreme cold environmental conditions as several patients still had a higher-than-normal PAWP.

In a case of HARHF reported with echocardiographic measurements, illustrated in Fig. 12.4, the right heart was minimally dilated but with postsystolic shortening and dilated inferior vena cava, suggesting pending RV-PA uncoupling [7]. Interestingly the clinical examination of this sub-

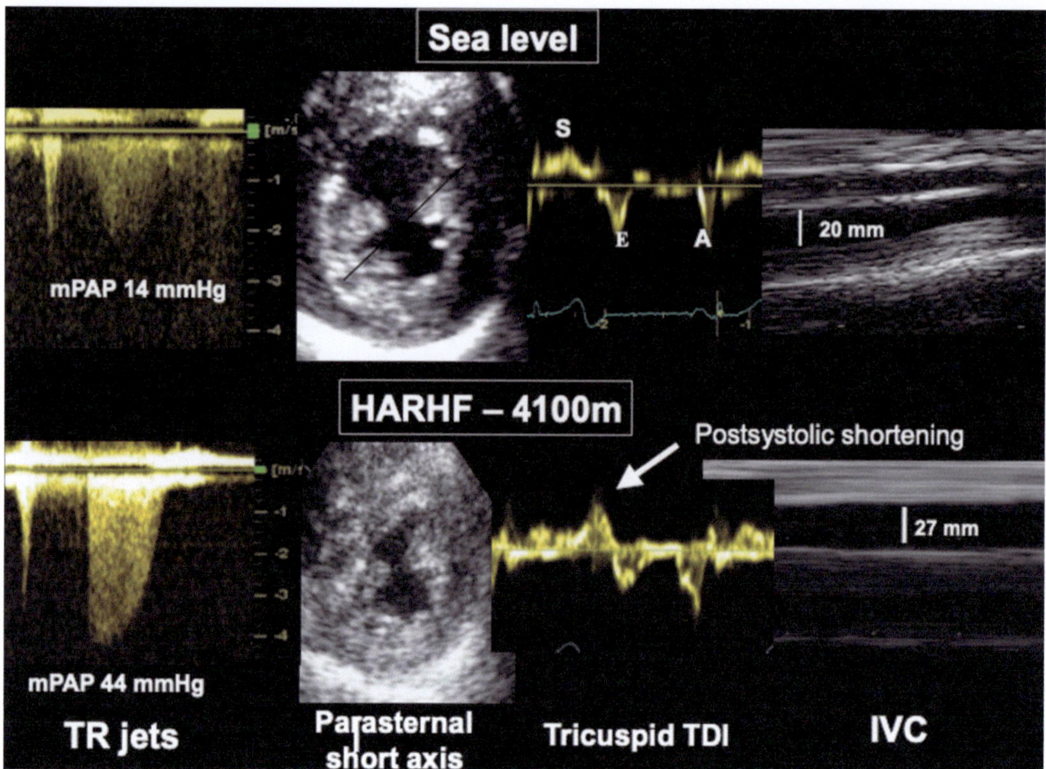

Fig. 12.4 High-altitude right-heart failure (HARHF) in a previously healthy subject after arrival in La Paz, 3600 m, and touring on the Bolivian altiplano at altitudes around 4000 m. Maximum velocity of tricuspid regurgitation is suggestive of severe pulmonary hypertension; there is a decreased eccentricity index, postsystolic shortening, and dilatation of the inferior vena cava with loss of inspiratory collapse. (From Ref. [7])

ject was unremarkable as systemic congestion symptomatology would likely appear in the presence of more markedly dilated right-heart structures and filling pressures. Imaging of the heart allows for an earlier diagnosis of HARHF. A more typically marked dilatation of right-heart chambers was recently reported in a Kyrgyz child with the so-called subacute infantile mountain sickness [70].

in remote places with not yet fully developed hospital equipment. While waiting for this to be done, the high-altitude experts should agree on updated definitions with improved dialogue with pulmonary hypertension and heart failure communities, and feasibility of large-scale prospective studies based on consensus phenotyping.

Perspective

High-altitude exposure may be a cause of severe PH and RHF. How often this happens is not exactly known. Progress in imaging of the right heart and the pulmonary circulation with easy-to-use portable echocardiography should make epidemiological studies of HARHF possible, even

References

1. Mosso A. La stanchezza del cuore. In: Fisiologia dell'uomo sulle Alpi. Molano: Fraztelli Treves, Editori; 1897.
2. Hecht HH, Kuida H, Lange RL, Thorne JL, Brown AM. Brisket disease II. Clinical features and hemodynamic observations in altitude-dependent right heart failure of cattle. Am J Med. 1962;32:171–83.
3. Anand IS, Malhotra R, Chandershekhar Y, Bali HK, Chauhan SS, Jindal SK, Bhandar RK, Wahi PL. Adult subacute mountain sickness: a syndrome of conges-

tive heart failure in man at very high altitude. Lancet. 1990;335:561–5.

4. Monge C. High altitude disease. Arch Int Med. 1937;59:32–40.

5. Pei SX, Chen XJ, Si Ren BZ, Liu YH, Chen XS, Harris EM, Anand IS, Harris PC. Chronic mountain sickness in Tibet. Q J Med. 1989;266:555–74.

6. Sui GJ, Lui YH, Cheng XS, Anand IS, Harris E, Harris P, Heath D. Subacute infantile mountain sickness. J Pathol. 1988;155:161–70.

7. Huez S, Faoro V, Vachiery JL, Unger P, Martinot JB, Naeije R. Images in cardiovascular medicine. High-altitude-induced right-heart failure. Circulation. 2007;115:308–9.

8. Naeije R. Physiological adaptation of the cardiovascular system to high altitude. Progr Cardiovasc Dis. 2010;52:456–66.

9. Soria R, Egger M, Scherrer U, Bender N, Rimoldi SF. Pulmonary artery pressure and arterial oxygen saturation in people living at high or low altitude: systematic review and meta-analysis. J Appl Physiol. 2016;121:1151–9.

10. Hoeper MM, Bogaard HJ, Condliffe R, Frantz R, Khanna D, Kurzyna M, Langleben D, Manes A, Satoh T, Torres F, Wilkins MR, Badesch DB. Definitions and diagnosis of pulmonary hypertension. J Am Coll Cardiol. 2013;62(25 Suppl):D45–50.

11. Simonneau G, Montani D, Celermajer DS, Denton CP, Gatzoulis MA, Krowka M, Williams PG, Souza R. Haemodynamic definitions and updated clinical classification of pulmonary hypertension. Eur Respir J. 2019;53:1801913. [Epub ahead of print].

12. Leon-Velarde F, Maggiorini M, Reeves JT, Aldashev A, Asmus I, Bernardi L, Ge RL, Hackett P, Kobayashi T, Moore LG, Penaloza D, Richalet JP, Roach R, Wu T, Vargas E, Zubieta-Castillo G, Zubieta-Calleja G. Consensus statement on chronic and subacute high altitude diseases. High Alt Med Biol. 2005;6:147–57.

13. Vanderpool R, Naeije R. Hematocrit-corrected pulmonary vascular resistance. Am Rev Respir Crit Care Med. 2018;198:305–9.

14. Naeije R, Vanderpool R. Pulmonary hypertension and chronic mountain sickness. High Alt Med Biol. 2013;14:117–25.

15. Campbell EJM, Short DS. The cause of oedema in "cor pulmonale". Lancet. 1960;1:1184–6.

16. Sanz J, Sánchez-Quintana D, Bossone E, Bogaard HJ, Naeije R. Anatomy, function, and dysfunction of the right ventricle: JACC state-of-the-art review. J Am Coll Cardiol. 2019;73:1463–82.

17. Reeves JT, Wagner WW Jr, McMurtry IF, Grover RF. Physiological effects of high altitude on the pulmonary circulation. Int Rev Physiol. 1979;20:289–310.

18. Sylvester JT, Shimoda LA, Aaronson PI, Ward JP. Hypoxic pulmonary vasoconstriction. Physiol Rev. 2012;92:367–520.

19. Grünig E, Weissmann S, Ehlken N, Fijalkowska A, Fischer C, Fourme T, Galié N, Ghofrani A, Harrison RE, Huez S, Humbert M, Janssen B, Kober J, Koehler R, Machado RD, Mereles D, Naeije R, Olschewski H, Provencher S, Reichenberger F, Retailleau K, Rocchi G, Simonneau G, Torbicki A, Trembath R, Seeger W. Stress-Doppler-echocardiography in relatives of patients with idiopathic and familial pulmonary arterial hypertension: results of a multicenter European analysis of pulmonary artery pressure response to exercise and hypoxia. Circulation. 2009;119:1747–57.

20. Motley HL, Cournand A, Werkö L, Himmelstein A, Dresdale D. The influence of short periods of induced acute anoxia upon pulmonary artery pressures in man. Am J Phys. 1947;150:315–20.

21. Naeije R, Mélot C, Mols P, Hallemans R. Effects of vasodilators on hypoxic pulmonary vasoconstriction in normal man. Chest. 1982;82:404–10.

22. Naeije R, Mélot C, Niset G, Delcroix M, Wagner PD. Improved arterial oxygenation by a pharmacological increase in chemosensitivity during hypoxic exercise in normal subjects. J Appl Physiol. 1993;74:1666–71.

23. Groves BM, Reeves JT, Sutton JR, Wagner PD, Cymerman A, Malconian MK, Rock PB, Young PM, Houston CS. Operation Everest II: elevated high altitude pulmonary resistance unresponsive to oxygen. J Appl Physiol. 1987;63:521–30.

24. Maggiorini M, Mélot C, Pierre S, Pfeiffer F, Greve I, Sartori C, Lepori M, Hauser M, Scherrer U, Naeije R. High altitude pulmonary edema is initially caused by an increased capillary pressure. Circulation. 2001;103:2078–83.

25. Dorrington KL, Clar C, Young JD, Jonas M, Tansley JG, Robbins PA. Time course of the human pulmonary vascular response to 8 hours of isocapnic hypoxia. Am J Phys. 1997;273:H1126–34.

26. Kronenberg RS, Safar P, Leej, Wright F, Noble W, Wahrenbrock E, Hickey R, Nemoto E, Severinghaus JW. Pulmonary artery pressure and alveolar gas exchange in man during acclimatization to 12,470 ft. J Clin Invest. 1971;50:827–37.

27. Sime F, Penaloza D, Ruiz L. Bradycardia, increased cardiac output and reversal of pulmonary hypertension in altitude natives at sea level. Br Heart J. 1971;33:647–57.

28. Penazola D, Arias-Stella J. The heart and pulmonary circulation at high altitudes. Healthy highlanders and chronic mountain sickness. Circulation. 2007;115:1132–46.

29. Faoro V, Huez S, Vanderpool RR, Groepenhoff H, de Bisschop C, Martinot JB, Lamotte M, Pavelescu A, Guénard H, Naeije R. Pulmonary circulation and gas exchange at exercise in Sherpas at high altitude. J Appl Physiol. 2014;116:919–26.

30. D'Alto M, Romeo E, Argiento P, D'Andrea A, Vanderpool R, Correra A, Bossone E, Sarubbi B, Calabrò R, Russo MG, Naeije R. Accuracy and precision of echocardiography versus right heart catheterization for the assessment of pulmonary hypertension. Int J Cardiol. 2013;168:4058–62.

31. Soria R, Egger M, Scherrer U, Bender N, Rimoldi SF. Pulmonary artery pressure at rest and during exercise in chronic mountain sickness: a meta-analysis.

Eur Respir J. 2019;53(6):1802040. [Epub ahead of print].

32. Banchero N, Sime F, Penaloza D, Cruz J, Gamboa R, Marticorena E. Pulmonary pressure, cardiac output, and arterial oxygen saturation during exercise at high altitude and at sea level. Circulation. 1966;33:249–62.

33. Bevegaard S, Holmgren A, Jonsson B. Circulatory studies in well trained athletes at rest and during heavy exercise, with special reference to stroke volume and the influence of body position. Acta Physiol Scand. 1963;57:26–50.

34. Bossone E, Rubenfire M, Bach DS, Ricciardi M, Armstrong WF. Range of tricuspid regurgitation velocity at rest and during exercise in normal adult men: implications for the diagnosis of pulmonary hypertension. J Am Coll Cardiol. 1999;33:1662–6.

35. Argiento P, Vanderpool RR, Mule M, Russo MG, D'Alto M, Bossone E, Chesler NC, Naeije R. Exercise stress echocardiography of the pulmonary circulation: limits of normal and sex differences. Chest. 2012;142:1158–65.

36. Groepenhoff H, Overbeek MJ, Mulè M, van der Plas M, Argiento P, Villafuerte FC, Beloka S, Faoro V, Macarlupu JL, Guenard H, de Bisschop C, Martinot JB, Vanderpool R, Penaloza D, Naeije R. Exercise pathophysiology in patients with chronic mountain sickness. Chest. 2012;142:877–84.

37. Groves BM, Droma T, Sutton JR, McCullough RG, McCullough RE, Zhuang J, Rapmund G, Sun S, Janes C, Moore LG. Minimal hypoxic pulmonary hypertension in normal Tibetans at 3,658 m. J Appl Physiol. 1993;74:312–8.

38. Lockhart A, Zelter M, Mensch-Dechene J, Antezana G, Paz-Zamora M, Vargas E, Coudert J. Pressure-flow-volume relationships in pulmonary circulation of normal highlanders. J Appl Physiol. 1976;41:449–56.

39. Vogel JHK, Weaver WF, Rose RL, Blount SG, Grover RF. Pulmonary hypertension on exertion in normal man living at 10150 feet (Leadville, Colorado). Med Thorac. 1962;19:269–85.

40. Penaloza D, Sime F. Chronic cor pulmonale due to loss of acclimatization (chronic mountain sickness). Am J Med. 1971;50:728–43.

41. Stuber T, Sartori C, Schwab M, Jayet PY, Rimoldi SF, Garcin S, Thalmann S, Spielvogel H, Salmòn CS, Villena M, Scherrer U, Allemann Y. Exaggerated pulmonary hypertension during mild exercise in chronic mountain sickness. Chest. 2010;137:388–92.

42. Grünig E, Mereles D, Hildebrandt W, Swenson ER, Kübler W, Kuecherer H, Bärtsch P. Stress Doppler echocardiography for identification of susceptibility to high altitude pulmonary edema. J Am Coll Cardiol. 2000;35:980–7.

43. Bärtsch P, Mairbäurl H, Maggiorini M, Swenson E. Physiologic aspects of high-altitude pulmonary edema. J Appl Physiol. 2005;98:1101–10.

44. Silverman HS, Wei S, Haigney MC, Ocampo CJ, Stern MD. Myocyte adaptation to chronic hypoxia and development of tolerance to subsequent acute severe hypoxia. Circ Res. 1997;80:699–707.

45. Noakes TD. Physiological models to understand exercise fatigue and the adaptations that predict or enhance athletic performance. Scand J Med Sci Sports. 2000;10:119–23.

46. Tucker CE, James WE, Berry MA, Johnstone CL, Grover RF. Depressed myocardial function in the goat at high altitude. J Appl Physiol. 1976;41:356–61.

47. Reeves JT, Groves BM, Sutton JR, Wagner PD, Cymerman A, Malconian MK, Rock PB, Young PM, Houston CS. Operation Everest II: preservation of cardiac function at extreme altitude. J Appl Physiol. 1987;63:531–9.

48. Suarez J, Alexander JK, Houston CS. Enhanced left ventricular systolic performance at high altitude during Operation Everest II. Am J Cardiol. 1987;60:137–42.

49. Lamia B, Muir JF, Molano LC, Viacroze C, Benichou J, Bonnet P, Quieffin J, Cuevelier A, Naeije R. Altered synchrony of right ventricular contraction in borderline pulmonary hypertension. Int J Cardiovasc Imaging. 2017;33:1331–9.

50. Pezzuto B, Forton K, Badagliacca R, Motoji Y, Faoro V, Naeije R. Right ventricular dyssynchrony during hypoxic breathing but not during exercise in healthy subjects a speckle tracking echocardiography study. Exp Physiol. 2018;103:1338–46.

51. Huez S, Retailleau K, Unger P, Pavelescu A, Vachiery JL, Derumeaux G, Naeije R. Right and left ventricular adaptation to hypoxia: a tissue Doppler imaging study. Am J Physiol Heart Circ Physiol. 2005;289:H1391–8.

52. Allemann Y, Stuber T, de Marchi SF, Rexhaj E, Sartori C, Scherrer U, Rimoldi SF. Pulmonary artery pressure and cardiac function in children and adolescents after rapid ascent to 3,450 m. Am J Physiol Heart Circ Physiol. 2012;302:H2646–53.

53. Huez S, Faoro V, Guénard H, Martinot JB, Naeije R. Echocardiographic and tissue Doppler imaging of cardiac adaptation to high altitude in native highlanders versus acclimatized lowlanders. Am J Cardiol. 2009;103:1605–9.

54. Dedobbeleer C, Hadefi A, Pichon A, Villafuerte F, Naeije R, Unger P. Left ventricular adaptation to high altitude: speckle tracking echocardiography in lowlanders, healthy highlanders and highlanders with chronic mountain sickness. Int J Cardiovasc Imaging. 2015;31:743–52.

55. Stembridge M, Ainslie PN, Hughes MG, Stöhr EJ, Cotter JD, Nio AQ, Shave R. Ventricular structure, function, and mechanics at high altitude: chronic remodeling in Sherpa vs. short-term lowlander adaptation. J Appl Physiol. 2014;117:334–43.

56. Ghofrani HA, Reichenberger F, Kohstall MG, Mrosek EH, Seeger T, Olschewski H, Seeger W, Grimminger F. Sildenafil increased exercise capacity during hypoxia at low altitudes and at Mount Everest base camp: a randomized, double-blind, placebo-controlled crossover trial. Ann Intern Med. 2004;141:169–77.

57. Faoro V, Lamotte M, Deboeck G, Pavelescu A, Huez S, Guenard H, Martinot JB, Naeije R. Effects of silde-

nafil on exercise capacity in hypoxic normal subjects. High Alt Med Biol. 2007;8:155–63.

58. Fischler M, Maggiorini M, Dorschner L, Debrunner J, Bernheim A, Kiencke S, Mairbäurl H, Bloch KE, Naeije R, Brunner-La Rocca HP. Dexamethasone but not tadalafil improves exercise capacity in adults prone to high altitude pulmonary edema. Am J Respir Crit Care Med. 2009;180:346–52.

59. Faoro V, Boldingh S, Moreels M, Martinez S, Lamotte M, Unger P, Brimioulle S, Huez S, Naeije R. Bosentan decreases pulmonary vascular resistance and improves exercise capacity in acute hypoxia. Chest. 2009;135:1215–22.

60. Naeije R, Huez S, Lamotte M, Retailleau K, Neupane S, Abramowicz D, Faoro V. Pulmonary artery pressure limits exercise capacity at high altitudes. Eur Respir J. 2010;36:1049–55.

61. Pavelescu A, Faoro V, Guenard H, De Bisschop C, Martinot JB, Melot C, Naeije R. Pulmonary vascular reserve and exercise capacity, at sea level and at high altitude. High Alt Med Biol. 2013;14:19–26.

62. Wagner PD. Reduced maximal cardiac output at altitude. Mechanisms and significance. Respir Physiol. 2000;120:1–11.

63. Naeije R. Pro: hypoxic pulmonary vasoconstriction is a limiting factor to exercise capacity at high altitudes. High Alt Med Biol. 2011;12:309–12.

64. Pratali L, Allemann Y, Rimoldi SF, Faita F, Hutter D, Rexhaj E, Brenner R, Bailey DM, Sartori C, Salmon CS, Villena M, Scherrer U, Picano E, Sicari R. RV contractility and exercise-induced pulmonary hypertension in chronic mountain sickness: a stress echocardiographic and tissue Doppler imaging study. JACC Cardiovasc Imaging. 2013;6:1287–97.

65. Brimioulle S, Wauthy P, Ewalenko P, Rondelet B, Vermeulen F, Kerbaul F, Naeije R. Single-beat estimation of right ventricular end-systolic pressure-volume relationship. Am J Physiol Heart Circ Physiol. 2003;284:H1625–30.

66. Rex S, Missant C, Claus P, Buhre W, Wouters PF. Effects of inhaled iloprost on right ventricular contractility, right ventriculo-vascular coupling and ventricular interdependence: a randomized placebo-controlled trial in an experimental model of acute pulmonary hypertension. Crit Care. 2008;12:R113.

67. Wauthy P, Pagnamenta A, Vassali F, Brimioulle S, Naeije R. Right ventricular adaptation to pulmonary hypertension. An interspecies comparison. Am J Physiol Heart Circ Physiol. 2004;286:H1441–7.

68. Naeije R. RV is doing well as high altitudes. Always? JACC Cardiovasc Imaging. 2013;6:1298–300.

69. Malherbe CR, Marquard J, Legg DE, Cammack KM, O'Toole D. Right ventricular hypertrophy with heart failure in Holstein heifers at elevation of 1,600 meters. J Vet Diagn Investig. 2012;24:867–77.

70. Muratali Uulu K, Cholponbaeva M, Duishobaev M, Toktosunova A, Maripov A, Sydykov A, Sarybaev A. A case of subacute infantile mountain sickness in a Kyrgyz child. High Alt Med Biol. 2018;19:208–10.

The Right Ventricle in Congenital Heart Diseases

13

Beatrijs Bartelds, Johannes M. Douwes, and Rolf M. F. Berger

Abbreviations

ACE	Angiotensin-converting enzyme
ARB	Angiotensin receptor blocker
ASD	Atrial septal defect
ccTGA	Congenitally corrected transposition of the great arteries
CHD	Congenital heart diseases
CMR	Cardiac magnetic resonance imaging
EF	Ejection fraction
FAC	Fractional area change
LV	Left ventricle
PAH	Pulmonary arterial hypertension
PH	Pulmonary hypertension
RV	Right ventricle
RVOT	Right ventricular outflow tract
TAPSE	Tricuspid annular plane systolic excursion
TGA-as	Transposition of the great arteries with atrial switch procedure
TI	Tricuspid insufficiency
TOF	Tetralogy of Fallot
VSD	Ventricular septal defect

B. Bartelds
Division of Pediatric Cardiology, Department of Pediatrics, Erasmus Medical Center, Sophia Children's Hospital, Rotterdam, The Netherlands
e-mail: b.bartelds@erasmusmc.nl

J. M. Douwes (✉) · R. M. F. Berger
Department of Pediatric and Congenital Cardiology, Center for Congenital Heart Diseases, Beatrix Children's Hospital, University Medical Center Groningen, Groningen, The Netherlands
e-mail: j.m.douwes@umcg.nl; r.m.f.berger@umcg.nl

Introduction

Right ventricular function is an important determinant of prognosis and outcome in congenital heart diseases [1]. Right ventricular adaptation to congenital heart diseases (CHD) has many faces as there is a wide variety in defects involving the right ventricle as well as in surgical corrections and treatment strategies. This results in a variety of RV loading conditions that can change over time as a result of surgical interventions, aging, or disease progression. Also, treatment practice has evolved, changing the nature and outcome of survivors of CHD. Lastly, several lesions also affect the left ventricle (LV) that may interact with RV function and thereby change the RV function.

Although in practice sometimes artificially, for educational and conceptual purposes the effects on the RV can be divided into three types of abnormal loading conditions, i.e., increased preload (e.g., shunts or valvular insufficiency), increased afterload (e.g., stenosis or connection to systemic circulation), or a mixture of both. During the process of maturation and aging and as a result of interventions loading conditions can

Table 13.1 Overview of lesions affecting the right ventricle in congenital heart diseases

Increased preload	Mixed		Increased afterload
Atrial septal defect (ASD)	ASD + PS	←	Pulmonary stenosis (PS)
	ASD + pulmonary hypertension	←	Pulmonary hypertension
Pulmonary insufficiency (PI)	PI and PS after correction of TOF	←	Tetralogy of Fallot (TOF)
Tricuspid insufficiency (TI)	ccTGA + TI	←	Congenitally corrected transposition of the great arteries (ccTGA)
	TGA-as + TI	←	Transposition of the great arteries after atrial switch procedure (TGA-as)
	HLHS + BT shunt	←	Hypoplastic left-heart syndrome (HLHS)
	HLHS + TI		

shift from increased afterload to increased preload (Table 13.1). A detailed description of cardiac morphology in CHD has been described in the several textbooks of CHD [2, 3]. In this chapter we describe the different faces of the RV with a focus on the functional capacity. We differentiate between lesions affecting preload, afterload, and a mixture of those.

Lesions Affecting Preload

Lesions leading to an isolated volume load of the RV can be divided into two major groups, lesions with a pre-tricuspid shunt (i.e., atrial septal defect (ASD)) or lesions with valvular insufficiency (e.g., tricuspid insufficiency, pulmonary insufficiency, Table 13.1). Pulmonary insufficiency as a result of treatment in patients with repaired tetralogy of Fallot will be discussed separately. The major difference between the two groups is the increased pulmonary blood flow in shunt lesions, which may induce increased pulmonary vascular resistance leading to pulmonary hypertension, thus inducing a shift from increased preload to increased afterload.

Atrial Septal Defect

Atrial septal defect (ASD) is a quite common lesion in CHD, with a female dominance [4]. There are several morphological variants depending upon the position of the ASD (Fig. 13.1a). The most common form is ASD II, and rare vari-

ants are sinus venosus defects. The latter differ in that they are frequently associated with a partially abnormal pulmonary venous return leading to an obligatory left-to-right shunt at the atrial level. Furthermore, sinus venosus defects induce a higher risk for the development of pulmonary arterial hypertension (PAH) than other types of atrial shunts.

Without association of other defects, an ASD will lead to a left-to-right shunt at atrial level, inducing an increased preload of the RV (Fig. 13.1b). The degree of shunting depends on

1. The size of the defect
2. The presence of partially abnormal pulmonary venous return
3. The orifice of the tricuspid and the mitral valve
4. The difference in compliance between the receiving right and left ventricles
5. The pulmonary hypertension or pulmonary stenosis affecting the RV compliance

Prenatally, the right and left ventricles together take care of the systemic circulation. A right-to-left flow across the foramen ovale is a natural phenomenon, allowing the passage of higher saturated blood into the left ventricle [5]. Also, pulmonary vascular resistance (PVR) is very high and this decreases rapidly at birth. Consequently, pulmonary blood flow increases, thereby increasing pulmonary venous return. These changes will cause the flap of the foramen to be pressed against the atrial septum and lead to closure of the foramen. In patients with an ASD, a left-to-right shunt will

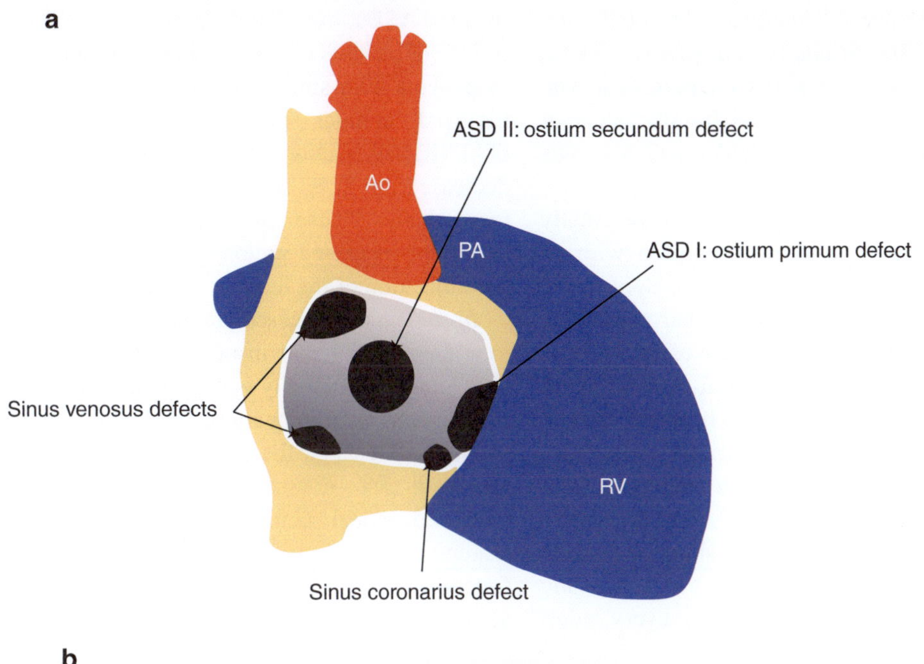

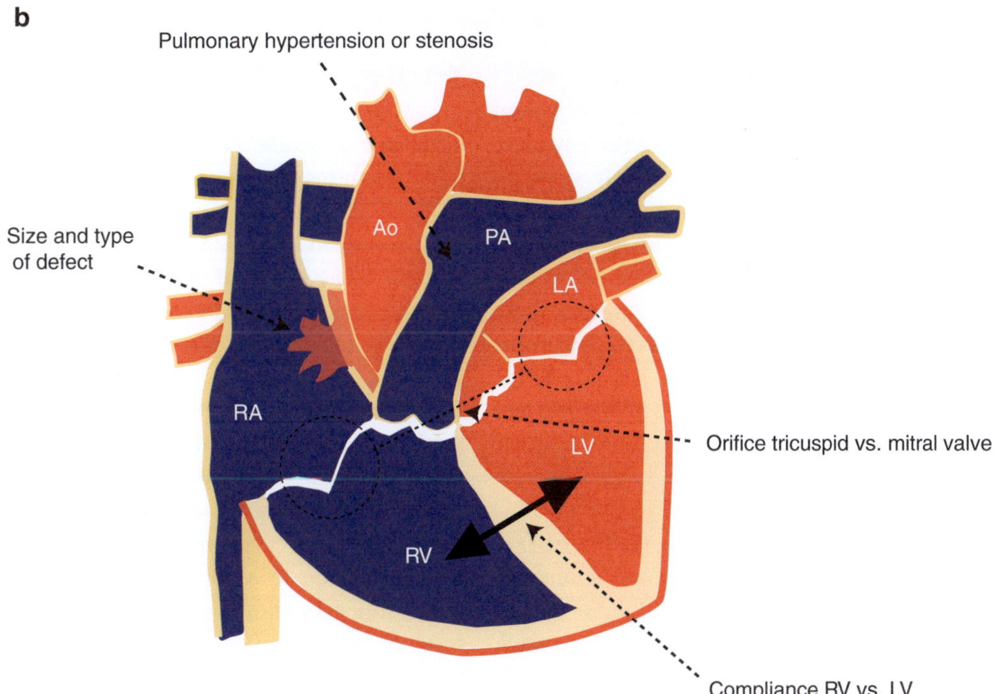

Fig. 13.1 (**a**) Different locations of atrial septal defects. (**b**) Factors influencing the degree of shunting in atrial septal defect. *Ao* Aorta, *PA* pulmonary artery, *RA* right atrium, *LA* left atrium, *RV* right ventricle, *LV* left ventricle

develop, the degree of which is dependent upon the decrease of pulmonary vascular resistance. Usually, no significant shunt develops in the first weeks, although in association of lesions affect- ing the inflow of the LV, such as a congenital mal- formation of the mitral valve or hypoplastic left heart, the shunt across the ASD may increase more rapidly. Alternatively, underdevelopment of the tricuspid valve will induce a right-to-left shunt across an ASD. Similarly, a restrictive RV in patients with corrected Fallot's tetralogy can lead to a right-to-left shunt, whereas diastolic failure of the LV, often observed in elder patients, may increase preexisting left-to-right shunt.

Since a volume load of the RV is usually well tolerated in childhood, children with an isolated ASD rarely present with symptoms. However, in association with other cardiac or pulmonary conditions, or in case of a very large ASD, clinical symptoms of left-to-right shunt may occur already early in life. In adult patients, in whom left ventricular diastolic properties change, e.g., in developing heart failure with preserved ejection fraction (EF) due to ischemic heart disease, the left-to-right shunt across the defect will increase. Indeed LV diastolic function should be assessed in every adult patient presenting with an ASD.

When left untreated, 10–20% of the patients with an ASD will develop pulmonary hypertension (PH), although usually not before their third decade of life. Patients with ASD-PH have less left-to-right shunt due to decreased right ventricular compliance, caused by an increased RV afterload due to PH. Adult patients with Eisenmenger syndrome have been reported to fare better than patients with other types of PAH; however these results may be due to a survival bias, as the survival in children with PAH-CHD is not better. Indeed, studies in animal models with a mixture of increased preload and afterload showed further deterioration of RV function as compared with isolated increased afterload only [6].

The RV adaptation to volume load in ASD is dilatation, which leads to increased strain and strain rates especially in the apical segments [7–9]. Also longitudinal motion is increased. Interestingly, in animal models of increased preload, no changes in elastance, and hence contractility, were noted, suggesting that only Frank-Starling mechanisms are responsible for the increased RV output [6]. After closure of the defects, strain and strain rates decrease [7], maybe to even lower than normal values [8]. In a long-term follow-up study of patients with

repaired ASDs, mild RV dysfunction was found in 25% of patients with secundum ASD and 50% of patients with sinus venosus ASD [10]. Also tricuspid annular plane systolic excursion (TAPSE) and fractional area change (FAC) were decreased in 22% and 10% of the patients, respectively. These data indicate long-term effects of increased preload on the RV despite normalization of the loading conditions.

In summary, increased preload of the RV due to a shunt or valvular insufficiency induces RV dilatation that is usually well tolerated for a long time. Increased pulmonary blood flow in cardiac shunts may change the phenotype to increased afterload. RV dilatation is associated with increased apical deformation during volume loading which decreases after unloading. RV function remains mildly impaired even years after closure of the defect.

Tetralogy of Fallot

Tetralogy of Fallot (TOF) is one of the most common forms of cyanotic CHD, accounting for 3.5% of infants born with CHD. TOF has first been described by Niels Stensen in 1661, but was recognized as its tetrad by Etienne-Louis Fallot in 1888 [11]. The tetrad consists of a pulmonary stenosis, ventricular septal defect, overriding of the aorta over the ventricular septal defect, and RV hypertrophy, due to the increased afterload of the RV (Fig. 13.2a). Although this description is straightforward, it should be recognized that the degree of pulmonary stenosis and subsequent development of the pulmonary artery varies widely, leading to a continuum of this disease with pulmonary atresia with VSD. The tetrad is a result of an anterior deviation of the outlet septum leading almost always to a combination of subvalvular muscular obstruction as well as underdeveloped pulmonary valve area. The morphological aspect of the RV outflow tract is being recognized increasingly as an important determinant of residual lesions after surgical correction. TOF may be associated with peripheral pulmonary stenosis of the PA branches.

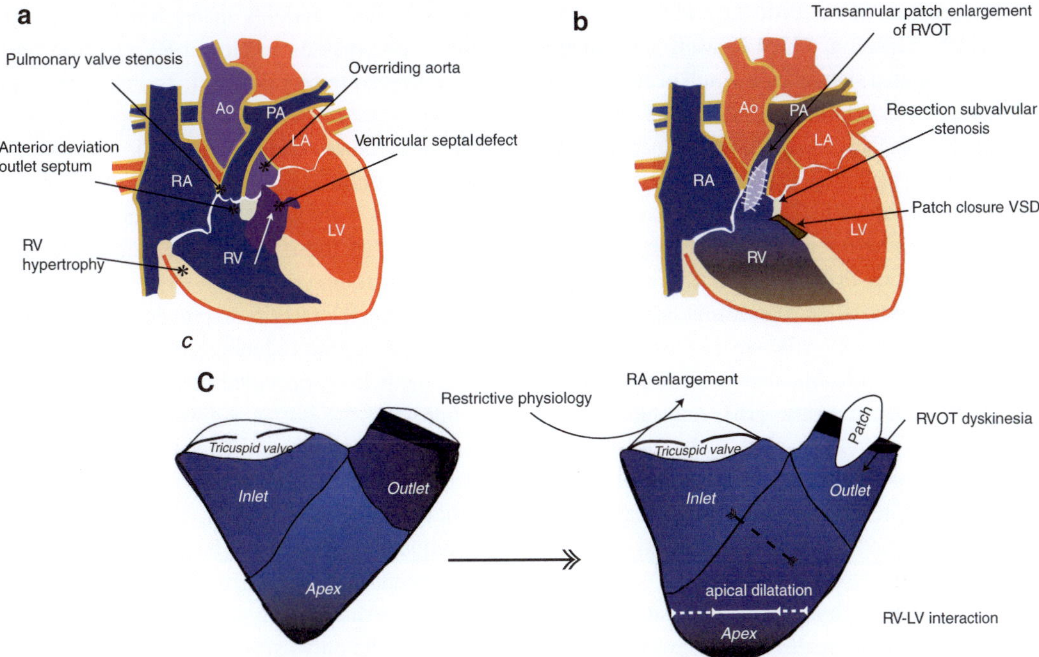

Fig. 13.2 (**a**) Characteristics of the tetralogy of Fallot. (**b**) Schematic representation of correction surgery leading to PI due to patch enlargement of the RV outflow tract. (**c**) Features of RV dysfunction in patients with corrected Fallot. *Ao* aorta, *PA* pulmonary artery, *RA* right atrium, *LA* left atrium, *RV* right ventricle, *LV* left ventricle

Historical Perspective

The majority of the current-age survivors were treated at later age as open-heart surgery was only available since the 1950s. Since then, with the improvement of perioperative cardiopulmonary bypass techniques and intensive care treatment, survival in the newborn period has increased to 98%. Also, the timing of surgery has shifted from 2–5 years of age in the 1980s to 3–9 months of age at present. With the growing numbers of adult survivors of TOF it became obvious that residual lesions with clinical relevance were associated predominantly with the right ventricular outflow tract (RVOT) reconstruction. The adult population should be divided according to the treatment era and age of surgical correction. The residual lesions and long-term follow-up are characterized by:

1. Pulmonary incompetence
2. RVOT dyskinesia
3. Restrictive RV
4. RV/LV interaction
5. Arrhythmias and risk of sudden death

Pulmonary Incompetence

Pulmonary regurgitation is a result of the need for relief of outflow tract obstruction caused by the subvalvular muscular obstruction, the stenosed pulmonary valve, and the supravalvular stenosis. To relief these obstructions a so-called transannular patch is used which immediately results in incompetence of the pulmonary valve (Fig. 13.2b). At first, the residual pulmonary regurgitation was thought to be innocent but long-term survival has shown that pulmonary regurgitation is not a benign lesion [12]. As an alternative, valve-sparing surgery can be performed in cases with adequate pulmonary artery size. Valve-sparing surgery was shown to result in less RV dilatation [13].

The response of the RV to the additional volume load is RV dilatation, which in itself is an adaptation rather than a sign of failure and occurs already shortly after Fallot repair (Table 13.2) [14]. RV dilatation is usually associated with increased trabeculation, which may complicate determination of RV volumes with CMR. Therefore, recently quantifications using a semiautomatic threshold-based algorithm excluding the trabeculae have been developed. These algorithms are quick and reliable in tracing RV volumes in corrected Fallot patients [15–17]. RV dilatation is invariably associated with worse outcome [18], reduced exercise performance [19–21], and arrhythmias [18]. Pulmonary regurgitation reduces power efficiency of the RV. The RV power loss increases with increasing RV end-diastolic volume [22].

There is increasing attention for sex differences in cardiac physiology and pathophysiology. In children, healthy boys were recently shown to have higher left and right ventricular volumes and mass compared to girls [23, 24]. Right ventricular adaptation to volume overloading is better in females compared to males. In corrected Fallot patients males have higher RV volumes and masses and lower RV ejection fraction compared to females [25]. To date, these sex differences are not accounted for in guidelines on congenital heart disease, including decision-making on pulmonary valve replacement in corrected Fallot patients. Current data ask for an amendment of these guidelines to include sex-specific treatment criteria.

Surprisingly, strategies to prevent RV dilatation using either volume-reducing surgery [35] or valve replacement have provided disappointing results in improving the outcome [36]. Also, treatment with angiotensin-converting enzyme antagonists or angiotensin receptor blockers did not change RV dilatation or outcome [30, 37]. Timing of volume reduction is thought to be an important factor in the potential to normalize RV function or outcome [36]. Alternatively, volume loading per se may not be the only aspect of the RV dysfunction in corrected Fallot. Other factors affecting RV dysfunction are RV deformation, dyssynchrony or chronotropic incompetence, restrictive physiology, and RV-LV interaction [38, 39] (Fig. 13.2c).

Table 13.2 CMR-derived RV volumes in patients with corrected tetralogy of Fallot

Author	N	Age at study	Age at surgery	RV EDVi	RV ESVi	RV SVi	RV EF (%)
Roest et al. [21]	15	17 ± 3	2 ± 2	132 ± 36	62 ± 26	69 ± 16	54 ± 9
Van Den Berg et al. [26]	36	17 (7–23)	0.9 ± 0.5	138 ± 40	64 (36–145)	66 ± 15	49 ± 7
Fernandes et al. [27]	33	12 ± 3	17 ± 16	157 ± 39	–	–	49 ± 9
Frigiola et al. [28]	60	22 ± 11	3 ± 5	142 ± 43	73 ± 33	40 ± 10	51 ± 10
Knauth et al. [29]	88	24 (10–57)	3 (0–30)	z-score 3.9 (3.2)	66 ± 33	–	48 ± 12
Babu-Narayan et al. [30]	32	29 ± 9	5 ± 6	123 ± 30	58 ± 21	65 ± 16	53 ± 9
Bonello et al. [31]	154	31 (22–40)	4.5 (2–8)	127 (102–148)	58 (45–75)	66 (55–76)	53 (47–58)
Greutmann et al. [32]	101	33 ± 12	5 (0.5–36)	158 ± 51	–	–	41 ± 8
Davlouros et al. [33]	85	33 ± 15	9 (0.5–50)	116 ± 33	56 ± 24	60 ± 18	52 ± 9
Kempny et al. [34]	21	36 (29–46)	7 (4–8)	140 ± 36	77 ± 26	42 ± 9	45 ± 10
Hagdorn et al. females [25]	157	24 [10–53]	1.4 [0–11.0]	114.4 [94–131.1]	52.5 [41.4–66.8]	–	52.3 [46.4–57.3]
Hagdorn et al. males [25]	163	23 [16–34]	1.3 [0–13.0]	122.5 [99.5–151.4]	64.4 [48.1–79.7]	–	47.7 [42.8–54.1]

Data are mean ± standard deviation or median and (range) or [interquartile range]. Age is in years. Volumes are in ml/m^2
EDV end-diastolic volume, *ESV* end-systolic volume, *SV* stroke volume, *EF* ejection fraction

RV Motion: A Gradient from Base to Apex

The wall motion of the RV can be described by echocardiography using longitudinal displacement and transversal displacement. Longitudinal displacement is reduced [40] already in childhood. Global longitudinal strain is also reduced and reduces further despite stable ejection fraction (EF) suggesting that this may be a marker for the timing of interventions, even though the effect of for instance pulmonary valve replacement on strain and myocardial deformation is uncertain [41–43]. Apart from a global decrease in longitudinal motion, there is also a gradient in transversal motion from base to apex. The RV can be divided into segments ranging from base to apex. Regional deformation imaging has shown reduced strain rates in all segments, in patients with Fallot as compared with controls or with, e.g., ASD [27, 44, 45]. However, in patients with Fallot, strain rates in the apex are more affected than those at base [46]. The apex of the RV contributes to more than half of the stroke volume and possibly failure of the apical region may contribute to RV failure.

RVOT Akinesia and Dyskinesia

Due to the extensive surgery the motion of the RVOT may be disturbed, leading to either RV akinesia or RV dyskinesia. RVOT akinesia is defined as the lack of thickening during systole, whereas dyskinesia ("aneurysm") is defined as an outward movement of the RVOT during systole. In a study of patients with "late repairs" (age of repair median 9 years), Davlouros et al. showed that RV akinesia/dyskinesia was present in ~55% of the patients and was an independent predictor for increased RV end-diastolic volume apart from pulmonary regurgitation [33]. RVOT dyskinesia may hamper proper interpretation of RV function [47]. The reduced performance of the RVOT may be the result of the reduced RV EF measured in many Fallot patients [48]. RV EF, however, is a poor prognosticator as it is the ratio of RV end-diastolic volume and stroke volume; hence even when SV is maintained or enhanced EF may be lower. RVOT dyskinesia not only hampers interpretation and volumetric assessment but also predicts the risk for ventricular arrhythmias [31], maybe due to scar tissue from surgery.

Dyssynchrony and RV-LV Interaction

RV dyssynchrony is almost always present after TOF correction due to the right bundle branch block related to VSD closure. The QRS duration prolongation caused by this block as well as residual volume loading has been shown to be an independent risk factor for the development of arrhythmias [49, 50]. Furthermore, RV dyssynchrony is associated with RV dilatation, reduced exercise capacity, and RV systolic dysfunction in children after Fallot repair [51, 52]. It should be noted that these studies include patients that were corrected at older age. It is unknown if these relations will hold in the cohort of patients corrected <1 year of age.

The QRS prolongation induces *inter*ventricular RV dyssynchrony although this effect may be limited. TOF is also invariably associated with *intra*ventricular dyssynchrony, of which as yet no uniform definition is given. However, so far studies looking at the contribution of *intra*ventricular dyssynchrony to RV dysfunction have yielded conflicting results [53–55]. Hence, although dyssynchrony is described in corrected Fallot's, its relation with RV adaptation and failure is yet unclear.

Adverse RV-LV interaction is an integral part of patients with TOF. It is hypothesized to arise from a combination of electrical dyssynchrony, shared septum and myocardial fibers, and geometric interactions leading to impaired LV function in Fallot patients. LV dysfunction has been associated with more severe pulmonary regurgitation and RV dilatation, possibly interfering with LV filling [13].

Restrictive RV Physiology

One of the hallmarks of the RV in patients after correction of TOF is the so-called restrictive physiology, first described by Gatzoulis [56]. A restrictive RV is defined as an antegrade flow in the pulmonary artery during diastole throughout the cardiac cycle. In the first description it was associated with less RV dilatation and improved exercise performance, although this view has been corrected by later research. Recently, long-term follow-up from the same group did not show an advantage of restrictive RV on the prevention of RV dilatation or exercise performance. Indeed, using dobutamine stress it has been shown that a restrictive RV leads to worsening of RV filling during cardiac stress [26]. The mechanisms of the diastolic dysfunction are unknown. It is suggested to be related to cardiac fibrosis, which is increased in patients with TOF [57]. Alternatively, it may be related to RV dilatation itself as dilated chambers operate at a steeper part of the pressure-volume relation leading to increased stiffness [58]. Restrictive RV physiology has recently also been associated with worse LV function, another component of patients with TOF [59]. It is speculated that it may interfere with LV filling, but further studies are necessary to elucidate the mechanisms of the restrictive RV.

Outcome and Risk Factors

In the tetralogy of Fallot, adverse outcomes include mortality and arrythmias, of which the latter is also associated with increased morbidity and mortality. Multiple risk factors for adverse outcome in TOF patients have been identified, including classical and newly identified predicting parameters. Among the classic parameters, prolonged QRS duration, RV dilatation, fibrosis, and mass have been associated with worse survival and occurrence of late arrhythmias [29, 49, 57]. Furthermore, LV dysfunction may be a predictor of adverse outcome and arrythmias, albeit a late one [27, 60–62]. Newer parameters include RV strain, LV fibrosis, LV strain, QRS fragmentation, and RV focal scar size [60, 63–66].

In summary, tetralogy of Fallot before correction imposes an increased afterload on the RV, but the majority of problems of RV dysfunction arise years after correction and are mainly associated with additional volume loading to the pulmonary regurgitation. Specific features adding to RV dysfunction in this lesion are RVOT dyskinesia, reduced apical deformation, dyssynchrony, and restrictive physiology.

The Systemic RV

In specific congenital heart diseases, the RV supports the systemic circulation rather than the low-resistance pulmonary circulation, phrased as a systemic RV. As the systemic circulation has a higher resistance, the RV has to increase its power in order to maintain cardiac output. Congenital heart defects associated with a systemic RV can be distinguished into two major phenotypes, i.e., the systemic RV in a biventricular circulation vs. the systemic RV in a univentricular circulation.

A systemic RV in a *biventricular* circulation either occurs naturally in the congenitally corrected transposition of the great arteries (ccTGA) or is a result of treatment in patients with a transposition of the great arteries after the atrial switch procedure (TGA-as) (Fig. 13.3a, b). Before the 1990s, palliation in TGA was achieved by rerouting the venous circulations using the procedure described by Senning or that by Mustard [3], leaving the RV coupled to the systemic circulation. In the 1990s, the *atrial* switch operation has been replaced by the *arterial* switch operation, which switches the pulmonary artery back to the RV and the aorta to the LV. The arterial switch operation creates a more physiological solution, as the LV is now again coupled to the systemic artery. However, at present there are still many adult survivors of the atrial switch procedure with a systemic RV.

A systemic RV in a *univentricular* circulation occurs in the growing group of survivors with a hypoplastic left-heart syndrome, or other univentricular malformations with a dominant RV.

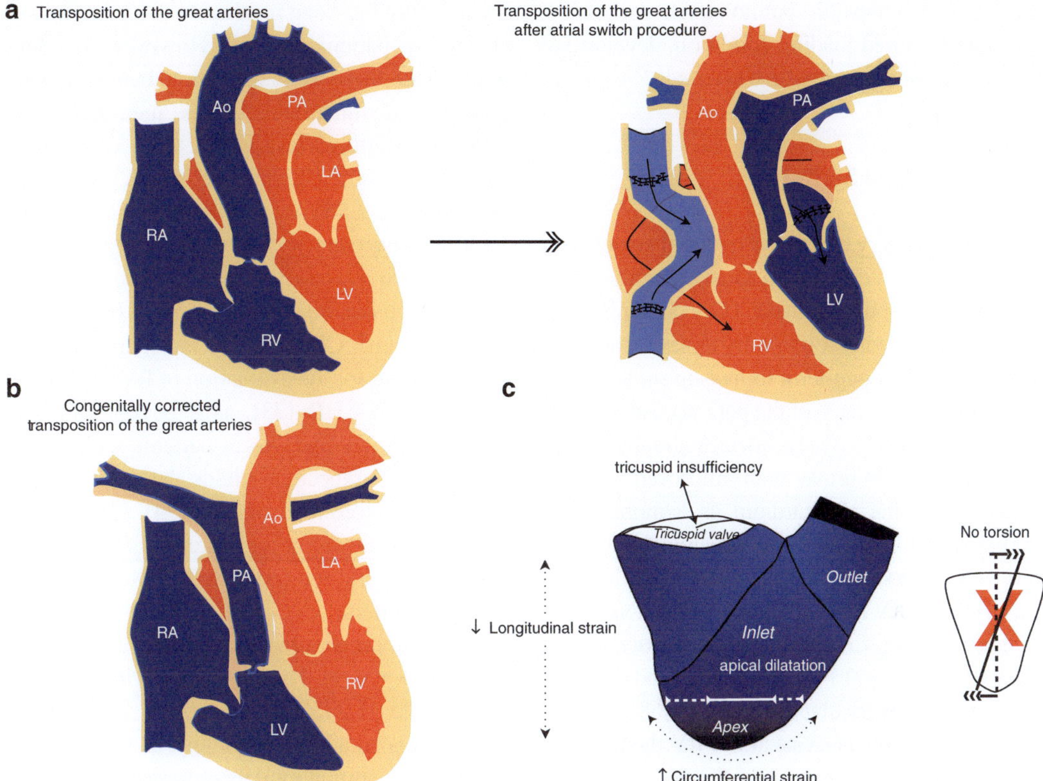

Fig. 13.3 (**a**) Transposition of the great arteries with subsequent atrial switch procedure leading to a systemic RV. (**b**) Congenitally corrected transposition of the great arteries. (**c**) Features of RV dysfunction in patients with a systemic RV. *Ao* aorta, *PA* pulmonary artery, *RA* right atrium, *LA* left atrium, *RV* right ventricle, *LV* left ventricle

The Systemic RV in a Biventricular Circulation: ccTGA and TGA-Senning/Mustard

ccTGA is frequently complicated by associated lesions, which profoundly affect clinical course. The most prevalent are pulmonary stenosis and/or a ventricular septal defect. Whereas a pulmonary stenosis (which in this situation forms an increased afterload for the LV) is generally well tolerated by the LV, a VSD leads to a volume load of the subaortic ventricle, which is the RV, and may cause signs and symptoms of congestive heart disease. Also, patients with ccTGA are prone to develop AV block, due to the anterior deviation of the atrioventricular node [2]. Atrioventricular block is prevalent without surgery and is a common complication of surgical procedures in patients with ccTGA [67, 68].

The natural history of ccTGA is characterized by a relatively long period of RV adaptation to the increased afterload which is present from birth, but eventually RV dysfunction appears in all patients [67]. However, RV dysfunction occurs earlier in patients with associated lesions. In the largest cohort series described so far, at the age of 45 years 67% of the patients with complex ccTGA vs. 25% of the patients with simple ccTGA had signs of RV dysfunction [67]. In other cohorts, primarily determined by surgical patients, the overall picture is similar [68]. It is yet unknown why patients with associated lesions have a worse prognosis but suggestions are chronotropic incompetence due to damage of AV node and myocardial damage during cardiac surgery. It should be noted though that patients with a systemic RV, hence an RV that has not been unloaded after birth, generally tolerate this pressure load quite long, while patients with idiopathic pulmonary hypertension, hence an acquired loading condition, develop RV failure in a much shorter time interval.

TGA and Atrial Switch

The natural history of TGA after atrial switch procedure (TGA-as) either via a Mustard or a Senning operation is like that of the ccTGA determined by RV dysfunction, albeit it usually arises earlier than in ccTGA [69]. Long-term follow-up studies show that after 25 years 61% of the patients had RV dysfunction shown by echocardiography [70]. Outcome may improve with improved surgical protection of the myocardium as a more recent study found that RV EF >40% was found in 98% of survivors with simple TGA-as. However, in complex TGA-as, RV EF >40% was found in only 58% of the survivors. Complicating factors are loss of sinus rhythm in >60% of the patients and development of supraventricular arrhythmias [68, 71].

In ccTGA and TGA-as alike, RV dysfunction is a final common pathway of the RV coupled to the systemic circulation. Factors associated with RV dysfunction are:

1. Tricuspid insufficiency
2. RV dyssynchrony
3. Response to exercise

RV Dysfunction in Systemic RV

Evaluation of RV failure is via clinical assessment of signs and symptoms. In adults with ischemic heart disease, the NYHA classification of heart failure has been invaluable in analyzing and stratifying patients at risk. However, in adults with CHD there is dissociation between complaints and functional values measured with CMR or exercise testing [72]. In adults with CHD, 15% of the patients in NYHA class I fulfill HF criteria defined as increased NT-proBNP and peak exercise capacity <25 ml/kg/min [72].

Apart from perceived status of heart failure, RV function can be serially assessed by echocardiography and CMR. CMR is regarded as the gold standard for the evaluation of RV function in patients with CHD [73], as it is best suited to quantify RV volume. As in patients with Fallot, exclusion of trabeculae yields the most reliable and reproducible RV volumes [74]. Care should be taken when comparing volumes between studies since scanning tools and protocols differ between centers.

A wide range of RV volumes and EF are reported when studying patients with systemic RVs (Table 13.3). The question is whether RV dilatation is an adaptive strategy, as is frequently described in animal models of increased pressure load [6, 9], or a sign of decompensation. At present there is no answer to that question, but in general severe RV dilatation is regarded as a sign of failure. Indeed, recently an RV end-diastolic volume of >150 ml/m^2 has been suggested to be a predictor for adverse events in a follow-up study of patients with both ccTGA and TGA-as [75]. The use of RV EF as predictor may be less accurate as it is influenced by tricuspid insufficiency and tricuspid insufficiency is invariably present in patients with systemic RVs [67].

Apart from CMR, 2D echocardiography of RV dimensions and wall motion has been used,

Table 13.3 RV volumes in systemic RVs

Author	N	Cohort	Age at study	RV EDVi	RV ESVi	RV SVi	RV EF (%)
Van Der Bom et al. [75]	88	All	33 ± 10	133 ± 35	86 ± 31	–	36 ± 7
Fratz et al. [76]	11	ccTGA	37 (6–59)	91 (60–208)	51 (14–96)	41 (28–59)	44 (20–75)
Grothoff et al. [69]	19	ccTGA	35 (19–49)	99 (65–134)	51 (37–56)	47 (36–65)	47 (43–55)
Fratz et al. [76]	12	TGA-as	20 (15–28)	98 (59–198)	54 (21–159)	45 (34–58)	47 (24–78)
Grothoff et al. [69]	31	TGA-as	22 (18–27)	95 (79–118)	49 (45–76)	36 (31–45)	41 (31–49)
Roest et al. [73]	27	TGA-as	26 ± 5	155 ± 55	70 ± 34	85 ± 26	56 ± 7
Pettersen et al. [77]	14	TGA-as	18 ± 1	119 ± 39	63 ± 26	–	47 ± 8

Data are mean ± standard deviation or median and (range). Age is in years. Volumes are in ml/m^2
EDV end-diastolic volume, *ESV* end-systolic volume, *SV* stroke volume, *EF* ejection fraction

reviewed in [42]. However, traditional measurements of RV motion, as TAPSE and FAC, correlate poorly with RV function in systemic RV as assessed by CMR [78].

Valuable insight into mechanisms of RV adaptation to increased afterload comes from studies combining both tissue Doppler imaging measurements by echocardiography and 3D volume measurements by CMR [77]. The contraction pattern in a normal RV shows a peristaltic wave beginning in the inflow region and moving toward the infundibulum [79, 80]. There are two major movements in a normal RV, an inward movement of the RV free wall, leading to a bellows effect, and a longitudinal movement from apex to base [81]. In the normal RV the longitudinal movement and strain exceed those of the circumferential fibers. In the systemic RV, this pattern is reversed, i.e., circumferential strain exceeds longitudinal strain, resembling normal LV movements (Fig. 13.3c). However, both strain and strain rates were lower than those in the LV. The reversal of strain patterns in the systemic RV vs. the normal RV has been confirmed by several echocardiographic studies [82]. Recently, a decrease in global RV strain by 10% has been shown to predict adverse events in adults with TGA-as [83].

Also, in contrast with the LV, the systemic RV does not develop torsion. Torsion, the angle between the rotation at the base vs. apex, contributes to LV emptying by producing a wringing motion as well as to LV filling during elastic recoil. The functional significance of these findings is not yet completely understood, since these observations were made in a population with relatively normal CMR measurements [77]. It is unclear whether these adaptation patterns are due to chronic abnormal loading or myocardial perfusion defects. In the normal RV myocardial perfusion via the right coronary artery occurs both during systole and diastole. However, in the systemic RV, myocardial perfusion is substantially changed which may affect function or induce fibrosis or scarring. Perfusion defects have been shown by several studies [84, 85]. Also, coronary flow reserve was reduced [86, 87]. The increased perfusion defects were associated with worse RV function [85], although these results have been debated in recent years [76].

It has been postulated that impaired perfusion together with increased demand may lead to ischemic events and subsequently scar forming and/or cardiac fibrosis. Cardiac fibrosis has been extensively shown in patients with systemic RVs [57, 88], and is related to decreasing RV function and worse outcome [89]. Fibrosis may also be the results of increased RV wall stress [85]. Whether these factors are amenable for therapeutic strategies remains to be determined.

Tricuspid Insufficiency

Tricuspid insufficiency (TI) is almost invariably present in late survivors with a systemic RV. The question is whether TI is either *a result of* RV dysfunction, due to annular dilatation, or *the cause for* RV dysfunction, leading to an additional volume load in an already pressure-loaded RV [6]. TI is influenced by the morphology of the valve, the annular dilatation, and the septal movement. In a systemic RV, where the septum bulges to the LV, the TI may increase. Indeed, patients with a subpulmonary stenosis have less TI. In ccTGA, the tricuspid valve is often dysplastic and in this setting TI precedes the development of RV dysfunction [90]. In TGA-as the relation between TI and RV dysfunction is less clear. Tricuspid valve surgery may stabilize RV function and results in better outcome than tricuspid valve replacement [91, 92]. However, tricuspid valve surgery is associated with an important risk of mortality.

Dyssynchrony

Deformation imaging has suggested that RV dysfunction is associated with RV dyssynchrony [93, 94]. Moreover, patients with dyssynchrony had more RV dilatation and reduced RV EF and exercise capacity. Increased dyssynchrony may provide treatment opportunities, such as resynchronization, which has been shown to improve right ventricular function, albeit in series with small numbers of patients with systemic RV [95–97].

Response to Exercise/Stress

More information may be derived from the RV response to stress such as exercise or dobutamine stress. Exercise capacity is generally lower in patients with CHD as compared with age-matched controls [39]. Likewise, in systemic RVs, though a wide range of peak VO_2 is reported, the average is about 66% of expected normal values [98]. There may be several reasons for the impaired exercise tolerance:

1. Impaired increase in contractility
2. Impaired RV filling
3. Chronotropic incompetence
4. Lung function

Several studies reported that patients with a systemic RV can increase cardiac output during exercise or dobutamine stress [73, 76, 99, 100]. The ability to increase contractility, measured by ESPVR, in the systemic RV appears to be normal. In contrast, the ventricular filling rate decreases in patients with TGA-as, whereas it increases in normal individuals [73, 99]. The reduced atrial filling rate during exercise/stress is more prominent in TGA-as than in ccTGA and is attributed to the extensive atrial surgery. During follow-up a mild baffle obstruction is frequently encountered [71], which may have profound effects on ventricular filling especially when heart rate increases.

Besides a reduced atrial filling, also chronotropic incompetence may play a role in reduced exercise capacity. Few patients with ccTGA or TGA-as are in normal sinus rhythm, there is a high rate of atrioventricular block, and many patients are chronotropic incompetent. Although these issues all may add, increasing chronotropic response via advanced pacing strategies did not improve exercise capacity [101]. In contrast, in a trial study using beta-blocker therapy, a lower heart rate during exercise was associated with better filling properties and improved exercise capacity [102], suggesting reverse relation between heart rate and output in systemic RVs. These observations underline the importance of abnormal filling patterns during stress in systemic RV, most prominent in TGA-as. The response to stress can be predictive for outcome in the systemic RV [75, 102]. Hence, exercise capacity is reduced and may reflect outcome though not directly related to intrinsic myocardial dysfunction.

Treatment Options

In the patient with heart failure due to ischemic heart disease, the cornerstones of treatment are angiotensin-converting enzyme (ACE) inhibitors or angiotensin receptor blockers (ARB), beta-blockers, and diuretics. In patients with heart failure due to systemic RV failure these therapies appear to be less effective.

Small series testing ACE inhibitors did not find any effects on RV EF, exercise capacity, or quality of life [103–105] (Table 13.4). The lack of effect was supposedly due to the relative lack of heart failure in these subjects and low levels of neurohormonal activation. Two small trials of angiotensin receptor blockade showed different results [106, 107]. However, in a recent large randomized trial, comprising 88 patients with ccTGA or TGA-as no significant effect was found on RV EF, the primary endpoint, after 3 years of follow-up [108]. Neither was there an effect on peak VO_2 or quality of life. The authors found a significant difference in the change of RV volumes, although RV volumes at the end of the study were not different between the groups (270 ± 77 ml in Valsartan vs. 259 ± 85 ml in placebo group). Hence there appears to be no benefit of ARB or ACE, findings that were recently also confirmed in an animal model of increased RV afterload [109]. A recent systematic review confirms no change in EF, ventricular dimensions, or peak VO_2 after 3 months of ACE or ARB treatment [110]. It was however noted that conclusive evidence is still lacking due to methodological limitations and small sample sizes in the currently available studies [110].

Beta-blocker therapy has not yet been evaluated in a large randomized trial. Beta-blocker therapy has been shown to be successful in rats with increased afterload [118]. In a small non-

Table 13.4 Effects of medical treatment in systemic RV

	ccTGA/ TGA-as	Medication	Study design	N	Follow-up (months)	RV EF	VO$_2$ peak	NYHA-class
Beta-blockers								
Lindenfeld et al. (2003) [111]	ccTGA	Carvedilol	Prospective	1	7	↑	NA	NA
Josephson et al. (2006) [112]	TGA-as	Various	Retrospective	8	36	NA	NA	↑
Giardini et al. (2007) [113]	Both	Carvedilol	Prospective	8	12	↑	=	↑
Doughan et al. (2007) [114]	TGA-as	Various	Retrospective	31	4	NA	NA	↑
Bouallal et al. (2010) [115]	Both	Various	Prospective	14	13	=	=	↑
ACE inhibitor								
Hechter et al. (2001) [103]	TGA-as	Various	Retrospective	14	24	=	=	NA
Robinson et al. (2002) [104]	TGA-as	Enalapril	Prospective	9	12	=[a]	=	NA
Therrien et al. (2008) [105]	TGA-as	Ramipril	Prospective	17	12	=	=	NA
Tutarel et al. (2012) [116]	TGA-as	Enalapril	Retrospective	14	13	NA	=	=
ATII antagonist								
Lester et al. (2001) [107]	TGA-as	Losartan	Prospective	7	2	↑	NA[b]	NA
Dore et al. (2005) [106]	Both	Losartan	Prospective	29	4	=[a]	=	NA
Van Der Bom et al. (2013) [108]	Both	Valsartan	Prospective	88	36	=	=	=

Data included from Winter et al. [117]
[a]EF determined by echocardiography instead of CMR
[b]Positive effect on exercise duration

randomized study in eight patients with systemic RVs, that were concomitantly treated with ACE inhibitors, Giardini et al. found an increase in exercise duration and RV EF and a decrease in RV volumes [113]. Possibly, lower heart rates improved RV filling, thereby accounting for the improvements. It should be noted though that all patients also received ACE, and that two patients did not tolerate the adequate dosage. One other small study also reported positive effects in the prevention of RV remodeling [114]. Further studies into the efficacy of beta-blockade in systemic RVs are warranted.

Pulmonary Artery Banding and Double Switch

Historically it was recognized that patients with a pulmonary stenosis in the setting of ccTGA fared better, maybe due to less TI or better RV performance when increasing septal pressure. Hence, pulmonary artery banding has been used as a strategy to support a failing circulation. Originally the idea was that after retraining the LV, the atrial switch procedure could be combined with an arterial switch procedure (double switch) so that the LV is again connected to the systemic circulation. However, many adult patients with heart failure did not reach the double-switch procedure, but were adequately supported by pulmonary artery banding. Indeed, in an animal model of increased RV afterload, additional aortic constriction also improved RV function [119]. The reason for this increase is incompletely understood, but the interaction of the ventricular septum with RV contraction appears to play a role.

The Systemic RV in Hypoplastic Left-Heart Syndrome

Before the introduction of the Norwood procedure, hypoplastic left-heart syndrome (HLHS) was generally fatal shortly after birth. Overall survival of children with HLHS has greatly improved over the last decades. The current 1-year survival rate has been reported to be around 60%, whereas 90% of the patients that have survived the first year are reported to survive up to 18 years of age [120]. These improved survival rates will lead to a growing number of patients with palliated HLHS. On the other hand, prenatal screening with the possibility of pregnancy termination could change the incidence of HLHS at live birth. Both these developments are expected to significantly affect HLHS epidemiology [121].

In a univentricular circulation the systemic ventricle is chronically volume overloaded, whereas after Fontan completion preload is significantly reduced. Both these phenomena lead to systemic ventricular systolic and diastolic dysfunction. In HLHS the right ventricle provides the systemic circulation and as such is additionally pressure overloaded. RV morphology in a univentricular circulation was shown to be a risk factor for worse outcome compared to LV morphology, due to RV failure [122].

Long-term morbidity for palliated HLHS includes exercise intolerance, high systemic venous pressures, hepatic dysfunction, thromboembolic events, protein-losing enteropathy, plastic bronchiolitis, and recurrent arrhythmias. Tricuspid valve insufficiency may develop due to congenital tricuspid valve abnormalities or malcoaptation due to right ventricular enlargement. Tricuspid valve regurgitation further compromises the systemic RV performance due to progressive RV dilatation and dysfunction [123]. Early in the disease course, larger RV end-diastolic and -systolic volumes and decreased RV function are associated with the failure of bidirectional cavopulmonary connection (stage 2 palliation) [124]. Furthermore, echocardiographic parameters reflecting RV function are predictive of mortality and are needed for heart transplantation during follow-up [125]. Due to the multifactorial etiology of Fontan failure, treatment of patients with failing Fontan remains difficult.

The RV in PAH Associated with CHD

PAH is a frequent and severe complication of CHD [126]. It is characterized by pulmonary vascular disease that is reversible at early stages, but in time progresses to intrinsically progressive disease [127]. According to current pulmonary hypertension guidelines, CHD-associated PAH (PAH-CHD) can be classified into four different subgroups: (1) Eisenmenger's syndrome, (2) PAH associated with systemic-to-pulmonary shunts, (3) PAH with small/coincidental defects, and (4) PAH after congenital heart defect correction [128]. PAH associated with systemic-to-pulmonary shunts (group 2) includes patients with significant intra- or extracardial left-to-right shunting leading to progressive pulmonary vascular disease. At a later disease stage, due to progressive pulmonary vascular disease, the pulmonary vascular resistance will supersede systemic vascular resistance. At that stage the left-to-right shunt will reverse to right-to-left shunting and is classified as Eisenmenger's syndrome (group 1 PAH-CHD). In contrast, persisting PAH in patients in whom the shunt defect is closed is classified as group 4 PAH (PAH after defect correction). Group 3 PAH-CHD includes patients with small/coincidental heart defects that do not account for the development of PAH.

In congenital heart disease patients with left-to-right shunting, we can distinguish pre-tricuspid versus post-tricuspid shunting. Pre-tricuspid shunts will lead to increased pulmonary blood flow and right ventricular volume overloading, whereas nonrestrictive post-tricuspid shunts lead to increased pulmonary blood flow with pulmonary arterial pressure overload and left ventricular volume overloading. PAH will develop more rapidly in nonrestrictive post-tricuspid shunts than in pre-tricuspid shunts. As PAH progresses the RV becomes more pressure loaded in both instances.

As pulmonary vascular resistance increases, left-to-right shunting (and ventricular volume overload) will decrease and eventually reverse to right-to-left shunting (Eisenmenger's syndrome). The right-to-left shunt provides a natural ability to unload the RV. In patients with pre-tricuspid shunts, right-to-left shunting reduces RV preload and volume overload, whereas right-to-left shunting in patients with post-tricuspid shunts (and suprasystemic pulmonary vascular resistance) reduces RV afterload. The effect of afterload reduction seems to be more beneficial, since Eisenmenger patients with post-tricuspid shunt have better outcome, compared to those with pre-tricuspid shunts.

In contrast, patients with corrected heart defects do not have the ability of RV unloading. In these patients PAH seems to be more rapidly progressive, with earlier RV failure and death. In PAH with small/coincidental defects there is usually no abnormal RV loading before PAH develops and these patients behave more like idiopathic PAH patients.

Another major difference between Eisenmenger's syndrome and all other forms of PAH in CHD is the long-lasting hypoxemia due to the right-to-left shunt. The hypoxemia induces polycythemia and hyperviscosity, an increased risk for thrombosis which in the presence of the shunt can give rise to arterial emboli and can induce systemic organ dysfunction [126, 129].

The increased afterload to the RV caused by PAH is generally well tolerated for many years in a subset of patients. Indeed, these survivors reaching adulthood have led to the impression that an Eisenmenger's syndrome is less severe of a loading condition than isolated pulmonary hypertension itself [130]. However, this observation is skewed by the survival bias, as in childhood 5-year survival of patients with PAH due to CHD does not differ much from iPAH [131, 132]. Other differences between PAH-CHD in pediatric versus adult cohorts are the better preserved RV function at diagnosis and less syncope at presentation [132, 133]. Again, the observation is that a RV that is not unloaded at birth (due to a congenital heart defect) may be better able to tolerate pressure and/or volume load than an unloaded RV that is suddenly confronted with increased afterload as iPAH. This suggests that the RV has a regenerative capacity that so far is unexplored.

ing to RV dysfunction, which is a main predictor of adverse outcome. Lesions with increased preload of the RV due to a shunt or valvular insufficiency induce RV dilatation that is usually well tolerated for a long time. Increased pulmonary blood flow in cardiac shunts leading to PAH may change the phenotype to increased afterload. RV dilatation is associated with increased apical deformation during volume loading which decreases after unloading. RV function remains mildly impaired even years after closure of the defect.

Tetralogy of Fallot before correction imposes an increased afterload on the RV, but the majority of the problems of RV dysfunction arise years after correction and are mainly associated with additional volume loading due to the pulmonary regurgitation. Specific features adding to RV dysfunction in this lesion are RVOT dyskinesia, reduced apical deformation, dyssynchrony, and restrictive physiology.

Lesions leading to increased afterload such as the systemic RV induce a switch to "LV-like" contraction pattern. However, the RV has no capability to develop torsion to support the adaptation. Although with a considerable "lag time," RV failure eventually ensues and is associated with additional volume load via tricuspid insufficiency, remodeling associated with perfusion defects and fibrosis, reduced filling especially at higher heart rates, and dyssynchrony.

Current treatment strategies have not been effective in preventing or reducing RV failure in the RV in CHD. New developments to support the RV may be resynchronization, supporting septal motion via pulmonary artery banding, and exploring the effects of beta-blocker therapy.

Summary

The RV in CHD poses a challenge for the cardiologist to evaluate and dissect the mechanism of RV adaptation and (dys)function as well as to treat RV failure. Many CHD lead to abnormal loading conditions of the RV, i.e., increased preload, increased afterload, or a mixture of both. Moreover, every lesion has specific features lead-

References

1. Norozi K, Wessel A, Alpers V, Arnhold JO, Geyer S, Zoege M, et al. Incidence and risk distribution of heart failure in adolescents and adults with congenital heart disease after cardiac surgery. Am J Cardiol. 2006;97:1238–43.

2. Anderson R, Baker E, Penny D, Redington A, Rigby M, Wernovsky G, editors. Pediatric cardiology. 3rd ed. Philadelphia: Churchill Livingstone; 2009.

3. Allen H, Driscoll D, Shaddy R, Feltes T, editors. Heart disease in infants, children, and adolescents. Philadelphia: Lippincott Williams & Wilkins; 2012.

4. Webb G, Gatzoulis MA. Atrial septal defects in the adult. Circulation. 2006;114:1645–53. https://doi.org/10.1161/CIRCULATIONAHA.105.592055.

5. Rudolph AM. Congenital diseases of the heart: clinical-physiological considerations. 3rd ed. New York: John Wiley & Sons; 2011.

6. Borgdorff MAJJ, Bartelds B, Dickinson MG, Steendijk P, de Vroomen M, Berger RMFF. Distinct loading conditions reveal various patterns of right ventricular adaptation. Am J Physiol Heart Circ Physiol. 2013;305:H354–64. Available from: https://pubmed.ncbi.nlm.nih.gov/23729212.

7. Eyskens B, Ganame J, Claus P, Boshoff D, Gewillig M, Mertens L. Ultrasonic strain rate and strain imaging of the right ventricle in children before and after percutaneous closure of an atrial septal defect. J Am Soc Echocardiogr. 2006;19:994–1000.

8. Van De Bruaene A, Buys R, Vanhees L, Delcroix M, Voigt JU, Budts W. Regional right ventricular deformation in patients with open and closed atrial septal defect. Eur J Echocardiogr. 2011;12:206–13.

9. Bartelds B, Borgdorff MA, Smit-van Oosten A, Takens J, Boersma B, Nederhoff MG, et al. Differential responses of the right ventricle to abnormal loading conditions in mice: pressure vs. volume load. Eur J Heart Fail. 2011;13:1275–82. Available from: https://pubmed.ncbi.nlm.nih.gov/22024026.

10. Cuypers JAAE, Opić P, Menting ME, Utens EMWJ, Witsenburg M, Helbing WA, et al. The unnatural history of an atrial septal defect: longitudinal 35 year follow up after surgical closure at young age. Heart. 2013;99:1346–52.

11. Apitz C, Webb GD, Redington AN. Tetralogy of Fallot. Lancet. 2009;374:1462–71.

12. Bouzas B, Kilner PJ, Gatzoulis MA. Pulmonary regurgitation: not a benign lesion. Eur Heart J. 2005;26:433–9. Available from: https://pubmed.ncbi.nlm.nih.gov/15640261/.

13. Annavajjhala V, Punn R, Tacy TA, Hanley FL, McElhinney DB. Serial assessment of postoperative ventricular mechanics in young children with tetralogy of Fallot: comparison of transannular patch and valve-sparing repair. Congenit Heart Dis. 2019;14:691–9. Available from: https://pubmed.ncbi.nlm.nih.gov/30989806/.

14. Hoelscher M, Bonassin F, Oxenius A, Seifert B, Leonardi B, Kellenberger CJ, et al. Right ventricular dilatation in patients with pulmonary regurgitation after repair of tetralogy of Fallot: how fast does it progress? Ann Pediatr Cardiol. 2020;13:294–300. Available from: https://pubmed.ncbi.nlm.nih.gov/33311917/.

15. Freling HG, Pieper PG, Vermeulen KM, van Swieten JM, Sijens PE, van Veldhuisen DJ, et al. Improved cardiac MRI volume measurements in patients with tetralogy of Fallot by independent end-systolic and end-diastolic phase selection. PLoS One. 2013;8:e55462.

16. Freling HG, Van Wijk K, Jaspers K, Pieper PG, Vermeulen KM, Van Swieten JM, et al. Impact of right ventricular endocardial trabeculae on volumes and function assessed by CMR in patients with tetralogy of Fallot. Int J Cardiovasc Imaging. 2013;29:625–31.

17. Jaspers K, Freling HG, Van Wijk K, Romijn EI, Greuter MJW, Willems TP. Improving the reproducibility of MR-derived left ventricular volume and function measurements with a semi-automatic threshold-based segmentation algorithm. Int J Cardiovasc Imaging. 2013;29:617–23.

18. Gatzoulis MA, Balaji S, Webber SA, Siu SC, Hokanson JS, Poile C, et al. Risk factors for arrhythmia and sudden cardiac death late after repair of tetralogy of Fallot: a multicentre study. Lancet. 2000;356:975–81.

19. Redington AN. Physiopathology of right ventricular failure. Pediatr Card Surg Annu. 2006;9:3–10.

20. Giardini A, Specchia S, Tacy TA, Coutsoumbas G, Gargiulo G, Donti A, et al. Usefulness of cardiopulmonary exercise to predict long-term prognosis in adults with repaired tetralogy of Fallot. Am J Cardiol. 2007;99:1462–7.

21. Roest AAW, Helbing WA, Kunz P, Van den Aardweg JG, Lamb HJ, Vliegen HW, et al. Exercise MR imaging in the assessment of pulmonary regurgitation and biventricular function in patients after tetralogy of Fallot repair. Radiology. 2002;223:204–11.

22. Fogel MA, Sundareswaran KS, De Zelicourt D, Dasi LP, Pawlowski T, Rome J, et al. Power loss and right ventricular efficiency in patients after tetralogy of Fallot repair with pulmonary insufficiency: clinical implications. J Thorac Cardiovasc Surg. 2012;143:1279–85.

23. Krupickova S, Risch J, Gati S, Caliebe A, Sarikouch S, Beerbaum P, et al. Cardiovascular magnetic resonance normal values in children for biventricular wall thickness and mass. J Cardiovasc Magn Reson. 2021;23:1. Available from: https://pubmed.ncbi.nlm.nih.gov/33390185/.

24. Van Der Ven JPG, Sadighy Z, Valsangiacomo Buechel ER, Sarikouch S, Robbers-Visser D, Kellenberger CJ, et al. Multicentre reference values for cardiac magnetic resonance imaging derived ventricular size and function for children aged 0–18 years. Eur Heart J Cardiovasc Imaging. 2020;21:102–13. Available from: /pmc/articles/PMC6923680/?report=abstract.

25. Hagdorn QAJ, Beurskens NEG, Gorter TM, Eshuis G, Hillege HL, Lui GK, et al. Sex differences in patients with repaired tetralogy of Fallot support a tailored approach for males and females: a cardiac magnetic resonance study. Int J Cardiovasc Imaging. 2020;36:1997–2005. Available from: https://pubmed.ncbi.nlm.nih.gov/32472300/.

26. Van Den Berg J, Wielopolski PA, Meijboom FJ, Witsenburg M, Bogers AJJC, Pattynama PMT, et al. Diastolic function in repaired tetralogy of Fallot at

rest and during stress: assessment with MR imaging. Radiology. 2007;243:212–9.

27. Fernandes FP, Manlhiot C, Roche SL, Grosse-Wortmann L, Slorach C, McCrindle BW, et al. Impaired left ventricular myocardial mechanics and their relation to pulmonary regurgitation, right ventricular enlargement and exercise capacity in asymptomatic children after repair of tetralogy of Fallot. J Am Soc Echocardiogr. 2012;25:494–503.

28. Frigiola A, Tsang V, Bull C, Coats L, Khambadkone S, Derrick G, et al. Biventricular response after pulmonary valve replacement for right ventricular outflow tract dysfunction: is age a predictor of outcome? Circulation. 2008;118:S182–90.

29. Knauth AL, Gauvreau K, Powell AJ, Landzberg MJ, Walsh EP, Lock JE, et al. Ventricular size and function assessed by cardiac MRI predict major adverse clinical outcomes late after tetralogy of Fallot repair. Heart. 2008;94:211–6.

30. Babu-Narayan SV, Uebing A, Davlouros PA, Kemp M, Davidson S, Dimopoulos K, et al. Randomised trial of ramipril in repaired tetralogy of Fallot and pulmonary regurgitation: the APPROPRIATE study (Ace inhibitors for Potential PRevention of the deleterious effects of Pulmonary Regurgitation in Adults with repaired TEtralogy of Fallot). Int J Cardiol. 2012;154:299–305.

31. Bonello B, Kempny A, Uebing A, Li W, Kilner PJ, Diller GP, et al. Right atrial area and right ventricular outflow tract akinetic length predict sustained tachyarrhythmia in repaired tetralogy of Fallot. Int J Cardiol. 2013;168:3280–6.

32. Greutmann M, Tobler D, Biaggi P, Mah ML, Crean A, Oechslin EN, et al. Echocardiography for assessment of right ventricular volumes revisited: a cardiac magnetic resonance comparison study in adults with repaired tetralogy of Fallot. J Am Soc Echocardiogr. 2010;23:905–11.

33. Davlouros PA, Kilner PJ, Hornung TS, Li W, Francis JM, Moon JCC, et al. Right ventricular function in adults with repaired tetralogy of Fallot assessed with cardiovascular magnetic resonance imaging: detrimental role of right ventricular outflow aneurysms or akinesia and adverse right-to-left ventricular interaction. J Am Coll Cardiol. 2002;40:2044–52.

34. Kempny A, Diller GP, Orwat S, Kaleschke G, Kerckhoff G, Bunck AC, et al. Right ventricular-left ventricular interaction in adults with tetralogy of Fallot: a combined cardiac magnetic resonance and echocardiographic speckle tracking study. Int J Cardiol. 2012;154:259–64.

35. Geva T, Gauvreau K, Powell AJ, Cecchin F, Rhodes J, Geva J, et al. Randomized trial of pulmonary valve replacement with and without right ventricular remodeling surgery. Circulation. 2010;122:S201–8.

36. Geva T. Indications for pulmonary valve replacement in repaired tetralogy of Fallot: the quest continues. Circulation. 2013;128:1855–7.

37. Bokma JP, Winter MM, Van Dijk AP, Vliegen HW, Van Melle JP, Meijboom FJ, et al. Effect of losartan on right ventricular dysfunction: results from the double-blind, randomized REDEFINE trial (right ventricular dysfunction in tetralogy of Fallot: inhibition of the renin-angiotensin-aldosterone system) in adults with repaired tetralogy of Fallot. Circulation. 2018;137:1463–71. Available from: https://www.ahajournals.org/doi/10.1161/CIRCULATIONAHA.117.031438.

38. Diller GP, Dimopoulos K, Okonko D, Uebing A, Broberg CS, Babu-Narayan S, et al. Heart rate response during exercise predicts survival in adults with congenital heart disease. J Am Coll Cardiol. 2006;48:1250–6.

39. Diller GP, Dimopoulos K, Okonko D, Li W, Babu-Narayan SV, Broberg CS, et al. Exercise intolerance in adult congenital heart disease: comparative severity, correlates, and prognostic implication. Circulation. 2005;112:828–35.

40. Koestenberger M, Nagel B, Ravekes W, Avian A, Heinzl B, Fandl A, et al. Tricuspid annular peak systolic velocity (S') in children and young adults with pulmonary artery hypertension secondary to congenital heart diseases, and in those with repaired tetralogy of Fallot: echocardiography and MRI data. J Am Soc Echocardiogr. 2012;25:1041–9.

41. Li VW-Y, Yu CK-M, So EK-F, Wong WH-S, Cheung Y-F. Ventricular myocardial deformation imaging of patients with repaired tetralogy of Fallot. J Am Soc Echocardiogr. 2020;33:788–801. Available from: https://pubmed.ncbi.nlm.nih.gov/32624088/.

42. Buechel ERV, Mertens LL. Imaging the right heart: the use of integrated multimodality imaging. Eur Heart J. 2012:949–60. Available from: https://pubmed.ncbi.nlm.nih.gov/22408035/.

43. Van den Eynde J, Sá MPBO, Vervoort D, Roever L, Meyns B, Budts W, et al. Pulmonary valve replacement in tetralogy of Fallot: an updated meta-analysis. Ann Thorac Surg. 2020. Available from: https://pubmed.ncbi.nlm.nih.gov/33378694/.

44. Dragulescu A, Grosse-Wortmann L, Fackoury C, Riffle S, Waiss M, Jaeggi E, et al. Echocardiographic assessment of right ventricular volumes after surgical repair of tetralogy of Fallot: clinical validation of a new echocardiographic method. J Am Soc Echocardiogr. 2011;24:1191–8.

45. Eyskens B, Brown SC, Claus P, Dymarkowski S, Gewillig M, Bogaert J, et al. The influence of pulmonary regurgitation on regional right ventricular function in children after surgical repair of tetralogy of Fallot. Eur J Echocardiogr. 2010;11:341–5. Available from: https://pubmed.ncbi.nlm.nih.gov/20085920/.

46. Bodhey NK, Beerbaum P, Sarikouch S, Kropf S, Lange P, Berger F, et al. Functional analysis of the components of the right ventricle in the setting of tetralogy of Fallot. Circ Cardiovasc Imaging. 2008;1:141–7.

47. Kutty S, Graney BA, Khoo NS, Li L, Polak A, Gribben P, et al. Serial assessment of right ventricular volume and function in surgically palliated hypoplastic left heart syndrome using real-time transthoracic three-dimensional echocardiography. J Am Soc Echocardiogr. 2012;25:682–9.

48. O'Meagher S, Munoz PA, Alison JA, Young IH, Tanous DJ, Celermajer DS, et al. Exercise capacity and stroke volume are preserved late after tetralogy repair, despite severe right ventricular dilatation. Heart. 2012;98:1595–9.

49. Beurskens NEG, Hagdorn QAJ, Gorter TM, Berger RMF, Vermeulen KM, van Melle JP, et al. Risk of cardiac tachyarrhythmia in patients with repaired tetralogy of Fallot: a multicenter cardiac MRI based study. Int J Cardiovasc Imaging. 2019;35:143–51. Available from: https://pubmed.ncbi.nlm.nih.gov/30094564.

50. Gatzoulis MA, Elliott JT, Guru V, Siu SC, Warsi MA, Webb GD, et al. Right and left ventricular systolic function late after repair of tetralogy of Fallot. Am J Cardiol. 2000;86:1352–7.

51. Lumens J, Fan CS, Walmsley J, Yim D, Manlhiot C, Dragulescu A, et al. Relative impact of right ventricular electromechanical dyssynchrony versus pulmonary regurgitation on right ventricular dysfunction and exercise intolerance in patients after repair of tetralogy of Fallot. J Am Heart Assoc. 2019;8. Available from: https://www.ahajournals.org/doi/10.1161/JAHA.118.010903.

52. Yim D, Hui W, Larios G, Dragulescu A, Grosse-Wortmann L, Bijnens B, et al. Quantification of right ventricular electromechanical dyssynchrony in relation to right ventricular function and clinical outcomes in children with repaired tetralogy of Fallot. J Am Soc Echocardiogr. 2018;31:822–30. Available from: https://pubmed.ncbi.nlm.nih.gov/29976349/.

53. Hui W, Slorach C, Bradley TJ, Jaeggi ET, Mertens L, Friedberg MK. Measurement of right ventricular mechanical synchrony in children using tissue doppler velocity and two-dimensional strain imaging. J Am Soc Echocardiogr. 2010;23:1289–96.

54. Roche SL, Grosse-Wortmann L, Redington AN, Slorach C, Smith G, Kantor PF, et al. Exercise induces biventricular mechanical dyssynchrony in children with repaired tetralogy of Fallot. Heart. 2010;96:2010–5.

55. Friedberg MK, Fernandes FP, Roche SL, Slorach C, Grosse-Wortmann L, Manlhiot C, et al. Relation of right ventricular mechanics to exercise tolerance in children after tetralogy of Fallot repair. Am Heart J. 2013;165:551–7.

56. Gatzoulis MA, Clark AL, Cullen S, Newman CGH, Redington AN. Right ventricular diastolic function 15 to 35 years after repair of tetralogy of Fallot: restrictive physiology predicts superior exercise performance. Circulation. 1995;91:1775–81.

57. Babu-Narayan SV, Kilner PJ, Li W, Moon JC, Goktekin O, Davlouros PA, et al. Ventricular fibrosis suggested by cardiovascular magnetic resonance in adults with repaired tetralogy of Fallot and its relationship to adverse markers of clinical outcome. Circulation. 2006;113:405–13.

58. Burkhoff D, Mirsky I, Suga H. Assessment of systolic and diastolic ventricular properties via pressure-volume analysis: a guide for clinical, translational, and basic researchers. Am J Physiol Heart Circ Physiol. 2005;289:H501–12.

59. Ahmad N, Kantor PF, Grosse-Wortmann L, Seller N, Jaeggi ET, Friedberg MK, et al. Influence of RV restrictive physiology on LV diastolic function in children after tetralogy of fallot repair. J Am Soc Echocardiogr. 2012;25:866–73.

60. Hagdorn QAJ, Vos JDL, Beurskens NEG, Gorter TM, Meyer SL, van Melle JP, et al. CMR feature tracking left ventricular strain-rate predicts ventricular tachyarrhythmia, but not deterioration of ventricular function in patients with repaired tetralogy of Fallot. Int J Cardiol. 2019;295:1–6. Available from: https://pubmed.ncbi.nlm.nih.gov/31402156.

61. Frigiola A, Redington AN, Cullen S, Vogel M. Pulmonary regurgitation is an important determinant of right ventricular contractile dysfunction in patients with surgically repaired tetralogy of Fallot. Circulation. 2004;110. Available from: https://pubmed.ncbi.nlm.nih.gov/15364855/.

62. Diller GP, Kempny A, Liodakis E, Alonso-Gonzalez R, Inuzuka R, Uebing A, et al. Left ventricular longitudinal function predicts life-threatening ventricular arrhythmia and death in adults with repaired tetralogy of Fallot. Circulation. 2012;125:2440–6.

63. de Alba CG, Khan A, Woods P, Broberg CS. Left ventricular strain and fibrosis in adults with repaired tetralogy of Fallot: a case-control study. Int J Cardiol. 2021;323:34–9. Available from: https://pubmed.ncbi.nlm.nih.gov/32882293/.

64. Diller GP, Orwat S, Vahle J, Bauer UMM, Bauer UMM, Urban A, et al. Prediction of prognosis in patients with tetralogy of Fallot based on deep learning imaging analysis. Heart. 2020;106:1007–14. Available from: https://pubmed.ncbi.nlm.nih.gov/32161041/.

65. Cochet H, Iriart X, Allain-Nicolaï A, Camaioni C, Sridi S, Nivet H, et al. Focal scar and diffuse myocardial fibrosis are independent imaging markers in repaired tetralogy of Fallot. Eur Heart J Cardiovasc Imaging. 2019;20:990–1003. Available from: https://pubmed.ncbi.nlm.nih.gov/30993335/.

66. Bokma JP, Winter MM, Vehmeijer JT, Vliegen HW, Van Dijk AP, Van Melle JP, et al. QRS fragmentation is superior to QRS duration in predicting mortality in adults with tetralogy of Fallot. Heart. 2016;103:666–71. Available from: https://pubmed.ncbi.nlm.nih.gov/27803032/.

67. Graham TP, Bernard YD, Mellen BG, Celermajer D, Baumgartner H, Cetta F, et al. Long-term outcome in congenitally corrected transposition of the great arteries. J Am Coll Cardiol. 2000;36:255–61.

68. Dobson R, Danton M, Nicola W, Hamish W. The natural and unnatural history of the systemic right ventricle in adult survivors. J Thorac Cardiovasc Surg. 2013;145:1493–503.

69. Grothoff M, Fleischer A, Abdul-Khaliq H, Hoffmann J, Lehmkuhl L, Luecke C, et al. The systemic right ventricle in congenitally corrected transposition of the great arteries is different from the right ventricle in dextro-transposition after atrial switch: a cardiac magnetic resonance study. Cardiol Young. 2013;23:239–47.

70. Roos-Hesselink JW, Meijboom FJ, Spitaels SEC, Van Domburg R, Van Rijen EHM, Utens EMWJ, et al. Decline in ventricular function and clinical condition after mustard repair for transposition of the great arteries (a prospective study of 22-29 years). Eur Heart J. 2004;25:1264–70.

71. Roubertie F, Thambo JB, Bretonneau A, Iriart X, Laborde N, Baudet E, et al. Late outcome of 132 Senning procedures after 20 years of follow-up. Ann Thorac Surg. 2011;92:2206–14.

72. Norozi K, Wessel A, Buchhorn R, Alpers V, Arnhold JO, Zoege M, et al. Is the ability index superior to the NYHA classification for assessing heart failure? Comparison of two classification scales in adolescents and adults with operated congenital heart defects. Clin Res Cardiol. 2007;96:542–7.

73. Roest AAW, Lamb HJ, Van Der Wall EE, Vliegen HW, Van Den Aerdweg JG, Kunz P, et al. Cardiovascular response to physical exercise in adult patients after atrial correction for transposition of the great arteries assessed with magnetic resonance imaging. Heart. 2004;90:678–84.

74. Winter MM, Bernink FJP, Groenink M, Bouma BJ, Van Dijk APJ, Helbing WA, et al. Evaluating the systemic right ventricle by CMR: the importance of consistent and reproducible delineation of the cavity. J Cardiovasc Magn Reson. 2008;10:40.

75. Van Der Bom T, Winter MM, Groenink M, Vliegen HW, Pieper PG, Van Dijk APJ, et al. Right ventricular end-diastolic volume combined with peak systolic blood pressure during exercise identifies patients at risk for complications in adults with a systemic right ventricle. J Am Coll Cardiol. 2013;62:926–36.

76. Fratz S, Hager A, Busch R, Kaemmerer H, Schwaiger M, Lange R, et al. Patients after atrial switch operation for transposition of the great arteries can not increase stroke volume under dobutamine stress as opposed to patients with congenitally corrected transposition. Circ J. 2008;72:1130–5.

77. Pettersen E, Helle-Valle T, Edvardsen T, Lindberg H, Smith HJ, Smevik B, et al. Contraction pattern of the systemic right ventricle. Shift from longitudinal to circumferential shortening and absent global ventricular torsion. J Am Coll Cardiol. 2007;49:2450–6.

78. Khattab K, Schmidheiny P, Wustmann K, Wahl A, Seiler C, Schwerzmann M. Echocardiogram versus cardiac magnetic resonance imaging for assessing systolic function of subaortic right ventricle in adults with complete transposition of great arteries and previous atrial switch operation. Am J Cardiol. 2013;111:908–13.

79. Kukulski T, Hübbert L, Arnold M, Wranne B, Hatle L, Sutherland GR. Normal regional right ventricular function and its change with age: a Doppler myocardial imaging study. J Am Soc Echocardiogr. 2000;13:194–204.

80. Haber I, Metaxas DN, Geva T, Axel L. Three-dimensional systolic kinematics of the right ventricle. Am J Physiol Heart Circ Physiol. 2005;289:H1826–33.

81. Haddad F, Doyle R, Murphy DJ, Hunt SA. Right ventricular function in cardiovascular disease, part II: pathophysiology, clinical importance, and management of right ventricular failure. Circulation. 2008;117:1717–31.

82. Eyskens B, Weidemann F, Kowalski M, Bogaert J, Dymarkowski S, Bijnens B, et al. Regional right and left ventricular function after the Senning operation: an ultrasonic study of strain rate and strain. Cardiol Young. 2004;14:255–64.

83. Kalogeropoulos AP, Deka A, Border W, Pernetz MA, Georgiopoulou VV, Kiani J, et al. Right ventricular function with standard and speckle-tracking echocardiography and clinical events in adults with D-transposition of the great arteries post atrial switch. J Am Soc Echocardiogr. 2012;25:304–12.

84. Millane T, Bernard EJ, Jaeggi E, Howman-Giles RB, Uren RF, Cartmill TB, et al. Role of ischemia and infarction in late right ventricular dysfunction after atrial repair of transposition of the great arteries. J Am Coll Cardiol. 2000;35:1661–8.

85. Giardini A, Lovato L, Donti A, Formigari R, Oppido G, Gargiulo G, et al. Relation between right ventricular structural alterations and markers of adverse clinical outcome in adults with systemic right ventricle and either congenital complete (after Senning operation) or congenitally corrected transposition of the great arteries. Am J Cardiol. 2006;98:1277–82.

86. Hauser M, Bengel FM, Hager A, Kuehn A, Nekolla SG, Kaemmerer H, et al. Impaired myocardial blood flow and coronary flow reserve of the anatomical right systemic ventricle in patients with congenitally corrected transposition of the great arteries. Heart. 2003;89:1231–5.

87. Singh TP, Humes RA, Muzik O, Kottamasu S, Karpawich PP, Di Carli MF. Myocardial flow reserve in patients with a systemic right ventricle after atrial switch repair. J Am Coll Cardiol. 2001;37:2120–5.

88. Broberg CS, Chugh SS, Conklin C, Sahn DJ, Jerosch-Herold M. Quantification of diffuse myocardial fibrosis and its association with myocardial dysfunction in congenital heart disease. Circ Cardiovasc Imaging. 2010;3:727–34.

89. Rydman R, Gatzoulis MA, Ho SY, Ernst S, Swan L, Li W, et al. Systemic right ventricular fibrosis detected by cardiovascular magnetic resonance is associated with clinical outcome, mainly new-onset atrial arrhythmia, in patients after atrial redirection surgery for transposition of the great arteries. Circ Cardiovasc Imaging. 2015;8. Available from: https://pubmed.ncbi.nlm.nih.gov/25948241/.

90. Prieto LR, Hordof AJ, Secic M, Rosenbaum MS, Gersony WM. Progressive tricuspid valve disease in patients with congenitally corrected transposition of the great arteries. Circulation. 1998;98:997–1005.

91. Saran N, Dearani JA, Said SM, Greason KL, Pochettino A, Stulak JM, et al. Long-term outcomes of patients undergoing tricuspid valve surgery. Eur J Cardio-thoracic Surg. 2019;56:950–8. Available from: https://pubmed.ncbi.nlm.nih.gov/30919898/.

92. Koolbergen DR, Ahmed Y, Bouma BJ, Scherptong RWC, Bruggemans EF, Vliegen HW, et al. Follow-up after tricuspid valve surgery in adult patients with systemic right ventricles. Eur J Cardio-thoracic Surg. 2016;50:456–63. Available from: https://pubmed.ncbi.nlm.nih.gov/26984988/.

93. Chow PC, Liang XC, Lam WWM, Cheung EWY, Wong KT, Cheung YF. Mechanical right ventricular dyssynchrony in patients after atrial switch operation for transposition of the great arteries. Am J Cardiol. 2008;101:874–81.

94. Friedberg MK, Mertens L. Deformation imaging in selected congenital heart disease: is it evolving to clinical use? J Am Soc Echocardiogr. 2012;25:919–31.

95. Filippov AA, Del Nido PJ, Vasilyev NV. Management of systemic right ventricular failure in patients with congenitally corrected transposition of the great arteries. Circulation. 2016;134:1293–302. Available from: https://pubmed.ncbi.nlm.nih.gov/27777298/.

96. Jauvert G, Rousseau-Paziaud J, Villain E, Iserin L, Hidden-Lucet F, Ladouceur M, et al. Effects of cardiac resynchronization therapy on echocardiographic indices, functional capacity, and clinical outcomes of patients with a systemic right ventricle. Europace. 2009;11:184–90. Available from: https://pubmed.ncbi.nlm.nih.gov/19038975/.

97. Dubin AM, Janousek J, Rhee E, Strieper MJ, Cecchin F, Law IH, et al. Resynchronization therapy in pediatric and congenital heart disease patients: an international multicenter study. J Am Coll Cardiol. 2005;46:2277–83. Available from: https://pubmed.ncbi.nlm.nih.gov/16360058/.

98. Kempny A, Dimopoulos K, Uebing A, Moceri P, Swan L, Gatzoulis MA, et al. Reference values for exercise limitations among adults with congenital heart disease. Relation to activities of daily life single centre experience and review of published data. Eur Heart J. 2012;33:1386–96. Available from: https://pubmed.ncbi.nlm.nih.gov/22199119/.

99. Derrick G, Narang I, White P, Kelleher A, Bush A, Penny D, et al. Failure of stroke volume augmentation during exercise and dobutamine stress is unrelated to load-independent indexes of right ventricular performance after the Mustard operation. Circulation. 2000;102:III154–9. Available from: https://www.ahajournals.org/doi/full/10.1161/circ.102.suppl_3.III-154.

100. Winter MM, Van Der Plas MN, Bouma BJ, Groenink M, Bresser P, Mulder BJM. Mechanisms for cardiac output augmentation in patients with a systemic right ventricle. Int J Cardiol. 2010;143:141–6.

101. Uebing A, Diller GP, Li W, Maskell M, Dimopoulos K, Gatzoulis MA. Optimised rate-responsive pacing does not improve either right ventricular haemodynamics or exercise capacity in adults with a systemic right ventricle. Cardiol Young. 2010;20:485–94.

102. Giardini A, Hager A, Lammers AE, Derrick G, Müller J, Diller GP, et al. Ventilatory efficiency and aerobic capacity predict event-free survival in adults with atrial repair for complete transposition of the great arteries. J Am Coll Cardiol. 2009;53:1548–55.

103. Hechter SJ, Fredriksen PM, Liu P, Veldtman G, Merchant N, Freeman M, et al. Angiotensin-converting enzyme inhibitors in adults after the Mustard procedure. Am J Cardiol. 2001;87:660–3.

104. Robinson B, Heise CT, Moore JW, Anella J, Sokoloski M, Eshaghpour E. Afterload reduction therapy in patients following intra-atrial baffle operation for transposition of the great arteries. Pediatr Cardiol. 2002;23:618–23.

105. Therrien J, Provost Y, Harrison J, Connelly M, Kaemmerer H, Webb GD. Effect of angiotensin receptor blockade on systemic right ventricular function and size: a small, randomized, placebo-controlled study. Int J Cardiol. 2008;129:187–92.

106. Dore A, Houde C, Chan KL, Ducharme A, Khairy P, Juneau M, et al. Angiotensin receptor blockade and exercise capacity in adults with systemic right ventricles: a multicenter, randomized, placebo-controlled clinical trial. Circulation. 2005;112:2411–6.

107. Lester SJ, McElhinney DB, Viloria E, Reddy GP, Ryan E, Tworetzky W, et al. Effects of Losartan in patients with a systemically functioning morphologic right ventricle after atrial repair of transposition of the great arteries. Am J Cardiol. 2001;88:1314–6.

108. Van Der Bom T, Winter MM, Bouma BJ, Groenink M, Vliegen HW, Pieper PG, et al. Effect of valsartan on systemic right ventricular function: a double-blind, randomized, placebo-controlled pilot trial. Circulation. 2013;127:322–30.

109. Borgdorff MA, Bartelds B, Dickinson MG, Steendijk P, Berger RMFF. A cornerstone of heart failure treatment is not effective in experimental right ventricular failure. Int J Cardiol. 2013;169:183–9. Available from: https://pubmed.ncbi.nlm.nih.gov/24067600.

110. Zaragoza-Macias E, Zaidi AN, Dendukuri N, Marelli A. Medical therapy for systemic right ventricles: a systematic review (part 1) for the 2018 AHA/ACC Guideline for the Management of Adults with Congenital Heart Disease: A Report of the American College of Cardiology/American Heart Association Task Force on Clinical Practice Guidelines. Circulation. 2019, 139:E801–13. Available from: https://pubmed.ncbi.nlm.nih.gov/30586770/.

111. Lindenfeld JA, Keller K, Campbell DN, Wolfe RR, Quaife RA. Improved systemic ventricular function after carvedilol administration in a patient with congenitally corrected transposition of the great arteries. J Hear Lung Transplant. 2003;22:198–201. Available from: https://pubmed.ncbi.nlm.nih.gov/12581770/.

112. Josephson CB, Howlett JG, Jackson SD, Finley J, Kells CM. A case series of systemic right ventricular dysfunction post atrial switch for simple D-transposition of the great arteries: the impact of beta-blockade. Can J Cardiol. 2006;22:769–72. Available from: https://pubmed.ncbi.nlm.nih.gov/16835671/.

113. Giardini A, Lovato L, Donti A, Formigari R, Gargiulo G, Picchio FM, et al. A pilot study on the effects of carvedilol on right ventricular remodelling and exercise tolerance in patients with systemic right ventricle. Int J Cardiol. 2007;114:241–6.

114. Doughan ARK, McConnell ME, Book WM. Effect of beta blockers (carvedilol or metoprolol XL) in patients with transposition of great arteries and dysfunction of the systemic right ventricle. Am J Cardiol. 2007;99:704–6.

115. Bouallal R, Godart F, Francart C, Richard A, Foucher-Hossein C, Lions C. Interest of β-blockers in patients with right ventricular systemic dysfunction. Cardiol Young. 2010;20:615–9. Available from: https://pubmed.ncbi.nlm.nih.gov/20519056/.

116. Tutarel O, Meyer GP, Bertram H, Wessel A, Schieffer B, Westhoff-Bleck M. Safety and efficiency of chronic ACE inhibition in symptomatic heart failure patients with a systemic right ventricle. Int J Cardiol. 2012;154:14–6. Available from: https://pubmed.ncbi.nlm.nih.gov/20843567/.

117. Winter MM, Bouma BJ, Groenink M, Konings TC, Tijssen JGP, Van Veldhuisen DJ, et al. Latest insights in therapeutic options for systemic right ventricular failure: a comparison with left ventricular failure. Heart. 2009;95:960–3.

118. Bogaard HJ, Natarajan R, Mizuno S, Abbate A, Chang PJ, Chau VQ, et al. Adrenergic receptor blockade reverses right heart remodeling and dysfunction in pulmonary hypertensive rats. Am J Respir Crit Care Med. 2010;182:652–60.

119. Apitz C, Honjo O, Humpl T, Li J, Assad RS, Cho MY, et al. Biventricular structural and functional responses to aortic constriction in a rabbit model of chronic right ventricular pressure overload. J Thorac Cardiovasc Surg. 2012;144:1494–501.

120. Siffel C, Riehle-Colarusso T, Oster ME, Correa A. Survival of children with hypoplastic left heart syndrome. Pediatrics. 2015;136:e864–70. Available from: https://pubmed.ncbi.nlm.nih.gov/26391936/.

121. Öhman A, El-Segaier M, Bergman G, Hanséus K, Malm T, Nilsson B, et al. Changing epidemiology of hypoplastic left heart syndrome: results of a national Swedish cohort study. J Am Heart Assoc. 2019;8. Available from: https://pubmed.ncbi.nlm.nih.gov/30661430/.

122. Erikssen G, Aboulhosn J, Lin J, Liestøl K, Estensen ME, Gjesdal O, et al. Survival in patients with univentricular hearts: the impact of right versus left ventricular morphology. Open Heart. 2018;5. Available from: https://pubmed.ncbi.nlm.nih.gov/30364544/.

123. Metcalf MK, Rychik J. Outcomes in hypoplastic left heart syndrome. Pediatr Clin N Am. 2020;67:945–62.

124. Hormaza VM, Conaway M, Schneider DS, Vergales JE. The effect of right ventricular function on survival and morbidity following stage 2 palliation: an analysis of the single ventricle reconstruction trial public data set. Congenit Heart Dis. 2019;14:274–9. Available from: https://pubmed.ncbi.nlm.nih.gov/30506893/.

125. Son JS, James A, Fan CPS, Mertens L, McCrindle BW, Manlhiot C, et al. Prognostic value of serial echocardiography in hypoplastic left heart syndrome. Circ Cardiovasc Imaging. 2018;11:e006983. Available from: https://pubmed.ncbi.nlm.nih.gov/30012823/.

126. D'Alto M, Mahadevan VS. Pulmonary arterial hypertension associated with congenital heart disease. Eur Respir Rev. 2012;21:328–37.

127. van der Feen DE, Bartelds B, de Boer RA, Berger RMF. Pulmonary arterial hypertension in congenital heart disease: translational opportunities to study the reversibility of pulmonary vascular disease. Eur Heart J. 2017;38:2034–41. Available from: https://pubmed.ncbi.nlm.nih.gov/28369399.

128. Galiè N, Humbert M, Vachiery J-L, Gibbs S, Lang I, Torbicki A, et al. 2015 ESC/ERS guidelines for the diagnosis and treatment of pulmonary hypertension: the joint task force for the diagnosis and treatment of pulmonary hypertension of the European Society of Cardiology (ESC) and the European Respiratory Society (ERS): Endor. Eur Heart J. 2016;37:67–119. Available from: http://www.ncbi.nlm.nih.gov/pubmed/26320113.

129. Dimopoulos K, Diller GP, Koltsida E, Pijuan-Domenech A, Papadopoulou SA, Babu-Narayan SV, et al. Prevalence, predictors, and prognostic value of renal dysfunction in adults with congenital heart disease. Circulation. 2008;117:2320–8.

130. Gatzoulis MA, Beghetti M, Galiè N, Granton J, Berger RMFF, Lauer A, et al. Longer-term bosentan therapy improves functional capacity in Eisenmenger syndrome: results of the BREATHE-5 open-label extension study. Int J Cardiol. 2008;127:27–32. Available from: https://pubmed.ncbi.nlm.nih.gov/17658633.

131. Van Loon RLE, Roofthooft MTRR, Hillege HL, ten Harkel ADJJ, van Osch-Gevers M, Delhaas T, et al. Pediatric pulmonary hypertension in the Netherlands: epidemiology and characterization during the period 1991 to 2005. Circulation. 2011;124:1755–64. Available from: https://pubmed.ncbi.nlm.nih.gov/21947294.

132. Barst RJ, McGoon MD, Elliott CG, Foreman AJ, Miller DP, Ivy DD. Survival in childhood pulmonary arterial hypertension: insights from the registry to evaluate early and long-term pulmonary arterial hypertension disease management. Circulation. 2012;125:113–22.

133. Berger RMFF, Beghetti M, Humpl T, Raskob GE, Ivy DD, Jing Z-CC, et al. Clinical features of paediatric pulmonary hypertension: a registry study. Lancet (London, England). 2012;379:537–46. Available from: https://pubmed.ncbi.nlm.nih.gov/22240409.

Pulmonary Embolism

Angel López-Candales and Srikanth Vallurupalli

Abbreviations

aPE	Acute pulmonary embolism
AUC	Appropriate use criteria
BP	Blood pressure
BNP	Brain natriuretic peptide
CDMT	Catheter-directed mechanical thrombectomy
CTEPH	Chronic thromboembolic pulmonary hypertension
CTPA	Computed tomographic pulmonary angiography
DVT	Deep venous thrombosis
DOACs	Direct-acting oral anticoagulants
ECG	Electrocardiogram
ESLD	End-stage liver disease
ESC	European Society of Cardiology
FAC	Fractional area change
IVS	Interventricular septum
LV	Left ventricle
LMWH	Low-molecular-weight heparin
OR	Odds ratio
PIOPED	Prospective investigation of pulmonary embolism diagnosis
PA	Pulmonary artery
PERC	Pulmonary Embolism Rule-out Criteria
PH	Pulmonary hypertension
PVR	Pulmonary vascular resistance
RHS	Right-heart strain
RV	Right ventricle
RVOT	RV outflow tract
TTE	Transthoracic echocardiogram
TAPSE	Tricuspid annular plane systolic excursion
TR	Tricuspid regurgitation
UFH	Unfractionated heparin
VTI	Velocity time integral
VTE	Venous thromboembolism
V/Q scan	Ventilation-perfusion scintigraphy
VKA	Vitamin K antagonist

A. López-Candales (✉)
Division of Cardiovascular Diseases, Truman Medical Center, Hospital Hill, University of Missouri-Kansas City, Kansas City, MO, USA
e-mail: angel.lopez-candales@tmcmed.org

S. Vallurupalli
Division of Cardiology, University of Arkansas for Medical Sciences, Little Rock, AR, USA

Introduction

Acute pulmonary embolism (aPE) has perennially been considered one of the great masqueraders in medicine. Even though PE might be considered both a common and ubiquitous disorder, presenting symptoms and signs are often nonspecific; therefore, a high index of clinical suspicion coupled with a detailed history and physical examination is invaluable when evaluating patients.

A wealth of clinical and laboratory data has linked the development of deep venous thrombosis (DVT) with thromboembolic potential that may result in aPE [1–11]. Representative duplex images of a normal popliteal vein (Fig. 14.1a, b) and acute DVT (Fig. 14.1c, d) as well as a chronic DVT (Fig. 14.2a, b) are shown for comparison. Even though DVT is the most common source of embolization resulting in aPE, additional sources for potential embolization are shown in Fig. 14.3. A more complete list of potential recognized sources of thromboembolism is given in Table 14.1.

Most patients with acute venous thromboembolism (VTE) present with thrombosis in the legs as well as pulmonary thrombus at the time of diagnosis [12]. A high index of suspicion is required to recognize which patients are at risk of this otherwise deadly clinical entity. VTE is clearly recognized as a significant healthcare problem in the United States. It is estimated that 900,000 cases of DVT and PE occur per year and approximately 300,000 deaths are attributed to VTE [13]. Therefore, better understanding of the mechanisms regulating venous thrombosis and clot resolution is critical.

Although thrombophlebitis or DVT of the lower limbs was first reported in ancient Hindu medicine writings around the year 800 BCE [14], subsequent descriptions of venous thrombogenesis were unclear and remained elusive. Our current understanding of thrombus formation revolves around the well-described interplay of factors such as venous stasis, changes in the vessel wall, and thrombogenic changes within the blood in order to result in VTE. Though Virchow coined the word embolism and made significant advances in our understanding of thrombosis, he never formally proposed this triad—a concept that first appeared in the medical literature almost 100 years after his death [15].

It is estimated that the incidence of VTE in industrialized countries is 1–3 individuals per 1000 per year [8, 16–18]. However, a dramatic increase in the risk of VTE then occurs in individuals older than 85 years to 8 per 1000 persons/ years, and for those over the age of 50 reaching as high as 1 in every 100 individuals annually [8]. These alarming statistics have led the United States Senate in 2005 to designate March as "DVT Awareness Month" followed by the Surgeon General's call to action in 2008 to prevent DVT and PE.

Anticoagulation is the mainstay of treatment of symptomatic VTE. Anticoagulation prevents further thrombus deposition, allows established thrombus to undergo stabilization and/or endogenous lysis, and reduces the risk of interval recurrent thrombosis [12]. This chapter focuses on not only the pathophysiological and hemodynamic alterations that occur with aPE, but also the mechanical abnormalities that these processes have on the right ventricle (RV). This review intends to highlight the importance of the pulmonary-circulation-ventricular circuit in mediating cardiac performance and how the latter is the most critical factor determining both morbidity and mortality.

Mechanisms Regulating Thrombosis

Even though the molecular and translational pathways that regulate the dynamic balance between clot formation and lysis are well beyond the scope of this chapter, it is important to have a basic understanding of the individual elements responsible for these processes.

A healthy vascular endothelium is critical in maintaining adequate hemostasis. Under normal conditions, intact endothelial cells promote vasodilatation and local fibrinolysis. Hence, blood coagulation, platelet adhesion and activation, as well as inflammation and leukocyte activation are suppressed resulting in normal blood fluidity. A list of specific elements that maintain the natural nonthrombogenic state of the endothelial surface can be found in Table 14.2 [19, 20].

In contrast, during periods of direct vascular trauma or as a result of activation of the coagulation cascade, a prothrombotic and proinflammatory state ensues [20]. The latter is mainly characterized by an enhanced production of von Willebrand factor, tissue factor, plasminogen activator inhibitor-1, and factor V that augment thrombosis [20]. In addition, release of substances such as platelet-activating factor and

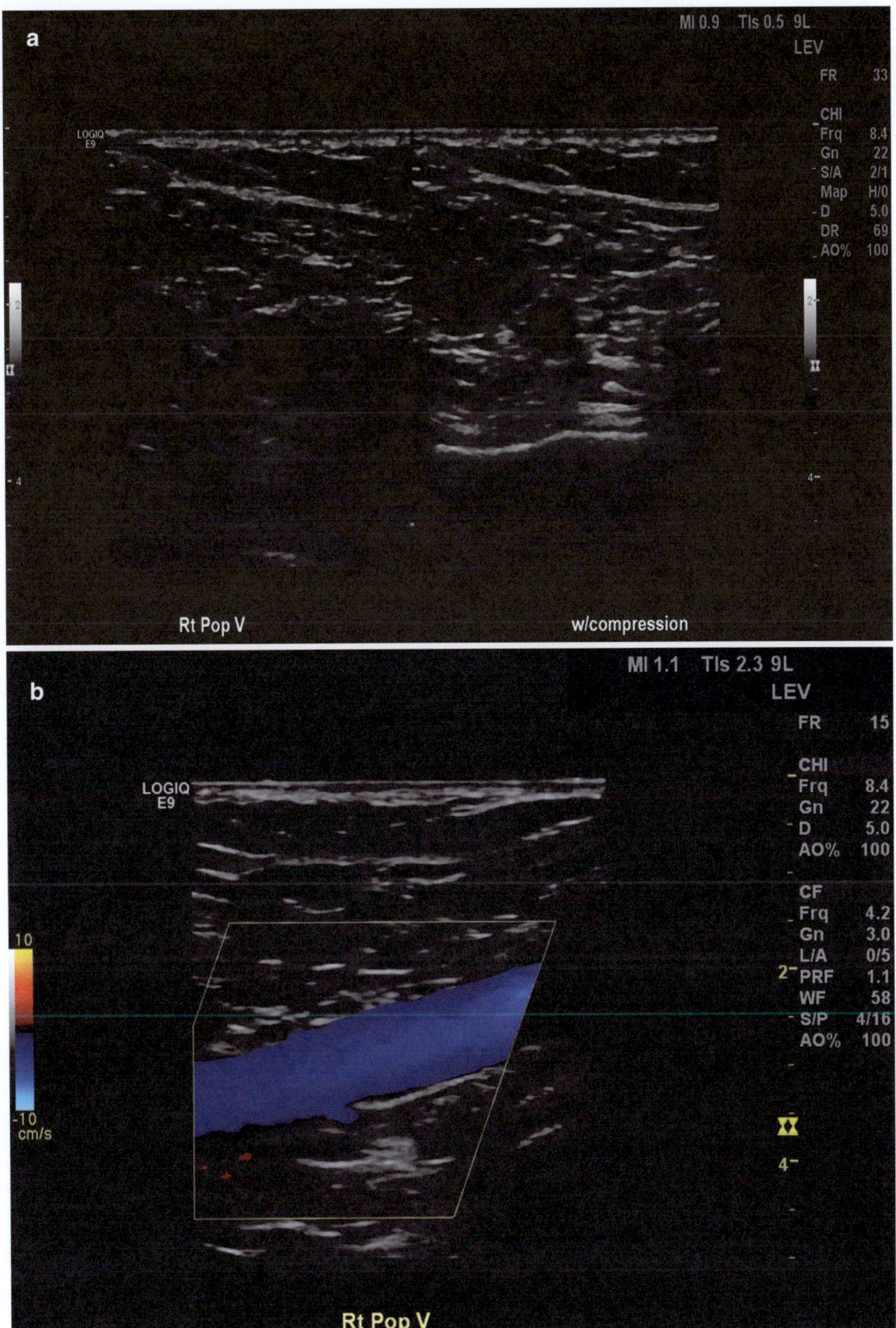

Fig. 14.1 (**a**) A representative duplex image showing a normal popliteal vein before and after manual compression. (**b**) Normal color duplex signal in a normal popliteal vein filling the whole-vein contour. (**c**) Case of an acute DVT showing a dilated popliteal vein that lacks compressibility. (**d**) Color is not found due to the proximal acute DVT that impedes flow

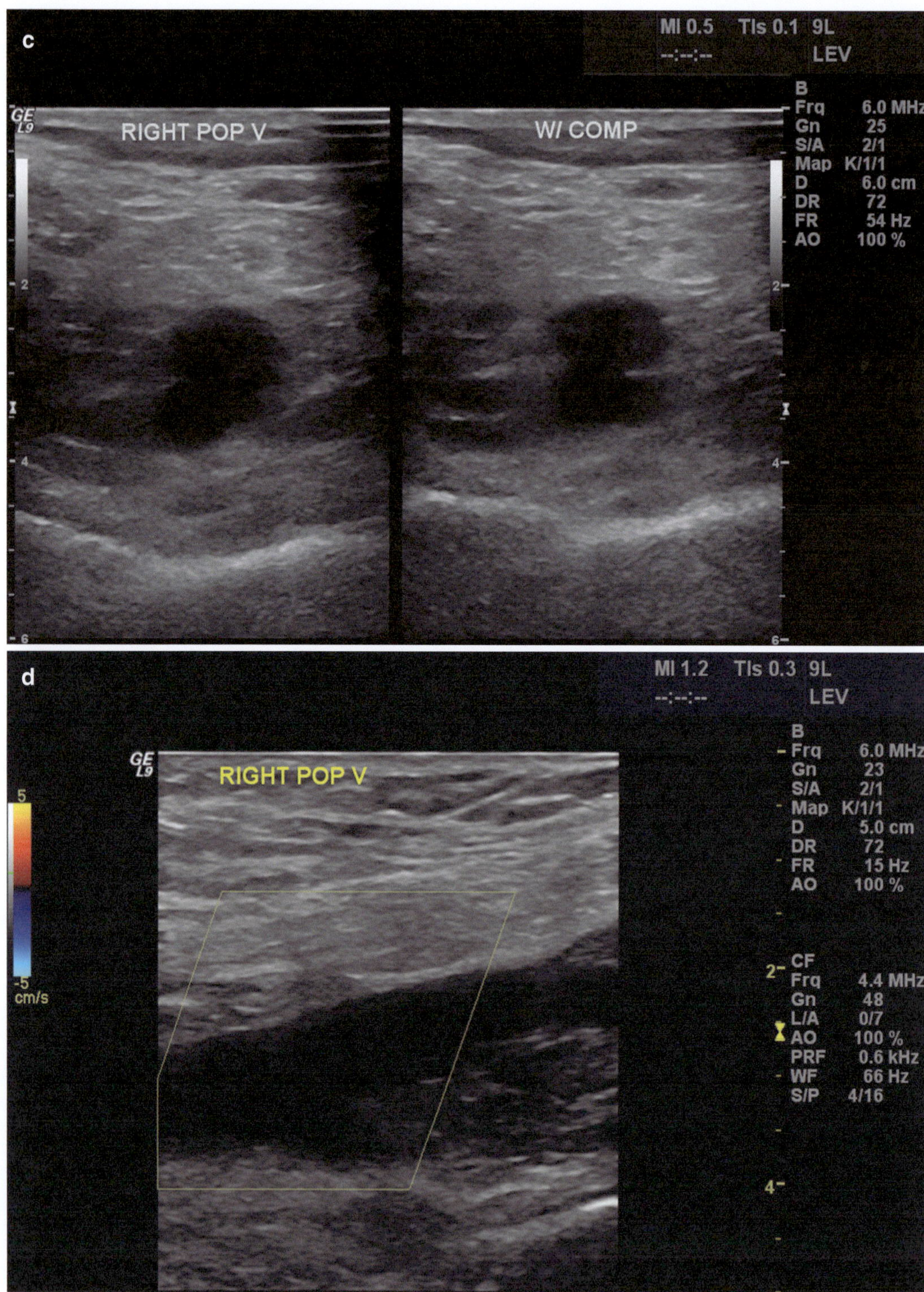

Fig. 14.1 (continued)

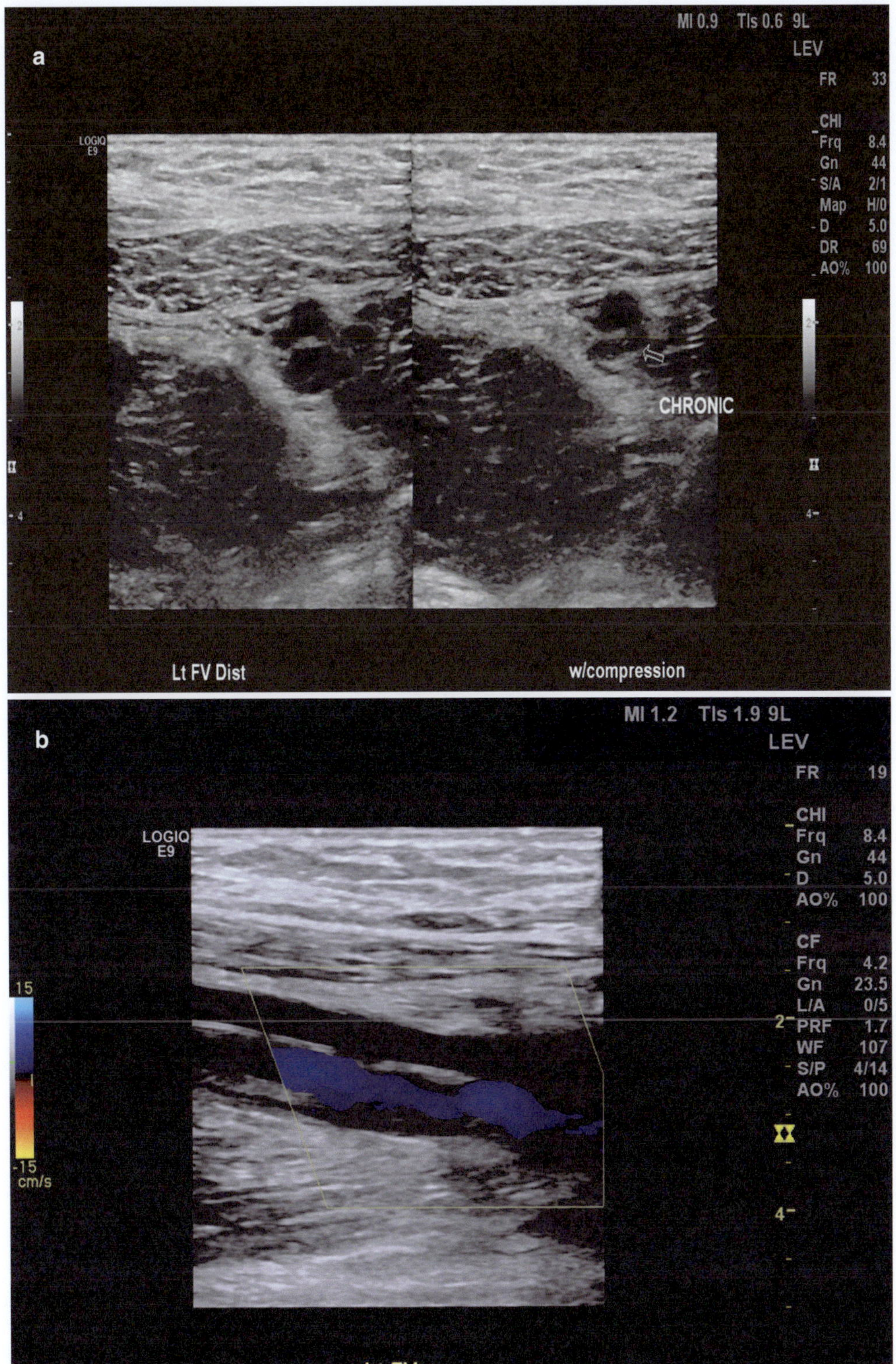

Fig. 14.2 (**a**) In sharp contrast, a chronic case of DVT is showing a visible organized clot. Please note that in most instances of a fresh clot as seen in (**a**), in acute DVT, the clot was not well visualized. (**b**) Color flow duplex signal within a popliteal vein with a partially filling clot that has distorted the main lumen

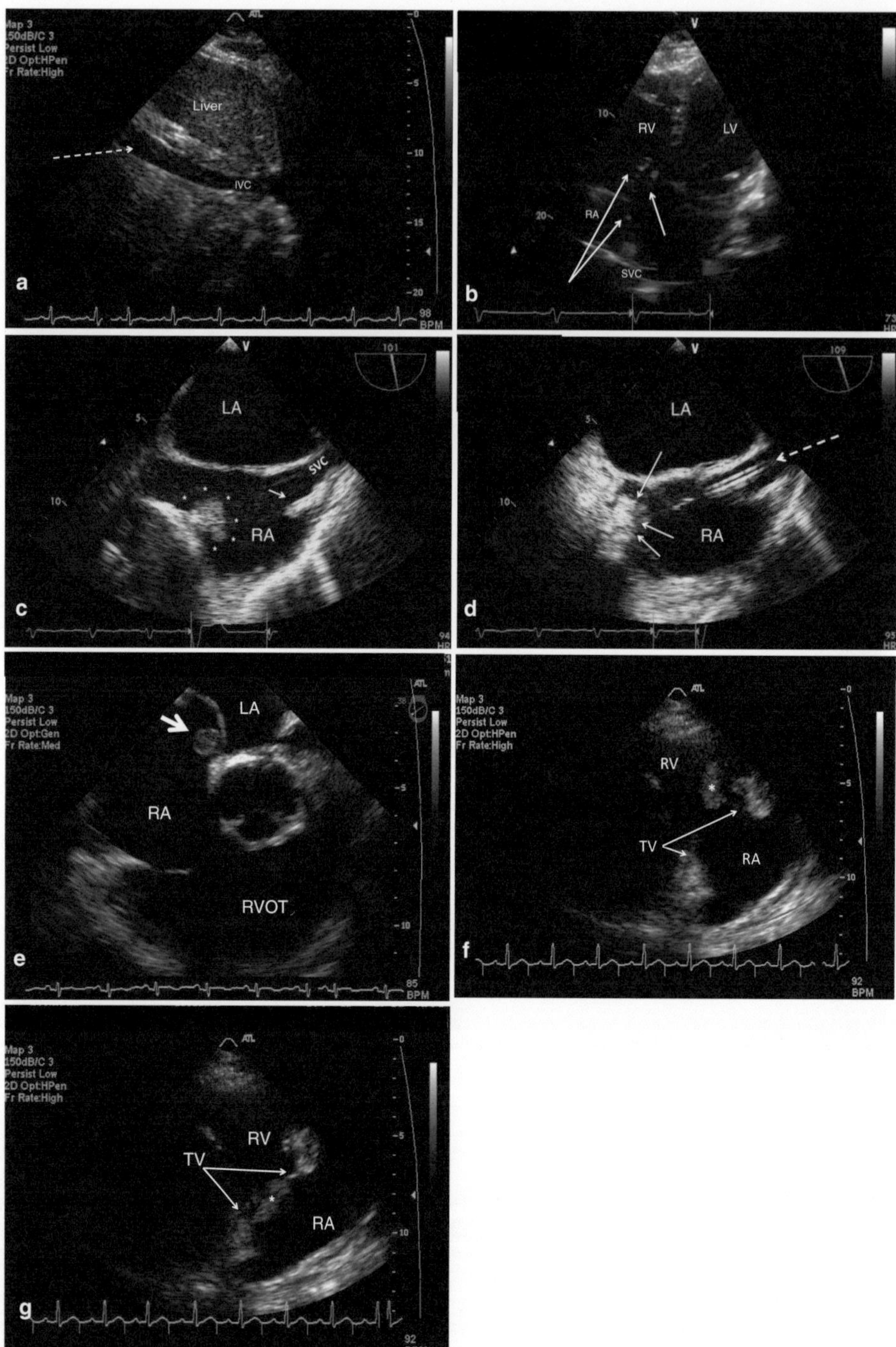

Fig. 14.3 (**a**) Representative subcostal echocardiographic image showing a homogeneous density filling the inferior vena cava (IVC) denoted by the white arrow. (**b**) Four-chamber apical echocardiographic image showing a rather large tubular thrombus cast within the right atrium (RA), crossing the tricuspid valve and into the right ventricle (RV). (**c**) Transesophageal view from the bi-caval view at 90° showing the right atrium (RA) and catheter (arrow) in the superior vena cava and a thrombus mass due to catheter-related trauma encircled by (*). (**d**) Improved visualization of the catheter seen in the SVC and the mural thrombus seen in the right atrium (RA). (**e**) Transesophageal view from 45° showing the right atrium (RA), RV outflow tract (RVOT), left atrium (LA), as well as a globular homogeneous mass (arrow) attached to the interatrial septum that was resected and found to be a myxoma. (**f**) Transthoracic view from the RV inflow showing the right atrium (RA), right ventricle (RV), and tricuspid valve (TV) as well as a homogeneous mass found to be a vegetation (*). (**g**) Additional view showing the same tricuspid valve vegetation as seen in (**f**)

Table 14.1 Potential mechanisms of thromboembolism

Venous clots originating from lower extremities (DVT)
Paget-Schroetter syndrome (spontaneous upper extremity venous thrombosis due to a compressive anomaly of the thoracic outlet)
May-Thurner syndrome (compression left common iliac vein)
Inferior vena cava abnormalities (agenesis, hypoplasia, or malformation that will cause DVT)
Massive microembolism during surgery
Air embolism
Carcinomatous tumor embolism
Cavitoatrial embolization of a renal carcinoma
Bone fat embolism after long-bone skeletal fracture
Body-sculpting fat embolism
Iatrogenic injections of various cements and coagulation materials
Embolization of a right-sided heart valve (tricuspid and pulmonic valves) vegetation

Table 14.2 Mechanisms responsible in maintaining non-thrombogenic state of endothelial surfaces

Endothelial production of thrombomodulin
Activation of protein C
Endothelial expression of heparan sulfate
Endothelial expression of dermatan sulfate
Constitutive expression of tissue factor pathway inhibitor
Local production of tissue plasminogen and urokinase-type plasminogen activators
Endothelium production of nitric oxide
Endothelium production of prostacyclin
Endothelium production of interleukin-10

endothelin-1 promotes vasoconstriction [21]. Finally, an exposed endothelial surface increases the expression of cell adhesion molecule, promoting accumulation and activation of leukocytes that further amplifies inflammation and thrombosis as shown in Fig. 14.4 [19, 22].

Thrombus contains a mixture of platelets, fibrin, and in some cases red blood cells [23, 24]. The composition of thrombus depends on flow and vessel characteristics. Arterial clots are formed under high shear stress, typically after rupture of an atherosclerotic plaque or other damage to the blood vessel wall, and are largely platelet rich (white clots) and thus generally treated with antiplatelet drugs [20, 25, 26]. Venous clots form under lower shear stress and are mostly rich in fibrin (red clots) and are hence treated with anticoagulant drugs [12, 20, 27–29].

The coagulation cascade is regulated at several levels. Interaction of tissue factor exposed by vascular injury with plasma factor VIIa results in the formation of small amounts of thrombin. This thrombin production is then amplified through the intrinsic pathway, resulting in the formation of the fibrin clot. These reactions take place on phospholipid surfaces, usually the activated platelet surface [30]. In case of venous thrombosis, changes in blood flow and in endothelial cell lining of blood vessels, as initially proposed by Virchow, increase the risk of VTE [31]. A series

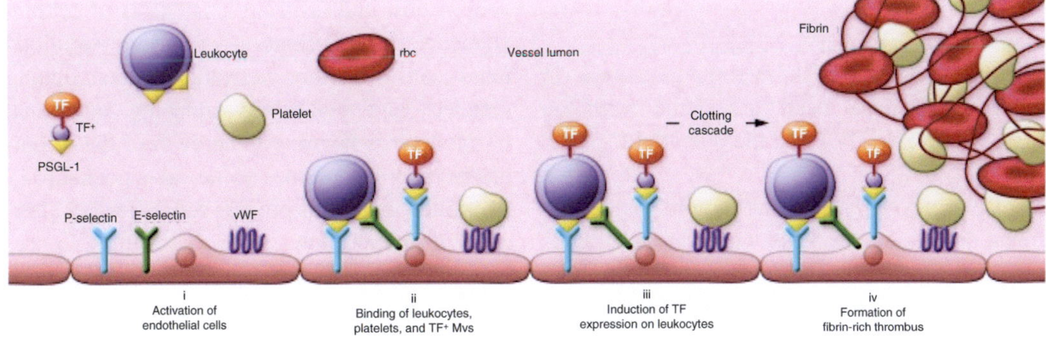

Fig. 14.4 Proposed mechanisms for venous thrombosis. It has been proposed that the formation of a venous thrombosis can be divided into distinct steps. First, the endothelium is activated by hypoxia and/or inflammatory mediators and expresses the adhesion proteins P-selectin, E-selectin, and vWF. Second, circulating leukocytes, platelets, and TF+ MVs bind to the activated endothelium. Third, the bound leukocytes become activated and express TF. The local activation of the coagulation cascade overwhelms the protective anticoagulant pathways and triggers thrombosis. The fibrin-rich clot also contains platelets and red blood cells. (Reproduced with permission from Mackman N. New insights into the mechanisms of venous thrombosis. J Clin Invest. 2012; 122: 2331–2336)

Table 14.3 Risk factors predisposing to deep venous thrombosis

Increasing age
Surgery (abdomen, pelvis, lower extremities)
Trauma (fractures of pelvis, hip, or lower extremities)
Obesity
Cancer and its treatment
Pregnancy and puerperium
Hormone-based contraceptives/hormone replacement therapy
Acute infection
Prolonged immobilization
Paralysis
Long-haul travel
Smoking
Prolonged hospitalization
Previous DVT
Congestive heart failure
Myocardial infarction
Indwelling central venous catheters
Inflammatory bowel syndrome
Nephrotic syndrome
Heparin-induced thrombocytopenia
Disseminated intravascular coagulation
Paroxysmal nocturnal hemoglobinuria
Thromboangiitis obliterans
Thrombotic thrombocytopenia purpura
Behçet's syndrome
Lupus anticoagulant (antiphospholipid antibody)
Antithrombin III deficiency
Protein C deficiency
Protein S deficiency
Factor V Leiden mutation
Prothrombin gene mutation
Dysfibrinogenemia
Factor XII deficiency

of well-recognized risk factors, as shown in Table 14.3, have been associated with an increased risk of DVT and the potential for VTE [32–51].

One group of patients that require some additional discussion are those with significant end-stage liver disease (ESLD). The previously held concept that ESLD patients are auto-anticoagulated as a result of a reduced hemostatic reserve given their reduced ability to synthesize procoagulant proteins and anticoagulation factors, hence at high risk for bleeding complications and consequently at a reduced risk for VTE, is no longer valid [51–53]. Close inspection

reveals that initial reports were simply based on data obtained from relatively small single-center studies [54, 55]. Subsequent emergences of more robust data from much larger national and international databases have shed more relevant clinical information [56–59]. Specifically, based on these results it is now recommended that hospitalized and immobilized cirrhotic patients, certainly at increased risk of thrombotic events, should receive VTE prophylaxis with either low-molecular-weight heparin or unfractionated heparin (Level III, Grade C) [51]. In contrast, cirrhotic patients with VTE should be treated with anticoagulation similar to other medical patients without a specific recommendation. Most importantly, therapy selection should be determined on a case-by-case analysis (Level III, Grade C) [51]. Certainly, additional prospective randomized trials are urgently needed to advance our understanding of this complex group of patients and better guide clinical practices.

Furthermore, in cases of compression of the left common iliac vein either by the presence of the fetus during pregnancy or in patients with May-Thurner syndrome [60, 61], the most likely site of thrombus formation in DVT is the pocket of the valve sinus [62–66]. These sites are particularly prone to thrombosis because of the disrupted and irregular blood flow patterns [62]. Initial formation of thrombus within the venous valve pocket further disrupts the architecture of these valve pockets, disrupting pulsatility of venous flow and favoring local stasis of cellular elements [67]. Formation of a semi-solidified mass causes further activation of circulating platelets and leukocytes inducing additional fibrinogenesis favoring the growth of the thrombus beyond the confines of the valve pocket [67]. Amplification of this process causes further alteration of luminal flow dynamics resulting in progressive occlusion of the vein lumen [67]. Intraluminal growth of the thrombus has also been shown to lower local oxygen tension, as oxygen is being consumed by trapped cells resulting in luminal hypoxemia favoring cell death and contributing to thrombus growth [67]. Notwithstanding the fact that the luminal linear velocity of the blood continues to decline and

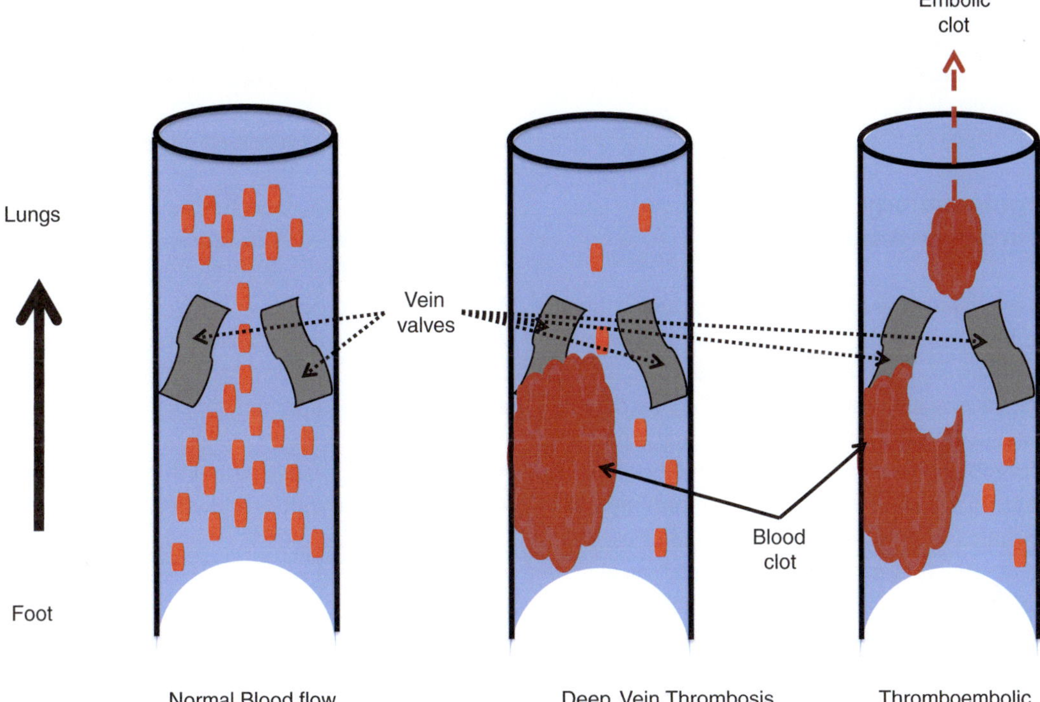

Fig. 14.5 Diagrammatic representation of a deep vein during normal flow, during acute thrombus formation (DVT), and during potential embolization (VTE). During normal flow blood cells freely move across vein valves. In the event of DVT, a clot forms on the underside of the vein valves. In the case of VTE, potential dislodgement of part of the clot material can be released into the venous circulation. Thrombosis is thought to be enhanced by a significant decline in oxygen tension in the region of the valve pocket sinus resulting in clot formation and the potential for VTE

further oxygen is being locally consumed, passing blood stream tugs additional layers of cells to the growing thrombus [67]. A graphic representation of this process is illustrated in Fig. 14.5 [62, 67–69].

Two simple anatomical considerations are important for understanding DVT and the potential for VTE. First, as the number of vein valves increases within any given vein segment, the risk of DVT increases. Second, during the stage of thrombus formation, not all portions of the thrombus anchor to the necrotic endothelium. Some portions of the growing thrombus are less strongly attached and can embolize in the direction of blood flow. Development of local symptoms of DVT depends on the extent of thrombosis, adequacy of collateral vessels, and also severity of associated vascular occlusion and inflamma-

tion. Phlegmasia cerulea and alba dolens refer to massive venous thrombus that can cause significant painful swelling of the calf and resultant pressure necrosis and gangrene. When the thrombus embolizes to the pulmonary vasculature, symptoms and hemodynamic adaptation largely depend on the underlying cardiopulmonary reserve of the individual [63–65]. A large thrombus is relatively well tolerated in the setting of normal cardiovascular reserve while a relatively smaller burden can cause hemodynamic compromise in those with limited reserve.

The early post-venous thrombosis stage is characterized by recruitments of neutrophils that are essential for thrombus resolution by promoting fibrinolysis and collagenolysis [70, 71]. This process then transitions over the course of a few days, peaking at approximately day 8, to a monocyte-predominant venous thrombus milieu that is then associated with plasmin and matrix metalloproteinase-mediated thrombus breakdown [72, 73].

Epidemiology of Venous Thromboembolism

It is important to realize that the current estimates of incidence of DVT and VTE represent an underestimate for several reasons. Milder cases may not be investigated and remain undiagnosed, while fatal undiagnosed events are never identified. The thrombosis cases treated outside the hospital setting (in the clinic or emergency room) are rarely included in studies. Since many studies use stringent validation criteria, patients with typical clinical findings but nondiagnostic radiologic studies are not reported. Finally, patients treated in long-term care facilities and cancer patients in hospice settings are usually not enrolled in clinical studies. It is also important to keep in mind that studies that include a large number of VTE cases diagnosed by autopsy have generally reported a higher proportion of PE than DVT cases likely due to the presence of asymptomatic PE.

Current estimates regarding incidence rates for VTE are recognized to be higher among African American populations when compared to Asian, Asian American, and Native American populations.

VTE is mostly seen in older individuals and is rare prior to late adolescence [74]. Even when incidence rates increase markedly for both men (130 per 100,000) and women (110 per 100,000) there is a clear difference that is important to be recognized [74]. Incidence rates of VTE are higher in women during childbearing years (16–44 years) compared to men of similar age; however, in individuals older than 45 years of age, VTE incidence rates are higher among men [74].

Interestingly, it has been reported that incident cases of VTE can occur without a specific recognizable trigger, in up to 40% of cases in populations of European and African origins [74].

Even when there is paucity of data relating VTE incidence, incidence rates for VTE, DVT,

and PE either remained constant or increased between 1981 and 2000 with a substantial increase rate for VTE noted between 2001 and 2009 based on PE cases, the latter likely reflecting the increased utilization of better imaging techniques.

Data largely obtained from a case-controlled study that included 726 women with incident VTE between 1988 and 2000 in Olmsted County, MN, USA, identified the following case particulars as significant risk factors for the development of VTE. These are presented in the decreasing order of clinical impact [75]:

- Major surgery (odds ratio (OR) 18.95)
- Active cancer with or without concurrent chemotherapy (OR 14.64)
- Neurological disease with leg paresis (OR 6.10)
- Hospitalization for acute illness (OR 5.07)
- Nursing-home confinement (OR 4.63)
- Trauma or fracture (OR 4.56)
- Pregnancy or puerperium (OR 4.24)
- Oral contraception (OR 4.03)
- Noncontraceptive estrogen plus progestin use (OR 2.53)
- Estrogen (OR 1.81)
- Progestin (OR 1.20)
- Body mass index (OR 1.08)

Interestingly previously held notions accounting for VTE risk factors such as age, varicose veins, and progestin were not significantly associated with incident VTE in this studied population when included in the multivariate analysis [75].

Hospitalization remains a well-recognized risk factor for VTE conferring a greater than 100-fold risk regardless of the fact that if this hospitalization is due to medical illness (VTE risk 22%) or surgically related (24%) [74].

Recognized VTE risk factors among medical illness patients include [74]:

- Age
- Obesity
- Previous VTE
- Thrombophilia
- Cancer

- Recent trauma or surgery
- Tachycardia
- Acute myocardial infarction or stroke
- Leg paresis or prolonged immobilization (bed rest)
- Congestive heart failure
- Acute infection
- Rheumatological disorders
- Hormone therapy
- Central venous catheter
- Admission to an intensive or coronary care unit
- White blood cell and platelet count

In the case of surgical patients, VTE risk factors include [74]:

- Age, particularly in those 65 years of age or older.
- Type of surgery such as neurosurgical, major orthopedic procedures of the leg, renal transplantation, cardiovascular surgery, and thoracic, abdominal, or pelvic surgical interventions for cancer. Furthermore, obesity and a poor physical status are well-recognized risk factors after total-hip arthroplasty.
- Smoking status.
- Presence or absence of active cancer.

Additional elements that should be considered known to increase VTE risk factors include [76–79]:

- Central venous catheters, particularly via femoral vein access
- Prior superficial vein thrombosis
- Long travels greater than 4 h
- Hypertriglyceridemia in postmenopausal women

The risk of DVT associated with varicose veins is uncertain and seems to vary with patient age [80].

However, we would like to point out that generalizations should be avoided as all these recommendations require further validation as the fluidity of medical and surgical care as well as the complexity of cases have evolved.

It is important to point out that nursing-home residents account for an ever-growing number of patients for VTE risk. In fact, hospitalization and being a resident of a nursing home account for 60% of incident VTE with nursing-home residence independently responsible for 1/10th of all VTE cases [74].

Traditionally, cancer increases VTE risk and currently accounts for 20% of all incident cases occurring in the community [74]. Specific cancers associated to the increased VTE risk include pancreas, ovaries, colon, stomach, lung, kidney, bone, and brain [81, 82]. Furthermore, when cancer patients receive immunosuppressive or cytotoxic chemotherapy, particularly L-asparaginase, thalidomide, lenalidomide, or tamoxifen, these medications place these patients at even higher risk [83, 84].

With regard to cancer patients, VTE risk is particularly increased [85, 86]:

- Gastric and pancreatic cancers
- Platelet counts $\geq 350 \times 10^9/l$
- Hemoglobin levels <100 g/l
- Use of red cell growth factors
- Leukocyte counts $\geq 11 \times 10^9/l$
- BMI 35 kg/m^2 or greater ≥ 35
- Elevated plasma-soluble P-selectin and D-dimers

Aside from all these recognized risk factors and clinical situations associated with VTE, true estimates of the total number of VTE events that are either incident or recurrent occurring each year vary widely. Despite some limitations, attack rates have been estimated between 91 and 255 for DVT and between 51 and 75 for PE per 100,000 person years [87, 88].

Recurrent VTE events occur in up to 30% of cases within 10 years of the initial event with a reported rate of 19–39 per 100,000 person years [87, 89]. Based on the data originally published by Heit et al. the estimated cumulative incidence of the first overall VTE recurrence was 1.6% at 7 days, 5.2% at 30 days, 8.3% at 90 days, 10.1% at 180 days, 12.9% at 1 year, 16.6% at 2 years, 22.8% at 5 years, and 30.4% at 10 years with the risk of first recurrence being the highest close to the incident event and then decreasing as time goes on [90]. Although prophylaxis is crucial, duration of this initial treatment does not appear to affect the rate of recurrence beyond the initial 3 months of recommended prophylactic anticoagulation suggesting that VTE is in fact a chronic disease with episodic recurrence [91–94].

Recognized independent predictors of VTE recurrence include [32, 90, 95–101]:

- Increasing age
- Increasing BMI
- Male sex
- Active cancer
- Neurological disease with leg paresis
- Idiopathic VTE
- Active lupus anticoagulant or antiphospholipid antibody
- Deficiency of antithrombin, protein C, or protein S
- Hyperhomocysteinemia
- Elevated plasma D-dimers
- In some cases, residual vein thrombosis
- Factor V Leiden mutations combined with deficiencies of antithrombin, protein S, or protein C
- Pancreatic, brain, lung, and ovarian cancer; myeloproliferative or myelodysplastic disorders; and stage IV cancers

Accurate assessments of case fatality rates after initial VTE are hindered by the nature of the analysis. First, retrospective data analysis is difficult to interpret when autopsy data is used because autopsies are not uniformly performed to confirm aPE diagnosis in patients dying unexpectedly. Second, prospective data collection is also difficult due to the declining rates of autopsies. Despite these limitations, it is believed that up to two-thirds of patients simply manifest DVT alone and death occurs in approximately 6% of these patients within a month of diagnosis, whereas a third of patients with symptomatic VTE develop PE and may experience up to a 12% mortality during the same time period [54]. Early mortality after VTE is strongly associated with presentation as PE, advanced age, cancer, and underlying cardiovascular disease [54, 102].

Finally, it is clear that VTE occurrence is not only influenced by multiple clinical factors and disease processes but also modified by several genetic-environmental interactions placing some individuals at greater risk than others and additional follow-up studies are certainly required.

Pulmonary Vasculature

The pulmonary vasculature consists of the arterial, venous, and bronchial arteries and to some extent albeit not a robust system the microvascular collateral circulation [103–106]. The pulmonary arterial (PA) system is the most relevant to a discussion of aPE and closely follows the bronchial pathways. From an anatomical perspective the main PA arises from the RV outflow tract (RVOT) and divides into the left and right pulmonary arteries. The left PA appears to be a continuation of the main PA as it arches over the left main stem bronchus and begins branching to supply the left upper and lower lobes. A representative view of the main PA with its main bifurcations is seen in Fig. 14.6.

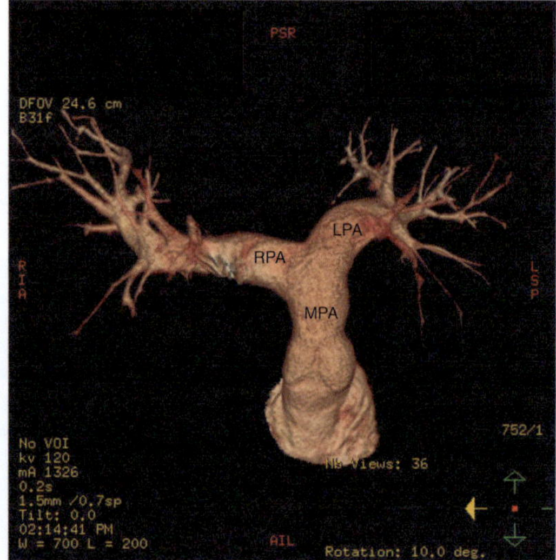

Fig. 14.6 Volume-rendered reconstructions of a multidetector-row computed tomographic scan elegantly showing the main pulmonary artery (*MPA*), left pulmonary artery (*LPA*), and right pulmonary artery (*RPA*) with proximal bifurcations. (Image reconstruction performed by Amy L. Smith, RT (R) (CT) and Dr. Robert O'Donnell, MD, University of Cincinnati Medical Center)

Typically, the right PA is longer and gives rise to the right upper lobe artery as it arches over the right main stem bronchus. It normally courses more caudal than the left, and its length is better visualized in chest radiography. The normal main PA caliber is less than 3 cm while both left and right PAs are usually 1.5 cm [107].

The right PA gives rise to an upper lobe artery, which then divides into an apical, a posterior, and an anterior segmental artery. The next right lobar artery branch is the middle lobe artery, which divides into a lateral and a medial lobe segmental artery. The right lower lobe artery divides into an apical, an anterior, a posterior, a medial, and a lateral segmental artery. Although this major branching pattern is typical and related to lobar and segmental lung development, other arterial branches may arise directly from the right and left PA [107]. In contrast,

a typical left PA gives rise to an upper and a lower lobe artery. The left upper lobe artery gives off the apicoposterior, anterior, and lingular arteries that further divide into a superior and an inferior segmental artery. The left lower lobe artery divides into a superior, an anteromedial, a lateral, and a posterior basal segmental artery [107].

Final diagnostic documentation of the involved segment is based on the highest branching order resolved by the imaging technique. Therefore, main PA arising from the RVOT is recognized as the first order. The right and left PA are considered as second order. Visualization of lobar artery segments is considered third order. Finally, segmental arteries are recognized as fourth order, subsegmental arteries are fifth order, and the first branches of subsegmental arteries are described as sixth order [107]. Figure 14.7

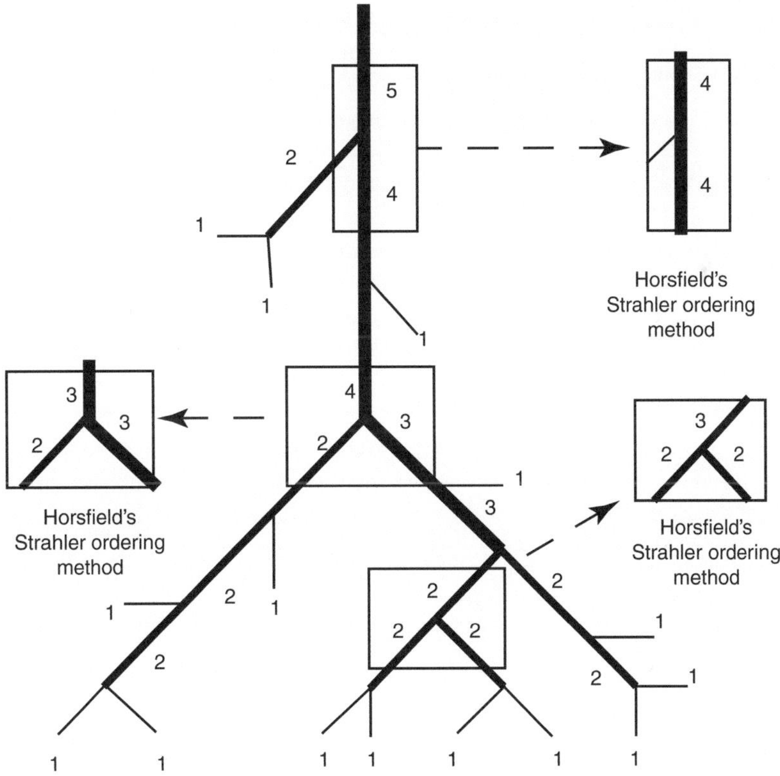

Fig. 14.7 Illustration of diameter-defined Strahler ordering system. Vessel order numbers are determined by their connection and diameters. Arteries with smallest diameters are of order 1. A segment is a vessel between two successive points of bifurcation. When two segments meet, order number of confluent vessel is increased by 1. Horsfield and diameter-defined systems apply to arterial and venous trees only. They are not applicable to capillary network, the topology of which is not treelike. Each group of segments of the same order connected in series is lumped together and called an element. (Reproduced with permission from Huang W et al. J Appl Physiol 1996; 81: 2123–2133)

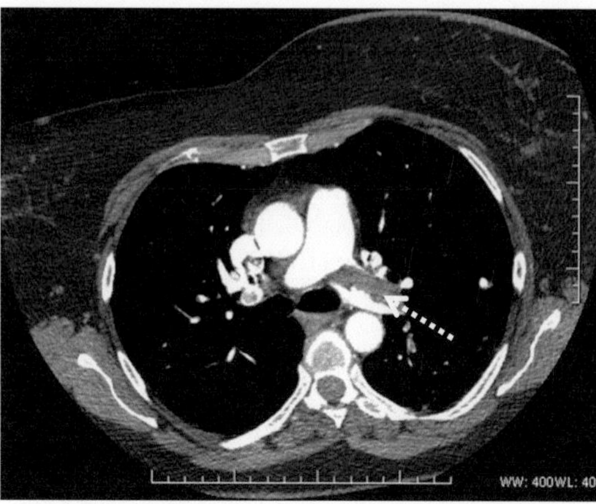

Fig. 14.8 Chest tomographic image showing a large filling defect suggestive of a large saddle embolus seen (broken arrow). (Image provided by Amy L. Smith, RT (R) (CT) and Dr. Robert O'Donnell, MD, University of Cincinnati Medical Center)

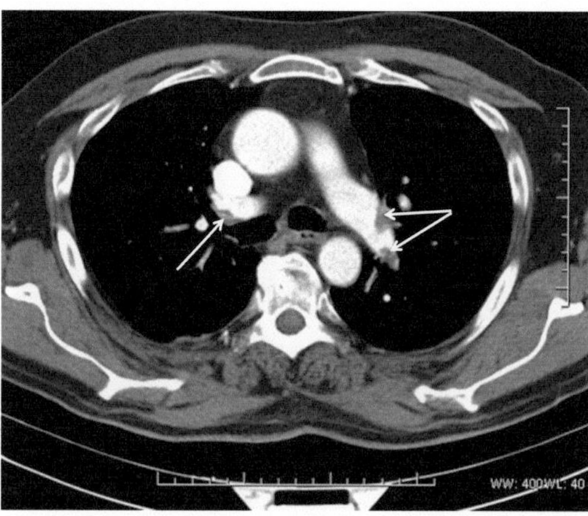

Fig. 14.9 Chest tomographic image showing two filling defects (shown by the arrows) on the left side and a defect on the right side representative of subsegmental regions of the PA vasculature. (Image provided by Amy L. Smith, RT (R) (CT) and Dr. Robert O'Donnell, MD, University of Cincinnati Medical Center)

demonstrates the proposed diameter-defined Strahler ordering system with regard to the PA system. Representative tomographic images of aPE cases are shown with a typical proximal saddle embolus shown in Fig. 14.8 and a subsegmental aPE shown in Fig. 14.9.

Pulmonary Arterial System Network and the Right Ventricle

In the normal state, the pulmonary artery vasculature acts as an elastic reservoir for the stroke volume ejected from the RV, with minimal resistance provided from the main PA all the way down to subsegmental arteries (approximately 0.5 mm diameter). Exquisite flow resistance regulation takes place at the level of the muscular arteriole capillaries, which exert the greatest arterial flow and pressure control [108–110]. The diameter of these artery segments closely parallels that of the accompanying bronchi [110–113]. In the normal state, this dynamic process is instrumental in matching perfusion to ventilation in real time and in regulating RV systolic function.

RV cardiac output depends on proper calibration between RV myocardial contractility and impedance to blood flow through the lungs. The RV can accommodate large volumes without significant compromise in systolic performance as long as there is no impedance to ejection or if the impedance occurs slowly over a period of time, such as in chronic pulmonary hypertension. However, it has limited contractile reserve to match even minor increases in impedance to ejection (acute pulmonary hypertension). Clinically, the degree of hemodynamic compromise depends on the magnitude and timing of pulmonary vascular obstruction [114–121]. A small embolism (even if recurrent and multiple) can be asymptomatic or present with mild dyspnea. Due to these differences in clinical presentation, case fatality rate for aPE ranges from <1% to about 60% [122]. A more recent data analysis using figures from the Nationwide Inpatient Sample from 1999 to 2008 showed that all-cause case fatality rate decrease was primarily driven by a decrease in case fatality rates for stable patients [123]. There was no reduction of case fatality rate in unstable patients receiving thrombolytic therapy [123]. Though it is important to highlight the fact that the general case

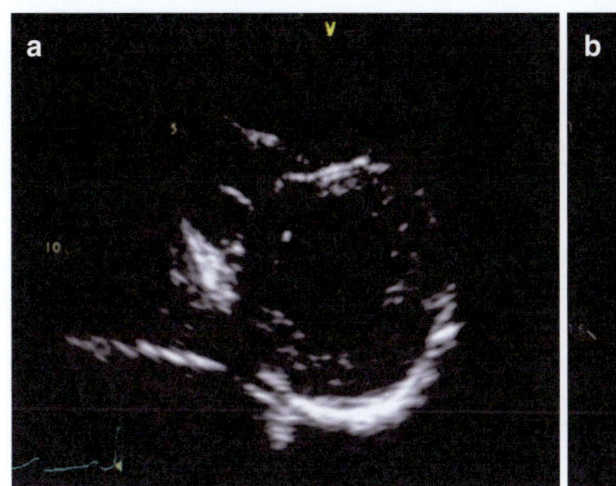
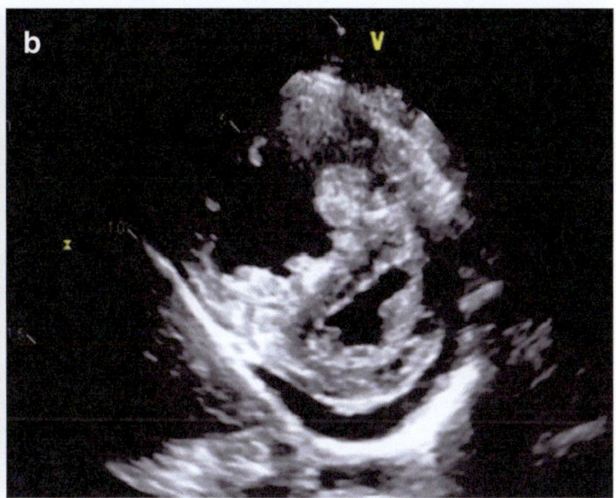

Fig. 14.10 (**a**) Echocardiographic short-axis view of the left ventricle at the papillary muscle level showing a normal curvature of the left ventricle in relationship to a normal-sized RV with normal wall thickness. (**b**) In contrast, a dilated and hypertrophied RV requires not only more energy to pump the same amount of blood as compared to the normal-sized RV but also the resultant higher wall tension and thus RV peak systolic pressure results in bowing of the interventricular septum causing systolic flattening during ventricular contraction

fatality rate for patients receiving thrombolytics and a vena cava filter was low, most of these unstable patients did not receive this combination therapy [123].

Even though the proposed pathways leading to RV injury are intrinsically different between chronic and acute pulmonary hypertension (PH) [124], RV dilatation and systolic dysfunction are common abnormalities shared by both clinical entities. These abnormalities in RV size and systolic performance are mainly explained by the Laplace relationship [125]. Specifically, an increased ratio between cavity radius and thickness will increase wall stress while a decrease in this ratio will decrease wall stress [126]. Acute elevations in PH (acute increase in impedance to flow in pulmonary artery, such as aPE) cause a sudden increase in cavity radius and since there is little time to compensate with increased wall thickness, wall stress increases. This principle is illustrated in Fig. 14.10 showing the relationship between RV wall dilatation and increased thickness and its effect on the left ventricle (LV).

The right and left ventricles differ in their ability to compensate for the increase in chamber size. In the case of the LV, wall thickness is greater than the RV. The LV can compensate both to physiologically acute increases in afterload (such as increased BP during exercise) or pathological, chronic causes such as systemic hypertension or valvular lesions (albeit by undergoing compensatory hypertrophy) [127]. Increase in thickness allows the LV to provide adequate stroke volume without an unacceptable reduction in myocardial performance [127]. In the more compliant RV, the thin walls allow it to accommodate larger volumes without hemodynamic stress (such as the increased preload during exercise), while at the same time allowing it to eject the same stroke volume as the LV against approximately 25% of the afterload the LV faces [128]. This increased compliance does not allow the RV to tolerate acute increases in afterload, such as in aPE [125]. Direct mechanical obstruction of the PA by thrombus or any other embolic material accompanied by potent release of local vasoconstrictors will result in hypoxemia causing a rapid increase in pulmonary vascular resistance (PVR) and the resultant increase in PVR [129–139]. The latter will ultimately determine the compromise in RV performance and the degree of hemodynamic collapse in accordance with the location and extent of the acute thromboembolic occlusion as well as the generation of local vasoconstrictive mediators along the PA system network in relation to underlying functional state of the myocardium. In cases of gradual increase in RV afterload, such as chronic PH, the RV should be able to handle these remodeling changes more efficiently, as there is time to assemble new sarcomeres in parallel in order to increase wall thickness and compensate for the hemodynamic stress [125].

Clinically, PVR can be assessed either invasively by catheter measurement or noninvasively by using transthoracic echocardiography (TTE). TTE estimation relies on measuring the maximum tricuspid regurgitation (TR) jet velocity using continuous-wave Doppler and the velocity time integral (VTI) of the pulsed Doppler signal across the RVOT. Thus, TTE calculation uses the following formula: PVR (Woods unit [WU]) = (TR velocity max/RVOT VTI) × 10 + 0.16 to approximate values that are obtained during invasive right-heart catheterization. Representative TTE Doppler signals are shown in Fig. 14.11 [140].

As mentioned earlier, this rise in PVR would depend on the location and extent of the acute thromboembolic occlusion and also generation of local vasoconstrictive mediators along the PA system network. In conjunction with the functional state of RV myocardium, the extent of increase of PVR is an important determinant of prognosis, particularly when aPE interferes with both the circulation and gas exchange.

While the presence of thrombus in the deep veins and pulmonary arteries has been discussed, it is not unusual to find intracardiac thrombi in those with suspected aPE. This finding signifies either a thrombus in transit from the leg veins to the pulmonary artery or a native intracardiac thrombus that can rarely cause aPE. Either way, presence of intracardiac thrombus is a poor prognostic sign. In the International Cooperative Pulmonary Embolism Registry (ICOPER), intracardiac thrombus was present in 42 of 1113 patients with a TTE at admission [141]. Patients with a demonstrable intracardiac thrombus at the time of the TTE were more hemodynamically compromised as suggested by lower systemic arterial pressure, higher prevalence of hypotension, faster heart rates, and frequent hypokinesis

of the RV as determined by TTE than patients without a demonstrable intracardiac thrombus at the time of diagnosis [141].

From a pathophysiological point of view, the cascade of events resulting in aPE can be simplistically explained not only by interference of both the circulation and gas exchange at the pulmonary level caused by the embolic material but also by the disturbance created by that material along the pulmonary-ventricular unit that ultimately results in some variable degree of RV mechanic disruption. Primary cause of death in severe aPE has been singled out as RV failure [142].

When occlusion of more than 30–50% of the total cross-sectional pulmonary arterial bed by thromboembolic material and local release of vasoconstriction substances occur, we see elevation in pulmonary artery pressures as a result of an increase in PVR [133, 143–145]. A marked and sudden increase in PVR will dilate an otherwise normal thin-wall RV that by the mechanisms previously described would not be able to generate a mean pulmonary pressure above 40 mmHg and consequently fail [125, 126, 143].

From a clinical point of view the estimated in-hospital or 30-day mortality risk determines the severity of an aPE event mainly determined by the patient's presentation. The latter will ultimately stratify patients into either high- (shock or persistent hypotension in the absence of arrhythmia, hypovolemia, or sepsis) or no high-risk PE with important diagnostic and therapeutic implications [143]. Differentiating patients based on this approach facilitates diagnostic and therapeutic strategies as reconciled on a recent guideline document that integrates previous knowledge into a more optimal and objective diagnostic and management strategies for those patients presenting with either a suspected or a confirmed aPE [143].

Clinical parameters based on severity index have shown to be quite useful in assessing prognosis and determining outcomes. The most validated score to date is the PESI in identifying patients' worse 30-day outcomes [146–149]. A simplified sPESI version is also available and has been validated [150, 151]. These clinical param-

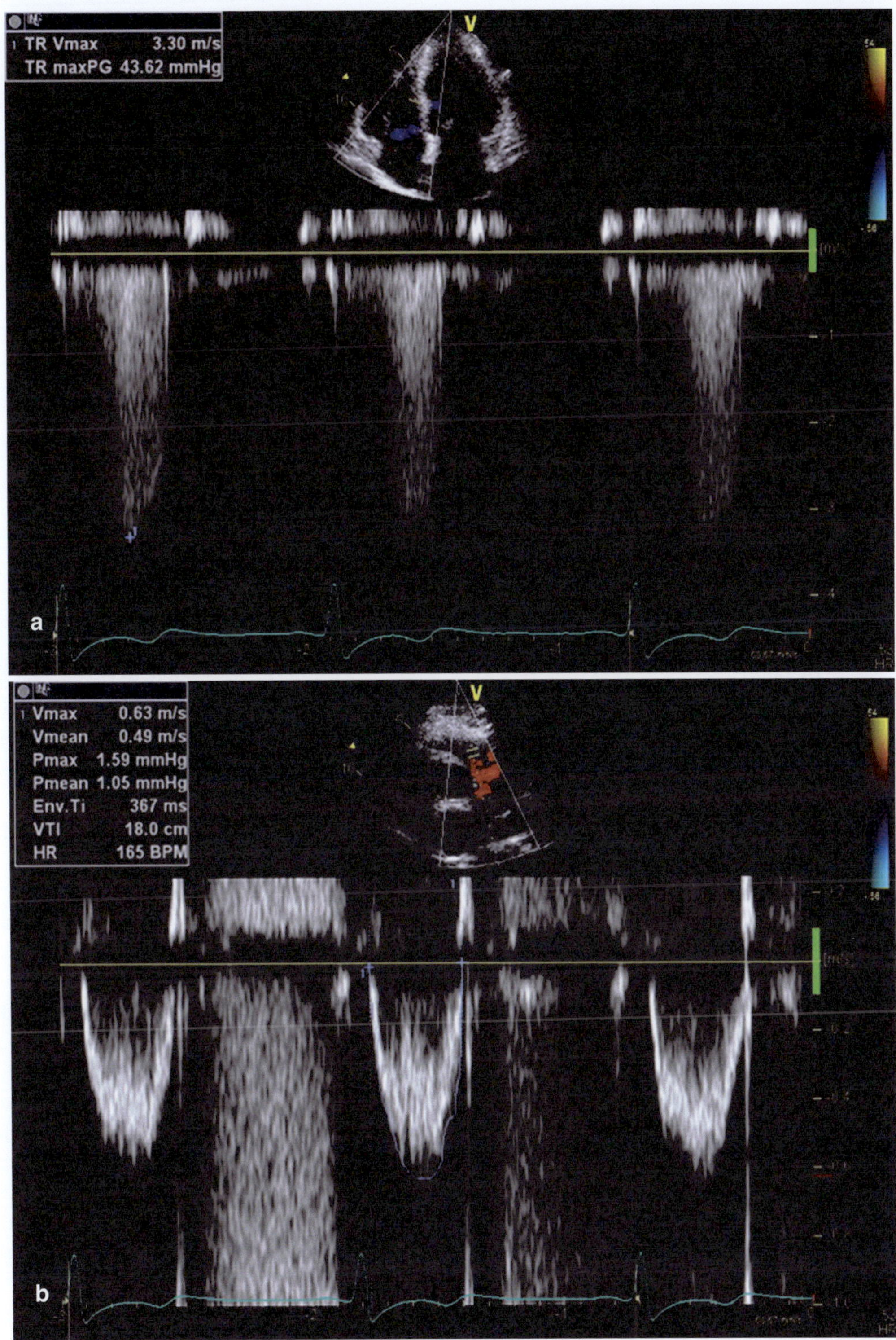

Fig. 14.11 Representative Doppler tracings used for PVR calculation using echocardiography. (**a**) Maximal TR velocity jet signal obtained from the apical four-chamber view measuring 3.3 m/s. (**b**) Pulsed Doppler signal across the RVOT showing a velocity time integral (VTI) of 18 cm resulting in a PVR of 2.0 WU. Echocardiographic estimation of PVR uses the following formula: PVR (Woods unit [WU]) = (TR velocity max/RVOT VTI) × 10 + 0.16

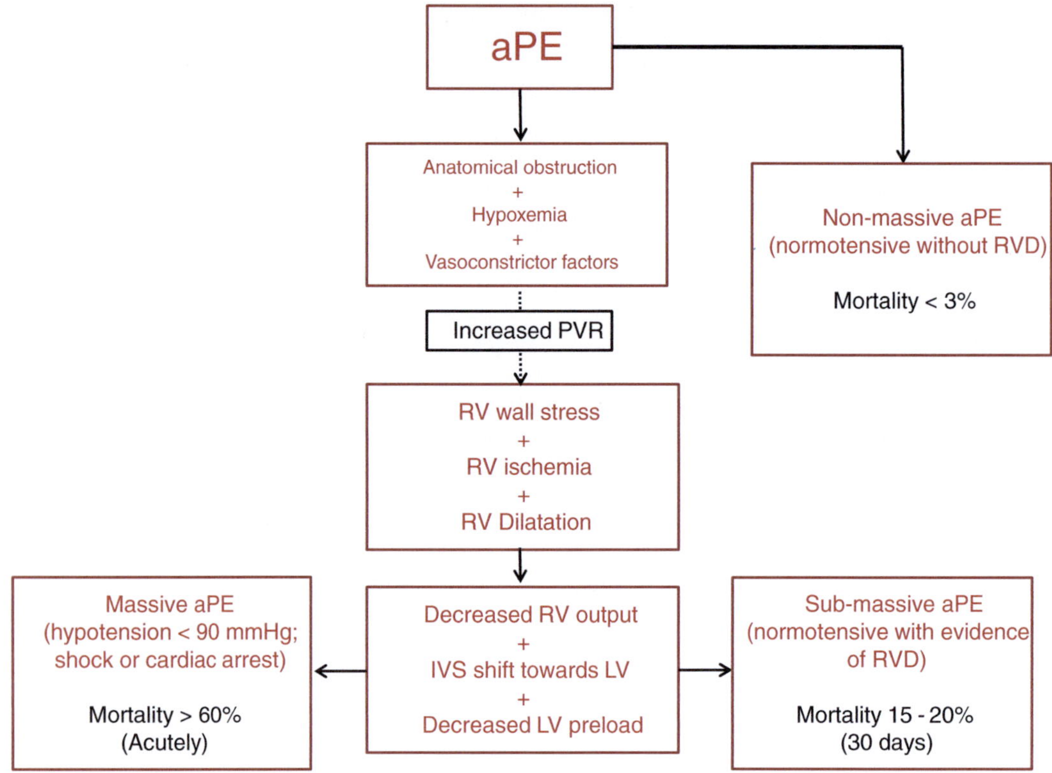

Fig. 14.12 Diagrammatic representation of the sequence of events during aPE and the potential clinical implications of the thrombotic occlusion and resultant hemodynamic implications with associated mortality rates

eters become clearly important in assessing the overall risk of adverse events and need for additional testing.

Traditionally, determination of the clinical magnitude of the thrombotic occlusion and its hemodynamic helps expedite therapeutic strategies [152]. A massive aPE is defined as a patient with hemodynamic compromise with significant RV dysfunction. Based on the location of thrombus, it is further categorized as saddle, main branch, or ≥2 lobar pulmonary emboli. It carries an estimated 60% mortality, two-thirds of which occur within the first hour after onset [122, 153, 154]. In contrast, sub-massive aPE occurs in hemodynamically stable patients who demonstrate evidence of right-heart strain, which is most commonly identified by TTE or elevation of cardiac enzymes [122, 154]. It carries an estimated 15–20% 30-day mortality rate and has been associated with chronic thromboembolic pulmonary hypertension and subsequent development of cor pulmonale [155]. Finally, a non-massive aPE is characterized by a normotensive patient with no evidence of RV dysfunction. A diagrammatic representation of this interrelationship is seen in Fig. 14.12. In summary, a high index of clinical suspicion is required to identify patients at risk as subtle findings can make the difference between life and death as shown in Fig. 14.13.

A recent publication by Jimenez and associates sheds light into most recent trends regarding hospital stay and 30-day mortality for aPE. Data from 23,858 patients from 2001 to 2013 taken from a large international aPE (RIETE) registry was used. For comparison purposes, results were divided into two time periods, first period between 2001 and 2005 and second period between 2010 and 2013. Using a multivariate regression model, these investigators found improvements in the overall length of stay (reduction from 13.6 to 9.3 days: 32% relative reduc-

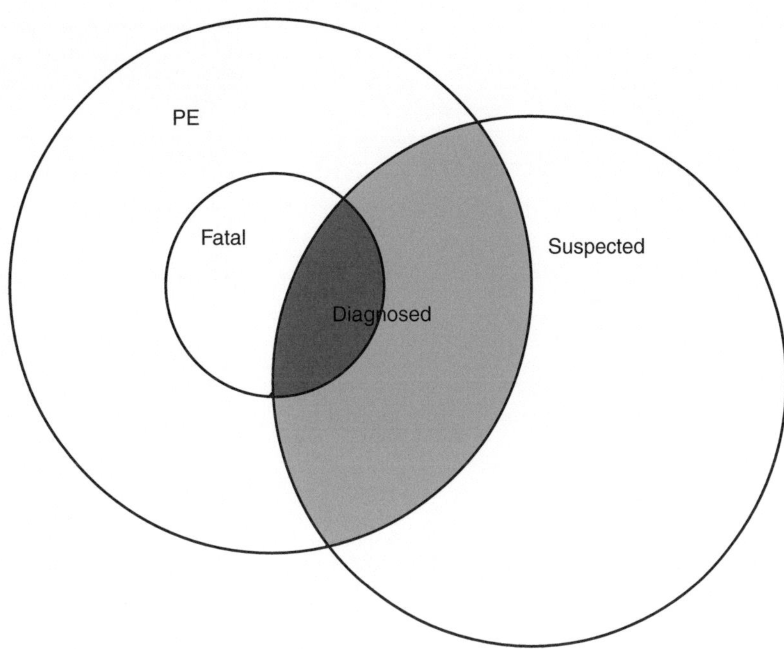

Fig. 14.13 Schema of relationship between suspected and actual cases of pulmonary embolism (PE). (From Ryu JH, Olson EJ, Pellikka PA. Clinical recognition of pulmonary embolism: problem of unrecognized and asymptomatic cases. Mayo Clin Proc 1998;73:877; with permission)

tion, $p < 0.001$) and reductions in mortality (risk-adjusted rates for all-cause mortality from 6.6% to 4.9% and rates for aPE-related mortality from 3.3% to 1.8%, $p < 0.01$) [156].

Acute Pulmonary Embolism, Right Ventricular Architecture, and Myocardial Mechanics

In addition to causing an obvious sudden increase in PVR, an acute occlusive pulmonary thrombus also disrupts normal RV ejection due to RV myocyte lysis and induction of a proinflammatory phenotype [157–159]. Experimental data of aPE in the rat model suggests that neutrophils are present in the RVOT region between 6 h and 18 h of the thrombotic insult. Current data suggests that this inflammation is independent of the damage caused by the obstructive thrombus and also amplifies the initial thrombotic injury [160, 161]. In humans, an elevated concentration of circulating myeloperoxidase as well as other inflammatory biomarkers has been demonstrated in the aPE setting [162–164]. Hence, it has been suggested that an inflammatory response might be a primary part of the development of acute RV dys-

function in the setting of aPE in both clinical and experimental models [134].

Advances in the understanding of myocardial fiber orientation have been instrumental in advancing our knowledge of how the RV responds to an increase in afterload in response to aPE. Specifically, the RV free wall is mainly comprised of transverse fibers while the LV is encircled by oblique fibers [165]. Oblique fibers from the interventricular septum (IVS) also extend into the RVOT [166]. A schematic representation of this fiber orientation is shown in Fig. 14.14. It is now well established that the comparison of varying fiber orientations shows marked differences in contractile performance. Helical or oblique fibers are responsible for twisting and untwisting, while transverse fibers exert a compressive bellows-like activity [166]. From a mechanical perspective, helical or oblique fibers are at a considerable mechanical advantage compared with transverse fibers [167].

In the healthy state, transverse fibers are the principal fiber group maintaining RV performance, with some assistance from the helical or oblique fibers from the LV (through the IVS) [168, 169]. In fact, left ventricular activity contributes to about 80% of the flow and up to two-

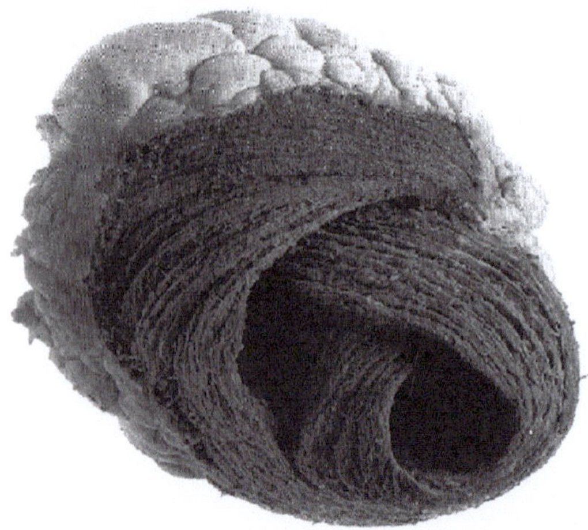

Fig. 14.14 Schematic representation of the myocardial fiber orientation relationship of the IVS, composed of oblique fibers that arise from the descending and ascending segments of the apical loop, surrounded by the transverse muscle orientation of the basal loop that comprises the free RV wall. (Reproduced with permission from Buckberg G D, and the RESTORE Group Eur J Cardiothorac Surg 2006; 29: S272–S278)

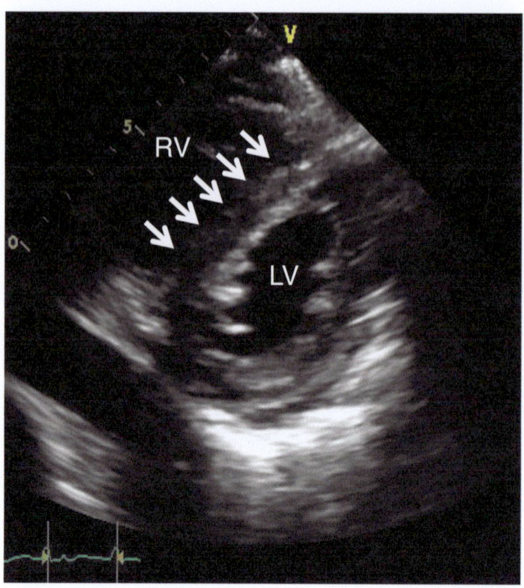

Fig. 14.15 Short-axis TTE view of the LV at the level of the papillary muscle showing a dilated RV that is causing significant flattening of the IVS as a result of an acute rise in PVR

thirds of the pressure generated by the RV during systole [168]. The influence of LV contractile function on RV contractile function via the shared IVS is part of the concept of ventricular interdependence.

However, in situations resulting in elevation in PVR, as it occurs in aPE, contribution from the IVS helical or oblique fibers becomes increasingly significant [170]. This contribution depends on the overall contractile state of the LV.

An acute increase in PVR results in systolic IVS flattening causing loss of the oblique orientation of the septal fibers as seen in Fig. 14.15 [24]. This contributes to the RV systolic dysfunction with aPE. In addition, the RV dilatation due to significant increases in PVR results in a shift of the IVS towards the LV causing LV underfilling [24–28]. This impaired LV performance and output add to the hemodynamic effects of aPE with catastrophic consequences as shown in Fig. 14.16.

Careful analysis of IVS in patients with chronic PH has led to the identification of two types of septal motions. Type A has been

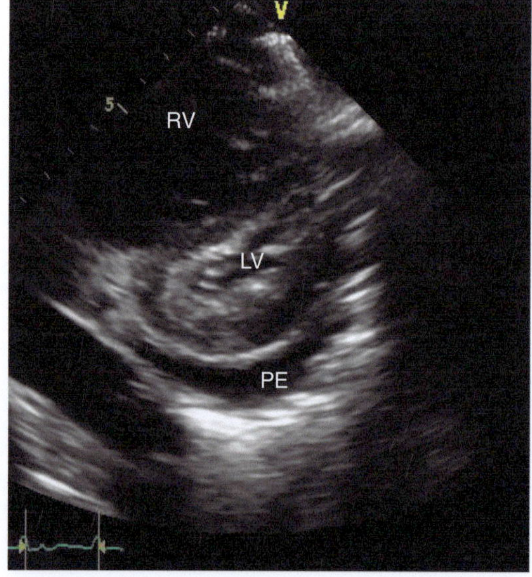

Fig. 14.16 Short-axis TTE view of the LV at the level of the papillary muscle showing a markedly dilated RV causing significant flattening of the IVS as a result of an acute rise in PVR resulting in both LV underfilling and impairing LV performance associated with hemodynamic compromise in cases of massive aPE. A pericardial effusion (PE) is also noted

described as marked anterior motion in early systole while type B shows marked posterior motion in early diastole [171]. Type A IVS motion is mainly seen in patients with worse hemodynamic profiles and worse clinical outcomes when compared to those with type B IVS motion [171]. Deviation of the IVS towards the LV can thus compromise LV systolic as well as diastolic function [172–174].

The study of RV mechanics and IVS motion highlights not only the intricate hemodynamic and mechanical interdependence of the RV-pulmonary circulation unit, but also the importance of identifying RV dysfunction, particularly since aPE mortality is indisputably dependent on the presence and magnitude of RV strain [116, 119, 122, 142, 172, 175–183].

Diagnosis and Assessment of Right Ventricular Function in Acute Pulmonary Embolism

Unfortunately, the limited sensitivity and specificity of some signs and symptoms in certain clinical situations hinder aPE recognition [184–187]. Henceforth, a keen clinical judgment is critical at all times. The latter has certainly proven useful on several large series but lacks standardization for which prediction models have been developed [188–195]. Most importantly, whenever clinical presentation raises the suspicion for aPE, prompt objective testing is urgently required.

Introduction of multi-detector computed tomographic (MDCT) angiography with high spatial and temporal resolution has certainly revolutionized the assessment of suspected aPE patients and cemented its status as the preferred imaging method of choice for these patients [196–198]. With a reported sensitivity of 83% and a specificity of 96%, data from PIOPED II also highlighted the importance of combining clinical probability based on the Wells rule with CT findings [199]. For example, patients presenting with a low or intermediate clinical probability of aPE and a negative CT had a high negative predictive value

for PE (96% and 89%, respectively) with only 60% in those with a high pretest probability [199]. On the other hand, the positive predictive value of a positive CT was high (92–96%) in patients with an intermediate or high clinical probability while it was only 58% in patients with a low pretest likelihood of aPE [199].

Additional CTPA findings in aPE are shown in Figs. 14.17, 14.18, and 14.19. In contrast, Figs. 14.20 and 14.21 show examples in which CTPA was useful to distinguish acute from chronic PE cases. Finally, Fig. 14.22 lists potential patient- and technique-related artifacts as well as anatomic mimickers that are important to be recognized when using multi-detector CT when evaluating patients with a presumptive diagnosis of aPE.

In other words, MDCT documentation at segmental or more proximal levels is sufficient proof for aPE diagnosis when the clinical suspicion is high and a negative MDCT should with confidence exclude aPE in cases with low clinical suspicion; however, what to do in cases of high clinical suspicion and a negative MDCT is less clear and there is paucity of data if additional testing is needed.

Lastly, three instances involving CT require our attention. First, isolated identification of subsegmental aPE on CT: this has been reported in 4.7% of patients when imaged by single-detector CT angiography and in 9.4% of those undergoing MDCT [200]. Based on the lower positive predictive value and poor inter-observer agreement when distal pulmonary segments are being evaluated, the use of compression venous ultrasonography might be considered to exclude the presence of DVT that might require treatment [201]. Second, combination of computed tomographic venography with CT angiography as a single procedure using one intravenous injection of contrast is an alternative being proposed based on the PIOPED II data [199, 202]. Though this combination increased sensitivity for aPE diagnosis from 83% to 90% with similar specificity (95%), there was no significant increase in its negative predictive value [199, 202].

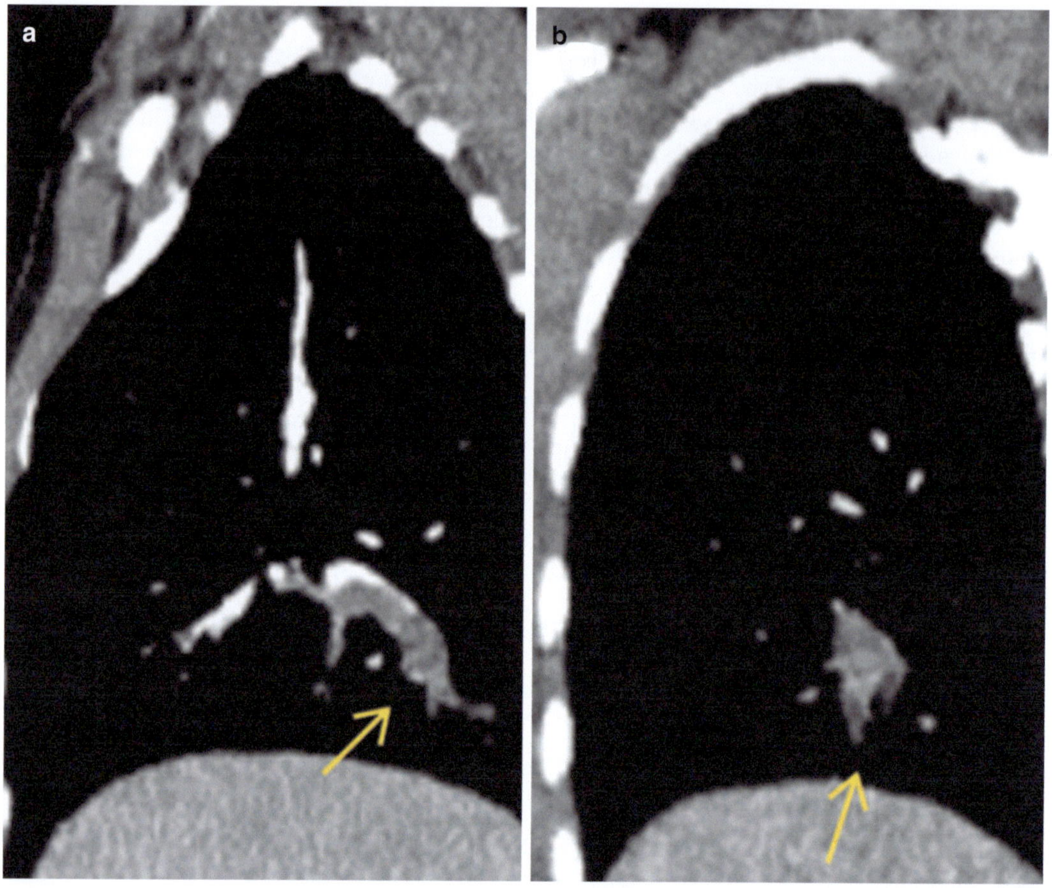

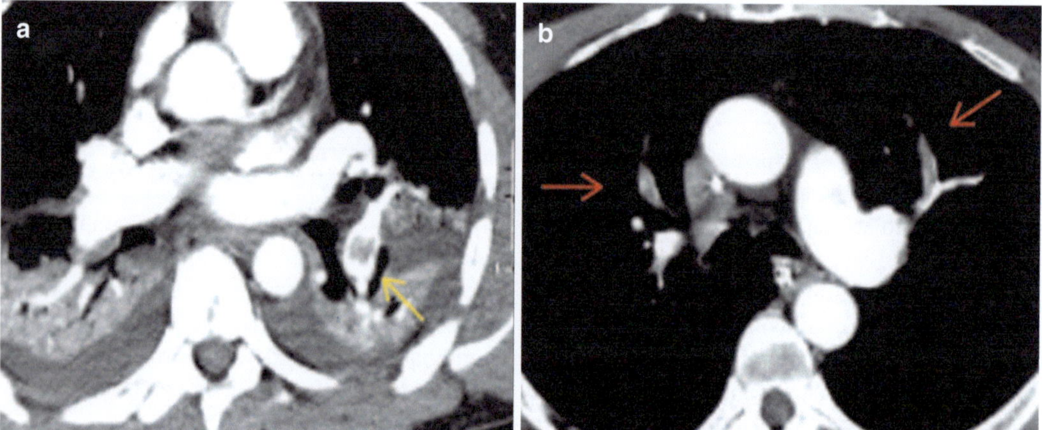

Fig. 14.17 (**a**) Sagittal and (**b**) coronal reformatted images in a 56-year-old man with chest pain and dyspnea reveal thrombosed lower lobe posterior basal segmental artery branches. Notice the relative associated abnormal vascular enlargement (arrows) as compared with the adjacent patent vessels. (Reproduced with permission from Chhabra A, et al. Applied Radiology 2007)

Fig. 14.18 (**a**) The donut sign in the left lower lobe pulmonary artery (arrow) and (**b**) tram track sign (arrows) in bilateral upper lobe segmental pulmonary arteries in cases of acute pulmonary emboli. (Reproduced with permission from Chhabra A, et al. Applied Radiology 2007)

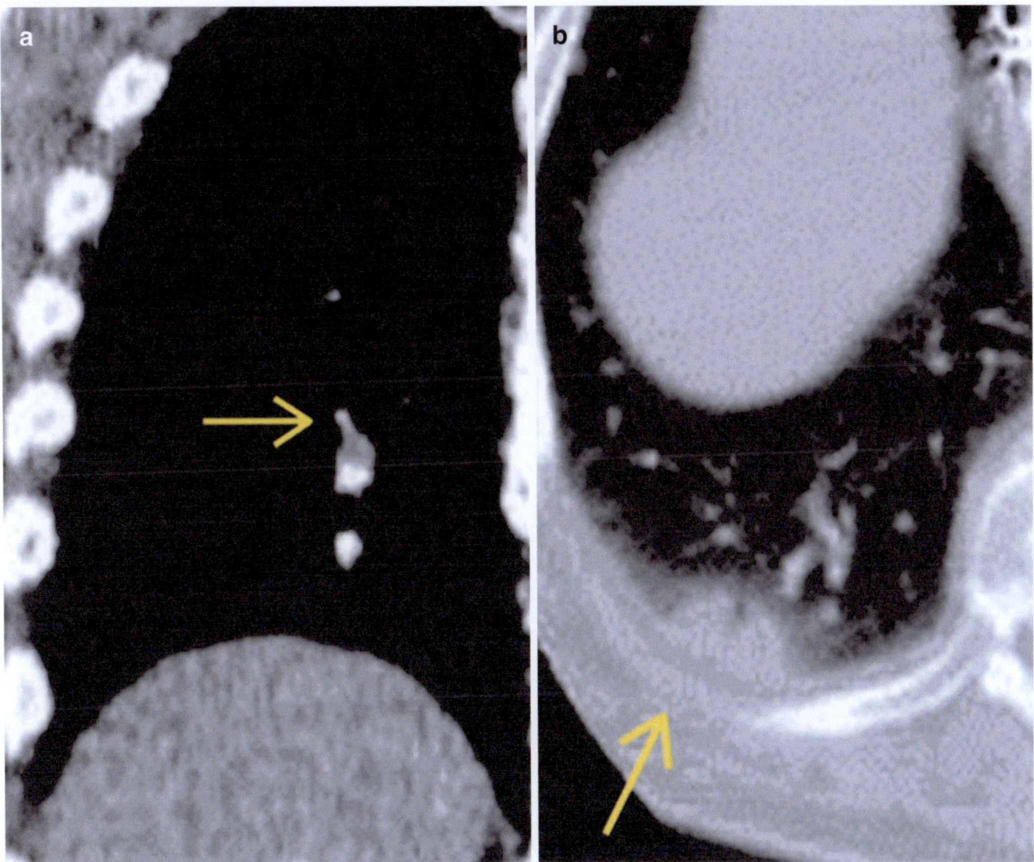

Fig. 14.19 (**a**, **b**) Acute right lower lobe subsegmental pulmonary embolus (arrows) in a 60-year-old man with peripheral pulmonary infarct. (Reproduced with permission from Chhabra A, et al. Applied Radiology 2007)

Furthermore, since CT venography yields similar results to the compression venous ultrasonography [202], the latter should be used instead as it would further reduce the total radiation dose. Finally, when an incidental pulmonary embolism is seen on CTs done among cancer, atrial fibrillation, and heart failure patients this might create some decision-making problem. Although accounting for only 1–2% of all CT cases [203–206], no robust treatment recommendations have been provided. However, it should be noted that most experts suggest that anticoagulation should be administered for incidental clots if found on lobar or more proximal level pulmonary circulation segments [207].

However, it is important to point out that the effectiveness of this imaging modality relies on identifying vascular obstruction and RV dilatation as a response of the former; however, it does not provide any information regarding RV function.

Ventilation–perfusion scintigraphy (V/Q scan) has been for some time a useful imaging modality used in the assessment of both acute and chronic PE considerations [208–210]. With lack of radiation and use of contrast material, V/Q scans have been preferentially used in outpatients with low clinical probability and for normal chest X-rays particularly among females, and in patients with a history of contrast-induced allergies, renal compromise, multiple myeloma, and paraproteinemic syndromes [211].

Though initial diagnostic criteria used for V/Q scan interpretation prompted revision into more useful management of high-probability scans and of normal perfusion V/Q scans, a high

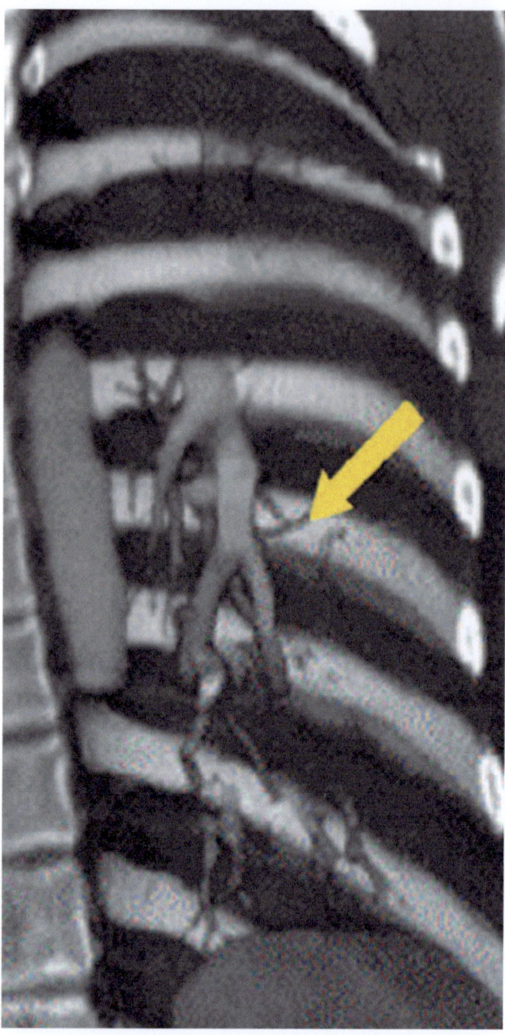

Fig. 14.20 A 56-year-old man with a history of treated pulmonary embolism in the left lower lobe segmental arteries presented with acute chest pain. No evidence of acute embolism was seen. This volume-rendered coronal image reveals an abrupt cutoff in the left lower lobe segmental arteries (yellow arrow) with visualization of dilated bronchial collaterals. (Reproduced with permission from Chhabra A, et al. Applied Radiology 2007)

number of nondiagnostic intermediate probability scans continue to be problematic as additional diagnostic testing is required [212–217]. This problem might have been solved by using single-photon emission computed tomography (SPECT) data acquisition imaging with or without low-dose CT [218–221]; however, large-scale prospective studies are required to validate this approach. Once again, V/Q scan imaging also falls short in providing any information regarding RV function.

For decades, pulmonary angiography was seen as the "gold standard" imaging modality tool when assessing aPE patients [222]. Though currently replaced by the less invasive and equally effective method in providing diagnostic accuracy as CT angiography technique, pulmonary angiography is still used when guiding percutaneous catheter-directed treatment for aPE.

Associated procedure-related mortality for pulmonary angiography has been reported at 0.5% while minor and major complications have been quoted at 5% and 1%, respectively [223]. As expected, deaths are most likely related to either hemodynamic compromise or respiratory failure and bleeding-related complications if thrombolysis follows a diagnostic pulmonary angiogram [224].

Digital subtraction angiography is a fluoroscopic technique that improves visualization for a better accurate depiction of blood vessels by eliminating surrounding structures. Though this technique improves peripheral visualization of pulmonary arterial branches with identification of thrombi as small as 1–2 mm, main trunk imaging is compromised by cardiac motion [225, 226]. Direct visualization of a filling defect or amputation of a pulmonary arterial branch constitutes the only validated diagnostic sign of aPE as none of the proposed indirect signs have been validated [187].

Obviously, a heightened clinical suspicion when we encounter a patient with the right risk profile sets in motion a series of diagnostic testing modalities that according to the situation allow to exclude or confirm aPE in order to institute appropriate treatment. At times, due to the critical nature of patients, a simple bedside ultrasound detection of a venous thrombus in the lower extremity is often enough to initiate the treatment for presumed aPE. However, absence of DVT by ultrasound does not preclude aPE diagnosis while the presence of DVT by ultrasound is not confirmatory of aPE [227].

Once a diagnosis of aPE is made, determining the RV response to this challenge by clinical, laboratory, and imaging methods influences clin-

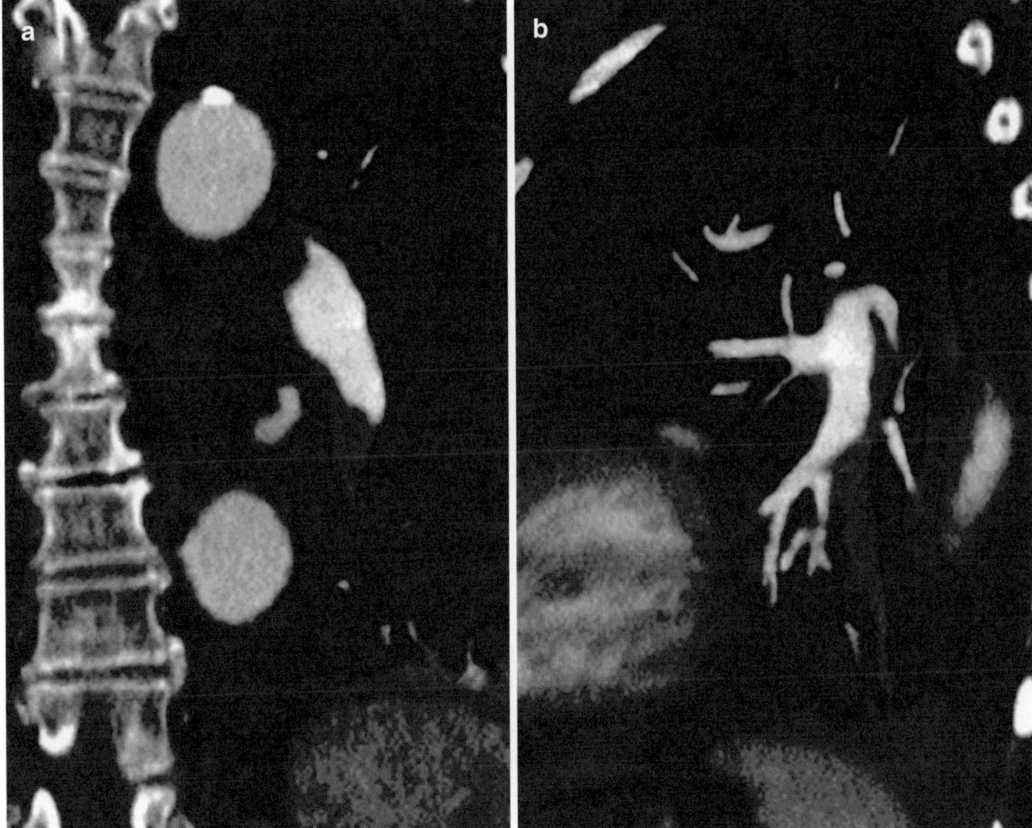

Fig. 14.21 (**a**) Coronal and (**b**) sagittal reconstructions in a 70-year-old man with a history of bilateral acute pulmonary embolism and a 6-month history of warfarin treatment. These scans show chronic pulmonary emboli forming obtuse angles with the vessel wall in the left lower lobe pulmonary artery and its posterior segmental branch. (Images courtesy of Dr. Drew A. Torigian, MD, Hospital of the University of Pennsylvania, Philadelphia, PA; Reproduced with permission from Chhabra A, et al. Applied Radiology 2007)

Artifacts and Mimics on Multidetector CT for aPE

- Patient-related artifacts:
  - Respiratory motion
  - Body habitus
  - Flow related Vascular resistance
- Anatomic pathologic mimics:
  - Peribronchial lymph node
  - Unopacified veins
  - Mucus-filled bronchi
  - Perivascular edema
- Technique-related artifacts:
  - Poor timing
  - Window setting
  - Patial voluming
  - Staristep

Reproduced with permission from Chhabra A, et al. Applied Radiology 2007

Fig. 14.22 List of potential patient- and technique-related artifacts as well as anatomic mimickers on multidetector CT for aPE. (Reproduced with permission from Chhabra A, et al. Applied Radiology 2007)

ical management and prognosis. Prompt hemodynamic stability and RV function assessment are critical.

Once a diagnosis of aPE is made, determining the RV response to this challenge by clinical, laboratory, and imaging methods influences clinical management and prognosis. Prompt hemodynamic stability and RV function assessment are critical. Risk stratification algorithms have been proposed to help physicians identify high-versus low-risk aPE patients in order to expedite diagnosis and treatment, as shown in Fig. 14.23.

While hemodynamic stability is often discernible by clinical examination, identification of high-risk features associated with significant RV strain and impending circulatory collapse with

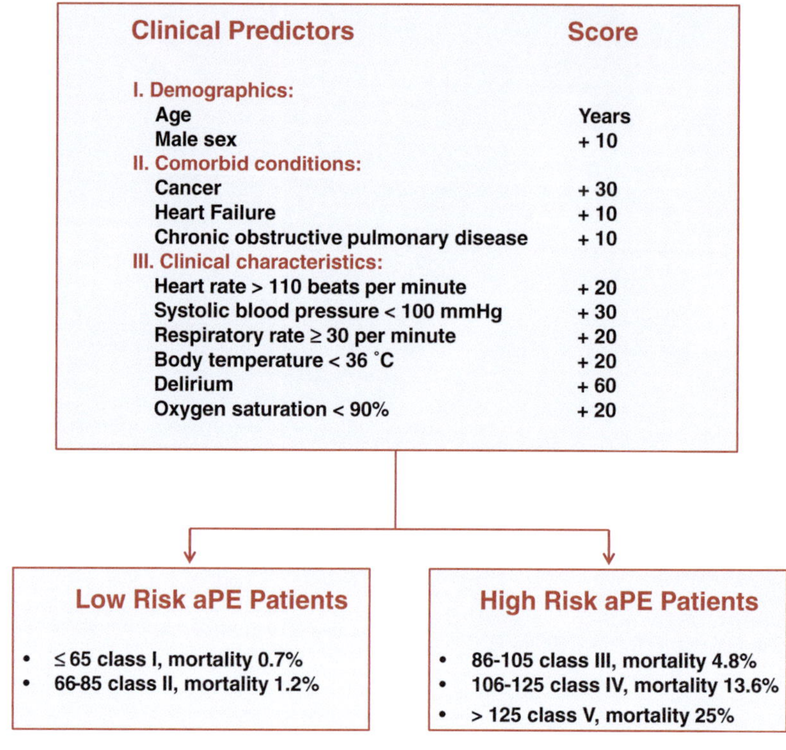

Fig. 14.23 Pulmonary embolism severity index (PESI). (Modified with permission from Aujesky D, Perrier A, Roy PM, et al. Validation of a clinical prognostic model to identify low-risk patients with pulmonary embolism. J Intern Med. 2007; 261: 597–604 and Masotti L, et al. Prognostic stratification of acute pulmonary embolism: focus on clinical aspects, imaging, and biomarkers. Vasc Health Risk Manag. 2009; 5: 567–575)

imaging can be challenging. Commonly used imaging modalities such as computed tomography and TTE are less than ideal in studying the true anatomic and functional derangements of the RV (Fig. 14.24) but are readily available and can detect simple markers that identify patients at risk of hemodynamic instability in aPE. Table 14.4 summarizes the most commonly associated variables currently used in the identification of abnormal RV strain. Figure 14.25 shows a pictorial representation of normal TTE RV findings that can be contrasted to abnormal RV strain findings as seen in Fig. 14.26.

Risk stratification algorithms have been proposed to help physicians identify high- versus low-risk aPE patients in order to expedite diagnosis and treatment [228–232]. While hemodynamic stability is often discernible by clinical examination, identification of high-risk features associated with significant RV strain and impending circulatory collapse with imaging can be challenging.

Although the electrocardiogram (ECG) has traditionally been one of the first diagnostic tests obtained from patients presenting with symptoms suggestive of aPE, it has not been incorporated into any risk stratification models. However, there are certain ECG findings in aPE that have been correlated with the presence of RHS [233–236]. Consequently, the American Heart Association has recommended risk stratification for aPE patients based on RHS [237]. Furthermore, in a study by Hariharan and associates, these investigators described 3-ECG findings that were independently associated with RHS [238]:

• TWI in leads V1 through V3 (5 points)
• S wave in lead I (2 points)
• Sinus tachycardia (3 points)

Using this score, these investigators were able to risk-stratify 85% of the aPE they studied [238]. Specifically, when the score was 5 or greater, it was 93% specific for RHS while a score of 2 or less excluded the presence of RHS with 85% sensitivity [238]. These results were similar to findings reported by other investigators [239, 240].

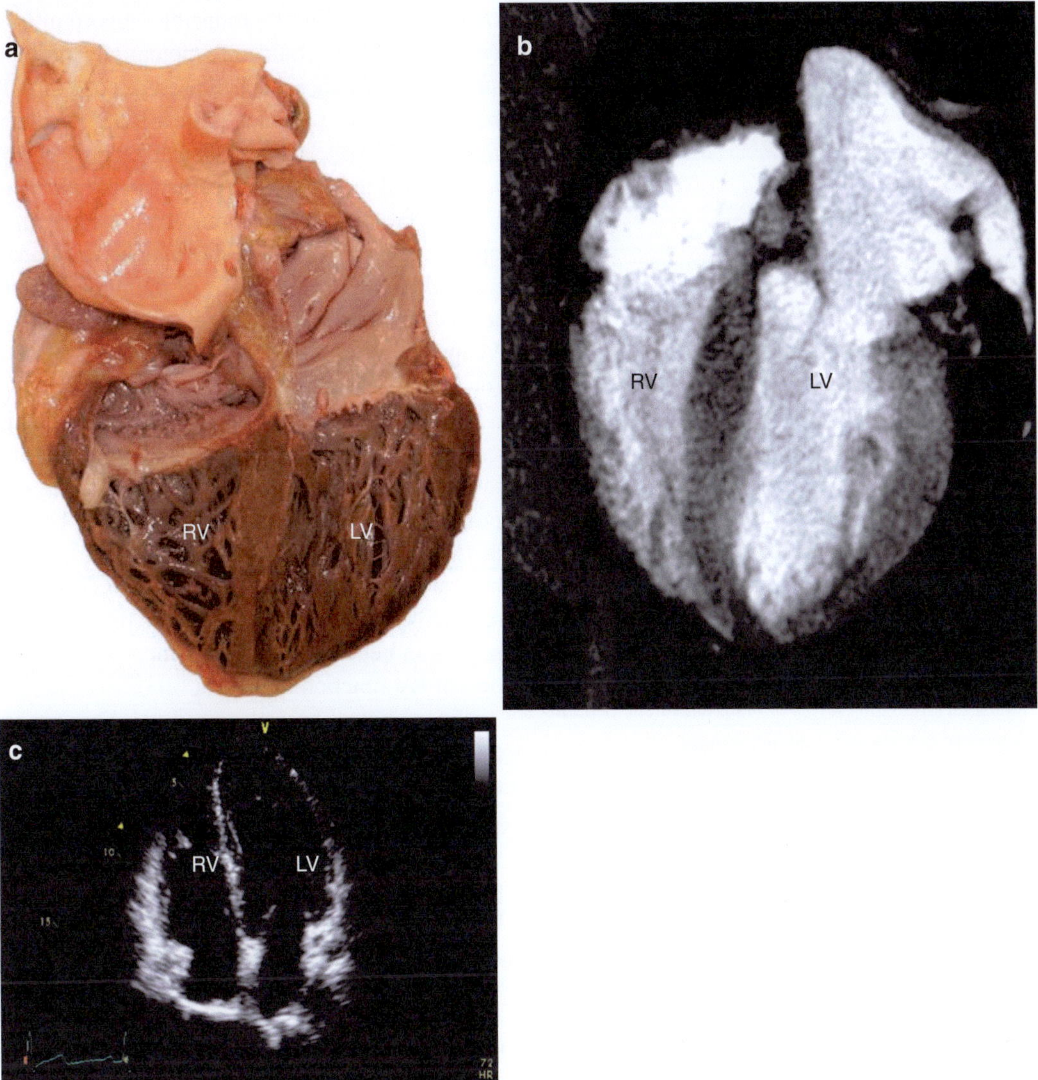

Fig. 14.24 (**a**) Open-cut macroscopic view of heart in a four-chamber view depicting the thin-walled RV in relation to the LV. (**b**) Computed tomographic view of a representative four-chamber view showing the same anatomical relationship of the macroscopic specimen. Image shows corresponding reformatted four-chamber contrast-enhanced ECG-gated MDCT scan. (Both (**a**) and (**b**) were reproduced with permission from Dupont MV, et al. Right ventricular function assessment by MKDCT. AJR 2011; 196: 77–86). (**c**) TTE representation of the RV and LV obtained from the same four-chamber apical view orientation as represented in (**a, b**)

Although these results might be encouraging further research should be undertaken not only to define the appropriate role of ECG in the assessment of RV involvement in aPE but also to clarify the potential role of ECG in aPE risk stratification models.

Biomarkers such as cardiac troponin, a well-known, reliable marker of injury, have been used in patients presenting with chest pain and dyspnea mainly with the aim of identifying an acute coronary syndrome; however, elevated cardiac troponins have been shown to occur in aPE as a result of acute RV dilatation and dysfunction [241]. Specifically, elevation in cardiac troponin levels can identify those aPE patients at higher risk of hemodynamic collapse [242]. Furthermore,

Table 14.4 Common markers of RV strain

RV end-systolic and end-diastolic dilatation
Increased RV-to-LV maximal diameter cavity ratio
Dilated RV apex
Dilated tricuspid annulus
Presence of IVS flattening
Increased pulmonary artery pressures
Increased PVR
Reduced measures of RV systolic function:
Fractional area change
TAPSE
Tricuspid annular TDI systolic velocity
Abnormal pulsed Doppler signal across RVOT
Reduced RVOT systolic excursion
Regional RV wall motion abnormalities
Reduced RV myocardial velocity generation
Reduced RV strain generation
Presence of RV dyssynchrony
Increased diameter of the superior vena cava
Reflux of contrast medium or color flow signal into the inferior vena cava
Increased circulating levels of troponin I in the absence of left-heart abnormalities
Increased circulating levels of brain natriuretic peptide
Abnormal electrocardiographic changes

the utility of cardiac troponin assessment among normotensive aPE patients has also been found useful to exclude RHS [243]. It is always important to keep in mind which clinical conditions affect cardiac troponin levels independently of cardiac injury [244].

In terms of the brain natriuretic peptide (BNP), a well-characterized peptide with numerous mechanistic actions known to primarily be secreted by the ventricles in response to stretching and wall tension, it is another biomarker with potential use in aPE patients [245–249]. Consequently, the value of measuring BNP levels in aPE patients with an initial stable hemodynamic status was considered. However, a meta-analysis of BNP levels found that while elevated BNP levels might be useful in identifying aPE at high risk of death and adverse outcome events, the high negative predictive value of a normal BNP level was certainly more useful in selecting those aPE patients with a likely uneventful follow-up [250].

In contrast to all the abovementioned imaging tools and blood markers, TTE provides a unique rapid, accurate, and reproducible opportunity to evaluate aPE. It could also potentially provide supportive evidence (such as presence of a thrombus in transit or presence of new RHS). As seen in Fig. 14.27 panels a and b depict the presence of a RV apical thrombus in a patient with biventricular dysfunction due to nonischemic cardiomyopathy. Two days later, the patient developed pleuritic chest pain and CTA of pulmonary arteries showed pulmonary embolism (Fig. 14.27c). Venous duplex of lower extremities was negative for thrombus.

In addition, it also aids in the hemodynamic evaluation of the extent and magnitude of the thrombotic burden that can be used to assess prognosis. Even though detection of clot burden in transit or identification of a proximal pulmonary artery thrombus is challenging by TTE on a regular basis, most routinely TTE's role basically resides in hemodynamic assessment and evaluation of RV function.

Since clinical hemodynamic stability appears to be dependent on RV function rather than the magnitude of clot burden in aPE, particularly within the first hour, confirmation and assessment of mechanical stability of RV function are promptly required once this diagnosis is entertained (Fig. 14.28).

While echocardiography is clinically used to suggest the presence of aPE (via the presence of RV dysfunction in a patient with suspected aPE but unable to obtain a diagnostic test), several pitfalls in this setting need to be borne in mind. First, presence of RV strain may represent a chronic finding (such as COPD or chronic pulmonary HTN). Thus, without a prior echocardiogram showing normal RV function, assuming that the RV dysfunction is due to aPE may result in unnecessary and potentially dangerous treatment for aPE. Second, new-onset RV dysfunction can occur with ARDS or other pulmonary injuries. Finally, in the supine, ventilated, critically ill patients, echocardiographic windows are often poor and a partially visualized RV can be considered normal in size and aPE be falsely ruled out. Despite past skepticism regarding the predictive value of TTE in assessing RV dysfunction among hemodynamically stable aPE patients, TTE

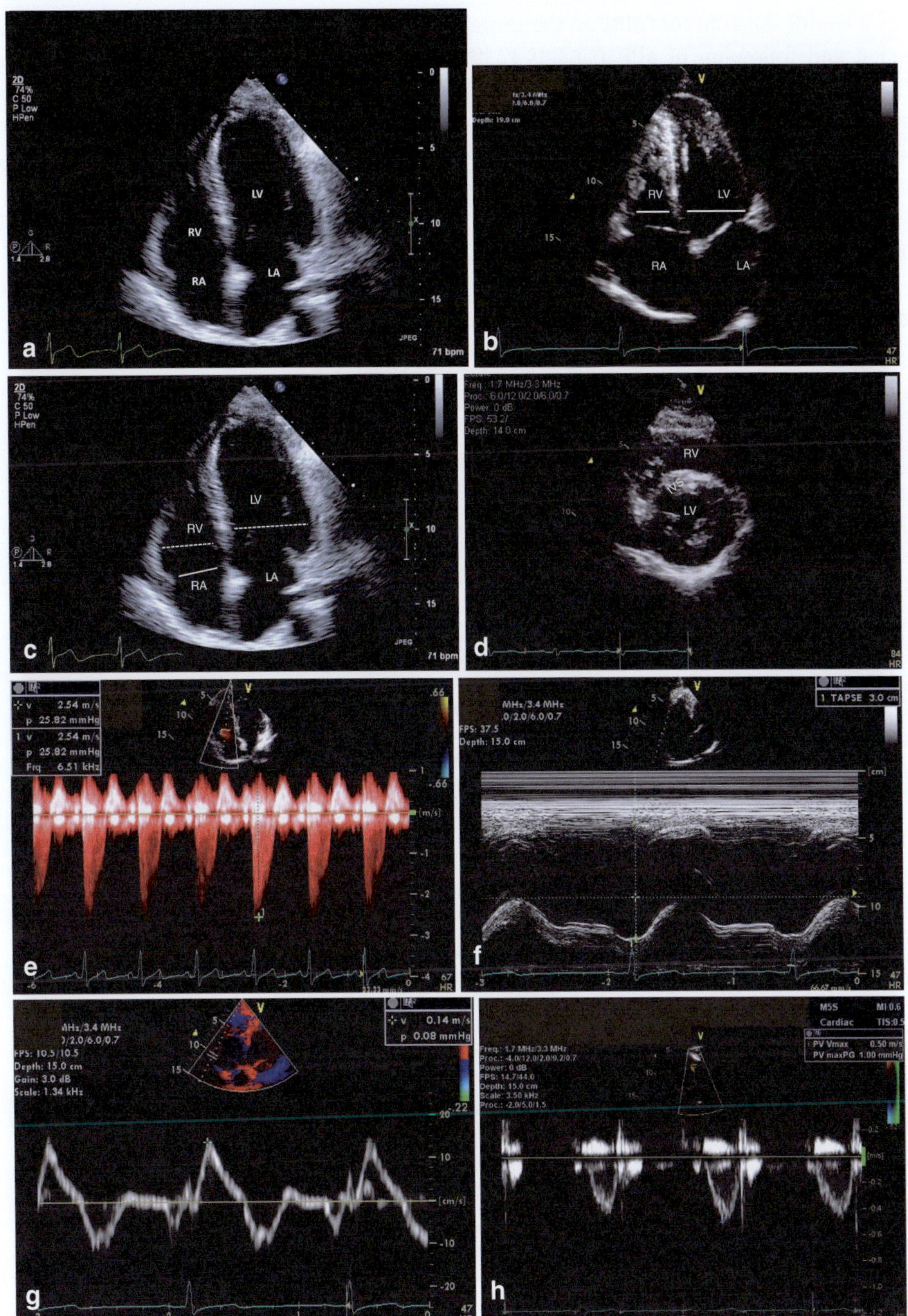

Fig. 14.25 Pictorial representation of normal TTE markers of RV size and systolic function. (**a**) Representative end diastolic four-chamber apical frame showing normal relation of RV size when compared to the LV; the right (RA) and left (LA) atria are also seen. (**b**) End-systolic four-chamber apical frame showing a normal-size relationship between the RV and LV denoted by straight white lines. (**c**) Representative end-diastolic four-chamber apical frame showing normal-size relationship between RV and LV (dashed lines) as well as a normal tricuspid annular size, denoted by the solid line. (**d**) Representative short-axis view at the level of the papillary muscles showing a normal relationship between RV and LV. Please note the crescent shape of the RV cavity at this level as well as the normal curvature of the IVS. (**e**) Representative tricuspid regurgitation signal that peaks early in systole with a peak velocity of 2.54 m/s. (**f**) Representative tricuspid annular plane systolic excursion from a normal patient with a maximum amplitude of 3 cm. (**g**) Representative tricuspid annular tissue Doppler imaging signal from a normal patient showing a normal systolic velocity of 0.14 m/s or 14 cm/s. (**h**) Representative pulsed Doppler signal across the pulmonic valve showing a normal RVOT envelope

remains a useful imaging modality in the initial evaluation and follow-up of aPE patients [239, 240]. In view of the above, the 2011 American Society of Echocardiography appropriate use criteria (AUC) assign TTE a score of 2 (inappropriate) for diagnosis of aPE while assigning a score of 8 (appropriate) to guide therapy [251].

To become a serious imaging contender, TTE has to offer critical data that surpasses rudimentary information based on subjective

interpretation of RV size and wall motions, abnormal IVS motion, presence of tricuspid regurgitation, and lack of collapse of the inferior vena cava during inspiration [252]. In general, RV systolic dysfunction can be easily quantified by measuring either tricuspid annular plane systolic excursion (TAPSE, <1.6 cm) or fractional area change (FAC <35%). In addition to these, other simple echo markers of RV strain have been described.

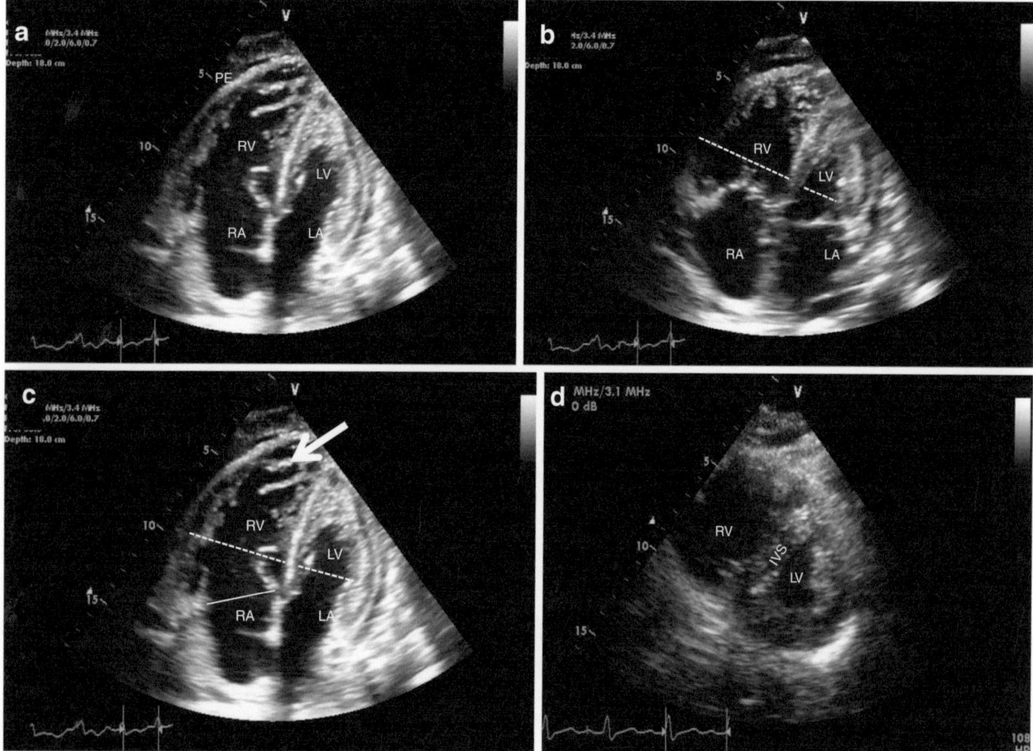

Fig. 14.26 Pictorial representation of abnormal TTE markers of RV strain. (**a**) Representative end-diastolic four-chamber apical frame from a patient with a confirmed aPE showing a dilated RV in comparison to the LV; a pericardial effusion (PE) is also appreciated. (**b**) End-systolic four-chamber apical frame showing a markedly dilated RV when compared to the LV denoted by the dashed white lines. (**c**) Representative end-diastolic four-chamber apical frame showing a dilated RV when compared to the LV. In addition, a dilated tricuspid annulus is also seen (solid line). Furthermore, stretched RV apex is also noted by the arrow and can be easily contrasted to the normal RV apex seen in Fig. 14.18b. (**d**) Representative short-axis view at the level of the papillary muscles showing a markedly dilated RV and small compressed LV. In addition, please note the flattened IVS that bows against

the LV. (**e**) Representative tricuspid regurgitation signal that peaks late in systole with a velocity of 2.98 m/s in a patient with aPE. (**f**) Representative tricuspid annular plane systolic excursion from a patient with hemodynamically significant aPE that is hypotensive. Please note the significant reduction in the maximum amplitude of less than 1 cm. (**g**) Representative tricuspid annular tissue Doppler imaging signal from a patient with a hemodynamically significant aPE showing significant reduction in the systolic velocity of 5 cm/s. (**h**) Representative pulsed Doppler signal across the pulmonic valve showing a markedly abnormal RVOT envelope from a hypotensive patient with a confirmed aPE; please note the narrow width (lines) of the signal and the mid-systolic indentation in the signal (arrows)

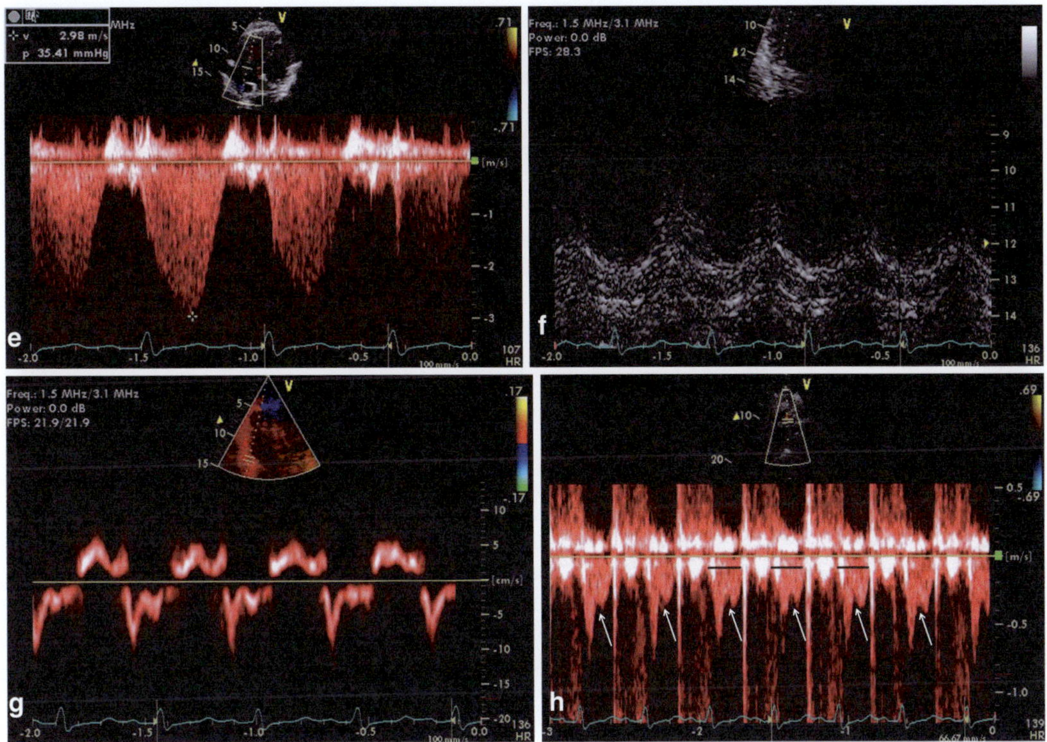

Fig. 14.26 (continued)

McConnell's sign has been traditionally used to describe regional RV dysfunction that spares the apex and was initially felt to aid both in the diagnosis of aPE and in the detection of RV strain. Initial studies reported sensitivity of 77%, specificity of 94%, positive predictive value of 71%, and negative predictive value of 96% to diagnose aPE [253]. However when applied in routine clinical practice for the diagnosis of aPE, McConnell's sign is not as reliable since similar pattern can be found in other right-heart pathologies such as acute RV infarct [254].

Doppler echocardiography is also useful in the evaluation of aPE patients. The acute increase in PVR often results in a rapid acceleration time and mid-systolic notching. An altered RVOT Doppler signal has been shown to be useful not only in characterizing PH severity, but also in overall RV systolic performance [255–257]. Representative RVOT images from a normal patient (Fig. 14.29a, b) and a patient with a confirmed aPE are shown (Fig. 14.30a, b).

The 60/60 sign refers to the presence of a short RVOT signal acceleration time (<60 ms) along with an estimated RV systolic pressure <60 mm of Hg [258]. This sign reflects the acute increase in PVR compared to a more chronic cause such as chronic pulmonary arterial hypertension. Similar to McConnell's, this sign is insensitive for the diagnosis of aPE.

As noted above, the clinical effects of aPE depend both on clot burden and the underlying cardiac reserve—some patients with a massive aPE but excellent cardiac reserve might behave similarly to patients with sub-massive aPE but compromised cardiac reserve [259, 260]. Untreated aPE can be fatal in up to 30% of patients largely depending on the degree of RV compromise [176, 261–263]. Since clinical hemodynamic stability appears to be dependent on the RV function rather than the magnitude of clot burden in aPE, particularly within the first hour, confirmation and assessment of mechanical stability of RV function are promptly required once this diagnosis is entertained [264–287].

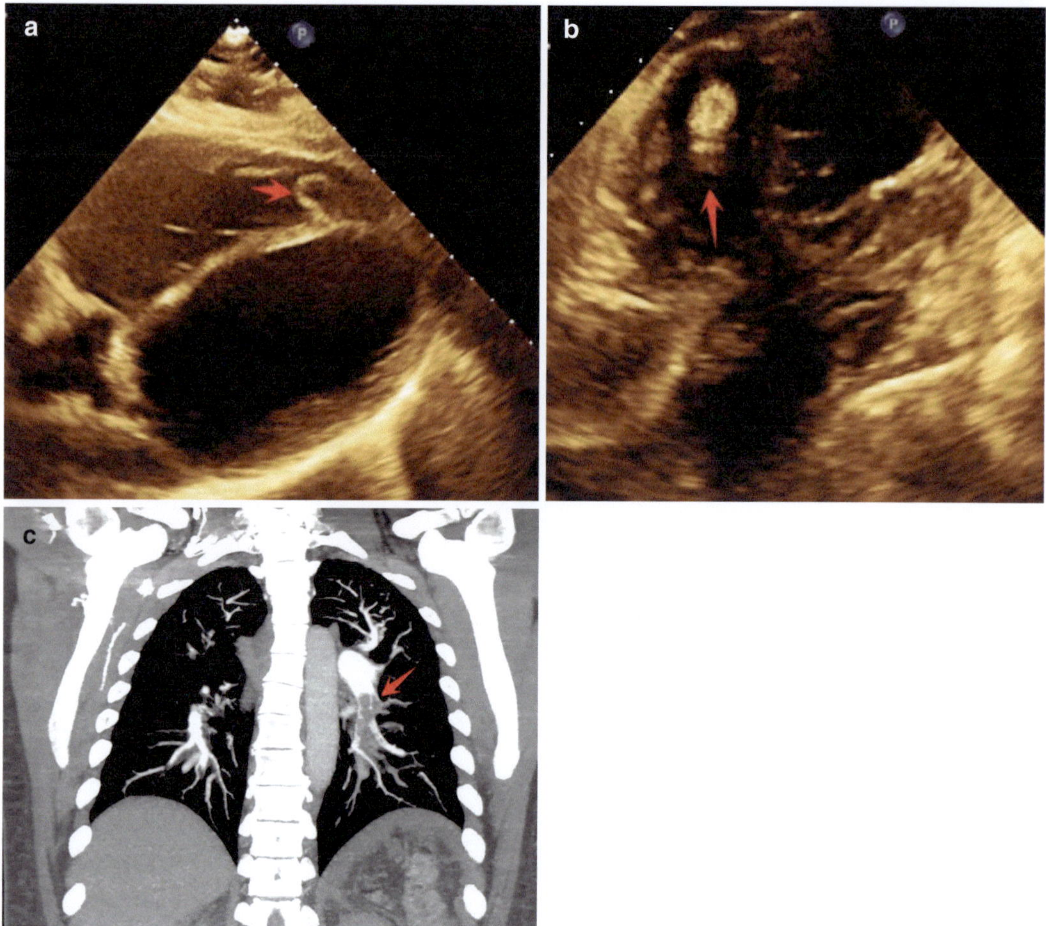

Fig. 14.27 (**a**, **b**) Depict the presence of a RV apical thrombus (red arrows) in a patient with biventricular dysfunction due to nonischemic cardiomyopathy. Two days later, the patient developed pleuritic chest pain and CTA of pulmonary arteries showed pulmonary embolism (**c**) as denoted by the red arrow. Venous duplex of lower extremities was negative for thrombus

New Frontiers in the Assessment of Right Ventricular Function in Acute Pulmonary Embolism

Integrity of RV function plays a pivotal role in determining the prognosis after aPE [124, 177, 179, 264–287]. Experimental data using healthy dogs has revealed that acute embolization using microbead injections induces dramatic stiffening of the PA leading to increased RV stroke work [288]. In this particular model, the use of both invasive and magnetic resonance imaging measures to assess PA stiffness and RV systolic function revealed that the RV was able to shift its working conditions, preserve function, and maintain hemodynamic coupling with the PA despite the acute insult [288]. This however occurs at the expense of a reduction in RV efficiency [288]. This interaction between RV and PA has clarified our understanding of RV function and it is now clear that RV systolic function cannot be studied in isolation, as both RV and PA work in series [289]. Evolution of RV pathology from normal to a decompensated state parallels the evolution of pulmonary vascular pathology; hence studying the RV and the PA as a unit will be critical to understanding the true performance of the RV [289].

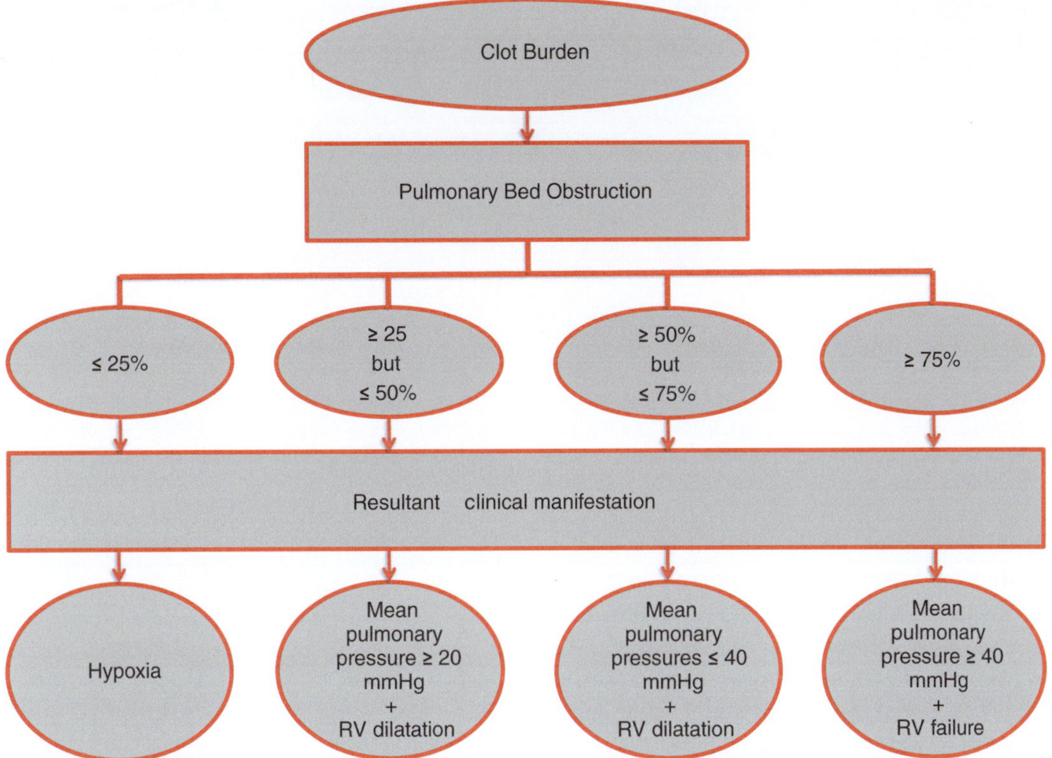

Fig. 14.28 Diagrammatic representation of the relationship between clot burden and approximate degree of pulmonary bed obstruction and corresponding clinical effect in the absence of previous cardiopulmonary history and normal RV reserve

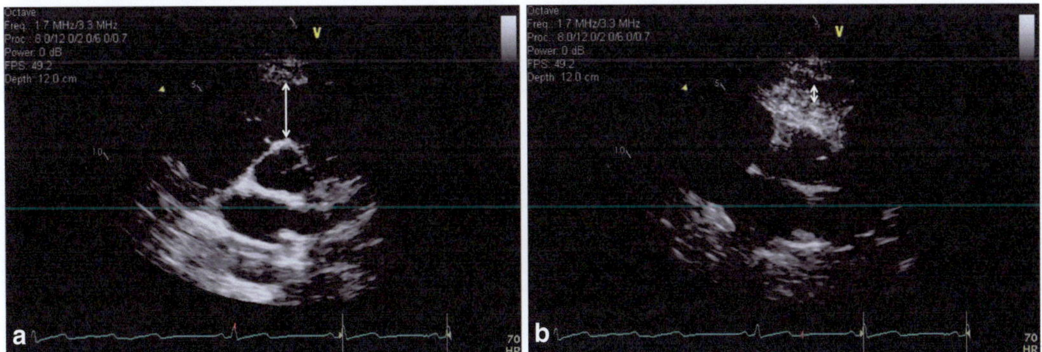

Fig. 14.29 Representative short-axis views at the level of the aortic valve demonstrating (**a**) RVOT end-diastolic length and (**b**) end-systolic length by the white arrows from a normal patient demonstrating excellent RVOT systolic function (RVOT end-diastolic length – RVOT end-systolic length)/RVOT end-diastolic length × 100

RV-PA coupling is critically important, and this relationship is best demonstrated by changes in hydraulic load occurring in the setting of PA stiffening as it will occur in aPE. As the RV is met with increased hydraulic wave reflection, its workload increases to maintain forward flow. It is important to remember that up to one-half of the hydraulic power in the main PA is contained in the pulsatile components of flow. Thus, acute changes in PA impedance, a measure of opposition to these pul-

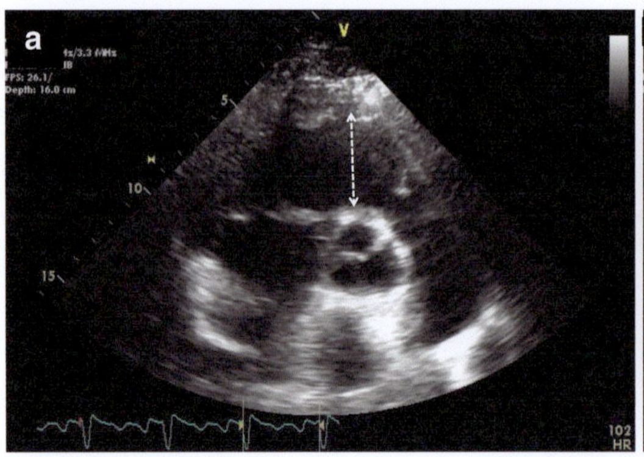
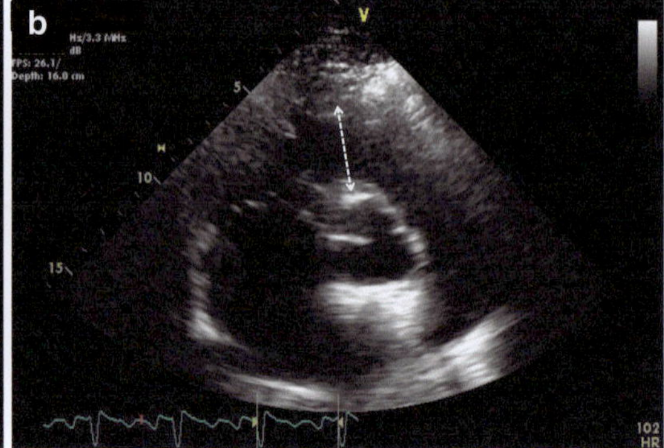

Fig. 14.30 Representative short-axis views at the level of the aortic valve demonstrating (**a**) RVOT end-diastolic length and (**b**) end-systolic length by the dashed white arrows from a patient with confirmed aPE. No significant difference between RVOT end-diastolic and end-systolic lengths corresponding to a reduced RVOT systolic excursion based on the formula listed in the figure legend of Fig. 14.29

satile components of flow, would be crucial to study, though unrealistic, unless they are measured in animal models. This is however unrealistic except when measured in animal models. The elastic properties of the pulmonary vasculature are vitally important as the heart would not be able to generate forward flow without them [290–292].

From a mechanistic perspective, RV ejection is dependent on PVR as well as on the oscillatory or pulsatile component of flow that is dissipated as wasted energy through the PA system with each RV ejection [292–295]. Hence, PA elasticity is crucial to maintain RV efficiency [292–295]. Since hemodynamic instability unmistakably predicts adverse outcomes and 30-day mortality in aPE patients when RV dysfunction is confirmed, a proposed scheme of high-risk features for the potential development of hemodynamic instability in aPE is listed in Fig. 14.31 [234, 265–287, 296–300].

As previously outlined above, the McConnell's sign suggests a regional rather than a global RV dysfunction in aPE [253, 254]. However, assessment of myocardial deformation with the use of velocity vector imaging often detects significant reduction in global myocardial strain generation of all main RV chamber segments, including the RV apex rather than regional abnormality [301]. Why only some patients present with regional compared to global RV dysfunction remains unknown and the role of the RV apex in aPE and its influence on overall prognosis have not been fully elucidated [301–303]. A representative velocity vector

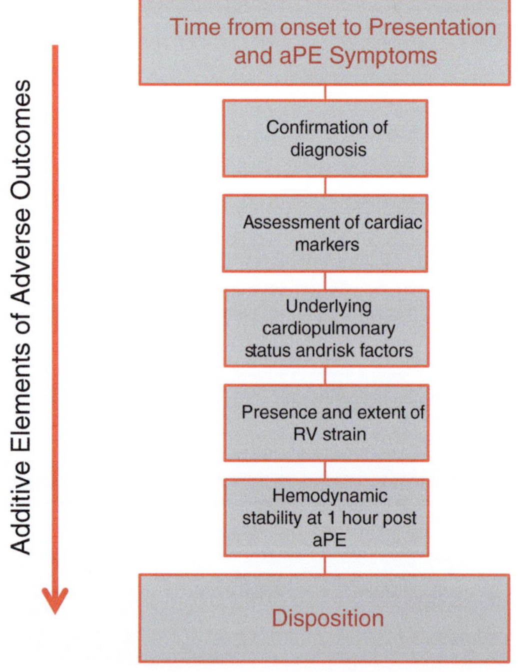

Fig. 14.31 Schematic diagram demonstrating high-risk features on admission that helps in the identification of poor prognosis in aPE

imaging sample from a normal RV showing normal longitudinal strain of all segments, including the RV apex, is shown in Fig. 14.32a–f. In sharp contrast, a representative velocity vector image is also shown from a patient with confirmed aPE (Fig. 14.33a–f) that shows significant reduction in overall systolic deformation from all segments, a very abnormal RV apical

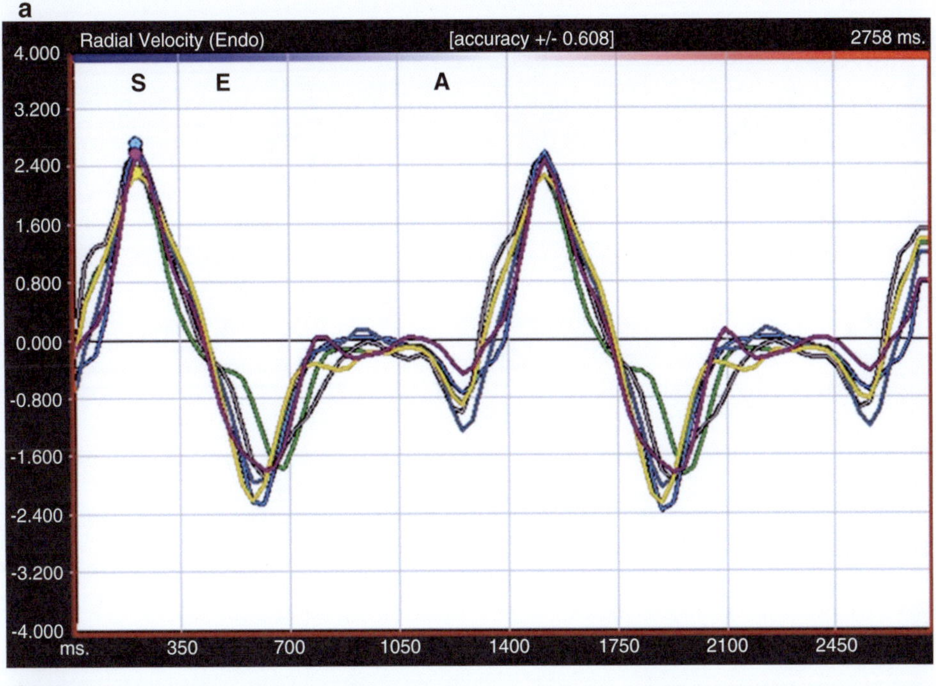

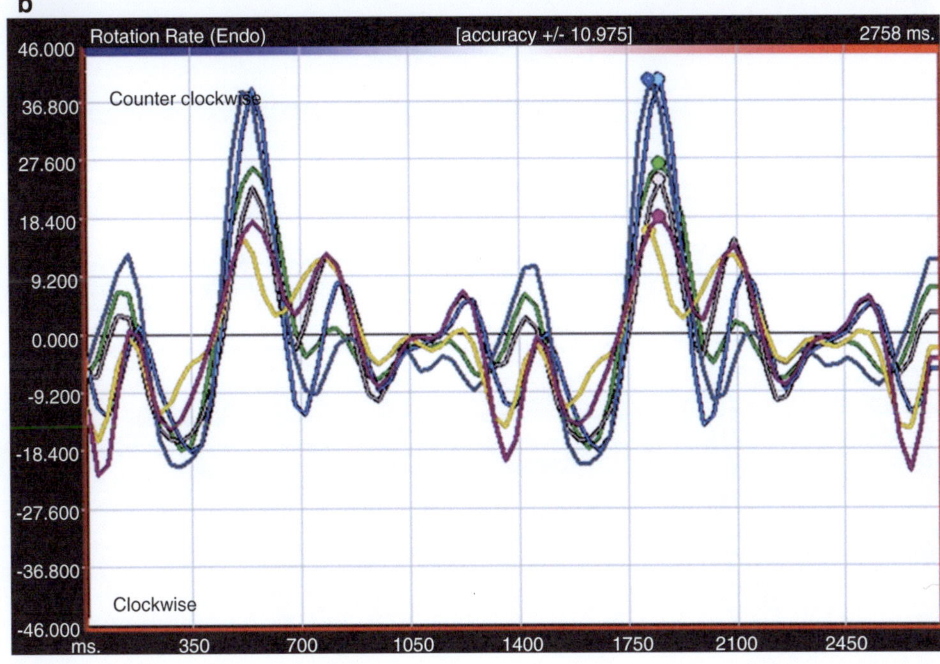

Fig. 14.32 Representative LV speckle tracking imaging signals obtained from the short-axis view at the level of the papillary muscles from an individual with normal biventricular systolic function. Color-coded representation is similar for all images and the green corresponds to the anterior septum; light purple to anterior wall; light blue to the lateral wall; dark blue to the posterior wall; yellow to the inferior wall; and deep purple to the inferior septum. (**a**) Radial velocity is shown for all six segments with the systolic component represented by S, early diastole by E, and late diastole by A. (**b**) Representative rotation rate showing normal synchronous counterclockwise as well as clockwise rotation of all segments. (**c**) Normal radial displacement curves of all six LV segments. (**d**) Representative radial rotation displacement curves showing normal synchronous counterclockwise as well as clockwise rotation of all segments. (**e**) Normal radial strain curves for all six LV segments. (**f**) Normal circumferential strain curves for all six LV segments

c

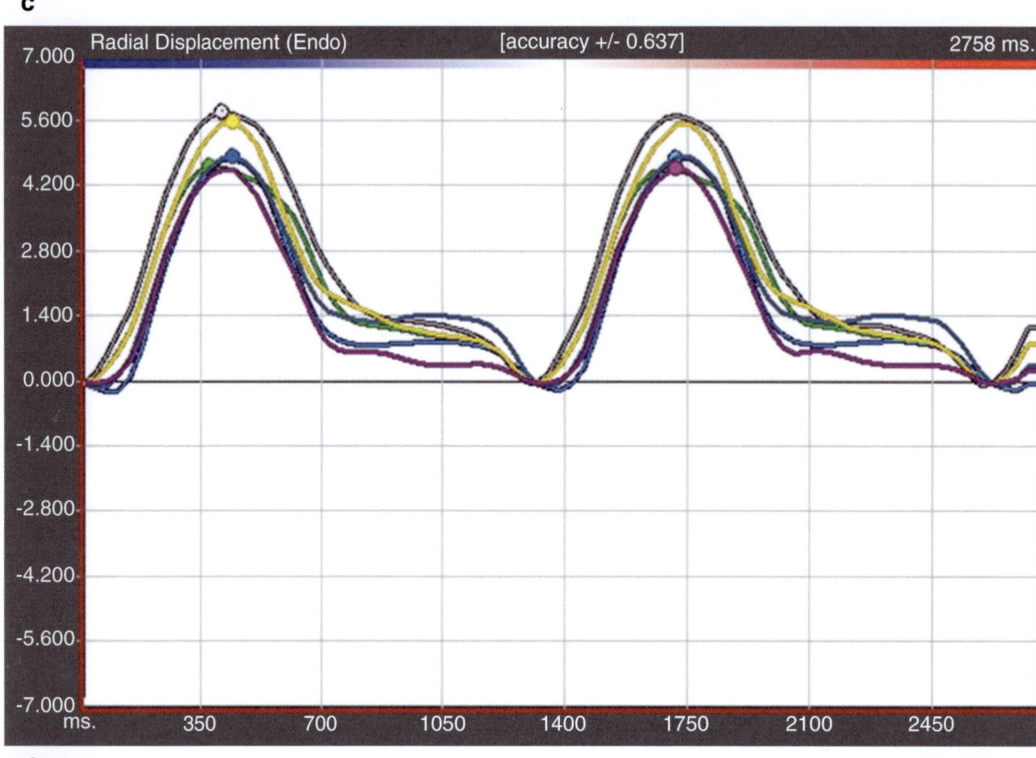

d

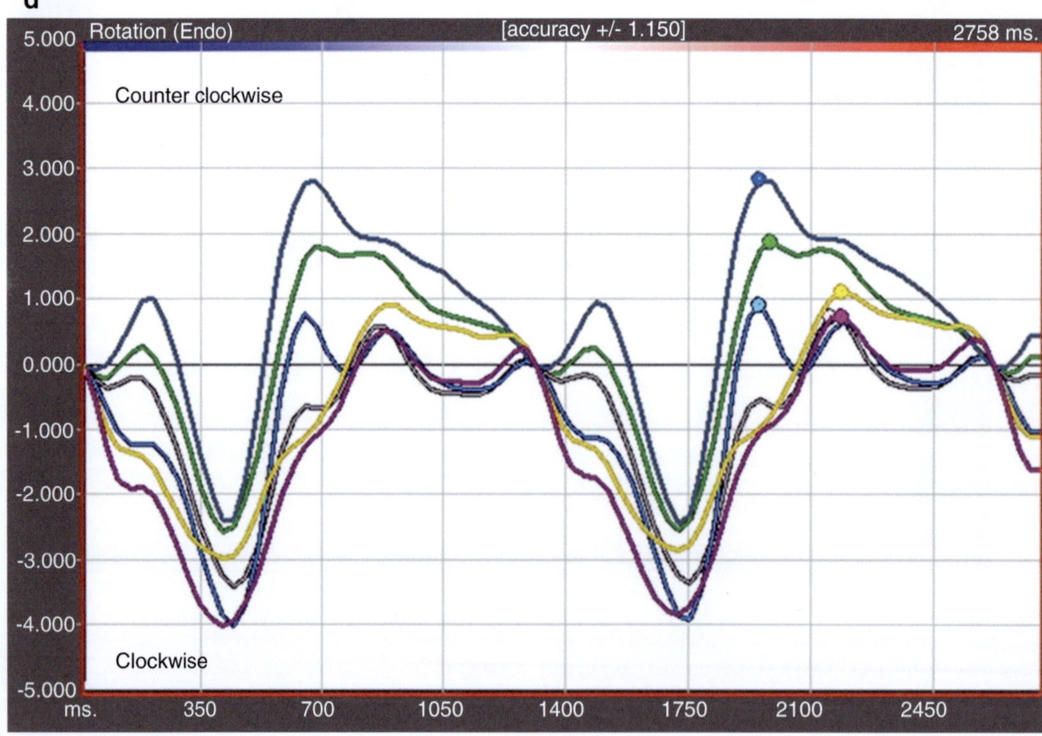

Fig. 14.32 (continued)

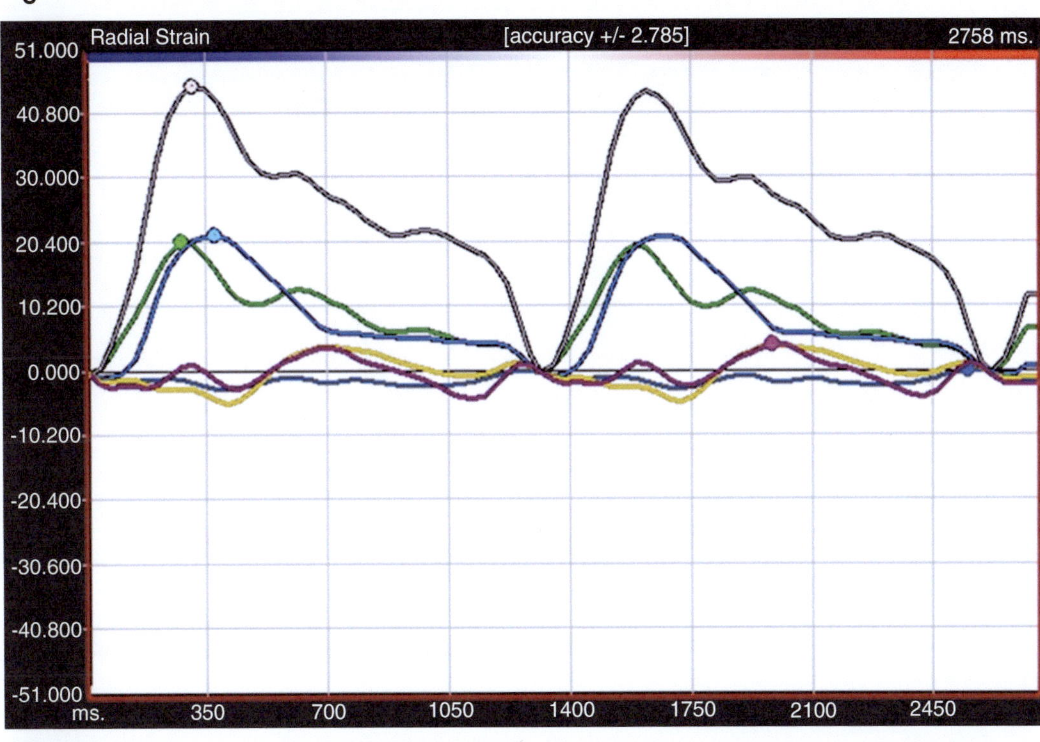

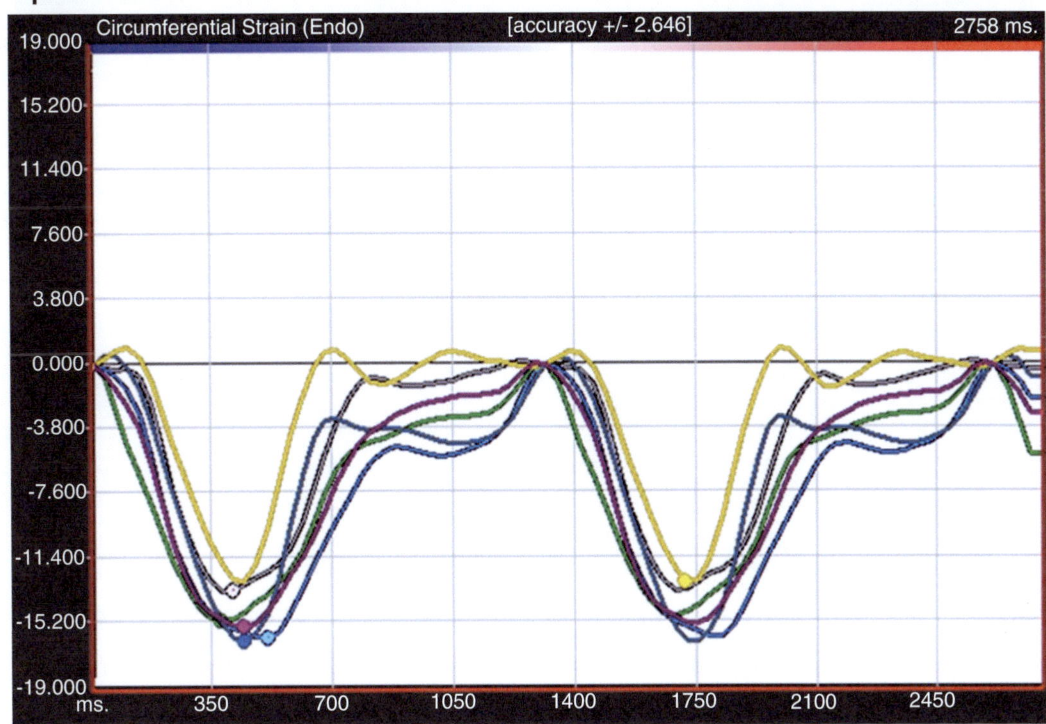

Fig. 14.32 (continued)

a

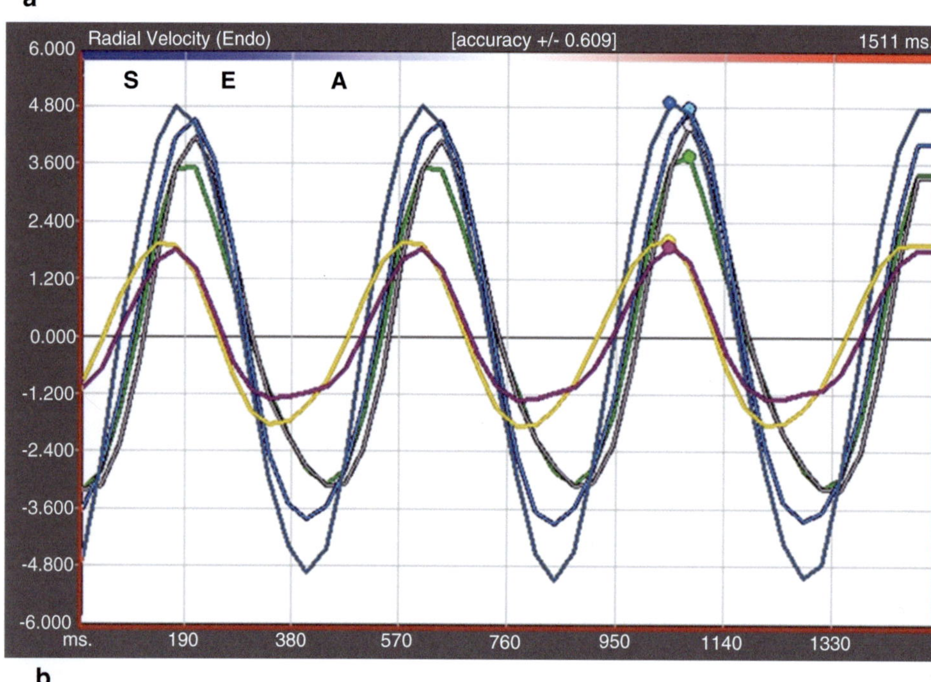

b

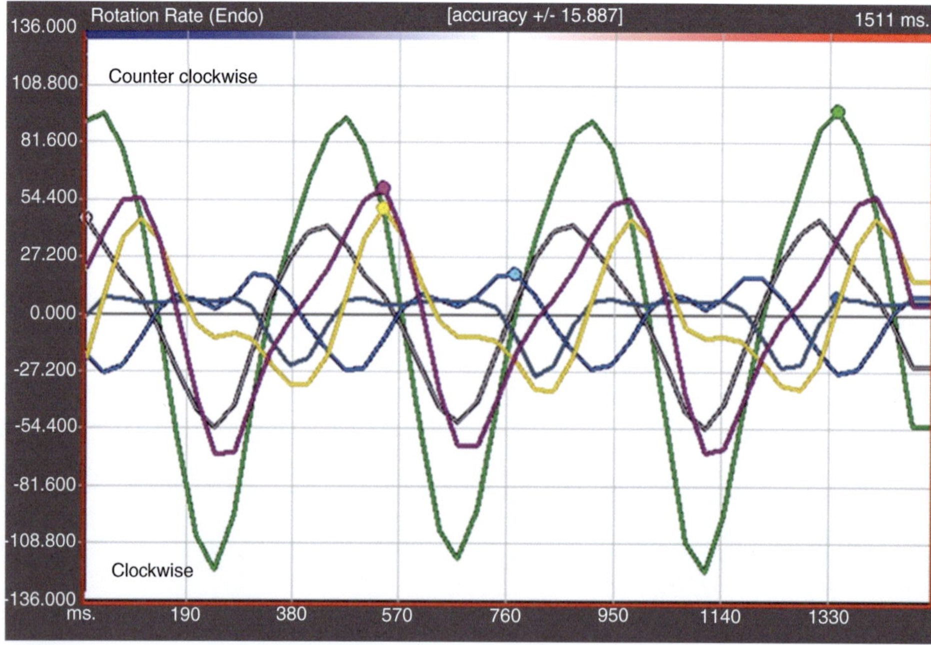

Fig. 14.33 Representative LV speckle tracking imaging signals obtained from the short-axis view at the level of the papillary muscles from a patient with confirmed aPE and RV dysfunction and abnormal strain. Color-coded representation is similar for all images as listed in Fig. 14.30. Green corresponds to the anterior septum; light purple to anterior wall; light blue to the lateral wall; dark blue to the posterior wall; yellow to the inferior wall; and deep purple to the inferior septum. (**a**) Radial velocity is shown for all six segments with the systolic component represented by S, early diastole by E, and late diastole by A. (**b**) Representative rotation rate showing dyssynchronous counterclockwise and clockwise rotation abnormalities of all segments. (**c**) Abnormal radial displacement curves of all six LV segments. (**d**) Representative radial rotation displacement curves showing dyssynchronous counterclockwise and clockwise rotation abnormalities of all segments. (**e**) Abnormal radial strain curves for all six LV segments. (**f**) Abnormal circumferential strain curves for all six LV segments

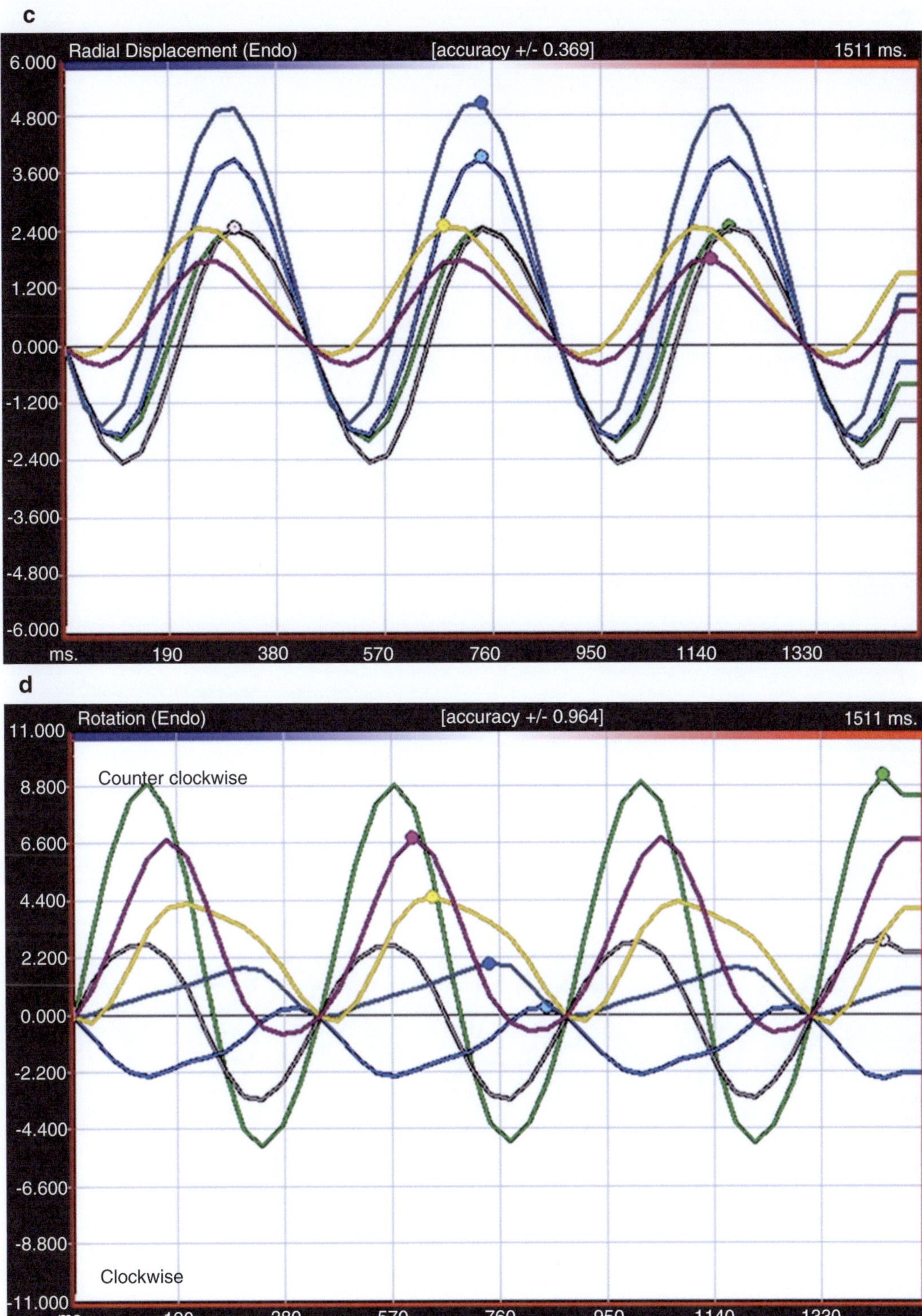

Fig. 14.33 (continued)

e

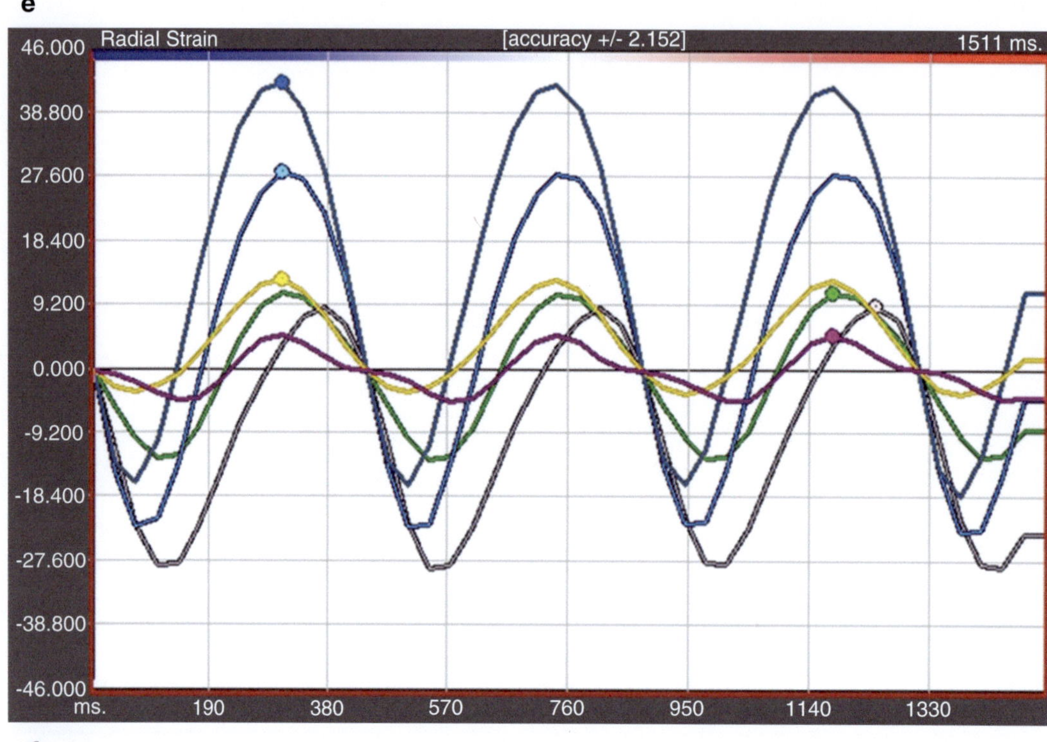

f

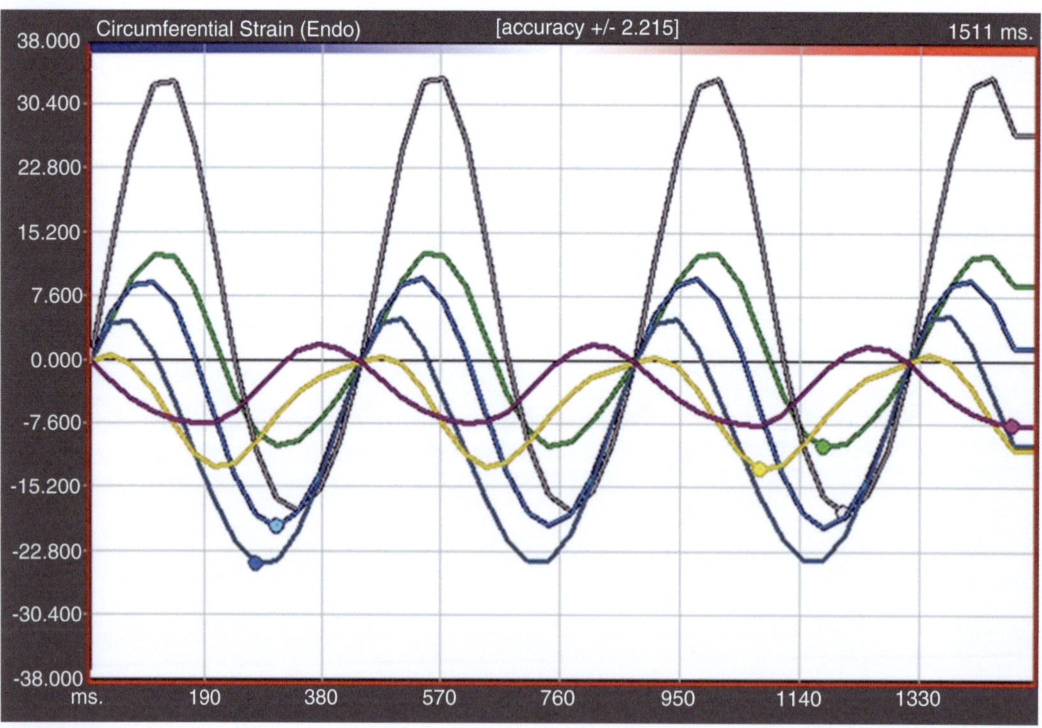

Fig. 14.33 (continued)

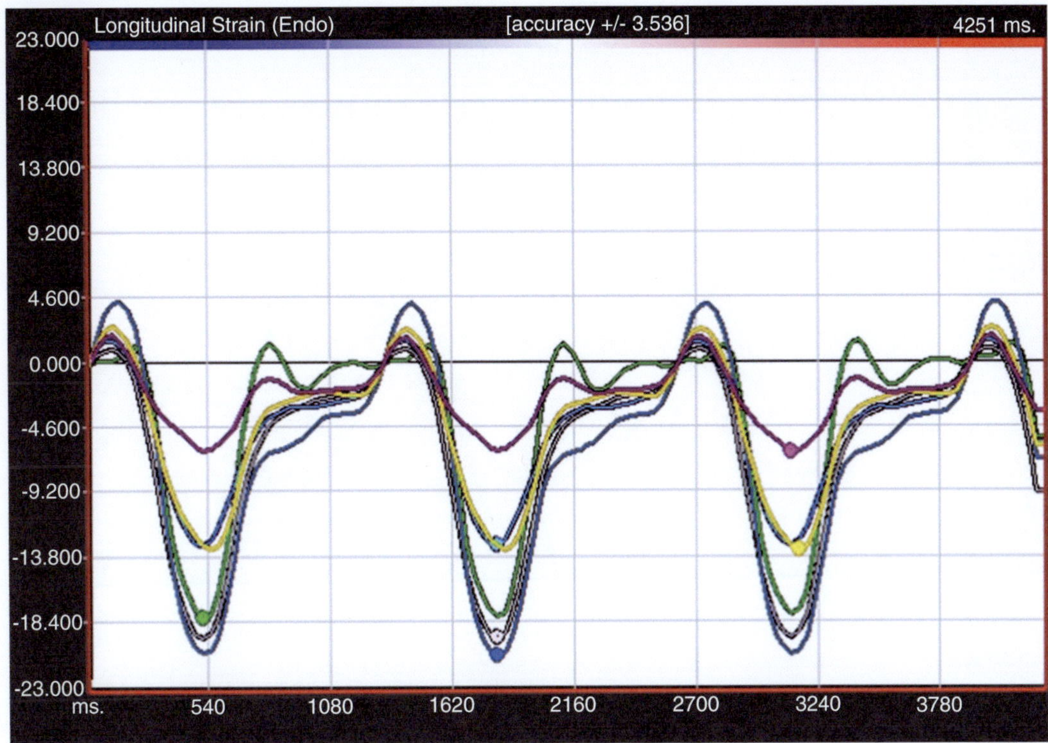

Fig. 14.34 Representative velocity vector imaging from a normal RV showing normal longitudinal strain curves from all six segments. Individual segment recognition is as follows: RV free wall annulus side is green; mid RV free wall is lilac; apical side of the RV wall is light blue; IVS base is dark blue; mid IVS is yellow; and apical side of the IVS is purple. Please note that all six segments have a normal negative deflection in systole with normal peak values of approximately −20%. Specifically, note the normal movement of the RV apical segment

segment signature, and significant temporal dys-synchrony among all six RV segments when compared to the well-coordinated peaking of all RV segments in Fig. 14.32.

As previously illustrated, RVOT systolic excursion has also been a useful echocardiographic variable used in estimating global impairment in RV contractility as well as acute hemodynamic derangement [304]. However, the ratio between main chamber RV fractional area change and RVOT systolic excursion appears to be markedly abnormal in patients with proven bilateral proximal embolus by CTPA. Furthermore, this ratio was also found to be a very useful TTE finding when trying to distinguish aPE from chronic PH [305].

Furthermore, speckle tracking strain imaging has been shown to be not only extremely accurate and reproducible, but also extremely useful in identifying subtle wall motion as well as systolic function abnormalities [306–309]. Tissue Doppler and speckle tracking imaging have been invaluable for assessing myocardial mechanics in chronic pulmonary hypertension [172, 310–314], especially in quantifying global as well as segmental longitudinal RV peak systolic strain and defining the presence of RV dyssynchrony in aPE patients [315]. Moreover, these abnormalities in RV heterogeneity and dyssynchrony resolve after the acute aPE insult and return to normal values [315]. Thus, speckle tracking as a portable, accurate, and reproducible imaging modality holds particular promise in offering prompt and reliable information that can be used not only at the bedside for diagnostic purpose, but also for follow-up of aPE patients once appropriate therapy is instituted. Representative speckle tracking images from a normal individual (Fig. 14.34) and

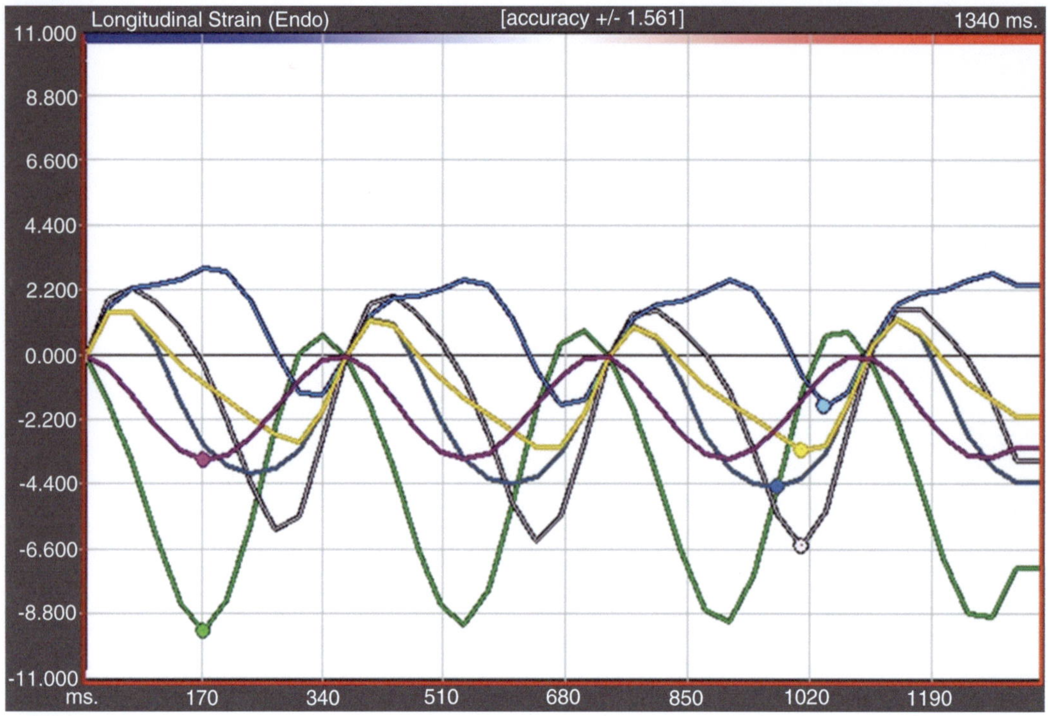

Fig. 14.35 Representative velocity vector imaging from an aPE patient showing abnormal longitudinal strain curves from all six segments. Individual segment recognition is similar as noted for Fig. 14.34. Please note that all six segments have significant reduction in the overall sys-tolic deformation. Specifically, note the very abnormal RV apical segment signature. Finally, a significant amount of dyssynchrony is also noted as time to peak of all six segments is different when compared to the well-coordinated peaking of all segments in Fig. 14.34

from a patient with confirmed aPE (Fig. 14.35) are shown.

In order to link the RV-PA unit with the LV, it will then be useful to review our current understanding of myocardial fiber direction. As proposed by the late Torrent-Guasp, if indeed there is a continuum of subepicardial RV muscle fibers forming a plane along the posterior LV to the region of the left fibrous trigone and these fibers do descend from the left fibrous trigone to the LV apex [316, 317], then whichever process affects the RV will certainly impact the LV. It has been shown that potential traction on this muscular band by RV dilatation adversely affects basal LV rotation in cases of chronic PH [172]. Whether this represents a functional continuity between the ventricles or is merely a static anatomical entity mediated by the IVS remains largely unknown. Therefore, it is reasonable to believe that similar interactions do occur with sudden increase in RV afterload in aPE. In addition, bow-ing of the IVS towards the LV has been shown to alter global LV kinetics in the rat model, even if intrinsic LV systolic function is normal [318]. In humans, aPE has shown to induce reversible global LV dysfunction; nonuniformity of LV contractility in the radial, longitudinal, and circumferential directions; and discoordination of radial LV wall motion [315]. Once again, all these abnormalities were found to be reversible and normalized with treatment after patient stabilization [315]. Recent evidence in experimental animal models suggests that aPE mainly impairs LV performance by primarily altering septal strain and apical rotation [319]. Similarly, even though mainly recognized in case of human chronic PH, abnormal LV diastolic function might be likely affected by the similar mechanisms during aPE [172, 173, 320, 321]. Unfortunately, to date none of these mechanisms that directly affect LV diastolic function in cases of aPE have been clinically investigated.

After Acute Pulmonary Embolism Diagnosis

In summary, it is clear that certain clinical conditions predispose to the development of DVT and also aPE; however, these conditions are also found in otherwise healthy people, and aggressive investigation for potential pulmonary embolism is likely to find an incidental clot without clinical consequence [322]. In fact, in up to 90% of autopsy reports an identifiable new or old PE might be found, particularly if microscopic examination is done on numerous blocks of lung tissue [323–325]. Therefore, it becomes sometimes difficult to determine how often any of these clots are clinically significant. Similarly, the advent of advanced diagnostic modalities has allowed detection of very small thrombi of otherwise unknown clinical significance [297], particularly when healthy outpatients present with severe pleuritic chest pain.

Several developments have taken place with regard to risk, diagnosis, and management of VTE since the last European Society of Cardiology (ESC) guidelines and update of the American College of Chest Physicians in 2016. In particular, it is important to take into consideration the very comprehensive 2019 ESC guidelines which were developed in collaboration with the European Respiratory Society [326]. Here are the most remarkable highlights:

Risk Assessment

1. Pretest probability scores include the revised Geneva score and the Wells rule [188, 327]. Based on the current data, aPE is expected to be confirmed according to pretest probability in 10% of cases when pretest probability is low compared to 30% in moderate and 65% in high pretest probability.
2. The Pulmonary Embolism Rule-out Criteria (PERC) score should be limited to patients seen in the emergency department with low pretest probability that any additional diagnostic testing is intended. This PERC score includes eight parameters [328]:
   (a) Age <50 years
   (b) Pulse <100 beats/min
   (c) Oxygen saturation >94%
   (d) No unilateral leg swelling
   (e) No hemoptysis
   (f) No recent trauma or surgery
   (g) No VTE history
   (h) No previous oral hormone use
3. D-dimer [329]:
   (a) Point-of-care D-dimers only to be used in patients with a low pretest probability due to their reduced sensitivity (88%) compared with the standard laboratory-based assay (95%).
   (b) In patients with low-to-intermediate clinical probability of aPE, D-dimer should be the initial test. If negative, no treatment is indicated. If positive, CTPA should be performed for definitive diagnosis.
   (c) Age-adjusted D-dimer (age × 10 mcg/l) for patients older than 50 years should be considered to identify low-risk patients (Class IIa).
   (d) D-dimer cutoff values adjusted for age or clinical probability can be used as an alternative to the fixed cutoff value.
4. Definition of hemodynamic instability:
   (a) Cardiac arrest
   (b) Obstructive shock (systolic blood pressure [BP] <90 mmHg or need for vasopressors to achieve BP ≥90 mmHg and end-organ hypoperfusion)
   (c) Persistent hypotension (systolic BP <90 mmHg or systolic BP drop ≥40 mmHg lasting longer than 15 min and not due to another identifiable cause)
5. Initial test to be obtained in patients deemed to be at a high clinical probability of PE is CTPA.

Imaging

1. Accepted diagnosis for VTE and aPE: Proximal DVT confirmed by compressive ultrasonography in a patient with clinical suspicion for aPE.
2. TTE alone cannot be used to rule out aPE. However, it is quite useful in suspected high-risk aPE, in which the absence of echocardiographic signs of RV overload or dys-

function essentially rules out aPE as the reason for hemodynamic instability.

3. Availability of imaging studies for aPE diagnosis:
   (a) CTPA is the most accessible not only with an excellent specificity (96%) but also helping to provide an alternative diagnosis. Main concerns are concern for breast radiation exposure (3–10 mSv) for young women, renal dysfunction, and iodinated contrast allergy.
   (b) Even though planar V/Q scan is inexpensive with few contraindications and relatively low radiation exposure (2 mSv), it is unable to provide an alternative diagnosis and it could be inconclusive in 50% of all cases.
   (c) V/Q single-photon emission CT provides the lowest rate of nondiagnostic tests (<3%), has few contraindications, and uses low radiation (2 mSv). Unfortunately, it does not provide an alternative diagnosis and to date there has been no validated outcome data.
   (d) Pulmonary angiography is the gold standard, but it is an invasive procedure with the highest radiation dose (10–20 mSv).

Prognosis

1. An initial risk stratification is to be performed in all patients with suspected or confirmed aPE. Prognostic assessment should include clinical parameters (simplified Pulmonary Embolism Severity Index [PESI] score, RV function, hemodynamics, and elevated biomarkers) [147, 149, 330, 331].
2. Markers associated with an unfavorable short-term prognosis in aPE have been associated with the presence of tachycardia, low systolic BP, respiratory insufficiency, and syncope.
3. TTE findings associated with a poor prognosis are an RV/left ventricular diameter ratio ≥1.0 and TAPSE <1.6 cm.
4. An RV/left ventricular diameter ratio ≥1.0 on CT is associated with a 2.5-fold increased risk of all-cause mortality and 5-fold increased aPE-related mortality.

5. High-sensitivity troponin has a 98% negative predictive value when <14 pg/mL for excluding an adverse in-hospital clinical outcome.
6. B-type natriuretic peptide, N-terminal pro-B-type natriuretic peptide, and troponin have low specificity and positive predictive value for early mortality for normotensive patients with PE.
7. Elevated lactate, high-serum creatinine, and hyponatremia are some of the other laboratory markers of adverse prognosis.
8. Prognostic assessment strategy is recommended for patients without hemodynamic instability:
   (a) Low risk (PESI Classes I–II, simplified PESI of 0)
   (b) Intermediate low risk (elevated PESI score with or without RV dysfunction or elevated troponin)
   (c) Intermediate high risk (elevated PESI score with both RV dysfunction and elevated troponin)
   (d) High risk (hemodynamic instability)

In addition, the 2019 ESC writing group also recommended the following regarding which patients are at increased risk of recurrence and how to institute follow-up of these patients [326].

Groups at Increased Risk of Recurrence (High at >8%/Year)

1. A strong (major) attributable transient or reversible risk factor, such as major surgery or trauma
2. Persistence of a weak (minor) transient or reversible risk factor or a nonmalignant risk factor for thrombosis
3. Index episode that occurred in the absence of any identifiable risk factor
4. One or more previous episodes of VTE
5. Major persistent prothrombotic condition
6. Active cancer

In terms of follow-up of these patients, the 2019 ESC authors recommend performing either the Medical Research Council Scale or the World Health Organization Functional Scale Assessment

3–6 months after aPE diagnosis with dyspnea (Class I) [332, 333]. Furthermore, a TTE should be ordered if the patient has persistent dyspnea at 3–6 months (Class IIa) post-aPE. Finally, a V/Q scan should be considered at 3–6 months if there are concerns for PH to be assessed for chronic thromboembolic PH (Class IIa), with referral to a PH or chronic thromboembolic PH specialist if abnormal (Class I).

Finally, treatment was also addressed by this 2019 document as follows [326]:

1. Prompt institution of anticoagulation is required in all high- or intermediate-probability aPE while awaiting results of diagnostic testing (Class I):
   (a) Low-molecular-weight heparin (LMWH) and fondaparinux are preferred over unfractionated heparin (UFH) given lower risks of major bleeding or heparin-induced thrombocytopenia (Class I).
   (b) UFH should be reserved for hemodynamically unstable patients or patients awaiting reperfusion therapy.
2. Oral anticoagulants:
   (a) Based on current data, direct-acting oral anticoagulants (DOACs) are noninferior to LMWH and vitamin K antagonist (VKA) with lower rates of major bleeding and are recommended over VKA in eligible patients (Class I).
   (b) Recommended dosing regimens:
      - Dabigatran parenteral anticoagulation for ≥5 days followed by dabigatran 150 mg BID
      - Rivaroxaban 15 mg BID for 3 weeks followed by 20 mg QD
      - Apixaban 10 mg BID for 7 days followed by 5 mg BID
      - Edoxaban UFH or LMWH for ≥5 days followed by 60 mg daily or 30 mg daily if creatinine clearance = 30–50 mL/min or body weight <60 kg
   (c) If VKA is given, UFH, LMWH, or fondaparinux should be continued for ≥5 days and until international normalized ratio is 2.5 (range 2.0–3.0) (Class I).
   (d) Recommended initial starting dose of warfarin may be 10 mg when <60 years in healthy patients while 5 mg could be used initially in all others.
   (e) Novel oral anticoagulants are contraindicated with severe renal impairment, during pregnancy and lactation, and in patients with antiphospholipid syndrome (Class III).
3. In terms of systemic thrombolytic therapy this should be reserved for high-risk, hemodynamically unstable patients (Class I). When thrombolytic therapy fails or patients are not considered adequate candidates, then surgical embolectomy should be recommended (Class I). Catheter-directed thrombolysis should be reserved for high-risk patients in whom thrombolysis has failed or is contraindicated (Class IIa).
4. Routine use of inferior vena cava filters is still not routinely recommended (Class III), though it could be considered if there are absolute contraindications to anticoagulation (Class IIa) or in cases of recurrent PE despite therapeutic anticoagulation (Class IIa).
5. Early discharge from hospital with continuation of home anticoagulation therapy should be considered in the following cases:
   (a) Use of the Hestia exclusion criteria that utilizes a checklist of clinical parameters or questions integrating aspects of aPE severity, comorbidity, and feasibility of home treatment. The use of this bedside tool gives the healthcare professional the ability of identifying that when one or more of the questions are answered with a "yes," then the patient cannot be discharged early. Consequently, when all Hestia criteria are negative, the risk of early aPE-related death or serious complication is low [326].
   (b) No serious comorbidity or aggravating conditions warranting hospitalization.
   (c) Logistically intact and identifiable proper outpatient care resources and follow-up ability.

Duration of Anticoagulation

1. Based on current data, all patients should receive 3 months of therapy (Class I).

2. Discontinuation of therapy is recommended after 3 months if index PE/DVT due to major transient or reversible risk factor (Class I).
3. The risk of recurrence is similar when therapy is withdrawn at 3–6 months versus 12–24 months.
4. Extended duration of anticoagulation increases bleeding risk but decreases recurrence risk by ≤90%.
5. Indefinite anticoagulation for recurrent VTE not related to a major transient or reversible risk factor (Class I).
6. Indefinite anticoagulation with VKA is recommended for patients with antiphospholipid syndrome (Class I).

Currently recommended algorithm for risk stratification, diagnostic, and treatment strategy to assess aPE is shown in Fig. 14.36 [179, 334–337]. As already reviewed it is critically important that objective imaging assessment of RV dysfunction (Fig. 14.37) or RV strain is done with the use of elevated cardiac biomarkers (Fig. 14.38) [334–343]. Pooled diagnostic sensitivities, specificities, and negative and positive predictive values for the use of TTE, CTPA, and cardiac biomarkers are shown in Fig. 14.39.

Chronic Pulmonary Embolism

It is important to now shift gears and discuss a prevalent clinical entity found in survivors of aPE: a condition known as chronic thromboembolic pulmonary hypertension (CTEPH). The latter results from either a single or a recurrent pulmonary embolism event(s) that for the most

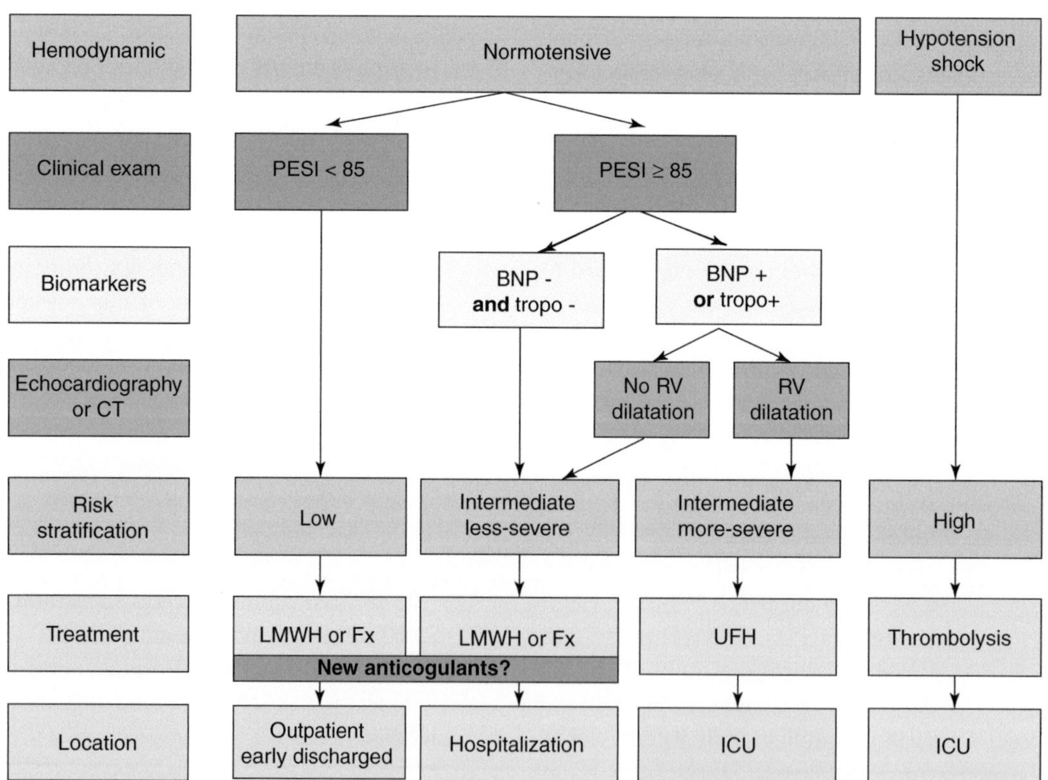

Fig. 14.36 Risk stratification, diagnostic, and treatment algorithm for patients with aPE. *BNP* brain natriuretic peptide, *Fx* fondaparinux, *ICU* intensive care unit, *LMWH* low-molecular-weight heparin, *PESI* pulmonary embolism severity index, *RV* right ventricle, *tropo* troponin, *UFH* unfractionated heparin. (Reprinted with permission from Penaloza A, et al. Curr Opin Crit Care. 2012; 18: 318–325)

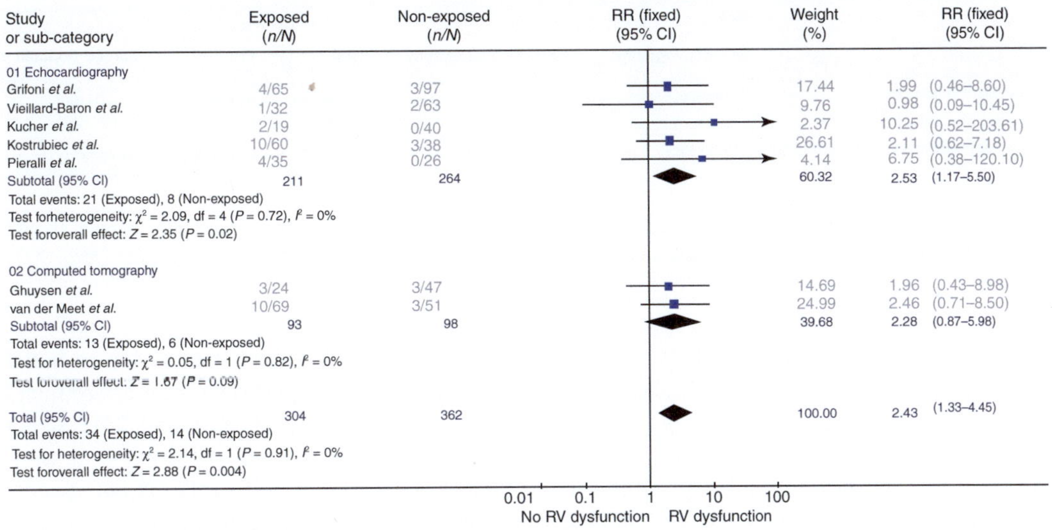

Study or sub-category	Exposed (n/N)	Non-exposed (n/N)	RR (fixed) (95% CI)	Weight (%)	RR (fixed) (95% CI)
01 Echocardiography					
Grifoni et al.	4/65	3/97		17.44	1.99 (0.46–8.60)
Vieillard-Baron et al.	1/32	2/63		9.76	0.98 (0.09–10.45)
Kucher et al.	2/19	0/40		2.37	10.25 (0.52–203.61)
Kostrubiec et al.	10/60	3/38		26.61	2.11 (0.62–7.18)
Pieralli et al.	4/35	0/26		4.14	6.75 (0.38–120.10)
Subtotal (95% CI)	211	264		60.32	2.53 (1.17–5.50)
Total events: 21 (Exposed), 8 (Non-exposed)					
Test for heterogeneity: $\chi^2 = 2.09$, df = 4 ($P = 0.72$), $I^2 = 0\%$					
Test for overall effect: $Z = 2.35$ ($P = 0.02$)					
02 Computed tomography					
Ghuysen et al.	3/24	3/47		14.69	1.96 (0.43–8.98)
van der Meet et al.	10/69	3/51		24.99	2.46 (0.71–8.50)
Subtotal (95% CI)	93	98		39.68	2.28 (0.87–5.98)
Total events: 13 (Exposed), 6 (Non-exposed)					
Test for heterogeneity: $\chi^2 = 0.05$, df = 1 ($P = 0.82$), $I^2 = 0\%$					
Test for overall effect: $Z = 1.67$ ($P = 0.09$)					
Total (95% CI)	304	362		100.00	2.43 (1.33–4.45)
Total events: 34 (Exposed), 14 (Non-exposed)					
Test for heterogeneity: $\chi^2 = 2.14$, df = 1 ($P = 0.91$), $I^2 = 0\%$					
Test for overall effect: $Z = 2.88$ ($P = 0.004$)					

0.01　0.1　1　10　100
No RV dysfunction　　RV dysfunction

Fig. 14.37 Prognostic value of right ventricular dysfunction for mortality in patients with pulmonary embolism without shock. The outcome was in-hospital mortality for all studies, except two: (*) 40-day mortality and (†) 90-day mortality. (Reprinted with permission from Sanchez, O, et al. Eur Heart J. 2008; 29: 1569–1577)

Study or sub-category	Exposed (n/N)	Non-exposed (n/N)	RR (fixed) (95% CI)	Weight (%)	RR (fixed) (95% CI)
01 BNP					
Tulevski et al.	0/3	0/11			Not estimable
Kucher et al.	2/21	0/38		14.41	8.86 (0.45–176.44)
ten Wolde et al.	9/36	2/74		52.30	9.25 (2.11–40.61)
Pieralli et al.	4/20	0/41		13.32	18.00 (1.02–318.87)
Tulevski et al.	2/14	0/14		19.98	5.00 (0.26–95.61)
Subtotal (95% CI)	94	178		100.00	9.51 (3.16–28.64)
Total events: 17 (Exposed), 2 (Non-exposed)					
Test for heterogeneity: $\chi^2 = 0.38$, df = 3 ($P = 0.95$), $I^2 = 0\%$					
Test for overall effect: $Z = 4.00$ ($P < 0.0001$)					
02 pro-BNP					
Pruszczyk et al.	11/56	0/14		23.91	6.05 (0.38–96.95)
Kostrubiec et al.	9/21	6/79		76.09	5.64 (2.26–14.08)
Subtotal (95% CI)	77	93		100.00	5.74 (2.18–15.13)
Total events: 20 (Exposed), 6 (Non-exposed)					
Test for heterogeneity: $\chi^2 = 0.00$, df = 1 ($P = 0.96$), $I^2 = 0\%$					
Test for overall effect: $Z = 3.53$ ($P = 0.0004$)					
03 Cardiac troponin					
Kucher et al.	2/16	0/43		10.43	12.94 (0.65–255.89)
Kostrubiec et al.	9/18	6/82		80.84	6.83 (2.78–16.78)
Tulevski et al.	2/6	0/22		8.73	16.43 (0.89–303.42)
Subtotal (95% CI)	40	147		100.00	8.31 (3.57–19.33)
Total events: 13 (Exposed), 6 (Non-exposed)					
Test for heterogeneity: $\chi^2 = 0.48$, df = 2 ($P = 0.79$), $I^2 = 0\%$					
Test for overall effect: $Z = 4.92$ ($P < 0.00001$)					

0.01　0.1　1　10　100
Low level　　Elevated level

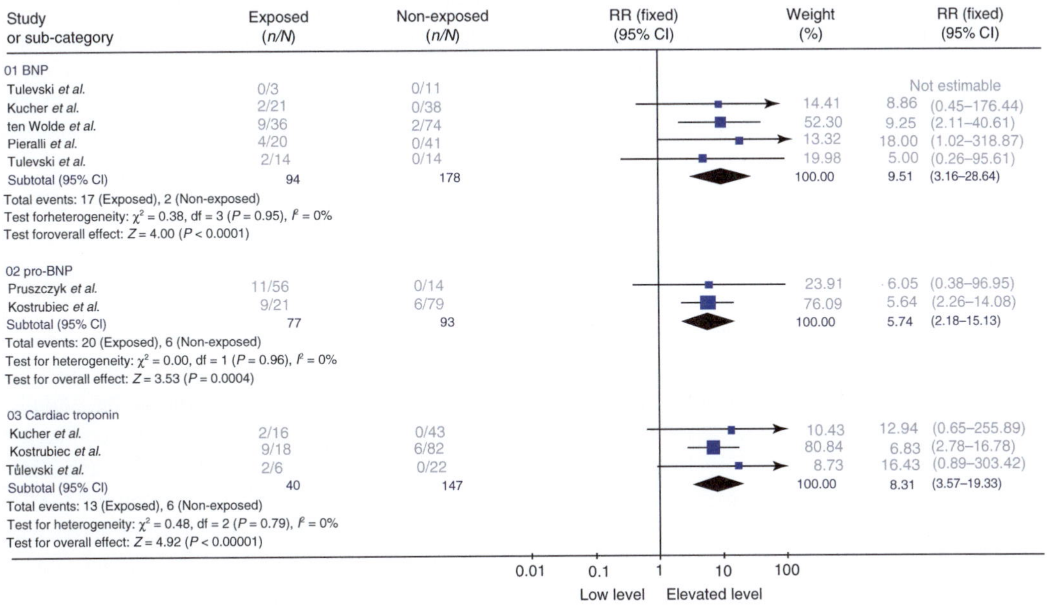

Fig. 14.38 Prognostic value of cardiac biomarkers for mortality in patients with pulmonary embolism without shock. The outcome was in-hospital mortality for all studies, except two: (*) 40-day mortality and (†) 90-day mortality. (Reprinted with permission from Sanchez, O, et al. Eur Heart J. 2008; 29: 1569–1577)

Test				
	Echocardiography	Computed tomography	BNP	Pro-BNP	Cardiac troponin
Sensitivity (%) (95% CI)	70 (46–86)	65 (35–85)	88 (65–96)	93 (14–100)	81 (23–100)
Specificity (%) (95% CI)	57 (47–66)	56 (39–71)	70 (64–75)	58 (14–92)	84 (77–90)
Negative predictive value (%) (95% CI)	60 (55–65)	58 (51–65)	76 (73–79)	81 (65–97)	73 (68–78)
Positive predictive value (%) (95% CI)	58 (53–63)	57 (49–64)	67 (64–70)	63 (50–76)	75 (69–80)

Fig. 14.39 Pooled diagnostic indexes for echocardiography, computed tomography, brain natriuretic peptide (BNP), pro-BNP, and cardiac troponin. (Reprinted with permission from Sanchez, O, et al. Eur Heart J. 2008; 29: 1569–1577)

part originates from a lower extremity vein DVT, although any venous thrombosis site can be responsible.

Even though the majority of aPE episodes typically resolve and restoration of normal pulmonary hemodynamics, gas exchange, and exercise tolerance occurs, in some patients there is incomplete embolic resolution with some residual degree of obstruction or significant narrowing of the central pulmonary vessels by organized scar tissue [344]. The latter would then result in CTEPH. When CTEPH is left untreated progressive RV failure and even death can occur [345].

Even though the full spectrum leading to CTEPH has not been fully defined, it appears that incomplete recovery of perfusion after the initial aPE insult is a common requisite. However, it is now known that changes in the distal pulmonary vascular bed, referred to as a secondary small-vessel vasculopathy, are also critically important for the evolution of this clinical entity in conjunction with a series of other characterized steps such as impaired fibrinolysis and fibrinogen mutations, endothelial dysfunction and defects in neoangiogenesis, differential gene expression, platelet dysfunction, and inflammation [346, 347]. However, it is important to point out that in approximately 25% of all CTEPH cases no identified preceding PE can be found [348].

As already established, for the majority of CTEPH cases to occur aPE patients must survive the initial event and complete adequate anticoagulation resulting in a whole spectrum of cases in which patients may have complete restoration of normal perfusion to significant residual chronic clot rising that raises the pulmonary pressures [349]. Recent data suggest that after 6 months of anticoagulation in patients treated for an initial aPE event, abnormal perfusion scans can be found between 30% and 50% of cases [350, 351]. So not only a persistent residual perfusion is a well-known requisite to develop CTEPH but also the larger the residual defect the more likely it is to progress to CTEPH [351]. Though the majority of patients with persistent perfusion defects after an aPE are for the most part either asymptomatic or mildly limited with no evidence of resting PH, in 10% of aPE patients with persistent perfusion defects, resting PH develops [350].

Even though there is paucity of data regarding true estimates of the incidence of aPE events, it has been suggested that approximately 300,000 aPE events occur yearly in the United States; of these aPE survivors some 3000 new cases of CTEPH should prospectively be diagnosed per year [352]. These estimates do not include the potential 25% of all CTEPH cases, not associated to a prior PE event [348], simply stating the fact that CTEPH is largely underdiagnosed.

To complicate matters even further, rates for identifying CTEPH patients might be complicated by the way studies have been conducted and what definition was employed in each clinical trial [353–356]. Specifically, estimates for the incidence of CTEPH using data from active surveillance studies following aPE patients range from 0.1% to 8.8% within 2 years of initial diagnosis [353–356].

Based on current data, CTEPH patients could be divided into those who survive aPE and those patients in whom a particular profile is seen more frequently with CTEPH rather than with idiopathic pulmonary arterial hypertension. Consequently, CTEPH has been associated with the following [357–360]:

- Unprovoked aPE cases (odds ratio [OR]: 20.0; 95% CI: 2.7–100)
- When there is a delay in diagnosis of greater than 2 weeks from symptom onset (OR: 7.9; 95% CI: 3.3–19.0) (28)
- RV dysfunction at the time of aPE
- Initial estimated RV systolic pressure by TTE >50 mmHg (3.3 times higher odds of persistent PH at 12 months)
- Antiphospholipid antibodies or the lupus anticoagulant is the only hypercoagulable state more commonly seen in CTEPH
- Infected ventriculoatrial shunts
- Splenectomy
- History of malignancy
- Hypothyroidism

In terms of diagnosing CTEPH, identification of chronic thromboembolic material obstructing the pulmonary arteries is required with a precapillary PH mean pulmonary artery pressure >20 mmHg and a PVR >3 Wood units in the setting of a pulmonary artery occlusion pressure <15 mmHg [361].

However, in order to get diagnosed a high index of suspicion is required from the onset. Unfortunately, the current median time between symptom onset and final CTEPH diagnosis is 14.1 months [348, 360]. A delay that likely contributes is secondary vasculopathy [362]. Therefore, it is important that once signs and/or symptoms of pulmonary hypertension are encountered in patients (regardless of a prior history of PE or not), obtain a TTE. This imaging modality, as previously mentioned, will not only provide objective evidence of PH while giving an estimate of RV size and function but also give an overall assessment of left ventricular size and function, valvular structures, and presence of intracardiac shunts [362].

If PH is identified, a V/Q scan continues to be a very useful imaging modality in the continued evaluation of these patients with suspected CTEPH. Diagnosis requires identification of at least one but more commonly several segmental or larger mismatched perfusion defects. Unfortunately, V/Q scans might underestimate the extent of pulmonary artery obstruction if recanalization of previously occluded segments has occurred [363]. If no mismatched segmental segment is identified, the patient might be referred for further evaluation to a pulmonary hypertension center for additional management. If, on the other hand, with mismatched defects, a CTPA should be considered unless a nonthrombotic condition is identified as the cause of the PH. CTPA is an excellent diagnostic modality for detecting CTEPH when performed at specialized centers as interpretive scanning difficulties are known to occur otherwise leading to a falsely low sensitivity for CT-PA [364–366]. However, even when properly interpreted, a negative CT-PA scan cannot exclude the possibility of CTEPH and consequently a V/Q scan remains as the preferred initial imaging test for screening [362].

Final CTEPH confirmation requires a right-heart catheterization with selective digital subtraction pulmonary angiography (DS-PA) that not only provides a comprehensive radiographic and hemodynamic assessment but can also be done with or without exhaled gas analysis.

Once CTEPH has been diagnosed, surgical consideration is given to every patient with the intention of offering the potential for cure with a low perioperative mortality (<5%) at experienced surgical centers [367].

Surgical resection of the occluding thromboembolic material to re-establish flow requires experienced surgeons that can result in significant improvement for most patients immediately post-surgery; however, the presence of residual PH can result in significant postoperative morbidity for which a number of pharmacological treatment options remain available for those patients and for inoperable CTEPH [362].

Conclusion

Acute pulmonary embolism encompasses a very heterogeneous patient population whose management continues to evolve with not only several unresolved issues to be answered by future or ongoing research but also better risk stratification strategies. Considerable progress has been made regarding identification of intermediate-high-risk patients, but ongoing discussion still debates whether patients classified as low risk based on clinical parameters should undergo additional imaging, particularly testing for RV function. Surely many will argue one way or another; some opponents will state that routine testing has not been shown to have therapeutic implications while others will cite time- and cost-intensive data. The fact of the matter is that this is still a fluid field and as new data continues to be collected, we should be able to change our position, if needed.

For the time being it is thoroughly clear that aPE is as much a disease of the RV as it is of the pulmonary arteries. While the pulmonary burden may predict the severity of symptoms, it is the RV that determines hemodynamic response and survival. Prompt assessment of RV function can direct treatment and influence prognosis.

References

1. Geerts WH, Pineo GF, Heit JA, Bergqvist D, Lassen MR, Colwell CW, Ray JG. Prevention of venous thromboembolism: the seventh ACCP conference on antithrombotic and thrombolytic therapy. Chest. 2004;126(Suppl. 3):338–400S.
2. Den Heijer M, Rosendaal FR, Blom HJ, Gerrits WB, Bos GM. Hyperhomocysteinemia and venous thrombosis: a meta-analysis. Thromb Haemost. 1998;80:566–9.
3. Martinelli I, Mannucci PM, De Stefano V, Taioli E, Rossi V, Crosti F, Paciaroni K, Leone G, Faioni EM. Different risks of thrombosis in four coagulation defects associated with inherited thrombophilia: a study of 150 families. Blood. 1998;92:2353–8.
4. Heit JA, Silverstein MD, Mohr DN, Petterson TM, Lohse CM, O'Fallon WM, Melton LJ 3rd. The epidemiology of venous thromboembolism in the community. Thromb Haemost. 2001;86:452–63.
5. Galli M, Luckiani D, Bertolini G, Barbui T. Lupus anticoagulants are stronger risk factors for thrombosis than anticardiolipin antibodies in the antiphospholipid syndrome: a systematic review of the literature. Blood. 2003;101:1827–32.
6. White RH, Zhou H, Romano PS. Incidence of symptomatic venous thromboembolism after different elective or urgent surgical procedures. Thromb Haemost. 2003;90:446–55.
7. Alikhan R, Cohen RT, Combe S, Samama MM, Desjardins L, Eldor A, Janbon C, Leizorovicz A, Olsson CG, Turpie AG. Risk factors for venous thromboembolism in hospitalized patients with acute medical illness: analysis of the MEDENOX Study. Arch Intern Med. 2004;164:963–8.
8. Hoffman M, Monroe DM. Coagulation 2006: a modern view of hemostasis. Hematol Oncol Clin North Am. 2007;21(1):1–11. https://doi.org/10.1016/j.hoc.2006.11.004.
9. Cina G, Marra R, Di Stasi C, Macis G. Epidemiology, pathophysiology and natural history of venous thromboembolism. Rays. 1996;21:315–27.
10. Wilkins RW, Stanton JR. Elastic stockings in the prevention of pulmonary embolism: a progress report. N Engl J Med. 1953;248:1087–90.
11. Ramzi DW, Leeper KV. DVT and pulmonary embolism: part II. Treatment and prevention. Am Fam Physician. 2004;69:2841–8.
12. Kearon C. Natural history of venous thromboembolism. Circulation. 2003;107(23 Suppl 1):I22–30.
13. Heit JA, Cohen AT, Anderson FJ. Estimated annual number of incident and recurrent, non-fatal venous thromboembolism (VTE) events in the US. Blood. 2005;106:11.
14. Boulay F, Berthier F, Schoukroun G, et al. Seasonal variations in hospital admission for deep vein thrombosis and pulmonary embolism: analysis of discharge data. BMJ. 2001;323:601–2.
15. Cervantes J, Rojas G. Virchows legacy: deep vein thrombosis and pulmonary embolism. World J Surg. 2005;29:S30–4.
16. Naess IA, Christiansen SC, Romundstad P, Cannegieter SC, Rosendaal FR, Hammerstrom J. Incidence and mortality of venous thrombosis: a population based study. J Thromb Haemost. 2007;5:692–9.
17. Cushman M, Tsai AW, White RH, Heckbert SR, Rosamond WD, Enright P, Folsom AR. Deep vein thrombosis and pulmonary embolism in two cohorts: the longitudinal investigation of thromboembolism etiology. Am J Med. 2004;117:19–25.
18. Rosendaal FR, Reitsma PH. Genetics of venous thrombosis. J Thromb Haemost. 2009;7(suppl 1):301–4.
19. Wakefield TW, Myers DD, Henke PK. Mechanisms of venous thrombosis and resolution. Arterioscler Thromb Vasc Biol. 2008;28:387–91.
20. Becker BF, Heindl B, Kupatt C, Zahler S. Endothelial function and hemostasis. Z Kardiol. 2000;89:160–7.
21. Gross PL, Aird WC. The endothelium and thrombosis. Semin Thromb Hemost. 2000;26:463–78.
22. Mackman N. New insights into the mechanisms of venous thrombosis. J Clin Invest. 2012;122:2331–6.
23. Mackman N. Triggers, targets and treatments for thrombosis. Nature. 2008;451:914–8.
24. Furie B, Furie BC. Mechanisms of thrombus formation. N Engl J Med. 2008;359:938–49.
25. Lippi G, Franchini M, Targher G. Arterial thrombus formation in cardiovascular disease. Nat Rev Cardiol. 2011;8:502–12.
26. Jackson SP. Arterial thrombosis-insidious, unpredictable and deadly. Nat Med. 2011;17:1423–36.

27. Undas A, Ariëns RA. Fibrin clot structure and function: a role in the pathophysiology of arterial and venous thromboembolic diseases. Arterioscler Thromb Vasc Biol. 2011;31:e88–99.

28. Wolberg AS. Plasma and cellular contributions to fibrin network formation, structure, and stability. Haemophilia. 2010;16(Suppl 3):7–12.

29. Mackman N. Role of tissue factor in hemostasis, thrombosis, and vascular development. Arterioscler Thromb Vasc Biol. 2004;24:1015–22.

30. Hoffbrand AV, Pettit JE. Essential hematology. 3rd ed. Oxford: Blackwell Scientific Publications; 1993.

31. Virchow RLK. Gesammelte Abhandlungen zur wissenschaftlichen Medicin. Von Meidinger & Sohn: Frankfurt; 1856.

32. Iorio A, et al. Risk of recurrence after a first episode of symptomatic venous thromboembolism provoked by a transient risk factor: a systematic review. Arch Intern Med. 2010;170:1710–6.

33. Rosendaal FR, van Hylckama VA, Doggen CJ. Venous thrombosis in the elderly. J Thromb Haemost. 2007;5(suppl 1):310–7.

34. Lowe GD, et al. Epidemiology of coagulation factors, inhibitors and activation markers: the Third Glasgow MONICA Survey. I. Illustrative reference ranges by age, sex and hormone use. Br J Haematol. 1997;97:775–84.

35. Li C, Ford ES, McGuire LC, Mokdad AH. Increasing trends in waist circumference and abdominal obesity among US adults. Obesity (Silver Spring). 2007;15:216–24.

36. Smeeth L, Cook C, Thomas S, Hall AJ, Hubbard R, Vallance P. Risk of deep vein thrombosis and pulmonary embolism after acute infection in a community setting. Lancet. 2006;367:1075–9.

37. Osterud B, Due J Jr. Blood coagulation in patients with benign and malignant tumours before and after surgery. Special reference to thromboplastin generation in monocytes. Scand J Haematol. 1984;32:258–64.

38. Johnson GJ, Leis LA, Bach RR. Tissue factor activity of blood mononuclear cells is increased after total knee arthroplasty. Thromb Haemost. 2009;102:728–34.

39. White RH, Romano PS, Zhou H, Rodrigo J, Bargar W. Incidence and time course of thromboembolic outcomes following total hip or knee arthroplasty. Arch Intern Med. 1998;158:1525–31.

40. James AH. Venous thromboembolism in pregnancy. Arterioscler Thromb Vasc Biol. 2009;29:326–31.

41. Bremme KA. Haemostatic changes in pregnancy. Best Pract Res Clin Haematol. 2003;16:153–68.

42. James AH, Jamison MG, Brancazio LR, Myers ER. Venous thromboembolism during pregnancy and the postpartum period: incidence, risk factors, and mortality. Am J Obstet Gynecol. 2006;194:1311–5.

43. Middeldorp S, et al. Effects on coagulation of levonorgestrel- and desogestrel-containing low dose oral contraceptives: a cross-over study. Thromb Haemost. 2000;84:4–8.

44. Vandenbroucke JP, et al. Oral contraceptives and the risk of venous thrombosis. N Engl J Med. 2001;344:1527–35.

45. Abdollahi M, Cushman M, Rosendaal FR. Obesity: risk of venous thrombosis and the interaction with coagulation factor levels and oral contraceptive use. Thromb Haemost. 2003;89:493–8.

46. Ayer JG, Song C, Steinbeck K, Celermajer DS, Ben Freedman S. Increased tissue factor activity in monocytes from obese young adults. Clin Exp Pharmacol Physiol. 2010;37:1049–54.

47. Khorana AA. Venous thromboembolism and prognosis in cancer. Thromb Res. 2010;125:490–3.

48. Caine GJ, Stonelake PS, Lip GY, Kehoe ST. The hypercoagulable state of malignancy: pathogenesis and current debate. Neoplasia. 2002;4:465–73.

49. Allman-Farinelli MA. Obesity and venous thrombosis: a review. Semin Thromb Hemost. 2011;37:903–7.

50. Noble S, Pasi J. Epidemiology and pathophysiology of cancer-associated thrombosis. Br J Cancer. 2010;102:S2–9.

51. Verbeek TA, Jonathan SG, Saner FH, et al. Hypercoagulability in end-stage liver disease: review of epidemiology, etiology, and management. Transplant Direct. 2018;4(11):e403. https://doi.org/10.1097/TXD.0000000000000843.

52. Silverstein MD, Heit JA, Mohr DN, et al. Trends in the incidence of deep vein thrombosis and pulmonary embolism: a 25-year population-based study. Arch Intern Med. 1998;158:585–93.

53. Northup PG, McMahon MM, Ruhl AP, et al. Coagulopathy does not fully protect hospitalized cirrhosis patients from peripheral venous thromboembolism. Am J Gastroenterol. 2006;101:1524–8.

54. Heit JA, Silverstein MD, Mohr DN, et al. Risk factors for deep vein thrombosis and pulmonary embolism: a population-based case-control study. Arch Intern Med. 2000;160:809–15.

55. Huerta C, Johansson S, Wallander MA, et al. Risk factors and short-term mortality of venous thromboembolism diagnosed in the primary care setting in the United Kingdom. Arch Intern Med. 2007;167:935–43.

56. Gulley D, Teal E, Suvannasankha A, et al. Deep vein thrombosis and pulmonary embolism in cirrhosis patients. Dig Dis Sci. 2008;53:3012–7.

57. Wu H, Nguyen GC. Liver cirrhosis is associated with venous thromboembolism among hospitalized patients in a nationwide US study. Clin Gastroenterol Hepatol. 2010;8:800–5.

58. Northup PG, Caldwell SH. Coagulation in liver disease: a guide for the clinician. Clin Gastroenterol Hepatol. 2013;11:1064–74.

59. Dabbagh O, Oza A, Prakash S, et al. Coagulopathy does not protect against venous thromboembolism in hospitalized patients with chronic liver disease. Chest. 2010;137:1145–9.

60. Cockett FB, Thomas ML. The iliac compression syndrome. Br J Surg. 1965;52:816–21.

61. Moudgill N, Hager E, Gonsalves C, Larson R, Lombardi J, DiMuzio P. May-Thurner syndrome: case report and review of the literature involving modern endovascular therapy. Vascular. 2009;17:330–5.

62. Bovill EG, van der Vliet A. Venous valvular stasis-associated hypoxia and thrombosis: what is the link? Annu Rev Physiol. 2011;73:527–45.

63. Nicolaides AN, Kakkar VV, Field ES, et al. The origin of deep vein thrombosis: a venographic study. Br J Radiol. 1971;44:653–63.

64. Kakkar VV, Howe CT, Flanc C, et al. Natural history of postoperative deep-vein thrombosis. Lancet. 1969;2:230–2.

65. Cogo A, Lensing AWA, Prandoni P, et al. Distribution of thrombosis in patients with symptomatic deep-vein thrombosis: implications for simplifying the diagnostic process with compression ultrasound. Arch Intern Med. 1993;153:2777–80.

66. Moser KM, LeMoine JR. Is embolic risk conditioned by location of deep venous thrombosis? Ann Intern Med. 1981;94:439–44.

67. Malone PC, Agutter PS. The aetiology of deep venous thrombosis. QJM. 2006;99:581–93.

68. Hamer JD, Malone PC, Silver IA. The PO2 in venous valve pockets: its possible bearing on thrombogenesis. Br J Surg. 1981;68(3):166–70.

69. Liu GC, Ferris EJ, Reifsteck JR, Baker ME. Effect of anatomic variations on deep venous thrombosis of the lower extremity. Am J Roentgenol. 1986;146(4):845–8.

70. Varma MR, Varga AJ, Knipp BS, Sukheepod P, Upchurch GR, Kunkel SL, Wakefield TW, Henke PK. Neutropenia impairs venous thrombosis resolution in the rat. J Vasc Surg. 2003;38:1090–8.

71. Stewart GJ. Neutrophils and deep venous thrombosis. Haemostasis. 1993;23(Suppl 1):127–40.

72. Henke PK, Pearce CG, Moaveni DM, Moore AJ, Lynch EM, Longo C, Varma M, Dewyer NA, Deatrick KB, Upchurch GR Jr, Wakefield TW, Hogaboam C, Kunkel SL. Targeted deletion of CCR2 impairs deep vein thrombosis resolution in a mouse model. J Immunol. 2006;177:3388–97.

73. Henke PK, Varma MR, Moaveni DK, Dewyer NA, Moore AJ, Lynch EM, Longo C, Deatrick CB, Kunkel SL, Upchurch GR Jr, Wakefield TW. Fibrotic injury after experimental deep vein thrombosis is determined by the mechanism of thrombogenesis. Thromb Haemost. 2007;98:1045–55.

74. Heit JA. Epidemiology of venous thromboembolism. Nat Rev Cardiol. 2015;12(8):464–74. https://doi.org/10.1038/nrcardio.2015.83.

75. Barsoum MK, Heit JA, Ashrani AA, Leibson CL, Petterson TM, Bailey KR. Is progestin an independent risk factor for incident venous thromboembolism? A population-based case-control study. Thromb Res. 2010;126(5):373–8.

76. Merrer J, et al. Complications of femoral and subclavian venous catheterization in critically ill patients: a randomized controlled trial. JAMA. 2001;286:700–7.

77. Cogo A, et al. Acquired risk factors for deep-vein thrombosis in symptomatic outpatients. Arch Intern Med. 1994;154:164–8.

78. Kuipers S, et al. The absolute risk of venous thrombosis after air travel: a cohort study of 8,755 employees of international organisations. PLoS Med. 2007;4:e290.

79. Doggen CJ, et al. Serum lipid levels and the risk of venous thrombosis. Arterioscler Thromb Vasc Biol. 2004;24:1970–5.

80. Decousus H, et al. Superficial venous thrombosis and venous thromboembolism: a large, prospective epidemiologic study. Ann Intern Med. 2010;152:218–24.

81. Noboa S, Mottier D, Oger E, EPI-GETBO Study Group. Estimation of a potentially preventable fraction of venous thromboembolism: a community-based prospective study. J Thromb Haemost. 2006;4(12):2720–2.

82. Chew HK, Wun T, Harvey D, Zhou H, White RH. Incidence of venous thromboembolism and its effect on survival among patients with common cancers. Arch Intern Med. 2006;166:458–64.

83. Blom JW, et al. Incidence of venous thrombosis in a large cohort of 66,329 cancer patients: results of a record linkage study. J Thromb Haemost. 2006;4:529–35.

84. Heit JA, et al. Risk factors for deep vein thrombosis and pulmonary embolism: a population-based case-control study. Arch Intern Med. 2000;160:809–15.

85. Khorana AA, Kuderer NM, Culakova E, Lyman GH, Francis CW. Development and validation of a predictive model for chemotherapy-associated thrombosis. Blood. 2008;111:4902–7.

86. Ay C, et al. Prediction of venous thromboembolism in cancer patients. Blood. 2010;116:5377–82.

87. Huang W, Goldberg RJ, Anderson FA, Kiefe CI, Spencer FA. Secular trends in occurrence of acute venous thromboembolism: the Worcester VTE study (1985–2009). Am J Med. 2014;127:829.e5–39.e5.

88. Heit JA. Estimating the incidence of symptomatic postoperative venous thromboembolism: the importance of perspective. JAMA. 2012;307:306–7.

89. Spencer FA, et al. Incidence rates, clinical profile, and outcomes of patients with venous thromboembolism. The Worcester VTE study. J Thromb Thrombolysis. 2009;28:401–9.

90. Heit JA, et al. Predictors of recurrence after deep vein thrombosis and pulmonary embolism: a population-based cohort study. Arch Intern Med. 2000;160:761–8.

91. van Dongen CJ, Vink R, Hutten BA, Büller HR, Prins MH. The incidence of recurrent venous thromboembolism after treatment with vitamin K antagonists in relation to time since first event: a meta-analysis. Arch Intern Med. 2003;163:1285–93.

92. Schulman S, et al. Post-thrombotic syndrome, recurrence, and death 10 years after the first episode of venous thromboembolism treated with warfa-

rin for 6 weeks or 6 months. J Thromb Haemost. 2006;4:734–42.

93. Prandoni P, et al. Residual venous thrombosis as a predictive factor of recurrent venous thromboembolism. Ann Intern Med. 2002;137:955–60.

94. Kyrle PA, Eichinger S. The risk of recurrent venous thromboembolism: the Austrian Study on Recurrent Venous Thromboembolism. Wien Klin Wochenschr. 2003;115:471–4.

95. Baglin T, et al. Does the clinical presentation and extent of venous thrombosis predict likelihood and type of recurrence? A patient-level meta-analysis. J Thromb Haemost. 2010;8:2436–42.

96. Kovacs MJ, et al. Patients with a first symptomatic unprovoked deep vein thrombosis are at higher risk of recurrent venous thromboembolism than patients with a first unprovoked pulmonary embolism. J Thromb Haemost. 2010;8:1926–32.

97. Schulman S, Svenungsson E, Granqvist S. Anticardiolipin antibodies predict early recurrence of thromboembolism and death among patients with venous thromboembolism following anticoagulant therapy. Duration of Anticoagulation Study Group. Am J Med. 1998;104:332–8.

98. Garcia D, Akl EA, Carr R, Kearon C. Antiphospholipid antibodies and the risk of recurrence after a first episode of venous thromboembolism: a systematic review. Blood. 2013;122:817–24.

99. Jayakody Arachchillage D, Greaves M. The chequered history of the antiphospholipid syndrome. Br J Haematol. 2014;165:609–17.

100. Brouwer JL, et al. High long-term absolute risk of recurrent venous thromboembolism in patients with hereditary deficiencies of protein S, protein C or antithrombin. Thromb Haemost. 2009;101:93–9.

101. Chee CE, et al. Predictors of venous thromboembolism recurrence and bleeding among active cancer patients: a population-based cohort study. Blood. 2014;123:3972–8.

102. White RH, Gettner S, Newman JM, Trauner KB, Romano PS. Predictors of rehospitalization for symptomatic venous thromboembolism after total hip arthroplasty. N Engl J Med. 2000;343:1758–64.

103. Buckingham M, Meilhac S, Zaffran S. Building the mammalian heart from two sources of myocardial cells. Nat Rev Genet. 2005;6:826–35.

104. Bruneau BG. The developmental genetics of congenital heart disease. Nature. 2008;451:943–8.

105. Larsen WJ. Human embryology. New York: Churchill Livingstone; 1993. p. 111–204.

106. Moore KL, Persaud TV. The developing human: clinically oriented embryology. Philadelphia, PA: WB Saunders; 1998. p. 241–53, 329–80.

107. Murillo H, Cutalo MJ, Jones RP, Lane MJ, Fleischmann D, Restrepo CS. Pulmonary circulation imaging: embryology and normal anatomy. Semin Ultrasound CT MR. 2012;33:473–84.

108. Gao Y, Raj JU. Regulation of the pulmonary circulation in the fetus and newborn. Physiol Rev. 2010;90:1291–335.

109. Burri PH. Structural aspects of postnatal lung development—alveolar formation and growth. Biol Neonate. 2006;89:313–22.

110. Sylvester JT, Shimoda LA, Aaronson PI, Ward JP. Hypoxic pulmonary vasoconstriction. Physiol Rev. 2012;92:367–520.

111. Berrocal T, Madrid C, Novo S, et al. Congenital anomalies of the tracheobronchial tree, lung, and mediastinum: embryology, radiology, and pathology. Radiographics. 2003;24:e17.

112. Castañer E, Gallardo X, Rimola J, et al. Congenital and acquired pulmonary artery anomalies in the adult: radiologic overview. Radiographics. 2006;26:349–71.

113. Grosse C, Grosse A. CT findings in diseases associated with pulmonary hypertension: a current review. Radiographics. 2010;30:1753–77.

114. Ghio S, Gavazzi A, Campana C, Inserra C, Klersy C, Sebastiani R, et al. Independent and additive prognostic value of right ventricular systolic function and pulmonary artery pressure in patients with chronic heart failure. J Am Coll Cardiol. 2001;37:183–8.

115. Becattini C, Agnelli G. Predictors of mortality from pulmonary embolism and their influence on clinical management. Thromb Haemost. 2008;100:747–51.

116. Sanchez O, Trinquart L, Colombet I, et al. Prognostic value of right ventricular dysfunction in patients with haemodynamically stable pulmonary embolism: a systematic review. Eur Heart J. 2008;29:1569–77.

117. Stevinson BG, Hernandez-Nino J, Rose G, Kline JA. Echocardiographic and functional cardiopulmonary problems six months after first-time pulmonary embolism in previously healthy patients. Eur Heart J. 2007;28:2517–24.

118. Haddad F, Hunt SA, Rosenthal DN, Murphy DJ. Right ventricular function in cardiovascular disease, part I: anatomy, physiology, aging, and functional assessment of the right ventricle. Circulation. 2008;117:1436–48.

119. Voelkel NF, Quaife RA, Leinwand LA, Barst RJ, McGoon MD, Meldrum DR, et al. Right ventricular function and failure: report of a National Heart, Lung, and Blood Institute working group on cellular and molecular mechanisms of right heart failure. Circulation. 2006;114:1883–91.

120. Hemnes AR, Champion HC. Right heart function and haemodynamics in pulmonary hypertension. Int J Clin Pract. 2008;62(Suppl 160):11–9.

121. McLaughlin VV, Archer SL, Badesch DB, Barst RJ, Farber HW, Lindner JR, et al. ACCF/AHA 2009 expert consensus document on pulmonary hypertension: a report of the American College of Cardiology Foundation Task Force on Expert Consensus Documents and the American Heart Association: developed in collaboration with the American College of Chest Physicians, American Thoracic Society, Inc., and the Pulmonary Hypertension Association. Circulation. 2009;119:2250–94.

122. Goldhaber SZ, Visani L, De Rosa M. Acute pulmonary embolism: clinical outcomes in the

International Cooperative Pulmonary Embolism Registry (ICOPER). Lancet. 1999;353:1386–9.

123. Stein PD, Matta F, Alrifai A, Rahman A. Trends in case fatality rate in pulmonary embolism according to stability and treatment. Thromb Res. 2012;130(6):841–6.

124. Watts JA, Marchick MR, Kline JA. Right ventricular heart failure from pulmonary embolism: key distinctions from chronic pulmonary hypertension. J Card Fail. 2010;16:250–9.

125. Bristow MR, Zisman LS, Lowes BD, Abraham WT, Badesch DB, Groves BM, Voelkel NF, Lynch DM, Quaife RA. The pressure-overloaded right ventricle in pulmonary hypertension. Chest. 1998;114(1 Suppl):101S–6S.

126. Carabello BA. The relationship of left ventricular geometry and hypertrophy to left ventricular function in valvular heart disease. J Heart Valve Dis. 1995;4(Suppl 2):S132–8.

127. Konstam MA, Cohen SR, Salem DN, et al. Comparison of left and right ventricular end-systolic pressure-volume relations in congestive heart failure. J Am Coll Cardiol. 1985;5:1326–34.

128. Nakamura H, Adachi H, Sudoh A, Yagyu H, Kishi K, Oh-ishi S, et al. Subacute cor pulmonale due to tumor embolism. Intern Med. 2004;43:420–2.

129. Archer S, Michelakis E. The mechanism(s) of hypoxic pulmonary vasoconstriction: potassium channels, redox O(2) sensors, and controversies. News Physiol Sci. 2002;17:131–7.

130. Memtsoudis SG, Rosenberger P, Walz JM. Critical care issues in the patient after major joint replacement. J Intens Care Med. 2007;22:92–104.

131. Toledo LS, Mauad R. Complications of body sculpture: prevention and treatment. Clin Plastic Surg. 2006;33:1–11.

132. Mirski MA, Lele AV, Fitzsimmons L, Toung TJ. Diagnosis and treatment of vascular air embolism. Anesthesiology. 2007;106:164–77.

133. Smulders YM. Pathophysiology and treatment of haemodynamic instability in acute pulmonary embolism: the pivotal role of pulmonary vasoconstriction. Cardiovasc Res. 2000;48:23–33.

134. Jones AE, Watts JA, Debelak JP, Thornton LR, Younger JG, Kline JA. Inhibition of prostaglandin synthesis during polystyrene microsphere-induced pulmonary embolism in the rat. Am J Physiol Lung Cell Mol Physiol. 2003;284:L1072–81.

135. Reeves WC, Demers LM, Wood MA, Skarlatos S, Copenhaver G, Whitesell L, et al. The release of thromboxane A2 and prostacyclin following experimental acute pulmonary embolism. Prostagland Leukotrienes Med. 1983;11:1–10.

136. Todd MH, Forrest JB, Cragg DB. The effects of aspirin and methysergide, singly and in combination, on systemic haemodynamic responses to pulmonary embolism. Can Anaesth Soc J. 1981;28:373–80.

137. Breuer J, Meschig R, Breuer HW, Arnold G. Effects of serotonin on the cardiopulmonary circulatory system with and without 5-HT2-receptor blockade by ketanserin. J Cardiovasc Pharmac. 1985;7:64–6.

138. Battistini B. Modulation and roles of the endothelins in the pathophysiology of pulmonary embolism. Can J Physiol Pharmacol. 2003;81:555–69.

139. Kapsch DN, Metzler M, Silver D. Contributions of prostaglandin F2 alpha and thromboxane A2 to the acute cardiopulmonary changes of pulmonary embolism. J Surg Res. 1981;30:522–9.

140. Kim SH, Yi MZ, Kim DH, Song JM, Kang DH, Lee SD, Song JK. Prognostic value of echocardiographic estimation of pulmonary vascular resistance in patients with acute pulmonary thromboembolism. J Am Soc Echocardiogr. 2011;24:693–8.

141. Torbicki A, Galié N, Covezzoli A, Rossi E, De Rosa M, Goldhaber SZ, ICOPER Study Group. Right heart thrombi in pulmonary embolism: results from the International Cooperative Pulmonary Embolism Registry. J Am Coll Cardiol. 2003;41:2245–51.

142. Konstantinides SV, Torbicki A, Agnelli G, et al. 2014 ESC guidelines on the diagnosis and management of acute pulmonary embolism: the task force for the diagnosis and management of acute pulmonary embolism of the European Society of Cardiology (ESC). Endorsed by the European Respiratory Society (ERS). Eur Heart J. 2014;35(43):3033–80.

143. McIntyre KM, Sasahara AA. The hemodynamic response to pulmonary embolism in patients without prior cardiopulmonary disease. Am J Cardiol. 1971;28(3):288–94.

144. Delcroix M, Mélot C, Lejeune P, Leeman M, Naeije R. Effects of vasodilators on gas exchange in acute canine embolic pulmonary hypertension. Anesthesiology. 1990;72(1):77–84.

145. Lankhaar JW, Westerhof N, Faes TJ, Marques KM, Marcus JT, Postmus PE, Vonk-Noordegraaf A. Quantification of right ventricular afterload in patients with and without pulmonary hypertension. Am J Physiol Heart Circ Physiol. 2006;291(4):H1731–7.

146. Chan CM, Woods C, Shorr AF. The validation and reproducibility of the pulmonary embolism severity index. J Thromb Haemost. 2010;8(7):1509–14.

147. Donzé J, Le Gal G, Fine MJ, et al. Prospective validation of the Pulmonary Embolism Severity Index. A clinical prognostic model for pulmonary embolism. Thromb Haemost. 2008;100(5):943–8.

148. Vanni S, Nazerian P, Pepe G, et al. Comparison of two prognostic models for acute pulmonary embolism: clinical vs. right ventricular dysfunction-guided approach. J Thromb Haemost. 2011;9(10):1916–23.

149. Aujesky D, Obrosky DS, Stone RA, et al. Derivation and validation of a prognostic model for pulmonary embolism. Am J Respir Crit Care Med. 2005;172(8):1041–6.

150. Jimenez D, Aujesky D, Moores L, et al. Simplification of the pulmonary embolism severity index for prognostication in patients with acute symptomatic pulmonary embolism. Arch Intern Med. 2010;170(15):1383–9.

151. Righini M, Roy PM, Meyer G, et al. The Simplified Pulmonary Embolism Severity Index (PESI): vali-

dation of a clinical prognostic model for pulmonary embolism. J Thromb Haemost. 2011;9(10):2115–7.

152. Nassiri N, Jain A, McPhee D, Mina B, Rosen RJ, Giangola G, et al. Massive and submassive pulmonary embolism: experience with an algorithm for catheter-directed mechanical thrombectomy. Ann Vasc Surg. 2012;26(1):18–24.

153. Silverstein MD, Heit JA, Mohr DN, Petterson TM, O'Fallon WM, Melton LJ 3rd. Trends in the incidence of deep vein thrombosis and pulmonary embolism: a 25-year population-based study. Arch Intern Med. 1998;158:585–93.

154. Agnelli G, Becattini C. Acute pulmonary embolism. N Engl J Med. 2010;363:266–74.

155. Piazza G, Goldhaber SZ. Current concepts: chronic thromboembolic pulmonary hypertension. New Engl J Med. 2011;364:351–60.

156. Jiménez D, de Miguel-Díez J, Guijarro R, et al., RIETE Investigators. Trends in the management and outcomes of acute pulmonary embolism: analysis from the RIETE Registry. J Am Coll Cardiol. 2016;67(2):162–70.

157. Hsiao SH, Lee CY, Chang SM, Yang SH, Lin SK, Huang WC. Pulmonary embolism and right heart function: insights from myocardial Doppler tissue imaging. J Am Soc Echocard. 2006;19:822–8.

158. Iwadate K, Tanno K, Doi M, Takatori T, Ito Y. Two cases of right ventricular ischemic injury due to massive pulmonary embolism. Forensic Sci Int. 2001;116:189–95.

159. Begieneman MP, van de Goot FR, van der Bilt I, Noordegraaf AV, Spreeuwenberg MD, Paulus WJ, et al. Pulmonary embolism causes endomyocarditis in the human heart. Heart. 2008;94:450–6.

160. Zagorski J, Gellar MA, Obraztsova M, Kline JA, Watts JA. Inhibition of CINC-1 decreases right ventricular damage caused by experimental pulmonary embolism in rats. J Immunol. 2007;179:7820–6.

161. Watts JA, Zagorski J, Gellar MA, Stevinson BG, Kline JA. Cardiac inflammation contributes to right ventricular dysfunction following experimental pulmonary embolism in rats. J Molec Cell Cardiol. 2006;41:296–307.

162. Kline JA, Zeitouni R, Marchick MR, Hernandez-Nino J, Rose GA. Comparison of 8 biomarkers for prediction of right ventricular hypokinesis 6 months after submassive pulmonary embolism. Am Heart J. 2008;156:308–14.

163. Nordenholz KE, Mitchell AM, Kline JA. Direct comparison of the diagnostic accuracy of fifty protein biological markers of pulmonary embolism for use in the emergency department. Acad Emerg Med. 2008;15:795–9.

164. Mitchell AM, Nordenholz KE, Kline JA. Tandem measurement of D dimer and myeloperoxidase of C-reactive protein to effectively screen for pulmonary embolism in the emergency department. Acad Emerg Med. 2008;15:800–5.

165. Torrent-Guasp F, Whimster WF, Redmann K. A silicone rubber mould of the heart. Technol Health Care. 1997;5:13–20.

166. Buckberg GD, RESTORE Group. The ventricular septum: the lion of right ventricular function, and its impact on right ventricular restoration. Eur J Cardiothorac Surg. 2006;29(Suppl 1):S272–8.

167. Sallin EA. Fiber orientation and ejection fraction in the human left ventricle. Biophys J. 1969;9:954–64.

168. Damiano RJ Jr, La Follette P Jr, Cox JL, Lowe JE, Santamore WP. Significant left ventricular contribution to right ventricular systolic function. Am J Physiol. 1991;261(5 Pt 2):H1514–24.

169. Osculati G, Malfatto G, Chianca R, Perego GB. Left-to-right systolic ventricular interaction in patients undergoing biventricular stimulation for dilated cardiomyopathy. J Appl Physiol. 2010;109:418–23.

170. Schwarz K, Singh S, Dawson D, Frenneaux MP. Right ventricular function in left ventricular disease: pathophysiology and implications. Heart Lung Circ. 2013;22:507–11.

171. Mori S, Nakatani S, Kanzaki H, Yamagata K, Take Y, Matsuura Y, et al. Patterns of the interventricular septal motion can predict conditions of patients with pulmonary hypertension. J Am Soc Echocardiogr. 2008;21:386–93.

172. Ramani GV, Bazaz R, Edelman K, López-Candales A. Pulmonary hypertension affects left ventricular basal twist: a novel use for speckle-tracking imaging. Echocardiography. 2009;26:44–51.

173. López-Candales A, Edelman K. Chronic pulmonary hypertension causes significant interventricular spatiotemporal dyssynchrony when onset of diastolic flow signals are assessed by color M-mode. Echocardiography. 2012;29:653–60.

174. Piazza G. Submassive pulmonary embolism. JAMA. 2013;309(2):171–80.

175. Konstantinides S. Should thrombolytic therapy be used in patients with pulmonary embolism? Am J Cardiovasc Drugs. 2004;4:69–74.

176. Kasper W, Konstantinides S, Geibel A, Olschewski M, Heinrich F, Grosser KD, et al. Management strategies and determinants of outcome in acute major pulmonary embolism: results of a multicenter registry. J Am Coll Cardiol. 1997;30:1165–71.

177. Wood KE. Major pulmonary embolism: review of a pathophysiologic approach to the golden hour of hemodynamically significant pulmonary embolism. Chest. 2002;121:877–905.

178. Goldhaber SZ, Haire WD, Feldstein ML, Miller M, Toltzis R, Smith JL, et al. Alteplase versus heparin in acute pulmonary embolism: randomized trial assessing right-ventricular function and pulmonary perfusion. Lancet. 1993;314:507–11.

179. Grifoni S, Olivotto I, Cecchini P, Pieralli F, Camaiti A, Santoro G, et al. Short-term clinical outcome of patients with pulmonary embolism, normal blood pressure, and echocardiographic right ventricular dysfunction. Circulation. 2000;101:2817–22.

180. Frémont B, Pacouret G, Jacobi D, Puglisi R, Charbonnier B, de Labriolle A. Prognostic value of echocardiographic right/left ventricular end-diastolic diameter ratio in patients with acute pulmonary embolism: results from a monocenter registry of 1,416 patients. Chest. 2008;133:358–62.

181. Sanchez O, Trinquart L, Caille V, Couturaud F, Pacouret G, Meneveau N, et al. Prognostic factors for pulmonary embolism: the PREP Study, a prospective multicenter cohort study. Am J Respir Crit Care Med. 2010;181:168–73.

182. Kucher N, Rossi E, De Rosa M, Goldhaber SZ. Prognostic role of echocardiography among patients with acute pulmonary embolism and a systolic arterial pressure of 90 mm Hg or higher. Arch Intern Med. 2005;165:1777–81.

183. Stein PD, Henry JW. Prevalence of acute pulmonary embolism among patients in a general hospital and at autopsy. Chest. 1995;108:978–81.

184. Miniati M, Pistolesi M, Marini C, et al. Value of perfusion lung scan in the diagnosis of pulmonary embolism: results of the Prospective Investigative Study of Acute Pulmonary Embolism Diagnosis (PISA-PED). Am J Respir Crit Care Med. 1996;154(5):1387–93.

185. Musset D, Parent F, Meyer G, et al. Diagnostic strategy for patients with suspected pulmonary embolism: a prospective multicentre outcome study. Lancet. 2002;360(9349):1914–20.

186. Le Gal G, Righini M, Roy PM, et al. Prediction of pulmonary embolism in the emergency department: the revised Geneva score. Ann Intern Med. 2006;144(3):165–71.

187. PIOPED Investigators. Value of the ventilation/perfusion scan in acute pulmonary embolism. Results of the prospective investigation of pulmonary embolism diagnosis (PIOPED). JAMA. 1990;263(20):2753–9.

188. Wells PS, Anderson DR, Rodger M, et al. Derivation of a simple clinical model to categorize patients probability of pulmonary embolism: in- creasing the models utility with the SimpliRED D-dimer. Thromb Haemost. 2000;83(3):416–20.

189. Anderson DR, Kovacs MJ, Dennie C, et al. Use of spiral computed tomography contrast angiography and ultrasonography to exclude the diagnosis of pulmonary embolism in the emergency department. J Emerg Med. 2005;29(4):399–404.

190. Kearon C, Ginsberg JS, Douketis J, et al. An evaluation of D-dimer in the diagnosis of pulmonary embolism: a randomized trial. Ann Intern Med. 2006;144(11):812–21.

191. Sohne M, Kamphuisen PW, van Mierlo PJ, et al. Diagnostic strategy using a modified clinical decision rule and D-dimer test to rule out pulmonary embolism in elderly in- and outpatients. Thromb Haemost. 2005;94(1):206–10.

192. van Belle A, Buller HR, Huisman MV, et al. Effectiveness of managing suspected pulmonary embolism using an algorithm combining clinical probability, D-dimer testing, and computed tomography. JAMA. 2006;295(2):172–9.

193. Wells PS, Anderson DR, Rodger M, et al. Excluding pulmonary embolism at the bedside without diagnostic imaging: management of patients with suspected pulmonary embolism presenting to the emergency department by using a simple clinical model and d-dimer. Ann Intern Med. 2001;135(2):98–107.

194. Rodger MA, Maser E, Stiell I, et al. The interobserver reliability of pretest probability assessment in patients with suspected pulmonary embolism. Thromb Res. 2005;116(2):101–7.

195. Runyon MS, Webb WB, Jones AE, et al. Comparison of the unstructured clinician estimate of pretest probability for pulmonary embolism to the Canadian score and the Charlotte rule: a prospective observational study. Acad Emerg Med. 2005;12(7):587–93.

196. Ghaye B, Szapiro D, Mastora I, et al. Peripheral pulmonary arteries: how far in the lung does multidetector row spiral CT allow analysis? Radiology. 2001;219(3):629–36.

197. Patel S, Kazerooni EA, Cascade PN. Pulmonary embolism: optimization of small pulmonary artery visualization at multi-detector row CT. Radiology. 2003;227(2):455–60.

198. Remy-Jardin M, Remy J, Wattinne L, et al. Central pulmonary thromboembolism: diagnosis with spiral volumetric CT with the single-breath-hold technique: comparison with pulmonary angiography. Radiology. 1992;185(2):381–7.

199. Stein PD, Fowler SE, Goodman LR, et al. Multidetector computed tomography for acute pulmonary embolism. N Engl J Med. 2006;354(22):2317–27.

200. Carrier M, Righini M, Wells PS, et al. Subsegmental pulmonary embolism diagnosed by computed tomography: incidence and clinical implications. A systematic review and meta-analysis of the management outcome studies. J Thromb Haemost. 2010;8(8):1716–22.

201. Stein PD, Goodman LR, Hull RD, et al. Diagnosis and management of isolated subsegmental pulmonary embolism: review and assessment of the options. Clin Appl Thromb Hemost. 2012;18(1):20–6.

202. Goodman LR, Stein PD, Matta F, et al. CT venography and compression sonography are diagnostically equivalent: data from PIOPED II. AJR Am J Roentgenol. 2007;189(5):1071–6.

203. Farrell C, Jones M, Girvin F, et al. Unsuspected pulmonary embolism identified using multidetector computed tomography in hospital outpatients. Clin Radiol. 2010;65(1):1–5.

204. Jia CF, Li YX, Yang ZQ, et al. Prospective evaluation of unsuspected pulmonary embolism on coronary computed tomographic angiography. J Comput Assist Tomogr. 2012;36(2):187–90.

205. Palla A, Rossi G, Falaschi F, et al. Is incidentally detected pulmonary embolism in cancer patients less severe? A case-control study. Cancer Invest. 2012;30(2):131–4.

206. Sahut D'Izarn M, Caumont Prim A, Planquette B, et al. Risk factors and clinical outcome of unsuspected pulmonary embolism in cancer

patients: a case-control study. J Thromb Haemost. 2012;10(10):2032–8.

207. Kearon C, Akl EA, Comerota AJ, et al. Antithrombotic therapy for VTE disease: antithrombotic therapy and prevention of thrombosis, 9th ed: American College of Chest Physicians Evidence-Based Clinical Practice Guidelines. Chest. 2012;141(2 Suppl):e419S–94S.

208. Alderson PO. Scintigraphic evaluation of pulmonary embolism. Eur J Nucl Med. 1987;13(Suppl):S6–10.

209. Bajc M, Neilly JB, Miniati M, Schuemichen C, Meignan M, Jonson B, EANM Committee. EANM guidelines for ventilation/perfusion scintigraphy: part 1. Pulmonary imaging with ventilation/perfusion single photon emission tomography. Eur J Nucl Med Mol Imaging. 2009;36(8):1356–70.

210. Bajc M, Neilly JB, Miniati M, Schuemichen C, Meignan M, Jonson B. EANM guidelines for ventilation/perfusion scintigraphy: part 2. Algorithms and clinical considerations for diagnosis of pulmonary emboli with V/P(SPECT) and MDCT. Eur J Nucl Med Mol Imaging. 2009;36(9):1528–38.

211. Reid JH, Coche EE, Inoue T, et al. Is the lung scan alive and well? Facts and controversies in defining the role of lung scintigraphy for the diagnosis of pulmonary embolism in the era of MDCT. Eur J Nucl Med Mol Imaging. 2009;36(3):505–21.

212. Gottschalk A, Sostman HD, Coleman RE, et al. Ventilation-perfusion scintigraphy in the PIOPED study. Part II. Evaluation of the scintigraphic criteria and interpretations. J Nucl Med. 1993;34(7):1119–26.

213. Sostman HD, Coleman RE, DeLong DM, et al. Evaluation of revised criteria for ventilation-perfusion scintigraphy in patients with suspected pulmonary embolism. Radiology. 1994;193(1):103–7.

214. Bajc M, Olsson B, Palmer J, et al. Ventilation/perfusion SPECT for diagnostics of pulmonary embolism in clinical practice. J Intern Med. 2008;264(4):379–87.

215. Glaser JE, Chamarthy M, Haramati LB, et al. Successful and safe implementation of a trinary interpretation and reporting strategy for V/Q lung scintigraphy. J Nucl Med. 2011;52(10):1508–12.

216. Sostman HD, Stein PD, Gottschalk A, et al. Acute pulmonary embolism: sensitivity and specificity of ventilation-perfusion scintigraphy in PIOPED II study. Radiology. 2008;246(3):941–6.

217. Stein PD, Terrin ML, Gottschalk A, et al. Value of ventilation/perfusion scans vs. perfusion scans alone in acute pulmonary embolism. Am J Cardiol. 1992;69(14):1239–41.

218. Collart JP, Roelants V, Vanpee D, et al. Is a lung perfusion scan obtained by using single photon emission computed tomography able to improve the radionuclide diagnosis of pulmonary embolism? Nucl Med Commun. 2002;23(11):1107–13.

219. Corbus HF, Seitz JP, Larson RK, et al. Diagnostic usefulness of lung SPET in pulmonary thromboembolism: an outcome study. Nucl Med Commun. 1997;18(10):897–906.

220. Reinartz P, Wildberger JE, Schaefer W, et al. Tomographic imaging in the diagnosis of pulmonary embolism: a comparison between V/Q lung scintigraphy in SPECT technique and multislice spiral CT. J Nucl Med. 2004;45(9):1501–8.

221. Gutte H, Mortensen J, Jensen CV, et al. Detection of pulmonary embolism with combined ventilation-perfusion SPECT and low-dose CT: head-to-head comparison with multidetector CT angiography. J Nucl Med. 2009;50(12):1987–92.

222. van Beek EJ, Reekers JA, Batchelor DA, et al. Feasibility, safety and clinical utility of angiography in patients with suspected pulmonary embolism. Eur Radiol. 1996;6(4):415–9.

223. Stein PD, Athanasoulis C, Alavi A, et al. Complications and validity of pulmonary angiography in acute pulmonary embolism. Circulation. 1992;85(2):462–8.

224. Wan S, Quinlan DJ, Agnelli G, et al. Thrombolysis compared with heparin for the initial treatment of pulmonary embolism: a meta-analysis of the randomized controlled trials. Circulation. 2004;110(6):744–9.

225. Diffin DC, Leyendecker JR, Johnson SP, et al. Effect of anatomic distribution of pulmonary emboli on interobserver agreement in the interpretation of pulmonary angiography. AJR Am J Roentgenol. 1998;171(4):1085–9.

226. Stein PD, Henry JW, Gottschalk A. Reassessment of pulmonary angiography for the diagnosis of pulmonary embolism: relation of interpreter agreement to the order of the involved pulmonary arterial branch. Radiology. 1999;210(3):689–91.

227. Zhang Y, Xia H, Wang Y, et al. The rate of missed diagnosis of lower-limb DVT by ultrasound amounts to 50% or so in patients without symptoms of DVT: a meta-analysis [published correction appears in Medicine (Baltimore)]. Medicine (Baltimore). 2019;98(37):e17103. https://doi.org/10.1097/MD.0000000000017103.

228. Aujesky D, Perrier A, Roy PM, Stone RA, Cornuz J, Meyer G, Obrosky DS, Fine MJ. Validation of a clinical prognostic model to identify low-risk patients with pulmonary embolism. J Intern Med. 2007;261:597–604.

229. Barra SN, Paiva L, Providência R, Fernandes A, Marques AL. A review on state-of-the-art data regarding safe early discharge following admission for pulmonary embolism: what do we know? Clin Cardiol. 2013;36:507–15.

230. Barra S, Paiva L, Providência R, Fernandes A, Nascimento J, Marques AL. LR-PED rule: low risk pulmonary embolism decision rule—a new decision score for low risk pulmonary embolism. Thromb Res. 2012;130:327–33.

231. Jiménez D, Aujesky D, Moores L, Gómez V, Lobo JL, Uresandi F, Otero R, Monreal M, Muriel A, Yusen RD, RIETE Investigators. Simplification of the pulmonary embolism severity index for prognostication in patients with acute symptomatic pulmonary embolism. Arch Intern Med. 2010;170:1383–9.

232. Rudski LG, Lai WW, Afilalo J, Hua L, Handschumacher MD, Chandrasekaran K, et al. Guidelines for the echocardiographic assessment of the right heart in adults: a report from the American Society of Echocardiography endorsed by the European Association of Echocardiography, a registered branch of the European Society of Cardiology, and the Canadian Society of Echocardiography. J Am Soc Echocardiogr. 2010;23:685–713.

233. Choi BY, Park DG. Normalization of negative T-wave on electrocardiography and right ventricular dysfunction in patients with an acute pulmonary embolism. Korean J Intern Med. 2012;27:53–9.

234. Golpe R, Castro-Anon O, Perez-de-Llano LA, et al. Electrocardiogram score predicts severity of pulmonary embolism in hemodynamically stable patients. J Hosp Med. 2011;6:285–9.

235. Kukla P, Dlstrokugopolski R, Krupa E, et al. Electrocardiography and prognosis of patients with acute pulmonary embolism. Cardiol J. 2011;18:648–53.

236. Daniel KR, Courtney DM, Kline JA. Assessment of cardiac stress from massive pulmonary embolism with 12-lead ECG. Chest. 2001;120:474–81.

237. Jaff MR, McMurtry MS, Archer SL, et al. Management of massive and submassive pulmonary embolism, iliofemoral deep vein thrombosis, and chronic thromboembolic pulmonary hypertension: a scientific statement from the American Heart Association [published corrections appear in Circulation. 2012;125:e495 and Circulation. 2012;126:e104]. Circulation. 2011;123:1788–830.

238. Hariharan P, Dudzinski DM, Okechukwu I, et al. Association between electrocardiographic findings, right heart strain, and short-term adverse clinical events in patients with acute pulmonary embolism. Clin Cardiol. 2015;38(4):236–42. https://doi.org/10.1002/clc.22383.

239. Kukla P, Długopolski R, Krupa E, et al. The value of ECG parameters in estimating myocardial injury and establishing prognosis in patients with acute pulmonary embolism. Kardiol Pol. 2011;69:933–8.

240. Punukollu G, Gowda RM, Vasavada BC, et al. Role of electrocardiography in identifying right ventricular dysfunction in acute pulmonary embolism. Am J Cardiol. 2005;96:450–2.

241. Douketis JD, Crowther MA, Stanton EB, Ginsberg JS. Elevated cardiac troponin levels in patients with submassive pulmonary embolism. Arch Intern Med. 2002;162(1):79–81. https://doi.org/10.1001/archinte.162.1.79.

242. Andrews J, MacNee W, Murchison J. Measurement of cardiac troponin identifies patients with moderate to large pulmonary emboli and right ventricular strain. Eur Respir J. 2014;44:P2407.

243. Keller K, Beule J, Schulz A, Coldewey M, Dippold W, Balzer JO. Cardiac troponin I for predicting right ventricular dysfunction and intermediate risk in patients with normotensive pulmonary embolism. Neth Heart J. 2015;23(1):55–61. https://doi.org/10.1007/s12471-014-0628-7.

244. Tanindi A, Cemri M. Troponin elevation in conditions other than acute coronary syndromes. Vasc Health Risk Manag. 2011;7:597–603. https://doi.org/10.2147/VHRM.S24509.

245. Sudoh T, Kangawa K, Minamino N, Matsuo H. A new natriuretic peptide in porcine brain. Nature. 1988;332:78–81.

246. Holmes SJ, Espiner EA, Richards AM, Yandle TG, Frampton C. Renal, endocrine, and hemodynamic effects of human brain natriuretic peptide in normal man. J Clin Endocrinol Metab. 1993;76:91–6.

247. Levin ER, Gardner DG, Samson WK. Natriuretic peptides. N Engl J Med. 1998;339:321–8.

248. Yoshimura M, Yasue H, Morita E, Sakaino N, Jougasaki M, Kurose M, et al. Hemodynamic, renal, and hormonal responses to brain natriuretic peptide infusion in patients with congestive heart failure. Circulation. 1991;84:1581–8.

249. Yasue H, Yoshimura M, Sumida H, Kikuta K, Kugiyama K, Jougasaki M, et al. Localization and mechanism of secretion of B-type natriuretic peptide in comparison with those of A-type natriuretic peptide in normal subjects and patients with heart failure. Circulation. 1994;90:195–203.

250. Coutance G, Le Page O, Lo T, Hamon M. Prognostic value of brain natriuretic peptide in acute pulmonary embolism. Crit Care. 2008;12(4):R109. https://doi.org/10.1186/cc6996.

251. Douglas PS, Garcia MJ, Haines DE, Lai WW, Manning WJ, Patel AR, et al. ACCF/ASE/AHA/ASNC/HFSA/HRS/SCAI/SCCM/SCCT/SCMR 2011 appropriate use criteria for echocardiography. J Am Soc Echocardiogr. 2011;24:229–67.

252. Ten Wolde M, Söhne M, Quak E, Mac Gillavry MR, Büller HR. Prognostic value of echocardiographically assessed right ventricular dysfunction in patients with pulmonary embolism. Arch Intern Med. 2004;164:1685–9.

253. McConnell MV, Solomon SD, Rayan ME, Come PC, Goldhaber SZ, Lee RT. Regional right ventricular dysfunction detected by echocardiography in acute pulmonary embolism. Am J Cardiol. 1996;78:469–73.

254. Casazza F, Bongarzoni A, Capozi A, Agostoni O. Regional right ventricular dysfunction in acute pulmonary embolism and right ventricular infarction. Eur J Echocardiogr. 2005;6:11–4.

255. Lopez-Candales A, Eleswarapu A, Shaver J, Edelman K, Gulyasy B, Candales MD. Right ventricular outflow tract spectral signal: a useful marker of right ventricular systolic performance and pulmonary hypertension severity. Eur J Echocardiogr. 2010;11:509–15.

256. Lopez-Candales A, Edelman K, Gulyasy B, Candales MD. Differences in the duration of total ejection between right and left ventricles in chronic pulmonary hypertension. Echocardiography. 2011;28:509–15.

257. López-Candales A, Edelman K. Shape of the right ventricular outflow Doppler envelope and severity of pulmonary hypertension. Eur Heart J Cardiovasc Imaging. 2012;13:309–16.

258. Kurzyna M, Torbicki A, Pruszczyk P, Burakowska B, Fijałkowska A, Kober J, Oniszh K, Kuca P, Tomkowski W, Burakowski J, Wawrzyńska L. Disturbed right ventricular ejection pattern as a new Doppler echocardiographic sign of acute pulmonary embolism. Am J Cardiol. 2002;90(5):507–11.
259. Gorham LW. A study of pulmonary embolism: two the mechanism of death based on a clinical pathological investigation of 100 cases of massive and 285 cases of minor embolism of the pulmonary artery. Arch Intern Med. 1961;108:76–90.
260. Del Guercio LRM, Cohn JDFNR. Pulmonary embolism shock: physiologic basis of a bedside screening test. JAMA. 1960;196:751–6.
261. Urokinase Pulmonary Embolism Trial. Phase 1 results: a cooperative study. JAMA. 1970;214:2163–72.
262. Alpert JS, Smith R, Carlson J, et al. Mortality in patients treated for pulmonary embolism. JAMA. 1976;236:1477–80.
263. Calder KK, Herbert M, Henderson SO. The mortality of untreated pulmonary embolism in emergency department patients. Ann Emerg Med. 2005;45:302–10.
264. Golpe R, Testa-Fernández A, Pérez-de-Llano LA, Castro-Añón O, González-Juanatey C, Pérez-Fernández R, Fariñas MC. Long-term clinical outcome of patients with persistent right ventricle dysfunction or pulmonary hypertension after acute pulmonary embolism. Eur J Echocardiogr. 2011;12:756–61.
265. Lo A, Stewart P, Younger JF, Atherton J, Prasad SB. Usefulness of right ventricular myocardial strain in assessment of response to thrombolytic therapy in acute pulmonary embolism. Eur J Echocardiogr. 2010;11:892–5.
266. McIntyre KM, Sasahara AA. Correlation of pulmonary photoscan and angiogram as measures of the severity of pulmonary embolic involvement. J Nucl Med. 1971;12:732–8.
267. McDonald IG, Hirsh J, Hale GS, et al. Major pulmonary embolism, a correlation of clinical findings, haemodynamics, pulmonary angiography, and pathological physiology. Br Heart J. 1972;34:356–64.
268. Dalen JE, Haynes FW, Hoppin FG, et al. Cardiovascular responses to experimental pulmonary embolism. Am J Cardiol. 1967;20:3–9.
269. McIntyre KM, Sasahara AA. Hemodynamic and ventricular responses to pulmonary embolism. Prog Cardiovasc Dis. 1974;17:175–90.
270. Parker BM, Smith JR. Pulmonary embolism and infarction: a review of the physiologic consequences of pulmonary artery obstruction. Am J Med. 1958;24:402–27.
271. Stein M, Levy SE. Reflex and humoral responses to pulmonary embolism. Prog Cardiovasc Dis. 1974;17:167–74.
272. Malik AB. Pulmonary microembolism. Physiol Rev. 1983;63:1114–207.
273. Alpert JS, Godtfredsen J, Ockene IS, et al. Pulmonary hypertension secondary to minor pulmonary embolism. Chest. 1978;73:795–7.
274. Calvin JE Jr, Baer RW, Glantz SA. Pulmonary artery constriction produces a greater right ventricular dynamic afterload than lung microvascular injury in the open chest dog. Circ Res. 1985;56:40–56.
275. Stein PD, Sabbah HN, Anbe DT, et al. Performance of the failing and nonfailing right ventricle of patients with pulmonary hypertension. Am J Cardiol. 1979;44:1050–5.
276. Calvin JE, Quinn B. Right ventricular pressure overload during acute lung injury: cardiac mechanisms and the pathophysiology of right ventricular systolic dysfunction. J Crit Care. 1989;4:251–65.
277. Calvin JE Jr. Acute right heart failure: pathophysiology, recognition, and pharmacological management. J Cardiothorac Vasc Anesth. 1991;5:507–13.
278. Taylor RR, Covell JW, Sonnenblick EH, et al. Dependence of ventricular distensibility on filling of the opposite ventricle. Am J Physiol. 1967;213:711–8.
279. Stein PD, Fowler SE, Goodman LR, Gottschalk A, Hales CA, Hull RD, Leeper KV Jr, Popovich J Jr, Quinn DA, Sos TA, Sostman HD, Tapson VF, Wakefield TW, Weg JG, Woodard PK, PIOPED II Investigators. Multidetector computed tomography for acute pulmonary embolism. N Engl J Med. 2006;354:2317–27.
280. Martins SR. Pulmonary CT angiography in pulmonary embolism: beyond diagnosis. Rev Port Cardiol. 2012;31:697–9.
281. Apfaltrer P, Bachmann V, Meyer M, Henzler T, Barraza JM, Gruettner J, Walter T, Schoepf UJ, Schoenberg SO, Fink C. Prognostic value of perfusion defect volume at dual energy CTA in patients with pulmonary embolism: correlation with CTA obstruction scores, CT parameters of right ventricular dysfunction and adverse clinical outcome. Eur J Radiol. 2012;81:3592–7.
282. Kang DK, Sun JS, Park KJ, Lim HS. Usefulness of combined assessment with computed tomographic signs of right ventricular dysfunction and cardiac troponin T for risk stratification of acute pulmonary embolism. Am J Cardiol. 2011;108:133–40.
283. Becattini C, Vedovati MC, Agnelli G. Prognostic value of troponins in acute pulmonary embolism: a meta-analysis. Circulation. 2007;116:427–33.
284. Jiménez D, Uresandi F, Otero R, Lobo JL, Monreal M, Martí D, Zamora J, Muriel A, Aujesky D, Yusen RD. Troponin-based risk stratification of patients with acute nonmassive pulmonary embolism: systematic review and metaanalysis. Chest. 2009;136:974–82.
285. Hunt JM, Bull TM. Clinical review of pulmonary embolism: diagnosis, prognosis, and treatment. Med Clin North Am. 2011;95:1203–22.
286. Stergiopoulos K, Bahrainy S, Strachan P, Kort S. Right ventricular strain rate predicts clinical outcomes in patients with acute pulmonary embolism. Acute Card Care. 2011;13:181–8.

287. Jiménez D, Aujesky D, Moores L, Gómez V, Martí D, Briongos S, Monreal M, Barrios V, Konstantinides S, Yusen RD. Combinations of prognostic tools for identification of high-risk normotensive patients with acute symptomatic pulmonary embolism. Thorax. 2011;66:75–81.

288. Bellofiore A, Roldán-Alzate A, Besse M, Kellihan HB, Consigny DW, Francois CJ, Chesler NC. Impact of acute pulmonary embolization on arterial stiffening and right ventricular function in dogs. Ann Biomed Eng. 2013;41:195–204.

289. Champion HC, Michelakis ED, Hassoun PM. Comprehensive invasive and noninvasive approach to the right ventricle-pulmonary circulation unit: state of the art and clinical and research implications. Circulation. 2009;120:992–1007.

290. Kussmaul WG, Noordergraaf A, Laskey WK. Right ventricular-pulmonary arterial interactions. Ann Biomed Eng. 1992;20:63–80.

291. Parmley WW, Tyberg JV, Glantz SA. Cardiac dynamics. Annu Rev Physiol. 1977;39:277–99.

292. Piene H. Pulmonary arterial impedance and right ventricular function. Physiol Rev. 1986;66:606–52.

293. Milnor WR, Bergel DH, Bargainer JD. Hydraulic power associated with pulmonary blood flow and its relation to heart rate. Circ Res. 1966;19:467–80.

294. Piene H, Sund T. Flow and power output of right ventricle facing load with variable input impedance. Am J Physiol. 1979;237:H125–30.

295. O'Rourke MF. Vascular impedance in studies of arterial and cardiac function. Physiol Rev. 1982;62:570–623.

296. Giannitsis E, Muller-Bardorff M, Kurowski V, et al. Independent prognostic value of cardiac troponin T in patients with confirmed pulmonary embolism. Circulation. 2000;102:211–7.

297. Konstantinides S, Geibel A, Olschewski M, et al. Importance of cardiac troponins I and T in risk stratification of patients with acute pulmonary embolism. Circulation. 2002;106:1263–8.

298. Kucher N, Goldhaber SZ. Cardiac biomarkers for risk stratification of patients with acute pulmonary embolism. Circulation. 2003;108:2191–4.

299. Kucher N, Goldhaber SZ. Risk stratification of acute pulmonary embolism. Semin Thromb Hemost. 2006;32:838–47.

300. Meyer T, Binder L, Hruska N, Luthe H, Buchwald AB. Cardiac troponin I elevation in acute pulmonary embolism is associated with right ventricular dysfunction. J Am Coll Cardiol. 2000;36:1632–6.

301. López-Candales A, Edelman K, Candales MD. Right ventricular apical contractility in acute pulmonary embolism: the McConnell sign revisited. Echocardiography. 2010;27:614–20.

302. Platz E, Hassanein AH, Shah A, Goldhaber SZ, Solomon SD. Regional right ventricular strain pattern in patients with acute pulmonary embolism. Echocardiography. 2012;29:464–70.

303. Descotes-Genon V, Chopard R, Morel M, Meneveau N, Schiele F, Bernard Y. Comparison of right ventricular systolic function in patients with low risk and intermediate-to-high risk pulmonary embolism: a two-dimensional strain imaging study. Echocardiography. 2013;30:301–8.

304. López-Candales A, Edelman K. Right ventricular outflow tract systolic excursion: a distinguishing echocardiographic finding in acute pulmonary embolism. Echocardiography. 2013;30(6):649–57.

305. Lopez-Candales A. Marked reduction in the ratio of main right ventricular chamber to outflow tract function in patients with proximal bilateral acute pulmonary embolism. Int J Cardiol. 2013;168(1):592–3.

306. Gorcsan J 3rd, Tanaka H. Echocardiographic assessment of myocardial strain. J Am Coll Cardiol. 2011;58:1401–13.

307. Huang SJ, Orde S. From speckle tracking echocardiography to torsion: research tool today, clinical practice tomorrow. Curr Opin Crit Care. 2013;19:250–7.

308. Amundsen BH, Helle-Valle T, Edvardsen T, Torp H, Crosby J, Lyseggen E, Støylen A, Ihlen H, Lima JA, Smiseth OA, Slørdahl SA. Noninvasive myocardial strain measurement by speckle tracking echocardiography: validation against sonomicrometry and tagged magnetic resonance imaging. J Am Coll Cardiol. 2006;47:789–93.

309. Helle-Valle T, Crosby J, Edvardsen T, Lyseggen E, Amundsen BH, Smith HJ, Rosen BD, Lima JA, Torp H, Ihlen H, Smiseth OA. New noninvasive method for assessment of left ventricular rotation: speckle tracking echocardiography. Circulation. 2005;112:3149–56.

310. López-Candales A, Rajagopalan N, Gulyasy B, Edelman K, Bazaz R. Differential strain and velocity generation along the right ventricular free wall in pulmonary hypertension. Can J Cardiol. 2009;25:73–7.

311. López-Candales A, Dohi K, Bazaz R, Edelman K. Relation of right ventricular free wall mechanical delay to right ventricular dysfunction as determined by tissue Doppler imaging. Am J Cardiol. 2005;96:602–6.

312. López-Candales A, Dohi K, Rajagopalan N, Suffoletto M, Murali S, Gorcsan J 3rd, Edelman K. Right ventricular dyssynchrony in patients with pulmonary hypertension is associated with disease severity and functional class. Cardiovasc Ultrasound. 2005;3(1):23.

313. Rajagopalan N, Dohi K, Simon MA, Suffoletto M, Edelman K, Murali S, López-Candales A. Right ventricular dyssynchrony in heart failure: a tissue Doppler imaging study. J Card Fail. 2006;12:263–7.

314. Dohi K, Onishi K, Gorcsan J 3rd, López-Candales A, Takamura T, Ota S, Yamada N, Ito M. Role of radial strain and displacement imaging to quantify wall motion dyssynchrony in patients with left ventricular mechanical dyssynchrony and chronic right ventricular pressure overload. Am J Cardiol. 2008;101:1206–12.

315. Sugiura E, Dohi K, Onishi K, Takamura T, Tsuji A, Ota S, Yamada N, Nakamura M, Nobori T, Ito M. Reversible right ventricular regional non-

uniformity quantified by speckle-tracking strain imaging in patients with acute pulmonary thromboembolism. J Am Soc Echocardiogr. 2009;22:1353–9.

316. Taccardi B, Lux RL, Ershler PR, et al. Anatomical architecture and electrical activity of the heart. Acta Cardiol. 1997;52:91–105.

317. Torrent-Guasp F, Buckberg GD, Clemente C, et al. The structure and function of the helical heart and its buttress wrapping: I. The normal macroscopic structure of the heart. Semin Thorac Cardiovasc Surg. 2001;134:301–19.

318. Sullivan DM, Watts JA, Kline JA. Biventricular cardiac dysfunction after acute massive pulmonary embolism in the rat. J Appl Physiol. 2001;90:1648–56.

319. Chua JH, Zhou W, Ho JK, Patel NA, Mackensen GB, Mahajan A. Acute right ventricular pressure overload compromises left ventricular function by altering septal strain and rotation. J Appl Physiol. 2013;115:186–93.

320. Ichikawa K, Dohi K, Sugiura E, Sugimoto T, Takamura T, Ogihara Y, Nakajima H, Onishi K, Yamada N, Nakamura M, Nobori T, Ito M. Ventricular function and dyssynchrony quantified by speckle-tracking echocardiography in patients with acute and chronic right ventricular pressure overload. J Am Soc Echocardiogr. 2013;26:483–92.

321. López-Candales A, Bazaz R, Edelman K, Gulyasy B. Altered early left ventricular diastolic wall velocities in pulmonary hypertension: a tissue Doppler study. Echocardiography. 2009;26:1159–66.

322. Egermayer P, Town GI. The clinical significance of pulmonary embolism: uncertainties and implications for treatment: a debate. J Intern Med. 1997;241:5–10.

323. Freiman DG, Suyemoto J, Wessler S. Frequency of pulmonary thromboembolism in man. N Engl J Med. 1965;272:1278–80.

324. Havig O. Deep vein thrombosis and pulmonary embolism: an autopsy study with multiple regression analysis of possible risk factors. Acta Chir Scand. 1977;478(Suppl):1–108.

325. Wagenvoort CA. Pathology of pulmonary thromboembolism. Chest. 1995;107(Suppl):10S–7S.

326. Konstantinides SV, Meyer G, Becattini C, et al. 2019 ESC guidelines for the diagnosis and management of acute pulmonary embolism developed in collaboration with the European Respiratory Society (ERS): the task force for the diagnosis and management of acute pulmonary embolism of the European Society of Cardiology (ESC). Eur Respir J. 2019;54:1901647.

327. Klok FA, Mos IC, Nijkeuter M, et al. Simplification of the revised Geneva score for assessing clinical probability of pulmonary embolism. Arch Intern Med. 2008;168:2131–6.

328. Kline JA, Mitchell AM, Kabrhel C, et al. Clinical criteria to prevent unnecessary diagnostic testing in emergency department patients with suspected pulmonary embolism. J Thromb Haemost. 2004;2:1247–55.

329. Geersing GJ, Janssen KJ, Oudega R, et al. Excluding venous thromboembolism using point of care D-dimer tests in outpatients: a diagnostic meta-analysis. BMJ. 2009;339:b2990.

330. Elias A, Mallett S, Daoud-Elias M, et al. Prognostic models in acute pulmonary embolism: a systematic review and meta-analysis. BMJ Open. 2016;6:e010324.

331. Kohn CG, Mearns ES, Parker MW, et al. Prognostic accuracy of clinical prediction rules for early post-pulmonary embolism all-cause mortality: a bivariate meta-analysis. Chest. 2015;147:1043–62.

332. Guerin L, Couturaud F, Parent F, et al. Prevalence of chronic thromboembolic pulmonary hypertension after acute pulmonary embolism. Prevalence of CTEPH after pulmonary embolism. Thromb Haemost. 2014;112:598–605.

333. Galie N, Humbert M, Vachiery JL, Gibbs S, et al., ESC Scientific Document Group. 2015 ESC/ERS guidelines for the diagnosis and treatment of pulmonary hypertension: the joint task force for the diagnosis and treatment of pulmonary hypertension of the European Society of Cardiology (ESC) and the European Respiratory Society (ERS): Endorsed by: Association for European Paediatric and Congenital Cardiology (AEPC), International Society for Heart and Lung Transplantation (ISHLT). Eur Heart J. 2016;37:67–119.

334. Vonk Noordegraaf A, Marcus JT, Roseboom B, Postmus PE, Faes TJ, de Vries PM. The effect of right ventricular hypertrophy on left ventricular ejection fraction in pulmonary emphysema. Chest. 1997;112:640–5.

335. Pieralli F, Olivotto I, Vanni S, Conti A, Camaiti A, Targioni G, Grifoni S, Berni G. Usefulness of bedside testing for brain natriuretic peptide to identify right ventricular dysfunction and outcome in normotensive patients with acute pulmonary embolism. Am J Cardiol. 2006;97:1386–90.

336. Kostrubiec M, Pruszczyk P, Bochowicz A, Pacho R, Szulc M, Kaczynska A, Styczynski G, Kuch-Wocial A, Abramczyk P, Bartoszewicz Z, Berent H, Kuczynska K. Biomarker-based risk assessment model in acute pulmonary embolism. Eur Heart J. 2005;26:2166–72.

337. Ghuysen A, Ghaye B, Willems V, Lambermont B, Gerard P, Dondelinger RF, D'Orio V. Computed tomographic pulmonary angiography and prognostic significance in patients with acute pulmonary embolism. Thorax. 2005;60:956–61.

338. Tulevski II, ten Wolde M, van Veldhuisen DJ, Mulder JW, van der Wall EE, Büller HR, Mulder BJ. Combined utility of brain natriuretic peptide and cardiac troponin T may improve rapid triage and risk stratification in normotensive patients with pulmonary embolism. Int J Cardiol. 2007;116:161–6.

339. Tulevski II, Hirsch A, Sanson BJ, Romkcs II, van der Wall EE, van Veldhuisen DJ, Büller HR, Mulder BJ. Increased brain natriuretic peptide as a marker for right ventricular dysfunction in acute pulmonary embolism. Thromb Haemost. 2001;86:1193–6.

340. Vieillard-Baron A, Page B, Augarde R, Prin S, Qanadli S, Beauchet A, Dubourg O, Jardin F. Acute cor pulmonale in massive pulmonary embolism: incidence, echocardiographic pattern, clinical implications and recovery rate. Intensive Care Med. 2001;27:1481–6.

341. Kucher N, Printzen G, Doernhoefer T, Windecker S, Meier B, Hess OM. Low pro-brain natriuretic peptide levels predict benign clinical outcome in acute pulmonary embolism. Circulation. 2003;107:1576–8.

342. ten Wolde M, Tulevski II, Mulder JW, Sohne M, Boomsma F, Mulder BJ, Buller HR. Brain natriuretic peptide as a predictor of adverse outcome in patients with pulmonary embolism. Circulation. 2003;107:2082–4.

343. Pruszczyk P, Kostrubiec M, Bochowicz A, Styczynski G, Szulc M, Kurzyna M, Fijalkowska A, Kuch-Wocial A, Chlewicka I, Torbicki A. N-terminal pro-brain natriuretic peptide in patients with acute pulmonary embolism. Eur Respir J. 2003;22:649–53.

344. Moser KM, Auger WR, Fedullo PF. Chronic major-vessel thromboembolic pulmonary hypertension. Circulation. 1990;81:1735–43.

345. Matthews DT, Hemnes AR. Current concepts in the pathogenesis of chronic thromboembolic pulmonary hypertension. Pulm Circ. 2016;6:145–54.

346. Moser KM, Bloor CM. Pulmonary vascular lesions occurring in patients with chronic major vessel thromboembolic pulmonary hypertension. Chest. 1993;103:685–92.

347. Galiè N, Kim NH. Pulmonary microvascular disease in chronic thromboembolic pulmonary hypertension. Proc Am Thorac Soc. 2006;3:571–6.

348. Pepke-Zaba J, Delcroix M, Lang I, et al. Chronic Thromboembolic Pulmonary Hypertension (CTEPH): results from an international prospective registry. Circulation. 2011;124:1973–81.

349. Ende-Verhaar YM, Cannegieter SC, Vonk Noordegraaf A, et al. Incidence of chronic thromboembolic pulmonary hypertension after acute pulmonary embolism: a contemporary view of the published literature. Eur Respir J. 2017;49:1601972.

350. Sanchez O, Helley D, Couchon S, et al. Perfusion defects after pulmonary embolism: risk factors and clinical significance. J Thromb Haemost. 2010;8:1248–55.

351. Pesavento R, Filippi L, Palla A, et al. Impact of residual pulmonary obstruction on the long-term outcome of patients with pulmonary embolism. Eur Respir J. 2017;49:1601980.

352. Heit JA, Spencer FA, White RH. The epidemiology of venous thromboembolism. J Thromb Thrombolysis. 2016;41:3–14.

353. Pengo V, Lensing AWA, Prins MH, et al. Incidence of chronic thromboembolic pulmonary hypertension after pulmonary embolism. N Engl J Med. 2004;350:2257–64.

354. Becattini C, Agnelli G, Pesavento R, et al. Incidence of chronic thromboembolic pulmonary hypertension after a first episode of pulmonary embolism. Chest. 2006;130:172–5.

355. Klok FA, van Kralingen KW, van Dijk AP, et al. Prospective cardiopulmonary screening program to detect chronic thromboembolic pulmonary hypertension in patients after acute pulmonary embolism. Haematologica. 2010;95:970–5.

356. Dentali F, Donadini M, Gianni M, et al. Incidence of chronic pulmonary hypertension in patients with previous pulmonary embolism. Thromb Res. 2009;124:256–8.

357. Klok FA, Dzikowska-Diduch O, Kostrubiec M, et al. Derivation of a clinical prediction score for chronic thromboembolic pulmonary hypertension after acute pulmonary embolism. J Thromb Haemost. 2016;14:121–8.

358. Ribeiro A, Lindmarker P, Johnsson H, et al. Pulmonary embolism: one-year follow-up with echocardiography doppler and five-year survival analysis. Circulation. 1999;99:1325–30.

359. Bonderman D, Wilkens H, Wakounig S, et al. Risk factors for chronic thromboembolic pulmonary hypertension. Eur Respir J. 2009;33:325–31.

360. Klok FA, Barco S, Konstantinides SV, et al. Determinants of diagnostic delay in chronic thromboembolic pulmonary hypertension: results from the European CTEPH Registry. Eur Respir J. 2018;52:1801687.

361. Simonneau G, Montani D, Celermajer DS, et al. Haemodynamic definitions and updated clinical classification of pulmonary hypertension. Eur Respir J. 2018;53:1801913.

362. Papamatheakis GD, Poch DS, Fernandes TM, et al. Chronic thromboembolic pulmonary hypertension. J Am Coll Cardiol. 2020;76:2155–69.

363. Ryan KL, Fedullo PF, Davis GB, et al. Perfusion scan findings understate the severity of angiographic and hemodynamic compromise in chronic thromboembolic pulmonary hypertension. Chest. 1988;93:1180–5.

364. He J, Fang W, Lv B, et al. Diagnosis of chronic thromboembolic pulmonary hypertension: comparison of ventilation/perfusion scanning and multidetector computed tomography pulmonary angiography with pulmonary angiography. Nucl Med Commun. 2012;33:459–63.

365. Sugiura T, Tanabe N, Matsuura Y, et al. Role of 320-slice CT imaging in the diagnostic workup of patients with chronic thromboembolic pulmonary hypertension. Chest. 2013;143:1070–7.

366. Rogberg AN, Gopalan D, Westerlund E, et al. Do radiologists detect chronic thromboembolic disease on computed tomography. Acta Radiol. 2019;60:1576–83.

367. Hoeper MM, Madani M, Nakanishi N, et al. Chronic thromboembolic pulmonary hypertension. Lancet Respir Med. 2014;2:573–82.

Right Ventricular Cardiomyopathies

15

Riccardo Bariani, Giulia Mattesi, Alberto Cipriani, and Barbara Bauce

Even if the presence of a cardiomyopathy involving the right ventricle (RV) usually identifies mainly a specific cardiac disease initially called "arrhythmogenic right ventricular cardiomyopathy (ARVC)" and recently renamed "arrhythmogenic cardiomyopathy," it is important to emphasize that myocardial insults of various etiologies may involve the RV and lead to structural and functional abnormalities.

Thus, in this chapter besides describing in detail the pathologic basis and the clinical feature of AC, we also briefly analyze RV cardiomyopathic involvement of other cardiac or systemic diseases.

Arrhythmogenic Cardiomyopathy

Arrhythmogenic cardiomyopathy (AC) is an inherited form of heart disease characterized pathologically by myocardial necrosis with fibrofatty replacement and clinically by ventricular arrhythmias and impairment of ventricular systolic function [1, 2].

R. Bariani · G. Mattesi · A. Cipriani · B. Bauce (✉)
Department of Cardiac, Thoracic, Vascular Sciences and Public Health, University of Padua, Padua, Italy

Historical Notes and First Clinical Descriptions

The first historical description of the condition can be found in the book *De Motu Cordis et Aneurysmatibus*, published in 1736 by Giovanni Maria Lancisi, who described a large family with recurrence of heart failure and sudden death with presence on autopsy of RV aneurysms [3].

In 1961, Dalla Volta described a series of patients with a dilated right ventricle of nonischemic origin and in whom cardiac catheterization demonstrated the presence of auricularization (strong right atrial contraction) of the right ventricle pressure curve [4].

The first complete clinical description of the disease was done in 1982 by Marcus who reported a series of 24 adult patients with recurrent episodes of ventricular tachycardia with left bundle branch block morphology, inverted T waves on the right precordial leads at electrocardiogram (ECG), and RV dilatation [5]. Histology examination documented the presence of extensive substitution of the RV myocardium with fatty and fibrous tissue. Since that moment on, the disease has been called both "arrhythmogenic right ventricular dysplasia" or "arrhythmogenic right ventricular cardiomyopathy."

Few years later Thiene reported detailed pathologic features of the disease, consisting of myocyte necrosis with fibro-fatty substitution, and identified this disease as an important cause of sudden cardiac death (SCD) in young subjects, with particular regard to athletes [6].

It is noteworthy that initially AC was hypothesized to be a result of a congenital defect of myocardial development, while in the following years the description of familial recurrence was in favor of a genetic origin [7].

Epidemiology

The AC prevalence is difficult to estimate due to the frequent misdiagnoses, but it reasonably ranges from 1:1000 to 1:5000 [2, 8]. While in the past AC was considered to be an endemic disease in North East Italy ("Venetian disease"), now its presence is well recognized in different ethnicities [9]. The disease usually becomes clinically overt in the second–fourth decades of life and males result to be more frequently affected compared to females (up to 3:1) [8, 9]. Nonetheless, the disease is rarely diagnosed before puberty.

Pathological Findings

The AC pathologic basis consists of myocardial ventricular atrophy followed by fibro-fatty tissue replacement; this process is progressive, starting from the epicardium and then extending to the endocardium, eventually becoming transmural [10, 11] (Fig. 15.1). The progression of the pathologic process can lead to wall thinning and aneurysms, typically located at the inferior, apical, and infundibular walls of the RV (the so-called triangle of dysplasia, the hallmark of AC). Although in the original description the disease was characterized by an exclusive or at least predominant RV involvement, in the last years the improvement of imaging techniques and in particular the introduction of cardiac magnetic resonance (CMR) with contrast agent injection have demonstrated that the left ventricle (LV) is frequently involved. For this reason the current phenotypic classification of the disease considers the presence of three variants: "right dominant," characterized by the predominant RV involvement, with no or minor LV

abnormalities; "biventricular" with a parallel involvement of the RV and LV; and "left dominant" (also referred to as "arrhythmogenic left ventricular cardiomyopathy: ALVC") characterized by a predominant LV involvement, with no or minor RV abnormalities [12].

This fact has led over the last few years to use the broader term of "arrhythmogenic cardiomyopathy," which includes all these phenotypic expressions [1, 13].

In AC patients histological examination reveals the presence of islands of surviving myocytes interspersed with fibrous and fatty tissue. Fatty infiltration, that in original descriptions was one of the milestones of the disease histologic feature, is now not considered anymore a sufficient morphologic hallmark of the disease, as a replacement-type fibrosis and myocyte degenerative changes should always be identified [2, 14].

Genetic Background

Since the first description, the presence of an inheritable pattern of the disease with familial recurrence has been demonstrated. In addition, it became evident that in the majority of cases the disease was inherited through an autosomal dominant transmission with incomplete penetrance and variable expressivity [1]. Notably, in 1986 a disease variant characterized by the association between AC and palmoplantar keratoderma/woolly hair (cardiocutaneous syndrome) was described in Naxos Island of Greek and named Naxos syndrome [15]. Differently from isolated AC, Naxos syndrome is inherited in an autosomal recessive manner with full penetrance. In 2000 a deletion in desmosomal gene plakoglobin was identified as the underlying genetic cause of ACM [16].

Few years later, mutations in other genes encoding for main components of the desmosome were found to be linked to AC [17].

Thus, it has become evident that abnormalities in desmosome structure have a key role in AC pathogenesis and for this reason AC is now considered to be mainly a "disease of the desmosome."

Desmosomes are complex structures consisting of proteins and are responsible for cell adhe-

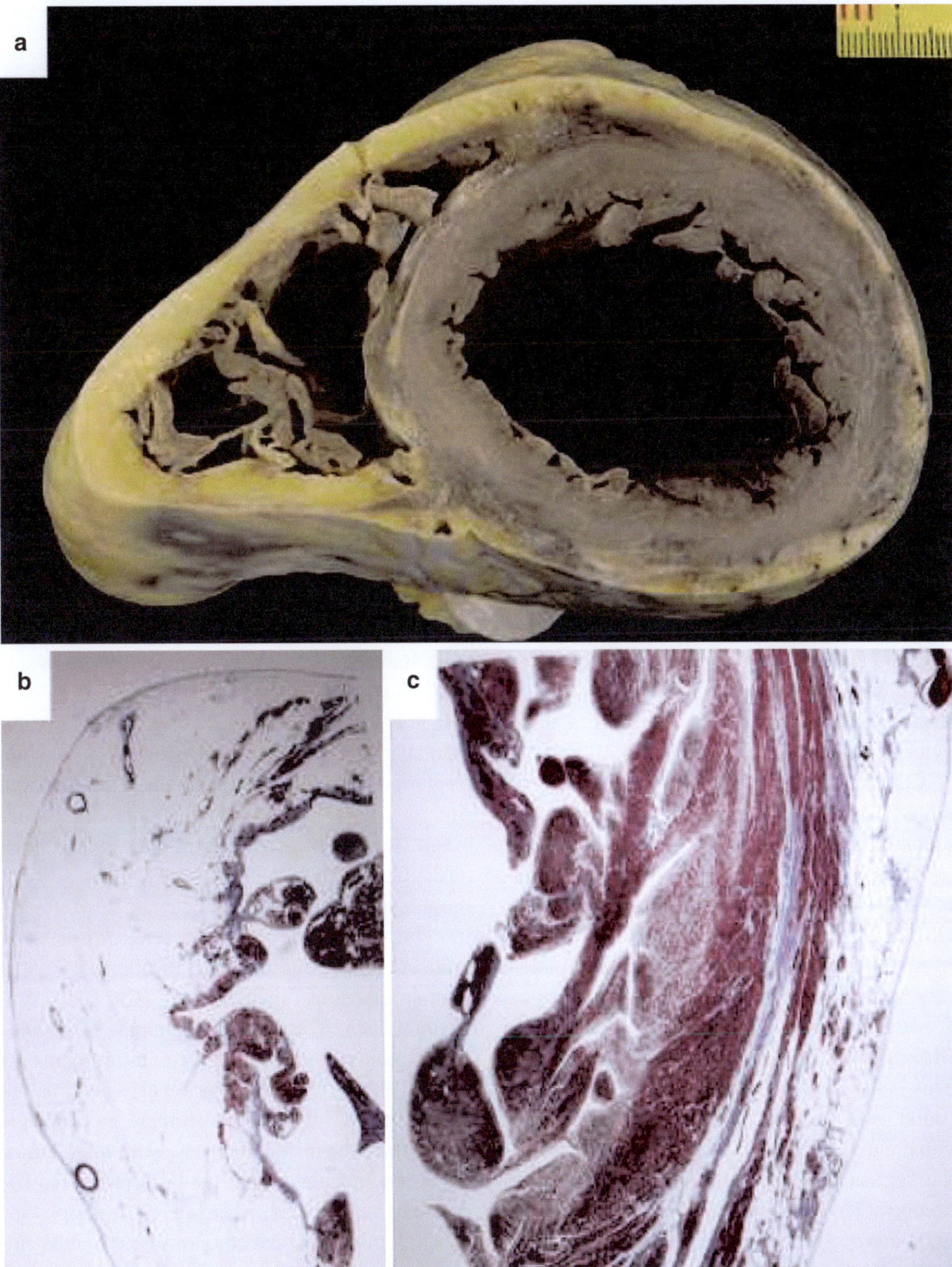

Fig. 15.1 Sudden death in AC patient 30 years after his clinical presentation with chest pain. At autopsy, the heart in cross section reveals diffuse biventricular involvement (**a**) with transmural fibro-fatty replacement of the RV free wall (**b**, trichrome staining ×3) and subepicardial mid-mural involvement of the LV free wall (**c**, trichrome stain-ing ×3). *AC* arrhythmogenic cardiomyopathy, *LV* left ventricle, *RV* right ventricle. (Reproduced form Bariani R et al., "'Hot phase' clinical presentation in arrhythmogenic cardiomyopathy". EP Eur 2020, under licence n. 5007620151917)

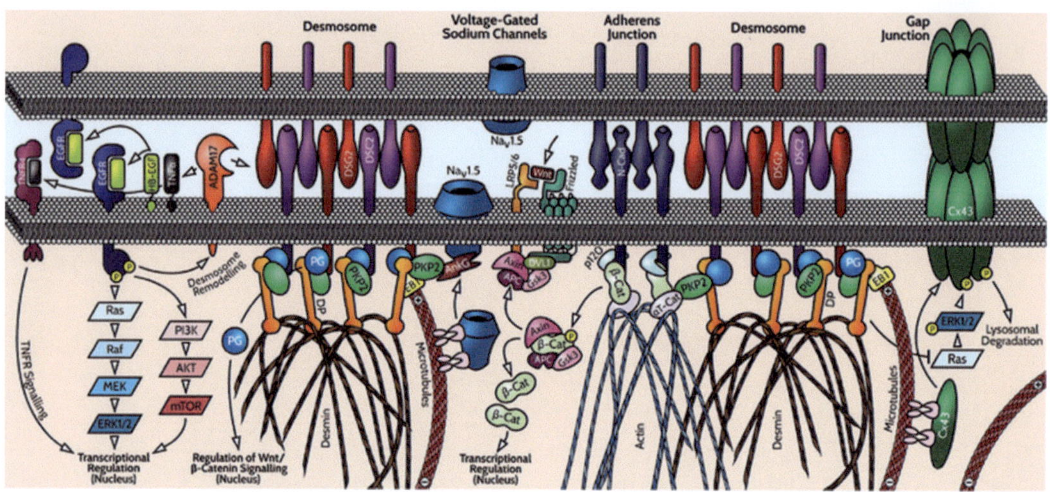

Fig. 15.2 Schematic representation of the complex integration of mechanical and electrochemical signaling at cardiac intercalated discs and it highlights the proposed remodeling of desmosomes, gap junctions, and ion channels in arrhythmogenic cardiomyopathy. (Reproduced under license (n. 5014280291051) from Elliott PM, Anastasakis A, Asimaki A, et al. Definition and treatment of arrhythmogenic cardiomyopathy: an updated expert panel report. Eur J Heart Fail. 2019;21(8):955–964. doi:https://doi.org/10.1002/ejhf.1534)

sion and signaling. One important function is to tether adjacent cells mechanically by joining their intermediate filaments to create a unified cytoskeletal network [1, 2] (Fig. 15.2).

Genetic studies demonstrated that approximately 30–50% of AC patients carry a pathogenic mutation in a desmosome gene.

The most frequent gene found in AC patients is PKP2 (19–46%) followed by DSP (1–16%), DSG2 (2.5–10%), DSC2 (1–8%), and JUP (1%). Moreover, approximately 10–25% of AC patients carry compound mutations.

Plakophilin 2 (PKP-2)

This is the most frequently mutated gene that is found in AC patients. The presence of heterozygous mutations in this gene is usually linked to the "classical" form of the disease with a predominant RV involvement. The majority of mutations have been identified in the C-terminal portion of the protein [18].

Desmoplakin (DSP)

Several mutations involving this gene have been identified so far, often leading to the synthesis of a truncated protein at the N-terminal or C-terminal side. Interestingly, these mutations can have different phenotypic expressions: if mutation involves N-terminal portion, the resulting phenotype is a classic form of AC with autosomal dominant transmission [19] while mutations on the C-terminal end (the one that interacts with intermediate filaments) are usually expressed with predominant LV involvement (ALVC) [19, 20]. Finally, the presence of a homozygous mutation can be characterized phenotypically by biventricular AC forms with almost exclusively fibrous infiltration associated with cutaneous involvement (Carvajal syndrome) [21]. The different clinical AC phenotypes linked to different protein domains of desmoplakin (N- or C-terminal) suggest the presence of distinct molecular mechanisms underlying the different disease variants. Thus, it has been speculated that the left-dominant variant may be secondary to an altered desmoplakin-desmin linkage, which compromises the integrity of the cytoskeleton in cardiomyocyte while an alteration in the relationship between desmoplakin and other components of desmosome would cause a classical disease phenotype [20]. Recently, a study compared clinical data of patients with truncating mutations in DSP and PKP-2 genes [22]. Authors concluded that LV involvement was exclusively present in patients with DSP mutations, which also had a preserved systolic function of both ventricles compared to PKP-2 patients. At CMR these patients frequently showed LGE on the LV, mainly located in lower and inferoseptal segments. Of note a frequent positive history of chest pain episodes in DSP patients was reported, both probands and family members; it has also been noted that acute episodes of myocardial damage can occur even in the presence of normal systolic function [22].

Desmoglein 2 (DSG-2)

Nine different mutations regarding this gene are currently known and are mainly located in the N-terminal region, responsible for a classical AC phenotype, even if in some cases a phenotypic overlap with dilated cardiomyopathy (DCM) has been reported [23].

Desmocollin 2 (DSC-2)

Mutations of this gene lead to premature truncation of desmocollin protein, with loss of its normal function, and they are associated with right-dominant forms. Both autosomal recessive and dominant transmission are reported [24].

Plakoglobin (JUP)

Deletion at the C-terminal end of this gene leads to formation of a truncated protein. Homozygous mutations are associated with Naxos cardio-cutaneous syndrome, with autosomal recessive transmission, while heterozygous mutations are expressed with only cardiac ventricular involvement [25].

Although less frequently found, mutations in non-desmosomal genes have also been linked to AC: desmin (DES), filamin C (FLNC), trans-membrane protein 43 (TMEM-43), lamin A/C (LMNA), titin (TTN), phospholamban (PLN), α-T-catenin (CTNNA-3), cadherin-2 (CDH2), transforming growth factor-β3 (TGF-β3), ryanodine receptor 2 (RYR2), and Na$_v$1.5 (SCN5A).

α-T-Catenin (CTNNA3)

This protein interacts with PKP-2 in the intercalated disc. Mutations in this gene lead to a decreased binding capacity to desmosomal components, resulting in impaired intercellular adhesion function. This form is usually characterized by incomplete penetrance [26].

Cadherin-2 (CDH2)

It is an integral glycoprotein that mediates cell adhesion in the presence of calcium. The intracellular domain is connected to actin filaments by catenins. Recently, in the worldwide cohort of patients affected by AC, previously negative at the genetic examination, mutations in CDH2 were detected. Moreover, these patients had an increased risk of ventricular arrhythmias, while evolution toward heart failure is rare [27].

Laminin (LMNA)

It is a nuclear matrix protein whose mutations are expressed with a wide phenotypic variety that may, although rarely, include cardiac involvement with an AC phenotype [28]. It is most frequently found in severe forms of the disease, with a dilated phenotype and high risk of sudden cardiac death [29].

Desmin (DES)

It is an intermediate filament protein that is essential for the organization of the cytoskeleton and structural maintenance of cardiomyocytes. Mutations in this gene, which often have complete penetrance, cause a group of skeletal myopathies associated with conduction blocks and cardiomyopathy, associated with a dilated or restrictive phenotype, and sometimes an AC forms [30]. It is interesting to underline that recently a mutation of this gene, compromising the binding between desmin and desmoplakin, has been described in AC subjects with a predominant and severe involvement of the LV [31].

Transmembrane Protein 43 (TMEM-43)

This is a nuclear protein that interacts with several other proteins in nucleus and with various transcription factors and it is reported to be responsible for a severe, full-penetrance phenotype of AC associated with a high risk of SCD [32].

Titin (TTN)

This giant protein is an important constituent of sarcomeres and one of the main pathogenic genes in cardiomyopathies with hypertrophic and dilated phenotype. A possible correlation between TTN and AC has been hypothesized considering its direct and close contact with intercalary discs. The AC phenotype linked to titin mutations is characterized by a biventricular involvement with high risk of heart failure, presence of arrhythmias (both supraventricular tachycardia and ventricular arrhythmias) and conduction blocks, configuring an "overlap syndrome" between different cardiomyopathies [33].

Filamin C (FLNC)

Filamins are a family of proteins that interconnect actin filaments, forming a network, and anchor membrane-associated proteins to the cytoskeleton, thus contributing both to structural stability and to signal transduction from cell membrane. FLNC is associated with sarcomere disc and mutations in the FLNC gene and mutations have been found in skeletal muscle myopathies and in dilated and restrictive cardiomyopathies. Truncated mutations of the FLNC gene have been associated with left-dominant forms of AC, with high prevalence of ventricular arrhythmias and signs of fibrosis on CMR and/or histological examination [34].

Ryanodine Receptor 2 (RYR2)

This was the first non-desmosomal gene to be described as associated with AC. RYR2 encodes for the cardiac ryanodine receptor, an important channel that allows calcium ions to pass from the sarcoplasmic reticulum to the cytoplasm during cardiac systole. This gene is usually associated with a primary nonstructural cardiomyopathy (catecholaminergic polymorphic ventricular tachycardia), but some mutations, probably due to a different molecular mechanism, are expressed with an AC phenotype characterized by frequent exercise-induced arrhythmias [35, 36].

Na$_v$1.5 (SCNA5)

Voltage-dependent sodium channels play a central role in the creation and propagation of the action potential through cardiomyocytes. Mutations in SCNA5 gene, which encodes for the pore-forming subunit of the Na$^+$ channel, have been associated with several arrhythmic diseases, including Brugada, long QT, and sick sinus node syndromes. They have also been found in a small percentage of AC patients, associated with an elongated QRS, but its role as disease gene has still to be elucidated [37].

Phospholamban (PLN)

This is a transmembrane protein of the sarcoplasmic reticulum involved in calcium transport by inhibiting the activity of the SERCA2 (sarcoplasmic/endoplasmic reticulum calcium ATPase) pump. Mutations in this gene are associated with restrictive, dilated, and arrhythmogenic cardiomyopathies; in the latter, a particularly severe phenotype is frequently found, with biventricular involvement and a peculiar electrocardiographic pattern (severe reduction of QRS voltages in limb leads) [38]. In a mouse model it was shown that a mutation in the PLN gene (Arg14del) leads to a high risk of developing DCM or AC with heart failure [39].

In the last 10 years, an increasing number of evidence and advances in molecular research have led to a change in the etiology of AC. From the initial idea of a monogenic disease, recent findings suggest rather a complex genetic condition, in which the phenotype is determined by the interaction of multiple genetic and environmental factors [1, 2]. The frequency of compound and digenic heterozygosity is reported to be 10–25% of cases depending on the study population. Noteworthy, genotype-phenotype correlation studies have shown that a higher mutational load correlates with an unfavorable clinical course, a higher risk of SCD, and frequent biventricular involvement [40–42].

Clinical Features and Natural History

In AC the presence of fibro-fatty tissue leads both to morphological ventricular abnormalities and circuits that constitute the anatomic basis of reentry ventricular arrhythmias. The diagnosis of the disease relies on the demonstration of anamnestic, clinical, morphological, and electrophysiological parameters which can be achieved from different instrumental tools. The phenotypic aspects of AC can variate in a considerable way, ranging from asymptomatic family members with mild forms of the disease to symptomatic patients who experienced life-threatening ventricular arrhythmias or refractory heart failure [1]. In affected families the presence of carriers of disease gene mutations has been demonstrated who do not show any signs of the disease (the so-called healthy carriers). The most common clinical presentation consists of arrhythmic symptoms such as palpitations, syncopal episodes, or cardiac arrest; unfortunately, SCD can be the first clinical manifestation of the disease in previously asymptomatic individuals, especially in the young and in competitive athletes [43, 44]. Classically, different clinical phases of the disease have been identified: (1) the initial "concealed phase" with absence of overt ventricular structural abnormalities, with or without minor ventricular arrhythmias; (2) the second phase of "clinically overt disease" characterized by the onset of ventricular arrhythmias and presence of ventricular functional and structural abnormalities; (3) the third phase that is due to progression of ventricular muscle disease leading to RV impairment with RV failure and relatively preserved LV function; and (4) the fourth phase "end stage" with biventricular pump failure. The prognosis in patients affected with AC is related to the degree of electric instability and of ventricular muscle disease. The overall mortality rate varies in literature, due to the different patients' selection. In a study on 37 AC families with a mean follow-up of 8.5 years, a mortality of 0.08% per year was found [8], while in a series of 61 AC patients with a mean follow-up of 4.6 years the mortality rate was estimated to be of 4% per year [45]. This high variability is probably in relation to the different populations and reflects the wide spectrum of AC clinical phenotype [2].

Sports Activity and Arrhythmogenic Cardiomyopathy

James et al. first reported in humans that a history of intense exercise was more often associated with desmosomal gene mutation carriers developing the disease and patients with overt AC suffering from major ventricular arrhythmias [46]. From then on, many other studies [47–53] confirmed that sports activity, especially if prolonged, promotes the development of AC in genotype-positive/phenotype-negative patients, deteriorates ventricular function in patients with overt AC, triggers ventricular arrhythmias, and increases the likelihood of ICD interventions. Indeed, the physical activity generates a mechanical stress at the level of a previously genetically impaired cell-cell adhesion, thus promoting myocyte death. In particular, Ruwald et al. showed that participation in competitive sport was associated with an absolute risk of potentially lethal arrhythmic events of 61% at 40 years of age in AC patients [49]. Sawant et al. and Lie et al. reported more severe RV dysfunction, LV dysfunction, and heart failure when endurance training was carried on [47, 50]. Animal studies demonstrated that in heterozygous plakoglobin-deficient (JUP+/−) mice endurance training (daily swimming) promoted the development of RV abnormalities such as dilatation and dysfunction and ventricular arrhythmias [54]. Moreover, the effect of endurance training in enhancing RV abnormalities was demonstrated in a mouse model overexpressing a nonsense plakophilin-2 (PKP2) gene mutation after adeno-associated virus injection [55]. Conversely, the risk of VAs and mortality both in AC patients and genotype-positive relatives can be reduced by lowering exercise [8, 49, 50]. Thus, on the one hand, preclinical genetic testing among asymptomatic gene carriers with the aim to educate about lifestyle changes can prevent the development of the disease in this category. On the other hand, the identification of early stages of the disease by preparticipation screening and disqualification from competitive sports activity may prevent disease progression and fatal arrhythmias [56]. Accordingly, both European and American guidelines recommend restriction from competitive sports activity of AC patients and at-risk relatives as a measure aimed to reduce the risk of SCD [57, 58]. However, considering the general physical and mental health benefits related to exercise, ESC guidelines allow a maximum of

150 min of low-moderate-intensity (3–6 metabolic 292 equivalent) exercise per week in all affected and at-risk subjects [57].

Disease Diagnosis

AC diagnosis is multiparametric as a single specific diagnostic marker does not exist, due to the wide clinical phenotype and a clinical overlap with other cardiac diseases. In 1994, an international task force proposed a diagnostic scoring system with major and minor criteria with the aim to uniform the diagnosis [59]. Definite AC diagnosis included two major criteria or one major and two minor criteria or four minor criteria from different categories. In the following years, clinical studies demonstrated these criteria to be highly specific but lacked sensitivity for the diagnosis in mild forms of the disease. For this reason, diagnostic criteria were revised in 2010, with addition of quantitative measurement of imaging tools and of new ECG parameters. Moreover, genetic analysis results entered among diagnostic criteria [60]. In 2019 an International Expert Report provided an extensive critical review of the clinical performance of AC ongoing diagnostic criteria with the aim to identify potential areas of improvement [60]. Major limitations of the 2010 Task Force criteria were considered to be the incomplete understanding of the genetic background of the disease and the absence of specific criteria for the diagnosis of the broader spectrum of the disease phenotypes, including ALVC forms [61, 62]. Moreover, 2010 criteria did not consider tissue characterization findings provided by CMR which offer the possibility to identify myocardial fibrosis and play a key role in the accurate diagnosis of the LV phenotype. For these reasons in 2020 a modification of diagnostic criteria, called "Padua criteria" (Table 15.1) which included also CMR findings and presence of ALVC forms, was proposed [13].

Table 15.1 "Padua criteria" for diagnosis of arrhythmogenic cardiomyopathy

Category	Right ventricle (upgraded 2010 ITF diagnostic criteria)	Left ventricle (new diagnostic criteria)
I. Morpho-functional ventricular abnormalities	By echocardiography, CMR, or angiography: *Major* • Regional RV akinesia, dyskinesia, or bulging, plus one of the following: – Global RV dilatation (increase of RV EDV according to the imaging test-specific nomograms) – Global RV systolic dysfunction (reduction of RV EF according to the imaging test-specific nomograms) *Minor* • Regional RV akinesia, dyskinesia, or aneurysm of RV free wall	By echocardiography, CMR, or angiography: *Minor* • Global LV systolic dysfunction (depression of LV EF or reduction of echocardiographic global longitudinal strain), with or without LV dilatation (increase of LV EDV according to the imaging test-specific nomograms for age, sex, and BSA) *Minor* • Regional LV hypokinesia or akinesia of LV free wall, septum, or both
II. Structural myocardial abnormalities	By CE-CMR: *Major* • Transmural LGE (stria pattern) of ≥1 RV region(s) (inlet, outlet, and apex in two orthogonal views) By EMB (limited indications): *Major* • Fibrous replacement of the myocardium in ≥1 sample, with or without fatty tissue	By CE-CMR: *Major* • LV LGE (stria pattern) of ≥1 bull's eye segment(s) (in two orthogonal views) of the free wall (subepicardial or midmyocardial), septum, or both (excluding septal junctional LGE)

Table 15.1 (continued)

Category	Right ventricle (upgraded 2010 ITF diagnostic criteria)	Left ventricle (new diagnostic criteria)
III. Repolarization abnormalities	*Major* • Inverted T waves in right precordial leads (V1, V2, and V3) or beyond in individuals with complete pubertal development (in the absence of complete RBBB) *Minor* • Inverted T waves in leads V1 and V2 in individuals with completed pubertal development (in the absence of complete RBBB) • Inverted T waves in V1, V2, V3, and V4 in individuals with completed pubertal development in the presence of complete RBBB	*Minor* • Inverted T waves in left precordial leads (V4–V6) (in the absence of complete LBBB)
IV. Depolarization abnormalities	*Minor* • Epsilon wave (reproducible low-amplitude signals between the end of QRS complex and the onset of the T wave) in the right precordial leads (V1–V3) • Terminal activation duration of QRS $\geq$55 ms measured from the nadir of the S wave to the end of the QRS, including R$'$, in V1, V2, or V3 (in the absence of complete RBBB)	*Minor* • Low QRS voltages (<0.5 mV peak to peak) in limb leads (in the absence of obesity, emphysema, or pericardial effusion)
V. Ventricular arrhythmias	*Major* • Frequent ventricular extrasystoles (>500 per 24 h), non-sustained or sustained ventricular tachycardia of LBBB morphology *Minor* • Frequent ventricular extrasystoles (>500 per 24 h), non-sustained or sustained ventricular tachycardia of LBBB morphology with inferior axis ("RVOT pattern")	*Minor* • Frequent ventricular extrasystoles (>500 per 24 h), non-sustained or sustained ventricular tachycardia with a RBBB morphology (excluding the "fascicular pattern")
VI. Family history/ genetics	*Major* • AC confirmed in a first-degree relative who meets diagnostic criteria • AC confirmed pathologically at autopsy or surgery in a first-degree relative • Identification of a pathogenic or likely pathogenetic AC mutation in the patient under evaluation *Minor* • History of AC in a first-degree relative in whom it is not possible or practical to determine whether the family member meets diagnostic criteria • Premature sudden death (<35 years of age) due to suspected AC in a first-degree relative • AC confirmed pathologically or by diagnostic criteria in a second-degree relative	

Modified from Corrado et al. "Diagnosis of arrhythmogenic cardiomyopathy: The Padua criteria", International Journal of Cardiology, Volume 319, 2020, Pages 106–114

AC arrhythmogenic cardiomyopathy, *BSA* body surface area, *EDV* end-diastolic volume, *EF* ejection fraction, *ITF* International Task Force, *LBBB* left bundle branch block

Diagnostic Tools in AC

As stated above, current AC diagnostic criteria take into consideration different parameters regarding anamnesis, electrophysiological features, and findings coming from imaging techniques.

Personal and Familial Anamnesis

Patients could be completely asymptomatic or complain about palpitations, dizziness, or syncopal episodes. In the presence of a severely reduced ventricular function, heart failure symptoms and signs could be present. A careful family history investigation with particular regard to SCD cases and presence of relatives showing arrhythmic diseases or presenting with arrhythmic symptoms should be performed. Finally, a family pedigree should be created.

Twelve-Lead Electrocardiogram (ECG)

ECG pattern plays a central role in AC diagnosis, as loss of electrical forces secondary to myocardial atrophy, conduction abnormalities caused by fibrofatty replacement and/or right ventricular dilatation, and presence of a transmural voltage gradient between injured and healthy myocytes lead to ventricular depolarization/repolarization

activities that can be appreciated on ECG [63]. Nonetheless, in a significant number of AC patients, ranging from 12% to 50% on different series, ECG can be normal [64–66]. The ECG patterns that can be found are the following (Figs. 15.3, 15.4, and 15.5):

- *Delay of terminal activation time*: It is defined as a slurring of the S wave in leads V1–V3 with the longest value from the nadir of the S wave to the end of all QRS ≥55 ms in the absence of r′ in leads V1–V3.
- *Right ventricular conduction delay:* Presence of conduction delay can be represented mainly by an incomplete right bundle branch block (RBBB) (rSr1 in lead V1 and QRS duration <120 ms) while a complete RBBB is less common.
- *QRS fragmentation:* It is defined as the presence of additional spikes within the QRS complex due to a regional delay of the normal ventricular conduction linked to fibro-fatty infiltration.
- *Negative T waves:* Inverted T waves on right precordial leads (V1, V2, and V3) in subjects older than 14 years are considered a diagnostic criterion for AC as they are related to the RV volumes. In addition, inverted T waves on

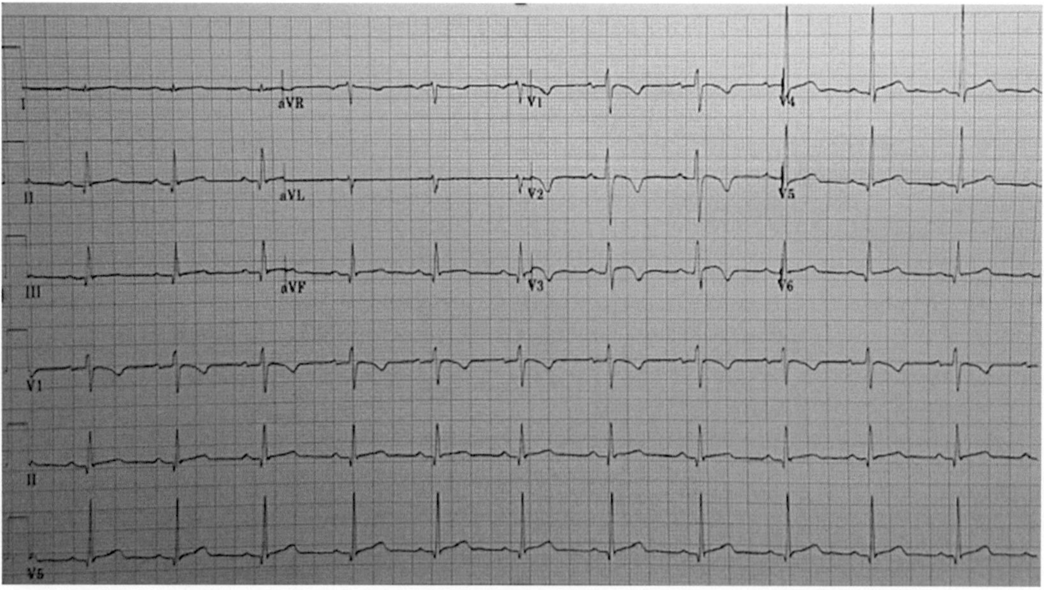

Fig. 15.3 ECG pattern of a patient affected by right-dominant arrhythmogenic cardiomyopathy. Presence of T-wave inversion right precordial leads (V1 through V3) secondary to the fibro-fatty replacement of the RV

inferior and lateral leads (V5–V6) can suggest a LV involvement.

- *Low QRS voltages:* Defined as a peak-to-peak QRS amplitude of less than 5 mm in the limb leads and/or less than 10 mm in the precordial leads [67]. The presence of low QRS voltages in limb leads has been demonstrated to be associated with the presence of LV late enhancement (LGE) and it is one of the criteria for ALVC diagnosis [13, 68].

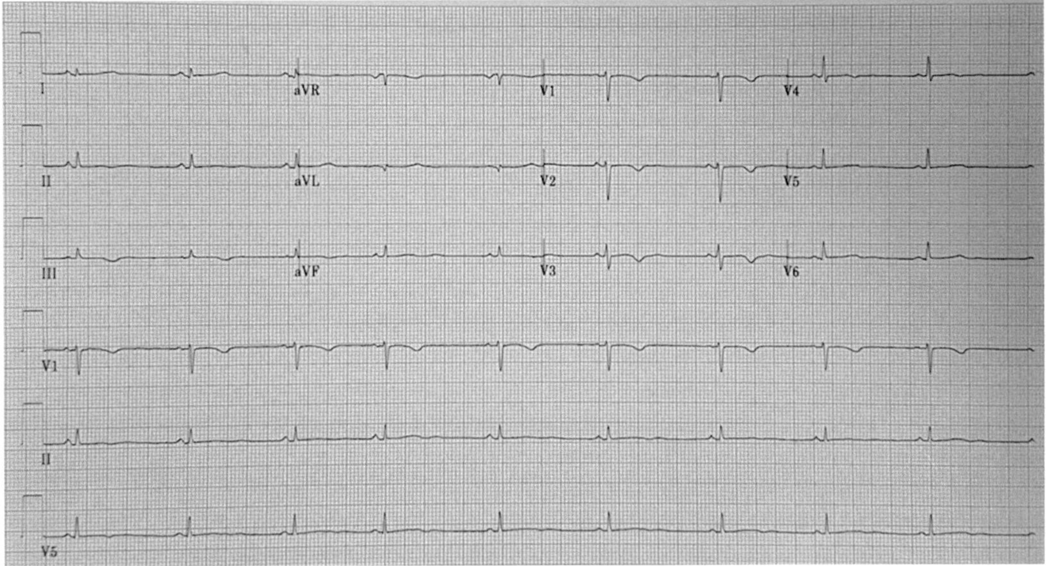

Fig. 15.4 ECG pattern of a patient affected by arrhythmogenic cardiomyopathy with biventricular involvement. Negative or flattening T waves are present in both precordial and limb leads. Moreover, QRS complex voltages are reduced in all leads as a result of extensive fibro-fatty replacement in both ventricles

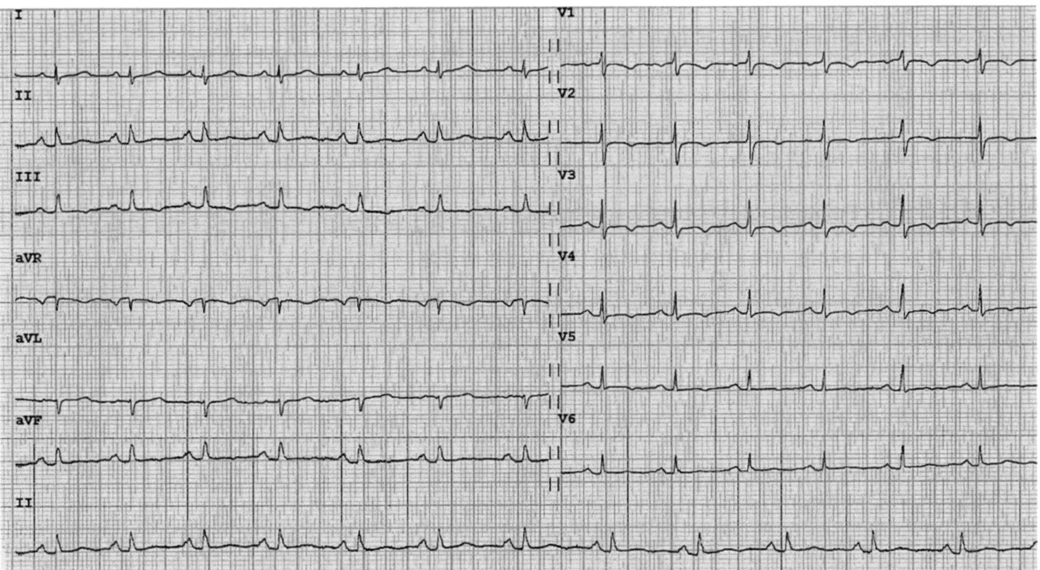

Fig. 15.5 ECG of a patient affected by left-dominant arrhythmogenic cardiomyopathy. T-wave inversion in lateral and limb lead is suggestive of left ventricular involvement

Ventricular Arrhythmia (VA) Detection

VAs linked to AC usually have a left bundle branch block (LBBB) pattern. While a left-axis deviation can lead to suspecting the presence of an AC form, the main problem is the differentiation from idiopathic ventricular arrhythmias with right-axis deviations originating from the RV infundibulum. The most sensitive parameters are a QRS duration in lead I ≥120 ms, a QRS transition in V6, notching on any complex, and early QRS onset in V1 [69, 70]. Regarding their complexity, ventricular arrhythmias can be isolated or organized in runs of non-sustained ventricular tachycardia (NSVT) or sustained ventricular tachycardia (sVT). Ventricular fibrillation (VF) is mostly reported in young patients during the earlier phases of AC, whereas sustained VTs occur more commonly later in the disease course [71]. Bhonsale et al. [72] demonstrated that AC patients who experienced ventricular fibrillation and SCD were significantly younger (median age 23 years) than those presenting with sustained monomorphic VTs (median age 36 years). In addition, in patients with late presentation (>50 years) sustained VT was the predominant arrhythmic event, while in young population VF was more common [73]. This age-related behavior of arrhythmic pattern could be explained by the progressive nature of the disease, considering that monomorphic VT is usually linked to reentry circuits around stable fibro-fatty myocardial scars that are the result from a long pathologic process, while VF may be the result of acute electrical instability, particularly in the context of myocarditis-mediated bouts of acute myocyte necrosis [71, 74].

Two-Dimensional Echocardiography

Echocardiography is the first-line imaging modality in AC, since it is a noninvasive, widely available technique which can provide information about volumes and systolic function of both ventricles. However, echocardiographic diagnosis in AC requires a specific expertise due to the retrosternal position, the complex geometry, and the load dependency of the RV [75]. In addition

to this, echocardiography shows a low sensitivity, especially in the early stages of the disease [76].

Regional wall motion abnormalities (RWMA), together with global RV dysfunction and dilation, represent the macroscopic results of the fibro-fatty changes at the histological level. The echocardiographic diagnosis of AC lies consequently in demonstrating their presence while performing the exam. Regional RV akinesia, dyskinesia, or aneurysm; right ventricle outflow tract (RVOT) diameter (measured from either parasternal long-axis [PLAX] view or parasternal short-axis [PSAX] view); and RV-fractional area change (FAC) are the only standard echocardiographic measures included in the 2010 Task Force criteria [60] (Table 15.2).

Moreover, even if not proved to raise the diagnostic sensibility, other parameters such as the RV basal diameter and those obtained by advanced echocardiographic methods have been proposed to strengthen the suspicion of AC in dubious cases [77].

Advanced Echo Modalities

Contrast echocardiography, Doppler tissue imaging, tissue deformation imaging, and 3D echocardiography are emerging tools in the echocardiographic assessment in AC.

Table 15.2 Diagnostic echocardiographic criteria in AC modified from Marcus et al. [60]

Echocardiographic criteria for AC from the 2010 Tasks Force Criteria:
Global or regional dysfunction and structural alterations
Major
Regional RV akinesia, dyskinesia, or aneurysm and one of the following measured at end diastole:
PLAX RVOT ≥32 mm
PSAX RVOT ≥36 mm
Fractional area change ≤33%
Minor
Regional RV akinesia or dyskinesia and one of the following measured at end diastole:
PLAX RVOT ≥29 to <32 mm
PSAX RVOT ≥32 to <36 mm
Fractional area change >33% to ≤40%

Contrast echocardiography can enhance the detection of RWMAs if the image quality is not satisfying [78]. Doppler tissue imaging for the measurement of the peak systolic annular velocity (s′) of the RV can provide additional information about the RV longitudinal systolic function. The latter can also be assessed by tissue deformation imaging that typically shows a reduced RV strain and an increased mechanical dispersion in AC patients [48, 79, 80]. Since these parameters are altered early before other macroscopic changes become evident, they appear particularly useful when early stages are suspected or when looking for the disease in relatives. 3D echocardiography allows a precise assessment of RV volumes and function, despite losing accuracy when end-stage forms with extremely enlarged ventricles are addressed [81].

Cardiac Magnetic Resonance

Cardiac magnetic resonance can allow a comprehensive evaluation of volumes, function, and tissue characterization in a single investigation. A standardized protocol is recommended when approaching AC patients, with cine images performed using steady-state free precession (SSFP) sequences and LGE images using phase-sensitive inversion recovery (PSIR) sequences [82]. Most of our knowledge about common findings as evidenced by CMR comes from studies carried out in patients affected by the classic right phenotype. Recognized CMR features associated with AC are RV wall thinning, RVOT enlargement, trabecular disarray, fibro-fatty replacement, ventricular dilatation, focal bulges, microaneurysms, and global or regional systolic dysfunction [82] (Fig. 15.6).

The CMR criteria in 2010 TF [60] included quantitative metrics, such as RV dilatation or global dysfunction, and qualitative findings, like akinesia, dyskinesia, and dyssynchronous contraction (i.e., RWMAs) (Table 15.3).

Besides these morpho-functional anomalies, CMR can show also structural alterations, such as fat infiltration by T1-weighted spin-echo images, and LGE by post-contrast sequences at the RV level. However, given the low reproducibility and inconsistency of these measures, neither of them was included into the 2010 TF criteria. As stated above in 2020 Padua criteria included also LGE among the criteria for diagnosis. Notably, detections of LGE at the RV level are hampered by the thin RV wall, which makes the LGE analysis less consistent than for the LV [83]. Moreover, LGE cannot distinguish between fat and fibrosis [82]. Also, LGE is a nonspecific finding that can be found in other diseases that mimic AC, such as myocarditis, sarcoidosis, and dilated cardiomyopathy. Likewise, intramyocardial fat has been demonstrated in older, obese patients and it is a common finding in autopsy cases dying for noncardiac causes [84–86]. Despite these limitations, contrast-enhanced CMR is currently the ideal technique to address the emerging biventricular and the left-dominant variants, thanks to its tissue characterization

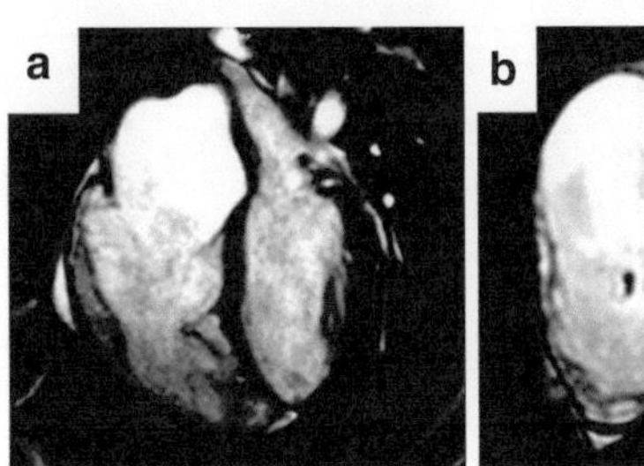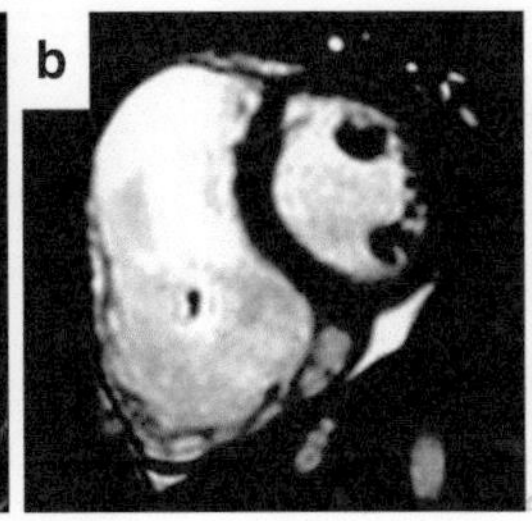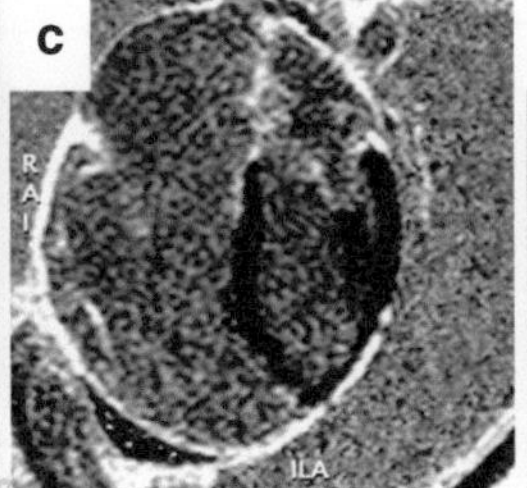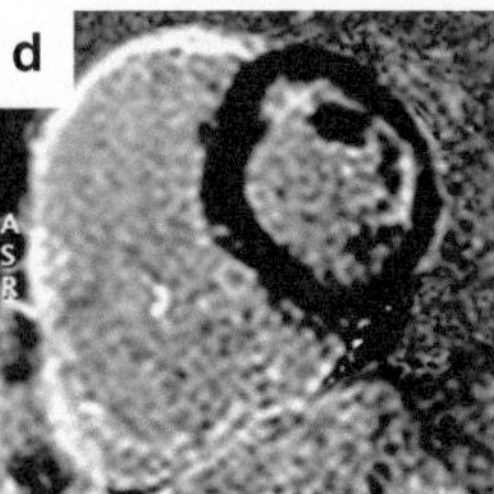

Fig. 15.6 CMR images of a patient affected by right-dominant arrhythmogenic cardiomyopathy. (**a**, **b**) Apical four-chamber view and mid short-axis view of cine images showing severe dilatation of the RV. (**c**, **d**) Apical four-chamber view and mid short-axis view of post-contrast sequences showing extensive LGE of the RV

capability that allows the detection of both fibrosis and fibro-fatty infiltration at the LV level (Fig. 15.7).

Endomyocardial Biopsy

It is an invasive procedure that is performed via venous access and catheterization of right heart and which allows the sampling of myocardium

Table 15.3 Diagnostic cardiac magnetic resonance-based criteria in AC modified from Marcus et al. [60]

Cardiac magnetic resonance-based criteria for AC form the 2010 Task Force Criteria:
Global or regional dysfunction and structural alterations
Major
Regional RV akinesia, dyskinesia, or dyssynchronous RV contraction and one of the following:
– Ratio of RV end-diastolic volume to BSA ≥110 mL/mq (male) or ≥110 mL/mq (female)
– RV ejection fraction ≤40%
Minor
Regional RV akinesia, dyskinesia, or dyssynchronous RV contraction and one of the following:
– Ratio of RV end-diastolic volume to BSA ≥100 to <110 mL/mq (male) or ≥90 to <100 mL/mq (female)
– RV ejection fraction >40% to ≤45%

AC arrhythmogenic cardiomyopathy, *BSA* body surface area, *RV* right ventricle

from free wall of the RV, which is then subjected to histological analysis. Although it is a part of the diagnostic 2010 Task Force criteria, this examination, due to its invasiveness, is reserved for selected AC patients, in which phenocopies (dilative cardiomyopathy, myocarditis, sarcoidosis) should be excluded [87]. As mentioned above, the sample is taken preferably from the free wall of the ventricle (the septum is rarely involved in classic variants of AC), and, in order to increase sensitivity and reduce risk of wall perforation, it should be guided by electro-anatomical mapping or CMR [14, 87]. Endomyocardial biopsy offers an in vivo characterization of the distinctive element of the disease, like fibro-fatty replacement and loss of myocytes. In details, according to the parameters of the International Task Force [88] if on morphometric analysis the residual myocytes are <60%, the major criterion is considered, and if between 65% and 70%, the minor criterion is considered. This method can help in the differential diagnosis between AC and so-called phenocopies of disease, such as DCM, myocarditis, sarcoidosis, or other conditions leading to myocardial tissue replacement. However, although endomyocardial biopsy can unequivocally detect the presence of fibrous or fibroadipose replacement and quantify the proportion of residual myocytes, it is severely limited by its poor sensitivity. Indeed, since pathological process affects the heart muscle focally and proceeds from epicardium through the endocardium, a negative his-

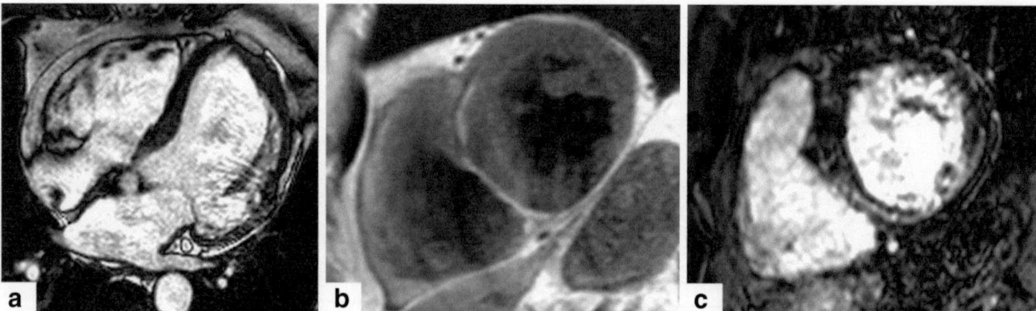

Fig. 15.7 CMR images of a patient affected by arrhythmogenic cardiomyopathy with biventricular involvement. (**a**) Apical four-chamber view of cine images showing dilatation of both ventricles with thinning of the LV lateral wall. (**b**) T1-weighted black blood sequences with fat suppression demonstrating fatty infiltration of septal and lateral walls. (**c**) Post-contrast sequences showing LGE in the same locations as in (**b**)

tological sample does not necessarily imply the absence of disease. Immunohistochemical analytical tests have recently been revised to evaluate on the sample the possible alteration in the distribution of desmosomal proteins [89]; unfortunately, specific findings for AC have not been yet identified.

Arrhythmogenic Left Ventricular Cardiomyopathy

Arrhythmogenic left ventricular cardiomyopathy (ALVC) is an AC form characterized by an early and predominant involvement of the left ventricle [12]. In contrast to the biventricular variant, where the degree of ventricular dysfunction is similar in the two ventricles, in this case right ventricular involvement, if present, has a minor significance. First evidence of ALVC came from autopsy reports and soon after from screening of families with mutations in the DSP gene [19, 90]. The first clinical description of the disease was made in 2008 [12] and unfortunately no validated diagnostic criteria for this AC form have been provided so far. In addition, 2010 TFC criteria have proved to be insensitive in the ALVC diagnosis [22]. Commonly, ECG shows T-wave inversion typically located in lower and/or lateral leads and presence of low QRS voltages in peripheral leads. It has been speculated that this may be secondary to fibro-fatty replacement of the left ventricle, but

conclusive studies are not yet available. Arrhythmias are characterized by a RBBB morphology and variable axis, frequently originating from the lateral wall of the LV. Notably, the degree of electrical instability seems not to correlate with the degree of LV, this being a distinguishing feature from DCM. CMR plays a pivotal role in diagnosis mostly through the possibility to highlight the presence of fibrous tissue by means of LGE detection. The peculiar pattern of LGE distribution is represented by LV subepicardial stria, most frequently located on inferolateral basal segments with variable extension and in some cases leading to a circumferential involvement of the entire ventricle (Fig. 15.8). Unfortunately, this pattern is not exclusive of AC and enters into differential diagnosis with other diseases such as myocarditis. Recent studies demonstrated that in patients with acute myocarditis LGE can be found in 41% of cases on subepicardial layers of LV inferior and lateral walls [91] with nonsignificant changes only in 30% of cases at 6 months' follow-up [92]. Conversely in ALVC, because of its progressive pathogenesis, LGE is unchanged or increased in almost all patients. For these reasons, the diagnosis cannot be based solely on instrumental examinations, but must take account of family history, genetic findings, and, in sporadic cases, endomyocardial biopsy. Similarly, DCM forms with clinical and instrumental features similar to those of ALVC have been described (so-called dilated cardiomyopathies with an arrhythmogenic pheno-

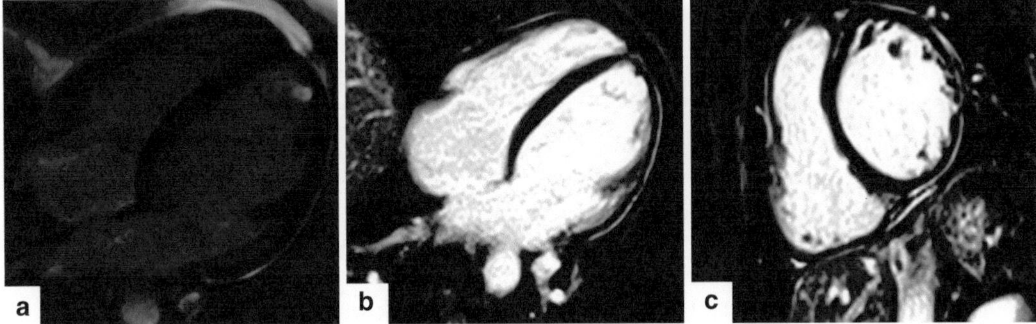

Fig. 15.8 CMR images of a patient affected by left-dominant arrhythmogenic cardiomyopathy. (**a**) Apical four-chamber view of cine images showing a mild dilated left ventricle with a thinned lateral wall compared to the septum. (**b, c**) Four-chamber view and short-axis view of post-contrast sequences showing subepicardial LGE in the form of stria of the anterolateral and inferolateral walls

type) [93]. However, studies comparing clinical and CMR characteristics of a group of DCM and AC patients demonstrated that the amount of LGE and its distribution are significantly different between the two groups. Interestingly, in AC gadolinium on the LV showed a peculiar pattern, as described above, while in DCM a common finding was an intramural stria at septal level. In addition, the amount of LGE was significantly higher in AC group. The explanation for these findings can be obtained by analyzing the different pathophysiology of the two cardiomyopathies. In DCM, fibrosis is a secondary phenomenon due to ventricular enlargement, while in AC it is a primary phenomenon resulting from the death of cardiomyocytes through necrosis and apoptosis [94]. Patients with ALVC may experience "hot phases" characterized by chest pain and enzymatic release. Unfortunately, differential diagnosis with acute myocarditis can be quite difficult. It is estimated that "hot phase" phenomenon has an incidence that ranges from 5% to 25% of patients in different series [22, 95]. In a recent paper our group analyzed clinical and instrumental findings of a series of 23 patients affected by AC, mainly with a ALVC or a biventricular phenotype, who experienced one or more episodes of myocardial injury [95]. From those data, myocarditis-like picture seems to be a rather uncommon clinical presentation of AC, often occurring in the pediatric age, and CMR is the first-choice examination for the differential diagnosis between AC and acute myocarditis. Moreover, in patients with this clinical presentation EMB can have a pivotal role in differential diagnosis as well as family screening and genetic test. As stated above, signs of myocardial injury that precede systolic dysfunction were found in a significant number of subjects carrying DSP truncating mutations [22]. To date, it is unclear why some AC patients develop episodes of myocardial injury and it has been speculated that this is in relation with the wall thickness considering that these episodes are more intense and symptomatic when involving the LV as in ALVC forms. Finally, their role in disease progression and arrhythmic risk remains to be elucidated. In contrast to classical variants, no conclusive data exist for ALVC as far as prognosis and arrhythmic

risk stratification are concerned. While parameters such as degree of RV dilatation and dysfunction, extension of T-wave inversion, and degree of electrical instability exist for right and biventricular variants [96], no validated predictors are present for ALVC forms to date. Recently, a risk score has been developed to help the clinician in the decision to implant an ICD in primary prevention [97]. However, it seems to lack sensitivity for left-dominant forms [98].

Therapeutic Strategies in AC

Physical Restriction

Sports activity enhances AC progression and worsens the disease arrhythmic substrate [44, 47, 49, 50, 54]. Conversely, the risk of ventricular arrhythmias (VAs) and mortality can be lowered by reducing exercise [8, 49, 50, 99].

Different categories of AC patients show a dose-dependent association between exercise exposure and disease penetrance. Genotype-positive relatives undergoing competitive sports and high-intensity physical exercise are affected by an increased risk of VAs and heart failure as documented by clinical studies [46, 100]. With this regard, pre-symptomatic genetic testing has a role because it can detect those individuals in whom a lifestyle change can reduce the risk of developing AC. Likewise, in patients with an overt phenotype, preparticipation screening and disqualification may prevent SCD [56].

Accordingly, both European and American guidelines recommend restriction from competitive sports activity of AC patients and at-risk relatives as a measure aimed to reduce the risk of SCD [57, 58].

Drug Therapy

Beta-Blockers

Ventricular arrhythmias and cardiac arrest in AC are usually promoted by adrenergic stimulation and occur typically during or early after a physical effort. Thus, beta-blockers are recommended in

AC patients symptomatic for frequent premature ventricular complex (PVCs) and non-sustained ventricular tachycardias (NSVT), patients with recurrent VT, appropriate ICD therapies, or inappropriate ICD interventions resulting from sinus tachycardia, supraventricular tachycardia, or atrial fibrillation/flutter with high ventricular rate.

In addition, since reducing the ventricular wall stress lowers the myocardial disease progression and is considered as a first-line medication in the management of heart failure, beta-blockers should be offered in all patients with a definite diagnosis of AC, irrespective of arrhythmias.

So far, in phenotype-negative gene carriers prophylactic use of these drugs is not justified [101, 102].

Antiarrhythmic Drugs

When beta-blockers alone are not sufficient to control the arrhythmic burden, anti-arrhythmic drug therapy is indicated for symptomatic patients with frequent PVCs and/or NSVT. In particular, sotalol and amiodarone (alone or associated with beta-blockers) are the most effective drugs with a relatively low proarrhythmic risk [101, 102].

Heart Failure Drugs

The standard pharmacological treatment for heart failure (angiotensin-converting enzyme inhibitors, angiotensin II receptor blockers, beta-blockers, and diuretics) is recommended in patients who develop right, left, or biventricular heart failure [102].

New Drugs

Therapeutic strategies targeting the Wtn/β and NFκB pathways appear to lower the disease in animal models and thus may be promising options in the future [103].

Catheter Ablation

Catheter ablation should be considered as a therapeutic option for patients symptomatic for PVCs or VT or frequent appropriate ICD interventions on VT despite optimal medical therapy, in order to improve symptoms and prevent ICD shocks, respectively [101]. The initial experience with this technique reported high acute success rates followed by high rates of recurrences due to the progressive nature of the disease leading to the development of multiple arrhythmogenic foci over time [104–106]. Moreover, regions of fibro-fatty replacement—that are regarded as arrhythmogenic substrate for VT—are mostly located in the subepicardial RV layers, thus partially explaining the failure of the traditional endocardial approach. Epicardial catheter ablation appears to be a feasible and more effective approach for patients in whom one or more endocardial procedures have been unsuccessful [102, 107]. Importantly, neither anti-arrhythmic drugs nor catheter ablation proved to reduce the risk of SCD. Thus, they should be considered as measures to reduce the frequency of arrhythmic episodes rather than to improve prognosis. The only effective therapy for the prevention of SCD in such patients is ICD implantation [102].

ICD Implantation

Regarding AC recommendation of ICD implantation in AC patients, three risk categories ("high," "moderate," and "low") have been defined. Those who have a history of cardiac arrest or hemodynamically unstable VT or who have severe ventricular dysfunction (either right or left or both ventricles) are considered "high-risk" subjects and receive a class I recommendation for ICD implantation.

Patients with major risk factors, such as syncope, non-sustained ventricular tachycardias, or moderate dysfunction of the right or left or both ventricles, are classified as "intermediate-risk" subjects, and receive a class IIa recommendation for ICD implantation. Recently, a score system including ECG, CMR, and degree of electrical instability has been proposed [97]. Since the presence of scars in AC may not affect the LV performance, but can still trigger adverse arrhythmic events, ICD implant for primary prevention should be considered in the presence of extensive LGE/fibrosis even if the LV systolic function is not severely depressed [102].

Heart Transplant

Heart transplant still represents the final therapeutic option for AC patients with advanced stages of the disease who suffer from refractory congestive heart failure and/or uncontrollable arrhythmic storms, despite previous attempts with catheter ablation and ICD therapy [102].

Right Ventricular Myocardial Changes in Specific Diseases

Different systemic or cardiac diseases can directly affect the right ventricle. A right ventricular involvement can be present in different cardiomyopathies having both genetic and non-inherited origin as hypertrophic cardiomyopathy, Fabry cardiomyopathy, DCM, or peripartum cardiomyopathy. Moreover, a RV involvement can be demonstrated in patients with systemic diseases as amyloidosis, sarcoidosis, or systemic sclerosis. Finally, RV physiologic changes can be detected in highly trained athletes.

Cardiac Sarcoidosis

The differential diagnosis between cardiac sarcoidosis and AC is often challenging because of both clinical and imaging features common to the two entities. In cardiac sarcoidosis life-threatening arrhythmias and heart failure can occur as a consequence of granulomatous infiltrates and fibrosis. The septum and the LV free wall are the most common locations at the LV level, while the RV free wall is involved in up to 40% of cases. Nevertheless, some peculiar features distinguish sarcoidosis from AC, and thus can help the diagnostic assessment. First, differently from AC, AV conduction delays are frequent because of the granulomatous infiltration of the interventricular septum. In addition to this, sarcoidosis is usually a systemic disease involving different organs such as lungs, skin, liver, and eyes. Conversely, cardiac isolated forms are less frequently found. Finally, advanced imaging

techniques can offer some useful tips for the diagnosis. Extracardiac findings can be evidenced during the exam. At post-contrast sequences, LGE shows an intramural or patchy appearance, localizes mostly at the basal lateral wall, and is responsive to immunosuppressive therapy. When combined with positron-emission tomography (PET), the fluorodeoxyglucose uptake can reveal active inflammatory lesions [108–110].

Dilated Cardiomyopathy

DCM is currently defined by the presence of left ventricular or biventricular systolic dysfunction and dilatation that are not explained by abnormal loading conditions or coronary artery disease [111]. In DCM patients RV function may be reduced due to the same process leading to LV cardiomyopathy or hemodynamic consequences of LV dilation, dysfunction, or increased filling pressure. At the same time, the reduced RV function may worsen LV preload. The prevalence of RV dysfunction in DCM ranges from 34% to 65% [112]. In DCM patients RV function has a relevant prognostic value and CMR studies confirmed that RV function strongly predicts cardiac mortality in patients with HF. Thus assessment of RV size and function in DCM patients appears to be crucial for providing relevant prognostic and therapeutic information [112].

Hypertrophic Cardiomyopathy

Even if in patients with hypertrophic cardiomyopathy (HCM) myocardial hypertrophy mainly involves the LV and RV hypertrophy and dysfunction can also be present. The degree of RV wall thickness has been found to correlate significantly with LV wall thickness, even if RV hypertrophy is not associated with a particular pattern of LV hypertrophy [113]. Of note, HCM patients with severe RV hypertrophy have a poor clinical outcome and CMR studies demonstrated that RV hypertrophy is associated with RV LGE and that it is an independent predictor of cardiovascular event occurrence [114, 115]. Even in the presence of RV hypertrophy, detection of RV outflow tract obstruction in HCM patients is quite uncommon, not dynamic, and mainly due to RV hypertrophy. Regarding non-sarcomeric HCM, RV hypertrophy has been described also in Anderson-Fabry disease and has been proved to correlate with disease severity and LV hypertrophy [112].

References

1. Corrado D, Basso C, Judge DP. Arrhythmogenic cardiomyopathy. Circ Res. 2017;121:784–802.
2. Basso C, Corrado D, Marcus FI, Nava A, Thiene G. Arrhythmogenic right ventricular cardiomyopathy. Lancet. 2009;373:1289–300.
3. Lancisi GM. Arrhythmogenic right ventricular cardiomyopathy, De Motu Cordis et Aneurysmatibus. Naples, 1728.
4. Dalla-Volta S, Battaglia G, Zerbini E. 'Auricularization' of right ventricular pressure curve. Am Heart J. 1961;61:25–33.
5. Marcus FI, et al. Right ventricular dysplasia: a report of 24 adult cases. Ann Noninvasive Electrocardiol. 1999;4:97–111.
6. Thiene G, et al. Right ventricular cardiomyopathy and sudden death in young people. N Engl J Med. 1988;318:129–33.
7. Nava A, et al. Familial occurrence of right ventricular dysplasia: a study involving nine families. J Am Coll Cardiol. 1988;12:1222–8.
8. Nava A, et al. Clinical profile and long-term follow-up of 37 families with arrhythmogenic right ventricular cardiomyopathy. J Am Coll Cardiol. 2000;36:2226–33.
9. Pilichou K, et al. Arrhythmogenic cardiomyopathy. Orphanet J Rare Dis. 2016;11:33.
10. Basso C, et al. Arrhythmogenic right ventricular cardiomyopathy: dysplasia, dystrophy, or myocarditis? Circulation. 1996;94:983–91.
11. Thiene G, Basso C. Arrhythmogenic right ventricular cardiomyopathy: an update. Cardiovasc Pathol. 2001;10:109–17.
12. Sen-Chowdhry S, et al. Left-dominant arrhythmogenic cardiomyopathy. An under-recognized clinical entity. J Am Coll Cardiol. 2008;52:2175–87.
13. Corrado D, et al. Diagnosis of arrhythmogenic cardiomyopathy: the Padua criteria. Int J Cardiol. 2020;319:106–14.
14. Basso C, et al. Quantitative assessment of endomyocardial biopsy in arrhythmogenic right ventricular cardiomyopathy/dysplasia: an in vitro validation of diagnostic criteria. Eur Heart J. 2008;29:2760–71.
15. Protonotarios N, et al. Cardiac abnormalities in familial palmoplantar keratosis. Br Heart J. 1986;56:321–6.
16. McKoy G, et al. Identification of a deletion in plakoglobin in arrhythmogenic right ventricular cardiomyopathy with palmoplantar keratoderma and woolly hair (Naxos disease). Lancet. 2000;355:2119–24.
17. Karmouch J, Protonotarios A, Syrris P. Genetic basis of arrhythmogenic cardiomyopathy. Curr Opin Cardiol. 2018;33:276–81.
18. Petros S, et al. Clinical expression of plakophilin-2 mutations in familial arrhythmogenic right ventricular cardiomyopathy. Circulation. 2006;113:356–64.
19. Bauce B, et al. Clinical profile of four families with arrhythmogenic right ventricular cardiomyopathy caused by dominant desmoplakin mutations. Eur Heart J. 2005;26:1666–75.
20. Sen-Chowdhry S, Syrris P, McKenna WJ. Genetics of right ventricular cardiomyopathy. J Cardiovasc Electrophysiol. 2005;16:927–35.
21. Norgett EE, et al. Recessive mutation in desmoplakin disrupts desmoplakin-intermediate filament interactions and causes dilated cardiomyopathy, woolly hair and keratoderma. Hum Mol Genet. 2000;9:2761–6.
22. Smith ED, et al. Desmoplakin cardiomyopathy, a fibrotic and inflammatory form of cardiomyopathy distinct from typical dilated or arrhythmogenic right ventricular cardiomyopathy. Circulation. 2020;141:1872–84.
23. Syrris P, et al. Desmoglein-2 mutations in arrhythmogenic right ventricular cardiomyopathy: a genotype–phenotype characterization of familial disease. Eur Heart J. 2007;28:581–8.
24. Heuser A, et al. Mutant desmocollin-2 causes arrhythmogenic right ventricular cardiomyopathy. Am J Hum Genet. 2006;79:1081–8.
25. Tsatsopoulou AA, Protonotarios NI, McKenna WJ. Arrhythmogenic right ventricular dysplasia, a cell adhesion cardiomyopathy: insights into disease pathogenesis from preliminary genotype-phenotype assessment. Heart. 2006;92:1720–3.
26. Van Hengel J, et al. Mutations in the area composita protein at-catenin are associated with arrhythmogenic right ventricular cardiomyopathy. Eur Heart J. 2013;34:201–10.
27. Alice G, et al. Cadherin 2-related arrhythmogenic cardiomyopathy: prevalence and clinical features. Circ Genomic Precis Med. 2021;14:e003097.
28. Quarta G, et al. Mutations in the Lamin A/C gene mimic arrhythmogenic right ventricular cardiomyopathy. Eur Heart J. 2012;33:1128–36.
29. Glöcklhofer CR, et al. A novel LMNA nonsense mutation causes two distinct phenotypes of cardiomyopathy with high risk of sudden cardiac death in a large five-generation family. Europace. 2018;20:2003–13.
30. Augusto JB, et al. Dilated cardiomyopathy and arrhythmogenic left ventricular cardiomyopathy: a comprehensive genotype-imaging phenotype study. Eur Heart J Cardiovasc Imaging. 2020;21:326–36.
31. Bermúdez-Jiménez FJ, et al. Novel Desmin mutation p.Glu401Asp impairs filament formation, disrupts

cell membrane integrity, and causes severe arrhythmogenic left ventricular cardiomyopathy/dysplasia. Circulation. 2018;137:1595–610.

32. Merner ND, et al. Arrhythmogenic right ventricular cardiomyopathy type 5 is a fully penetrant, lethal arrhythmic disorder caused by a missense mutation in the TMEM43 gene. Am J Hum Genet. 2008;82:809–21.

33. Matthew T, et al. Genetic variation in titin in arrhythmogenic right ventricular cardiomyopathy–overlap syndromes. Circulation. 2011;124:876–85.

34. Ortiz-Genga MF, et al. Truncating FLNC mutations are associated with high-risk dilated and arrhythmogenic cardiomyopathies. J Am Coll Cardiol. 2016;68:2440–51.

35. Tiso N, et al. Identification of mutations in the cardiac ryanodine receptor gene in families affected with arrhythmogenic right ventricular cardiomyopathy type 2 (ARVD2). Hum Mol Genet. 2001;10:189–94.

36. Austin KM, et al. Molecular mechanisms of arrhythmogenic cardiomyopathy. Nat Rev Cardiol. 2019; https://doi.org/10.1038/s41569-019-0200-7.

37. Te Riele ASJM, et al. Multilevel analyses of SCN5A mutations in arrhythmogenic right ventricular dysplasia/cardiomyopathy suggest non-canonical mechanisms for disease pathogenesis. Cardiovasc Res. 2017;113:102–11.

38. Van Rijsingen IAW, et al. Outcome in phospholamban R14del carriers results of a large multicentre cohort study. Circ Cardiovasc Genet. 2014;7:455–65.

39. Eijgenraam TR, et al. The phospholamban p.(Arg14del) pathogenic variant leads to cardiomyopathy with heart failure and is unresponsive to standard heart failure therapy. Sci Rep. 2020;10:9819.

40. Xu T, et al. Compound and digenic heterozygosity contributes to arrhythmogenic right ventricular cardiomyopathy. J Am Coll Cardiol. 2010;55:587–97.

41. Rigato I, et al. Compound and digenic heterozygosity predicts lifetime arrhythmic outcome and sudden cardiac death in desmosomal gene-related arrhythmogenic right ventricular cardiomyopathy. Circ Cardiovasc Genet. 2013;6:533–42.

42. Bauce B, et al. Multiple mutations in desmosomal proteins encoding genes in arrhythmogenic right ventricular cardiomyopathy/dysplasia. Heart Rhythm. 2010;7:22–9.

43. Corrado D, Thiene G, Nava A, Rossi L, Pennelli N. Sudden death in young competitive athletes: clinicopathologic correlations in 22 cases. Am J Med. 1990;89:588–96.

44. Corrado D, Basso C, Rizzoli G, Schiavon M, Thiene G. Does sports activity enhance the risk of sudden death in adolescents and young adults? J Am Coll Cardiol. 2003;42:1959–63.

45. Lemola K, et al. Predictors of adverse outcome in patients with arrhythmogenic right ventricular dysplasia/cardiomyopathy: long term experience of a tertiary care centre. Heart. 2005;91:1167–72.

46. James CA, et al. Exercise increases age-related penetrance and arrhythmic risk in arrhythmogenic right ventricular dysplasia/cardiomyopathy–associated desmosomal mutation carriers. J Am Coll Cardiol. 2013;62:1290–7.

47. Sawant AC, et al. Exercise has a disproportionate role in the pathogenesis of arrhythmogenic right ventricular dysplasia/cardiomyopathy in patients without desmosomal mutations. J Am Heart Assoc. 2014;3:e001471.

48. Saberniak J, et al. Comparison of patients with early-phase arrhythmogenic right ventricular cardiomyopathy and right ventricular outflow tract ventricular tachycardia. Eur Heart J Cardiovasc Imaging. 2017;18:62–9.

49. Ruwald A-C, et al. Association of competitive and recreational sport participation with cardiac events in patients with arrhythmogenic right ventricular cardiomyopathy: results from the North American multidisciplinary study of arrhythmogenic right ventricular cardiomyopathy. Eur Heart J. 2015;36:1735–43.

50. Lie ØH, et al. Harmful effects of exercise intensity and exercise duration in patients with arrhythmogenic cardiomyopathy. JACC Clin Electrophysiol. 2018;4:744–53.

51. Ruiz Salas A, et al. Impact of dynamic physical exercise on high-risk definite arrhythmogenic right ventricular cardiomyopathy. J Cardiovasc Electrophysiol. 2018;29:1523–9.

52. Müssigbrodt A, et al. Effect of exercise on outcome after ventricular tachycardia ablation in arrhythmogenic right ventricular dysplasia/cardiomyopathy. Int J Sports Med. 2019;40:657–62.

53. Paulin FL, et al. Exercise and arrhythmic risk in TMEM43 p.S358L arrhythmogenic right ventricular cardiomyopathy. *Hear*. Rhythm. 2020;17:1159–66.

54. Kirchhof P, et al. Age- and training-dependent development of arrhythmogenic right ventricular cardiomyopathy in heterozygous plakoglobin-deficient mice. Circulation. 2006;114:1799–806.

55. Cruz FM, et al. Exercise triggers ARVC phenotype in mice expressing a disease-causing mutated version of human plakophilin-2. J Am Coll Cardiol. 2015;65:1438–50.

56. Corrado D, et al. Trends in sudden cardiovascular death in young competitive athletes after implementation of a Preparticipation screening program. JAMA. 2006;296:1593–601.

57. Pelliccia A, et al. 2020 ESC guidelines on sports cardiology and exercise in patients with cardiovascular disease: the task force on sports cardiology and exercise in patients with cardiovascular disease of the European Society of Cardiology (ESC). Eur Heart J. 2021;42:17–96.

58. Maron BJ, et al. Eligibility and disqualification recommendations for competitive athletes with cardiovascular abnormalities: task force 3: hypertrophic cardiomyopathy, arrhythmogenic right ventricular cardiomyopathy and other cardiomyopathies, and myocarditis: a scientific statement from the

American Heart Association and American College of Cardiology. Circulation. 2015;132:e273–80.

59. McKenna WJ, et al. Diagnosis of arrhythmogenic right ventricular dysplasia/cardiomyopathy. Task Force of the Working Group Myocardial and Pericardial Disease of the European Society of Cardiology and of the Scientific Council on Cardiomyopathies of the International Society. Br Heart J. 1994;71:215–8.

60. Marcus FI, et al. Diagnosis of arrhythmogenic right ventricular cardiomyopathy/dysplasia: proposed modification of the task force criteria. Circulation. 2010;121:1533–41.

61. Elliott PM, et al. Definition and treatment of arrhythmogenic cardiomyopathy: an updated expert panel report. Eur J Heart Fail. 2019;21:955–64.

62. Corrado D, et al. Arrhythmogenic right ventricular cardiomyopathy: evaluation of the current diagnostic criteria and differential diagnosis. Eur Heart J. 2020;41:1414–29.

63. di Gioia CRT, et al. Nonischemic left ventricular scar and cardiac sudden death in the young. Hum Pathol. 2016;58:78–89.

64. Nunes de Alencar Neto J, Baranchuk A, Bayés-Genís A, Bayés de Luna A. Arrhythmogenic right ventricular dysplasia/cardiomyopathy: an electrocardiogram-based review. Europace. 2018;20:f3–f12.

65. Te Riele ASJM, et al. Malignant arrhythmogenic right ventricular dysplasia/cardiomyopathy with a normal 12-lead electrocardiogram: a rare but underrecognized clinical entity. Heart Rhythm. 2013;10:1484–91.

66. Steriotis AK, et al. Electrocardiographic pattern in arrhythmogenic right ventricular cardiomyopathy. Am J Cardiol. 2009;103:1302–8.

67. Borys Surawicz TK. Chou's electrocardiography in clinical practice: adult and pediatric—Borys Surawicz. Timothy Knilans—Google Libri.

68. De Lazzari M, et al. Relationship between electrocardiographic findings and cardiac magnetic resonance phenotypes in arrhythmogenic cardiomyopathy. J Am Heart Assoc. 2018; https://doi.org/10.1161/JAHA.118.009855.

69. Gandjbakhch E, Redheuil A, Pousset F, Charron P, Frank R. Clinical diagnosis, imaging, and genetics of arrhythmogenic right ventricular cardiomyopathy/dysplasia: JACC state-of-the-art review. J Am Coll Cardiol. 2018;72:784–804.

70. Hoffmayer KS, et al. Electrocardiographic comparison of ventricular arrhythmias in patients with arrhythmogenic right ventricular cardiomyopathy and right ventricular outflow tract tachycardia. J Am Coll Cardiol. 2011;58:831–8.

71. Mattesi G, Zorzi A, Corrado D, Cipriani A. Natural history of arrhythmogenic cardiomyopathy. J Clin Med. 2020;9:878.

72. Bhonsale A, et al. Impact of genotype on clinical course in arrhythmogenic right ventricular dysplasia/cardiomyopathy-associated mutation carriers. Eur Heart J. 2015;36:847–55.

73. Bhonsale A, et al. Cardiac phenotype and long-term prognosis of arrhythmogenic right ventricular cardiomyopathy/dysplasia patients with late presentation. Heart Rhythm. 2017;14:883–91.

74. Migliore F, et al. Prognostic value of endocardial voltage mapping in patients with arrhythmogenic right ventricular cardiomyopathy/dysplasia. Circ Arrhythmia Electrophysiol. 2013;6:167–76.

75. Yoerger DM, et al. Echocardiographic findings in patients meeting task force criteria for arrhythmogenic right ventricular dysplasia: new insights from the multidisciplinary study of right ventricular dysplasia. J Am Coll Cardiol. 2005;45:860–5.

76. Borguist R, et al. The diagnostic performance of imaging methods in ARVC using the 2010 task force criteria. Eur Heart J Cardiovasc Imaging. 2014; https://doi.org/10.1093/ehjci/jeu109.

77. Haugaa KH, et al. Comprehensive multi-modality imaging approach in arrhythmogenic cardiomyopathy—an expert consensus document of the European Association of Cardiovascular Imaging. Eur Heart J Cardiovasc Imaging. 2017;18:237–53.

78. López-Fernández T, Ángel García-Fernández M, Pérez David E, Moreno Yangüela M. Usefulness of contrast echocardiography in arrhythmogenic right ventricular dysplasia. J Am Soc Echocardiogr. 2004;17:391–3.

79. Sarvari SI, et al. Right ventricular mechanical dispersion is related to malignant arrhythmias: a study of patients with arrhythmogenic right ventricular cardiomyopathy and subclinical right ventricular dysfunction. Eur Heart J. 2011;32:1089–96.

80. Teske AJ, et al. Early detection of regional functional abnormalities in asymptomatic ARVD/C gene carriers. J Am Soc Echocardiogr. 2012;25:997–1006.

81. Prakasa KR, et al. Feasibility and variability of three dimensional echocardiography in arrhythmogenic right ventricular dysplasia/cardiomyopathy. Am J Cardiol. 2006;97:703–9.

82. te Riele ASJM, Tandri H, Bluemke DA. Arrhythmogenic right ventricular cardiomyopathy (ARVC): cardiovascular magnetic resonance update. J Cardiovasc Magn Reson. 2014;16:50.

83. Tandri H, et al. Magnetic resonance imaging findings in patients meeting task force criteria for arrhythmogenic right ventricular dysplasia. J Cardiovasc Electrophysiol. 2003;14:476–82.

84. Basso C, Thiene G. Adipositas cordis, fatty infiltration of the right ventricle, and arrhythmogenic right ventricular cardiomyopathy. Just a matter of fat? Cardiovasc Pathol. 2005;14:37–41.

85. Tandri H, et al. Magnetic resonance imaging of arrhythmogenic right ventricular dysplasia. Sensitivity, specificity, and observer variability of fat detection versus functional analysis of the right ventricle. J Am Coll Cardiol. 2006;48:2277–84.

86. Tansey DK, Aly Z, Sheppard MN. Fat in the right ventricle of the normal heart. Histopathology. 2005;46:98–104.

87. Angelini A, Basso C, Nava A, Thiene G. Endomyocardial biopsy in arrhythmogenic right ventricular cardiomyopathy. Am Heart J. 1996;132:203–6.
88. Marcus FI, et al. Diagnosis of arrhythmogenic right ventricular cardiomyopathy/dysplasia. Circulation. 2010;121:1533–41.
89. Asimaki A, et al. A new diagnostic test for arrhythmogenic right ventricular cardiomyopathy. N Engl J Med. 2009;360:1075–84.
90. Collett BA, Davis GJ, Rohr WB. Extensive fibrofatty infiltration of the left ventricle in two cases of sudden cardiac death. J Forensic Sci. 1994;39:1182–7.
91. Aquaro GD, et al. Cardiac MR with late gadolinium enhancement in acute myocarditis with preserved systolic function: ITAMY study. J Am Coll Cardiol. 2017;70:1977–87.
92. Aquaro GD, et al. Prognostic value of repeating cardiac magnetic resonance in patients with acute myocarditis. J Am Coll Cardiol. 2019;74:2439–48.
93. Spezzacatene A, et al. Arrhythmogenic phenotype in dilated cardiomyopathy: natural history and predictors of life-threatening arrhythmias. J Am Heart Assoc. 2015;4:e002149.
94. Cipriani A, et al. Arrhythmogenic right ventricular cardiomyopathy: characterization of left ventricular phenotype and differential diagnosis with dilated cardiomyopathy. J Am Heart Assoc. 2020; https://doi.org/10.1161/JAHA.119.014628.
95. Bariani R, et al. 'Hot phase' clinical presentation in arrhythmogenic cardiomyopathy. Europace. 2020; https://doi.org/10.1093/europace/euaa343.
96. Corrado D, Link MS, Calkins H. Arrhythmogenic right ventricular cardiomyopathy. N Engl J Med. 2017;376:61–72.
97. Cadrin-Tourigny J, et al. A new prediction model for ventricular arrhythmias in arrhythmogenic right ventricular cardiomyopathy. Eur Heart J. 2019;40:1850–8.
98. Aquaro GD, et al. Prognostic value of magnetic resonance phenotype in patients with arrhythmogenic right ventricular cardiomyopathy. J Am Coll Cardiol. 2020;75:2753–65.
99. Wang W, et al. Arrhythmic outcome of arrhythmogenic right ventricular cardiomyopathy patients without implantable defibrillators. J Cardiovasc Electrophysiol. 2018;29:1396–402.
100. Saberniak J, et al. Vigorous physical activity impairs myocardial function in patients with arrhythmogenic right ventricular cardiomyopathy and in mutation positive family members. Eur J Heart Fail. 2014;16:1337–44.
101. Priori SG, et al. ESC guidelines for the management of patients with ventricular arrhythmias and the prevention of sudden cardiac death the task force for the management of patients with ventricular arrhythmias and the prevention of sudden cardiac death of the European Society of Cardiology (ESC) Endorsed by: Association for European Paediatric and Congenital Cardiology (AEPC). Eur Heart J. 2015;36:2793–867.
102. Corrado D, et al. Treatment of arrhythmogenic right ventricular cardiomyopathy/dysplasia: an international task force consensus statement. Circulation. 2015;132:441–53.
103. Van Der Voorn SM, et al. Arrhythmogenic cardiomyopathy: pathogenesis, pro-arrhythmic remodelling, and novel approaches for risk stratification and therapy. Cardiovasc Res. 2020;116:1571–84.
104. Marchlinski FE, et al. Electroanatomic substrate and outcome of catheter ablative therapy for ventricular tachycardia in setting of right ventricular cardiomyopathy. Circulation. 2004;110:2293–8.
105. Verma A, et al. Short- and long-term success of substrate-based mapping and ablation of ventricular tachycardia in arrhythmogenic right ventricular dysplasia. Circulation. 2005;111:3209–16.
106. Dalal D, et al. Morphologic variants of familial arrhythmogenic right ventricular dysplasia/cardiomyopathy. A genetics-magnetic resonance imaging correlation study. J Am Coll Cardiol. 2009;53:1289–99.
107. Assis FR, Tandri H. Epicardial ablation of ventricular tachycardia in arrhythmogenic right ventricular cardiomyopathy. Card Electrophysiol Clin. 2020;12:329–43.
108. Vita T, et al. Complementary value of cardiac magnetic resonance imaging and positron emission tomography/computed tomography in the assessment of cardiac sarcoidosis. Circ Cardiovasc Imaging. 2018;11:e007030.
109. Philips B, et al. Arrhythmogenic right ventricular dysplasia/cardiomyopathy and cardiac sarcoidosis. Circ Arrhythmia Electrophysiol. 2014;7:230–6.
110. Yatsynovich Y, Dittoe N, Petrov M, Maroz N. Cardiac sarcoidosis: a review of contemporary challenges in diagnosis and treatment. Am J Med Sci. 2018;355:113–25.
111. Pinto YM, et al. Proposal for a revised definition of dilated cardiomyopathy, hypokinetic non-dilated cardiomyopathy, and its implications for clinical practice: a position statement of the ESC working group on myocardial and pericardial diseases. Eur Heart J. 2016;37:1850–8.
112. Cavigli L, et al. The right ventricle in "left-sided" cardiomyopathies: the dark side of the moon. Trends Cardiovasc Med. 2020; https://doi.org/10.1016/j.tcm.2020.10.003.
113. Maron MS, et al. Right ventricular involvement in hypertrophic cardiomyopathy. Am J Cardiol. 2007;100:1293–8.
114. Guo X, et al. The clinical features, outcomes and genetic characteristics of hypertrophic cardiomyopathy patients with severe right ventricular hypertrophy. PLoS One. 2017;12:e0174118.
115. Nagata Y, et al. Right ventricular hypertrophy is associated with cardiovascular events in hypertrophic cardiomyopathy: evidence from study with magnetic resonance imaging. Can J Cardiol. 2015;31: 702–8.

Part IV

Treatment of Right Heart Dysfunction

Right-Heart Reverse Remodeling During Treatment for Pulmonary Hypertension

Roberto Badagliacca, Giovanna Manzi, and Carmine Dario Vizza

The Heart Remodeling

The complex process of heart remodeling consists of progressive changes in cardiac dimensions, mass, shape, and cellular and extracellular composition occurring in response to cardiac injury (e.g. myocardial loss) or mechanical stress (e.g. pressure/volume overload) [1]. These structural changes are initially compensatory aiming at maintaining a normal stroke volume but with the progression of the disease become deleterious, leading to ventricular dysfunction and poor prognosis. Indeed, to some extent different therapeutic approaches can induce reverse remodeling (RR), restoring chamber geometry, reducing ventricular volumes and improving function. Therefore, the main goal of treatment is to prevent or reverse the maladaptive remodeling process improving patients' outcomes [2, 3].

Right Ventricle Response to Chronic Pressure Overload

Pulmonary arterial hypertension (PAH) is an obstructive vasculopathy with patient's functional status and prognosis depending mostly on the ability of the right ventricle (RV) to adapt to the increased afterload. In the earlier stages, increased contractility occurs in order to improve RV-to-pulmonary artery coupling (*homeometric adaptation*) and to preserve cardiac output. In the later stages, chronic exposure to increased afterload leads to the failure of the *homeometric adaptation* with RV dilation [4–6]. Through *heterometric adaptation*, stroke volume is maintained by progressive increase in RV end-diastolic volume. Functional tricuspid regurgitation usually occurs because of annular valve dilatation resulting in additional RV volume overload. Both pressure and volume overloads determine the progressive reduction of cardiac output, complicated by the leftward ventricular septum shift due to ventricular interdependence, determining further underfilling of the left ventricle (LV) finally leading to the clinical syndrome of heart failure.

Therefore, RV dimensions, RV-pulmonary artery coupling, stroke volume, systolic function, filling pressures and potentially RV fibrosis draw the line between adapted and maladapted RV.

In PAH the RV may adapt to increased afterload through two different patterns (concentric vs eccentric hypertrophy), easily assessed through the RV mass-to-volume (M/V) ratio by cardiovascular magnetic resonance (CMR). Higher M/V ratio, indicative of a concentric remodeling pattern, is associated with a better systolic function and a more suitable RV-pulmonary artery coupling, compared with a low RV M/V ratio, and emerged as an independent predictor of clinical worsening in PAH [7, 8].

R. Badagliacca (✉) · G. Manzi · C. D. Vizza
Department of Clinical, Anesthesiological and Cardiovascular Sciences, Sapienza University of Rome, Rome, Italy
e-mail: roberto.badagliacca@uniroma1.it; giovanna.manzi@uniroma1.it; dario.vizza@uniroma.it

The heterogeneity of RV response to afterload is reflected in the different clinical presentation: some PAH patients remain well compensated while others rapidly decompensate, developing RV failure. The mechanisms influencing the type of RV adaptation are largely unknown but genetic factors and the timing of increased afterload onset (e.g. congenital heart diseases versus acquired PAH) seem to play an active role.

The Concept of Reverse Remodeling

Increasing evidence shed light on the possibility to induce RR of the pathologic ventricle removing the pathophysiologic trigger with medical or surgical treatments, restoring chamber dimensions, shape and contractility, and potentially improving morbidity and mortality.

In this field, the greatest knowledge comes from diseases affecting the left side of the heart, especially ischemic chronic heart failure.

In patients with chronic heart failure, changes in left-heart size and ejection fraction (EF) can be observed with pharmacological and non-pharmacological therapies [9, 10]. Beta-blockers have demonstrated to induce a more pronounced reversal of LV dilation associated with increased EF than other drugs, as ACE inhibitors [1]. Indeed, studies testing the anti-remodeling effects of metoprolol [11], carvedilol [12] and bisoprolol [13] showed a significant increase in LVEF (on average + 8–10%) and a trend toward reduction in end-diastolic and end-systolic volumes (range 20–30%) after 6–12 months of therapy.

In patients with left bundle branch block and ventricular dyssynchrony, LVRR can be achieved by cardiac resynchronization therapy (CRT). Resynchronization of right and left ventricular contraction by CRT usually increases LVEF by 20% and reduces LV volumes by 15%, consequently improving WHO functional class, exercise capacity and quality of life [14]. Most of the clinical trials define CRT-induced LVRR as a 15% reduction in LV end-systolic volume after a 6-month treatment period [15–17]. Indeed, LV end-systolic volume is the most used echocardiographic measurement in this setting, reflecting both chamber morphology and LV systolic function and showing superior predictive value for survival after myocardial infarction compared with LVEF and LV end-diastolic volume.

Left ventricular assist devices (LVADs) may also induce LVRR, greatly unloading the LV, shifting leftward the LV end-diastolic pressure-volume relationship and restoring blood pressure and flow to near-normal levels [18, 19]. As reported in a large cohort study, immediately after LVAD implantation, LV dimensions decrease by 20–30% and LVEF improves reaching a value above 40% in nearly a third of patients [20, 21]. However, original LV function may deteriorate over time with LVAD support potentially inducing disuse atrophy [22].

Despite the arbitrary and heterogeneous cut-off values used across studies to define LVRR, the proposed definitions all include the improvement of LV dimensional and/or functional parameters. Greater evidence has been collected for patients with idiopathic dilated cardiomyopathy, where some studies defined LVRR using increased LVEF of at least 10 percentage points from baseline or above a threshold value set at 50%, while others considered the increase in LV fractional shortening >25% [23–25]. Moreover, some studies included in the definition of RR the improvement of both LV systolic function and LV size, the latter as the decrease in the indexed LV end-diastolic diameter of at least 10% from baseline [26] or the achievement of an absolute value below 33 mm/m^2 [27].

The crucial role of LVRR and its impact on survival [28] highlight the clinical need of a common standardized definition, currently missing.

Reverse Right Ventricular Remodeling in Patients with Pulmonary Hypertension: The Effect of Ventricular Unloading

Recent studies on patients undergoing lung transplantation, pulmonary endarterectomy (PEA) and balloon pulmonary angioplasty have clearly shown the ability of the RV to regain physiologic morphology and function when significantly unloaded. Studies including patients with end-stage PAH refractory to medical treatment undergoing isolated lung transplantation showed a postoperative complete reverse cardiac remodeling, with RV function and size normalization (range of reduction in RV basal and mid-diameter 35–40% at 3 months), improvement of tricuspid regurgitation and restoring of interventricular septum in its physiologic position [29, 30].

RVRR has been observed also in patients with chronic thromboembolic pulmonary hypertension after a hemodynamically successful PEA. Indeed, as reported in different studies with CMR imaging-derived RV metrics, PEA can induce RVRR, significantly decreasing RV volumes within 3 months (on average −30%) and improving RV ejection fraction between 9% and 19% [31–33]. While PEA is the therapy of choice for eligible chronic thromboembolic pulmonary hypertension, inoperable patients or those with residual PH after PEA have a clear indication to balloon pulmonary angioplasty. As well as with PEA, recent studies have demonstrated RVRR after multiple sessions of balloon pulmonary angioplasty, able to induce significant improvement in pulmonary vascular resistance and cardiac output, leading to consequent reduction in RV volumes (range −35% to −40%) and mass and improvement in RVEF (mean +20%), without significantly affecting LV volumes and function [34, 35].

The Evaluation of Right Ventricular Reverse Remodeling

Although heterogeneous, the various definitions of LVRR resulting from different studies conducted in this field all included variations in LV size and function as a hallmark. Conversely, few studies focused on the RR of the RV, with a consequent lack of a potential definition. As a critical issue further studies are required to understand if including in the definition merely changes in right-heart morphological and functional parameters would be appropriate or the association with patient's outcome would be desirable.

Concerning the correct way to face with right-heart RR assessment, the use of a multiparametric approach (i.e. echocardiography and CMR) would allow to overcome reproducibility limitations and provide a more integrated assessment of the interplay between cardiac physiology and pathophysiology.

The complex shape and geometry of the RV make the evaluation of its volumes, mass and function difficult using echocardiographic two-dimensional imaging modalities. Thanks to the unique myocardial magnetic properties allowing an accurate planimetry interface easily reproducible, CMR is considered the reference technique for RV volumetric measurement and derived-ejection phase metrics [36]. Indeed, reproducibility of CMR-derived RV volumetric parameters is recognized to be superior to echocardiography [37].

Despite these advantages, CMR requires adequate standardization in postprocessing (i.e. manual contouring with the inclusion or exclusion of the RV trabeculations) and suffers from some limitations hampering its widespread use in clinical practice (availability, limited access, long testing time, feasibility for high-risk patients and high costs) [38]. Conversely, echocardiography is widely available, low cost, and safe, remaining crucial as the first-line modality for RV structure and function assessment [39].

A complete echocardiographic assessment of the RV should include two-dimensional and three-dimensional (3D) imaging, tissue Doppler imaging and speckle tracking techniques for myocardial strain metrics. Echocardiographic measurements of tricuspid annular peak systolic excursion, RV fractional area change, 3D RVEF, free-wall RV longitudinal strain and tricuspid peak myocardial contraction velocity (S′) have all shown good correlation with CMR-derived RVEF [40–42]. According to the higher temporal resolution compared with CMR, echo-derived RV strain evaluation should be considered more appropriate for patients' assessment [43].

Considering advantages and disadvantages of each imaging modality, right-heart RR assessment should potentially combine both echocardiography and CMR to allow the highest temporal and spatial resolution in the same patient.

Among right-heart dimensional parameters tightly related to pressure overload, relative RV areas and volumes, eccentricity indices of the LV, and right atrial areas and volumes may all be considered as valuable afterload-dependent variables for reverse remodeling assessment. Additionally, RV fractional area change and EF, tissue Doppler imaging-S', longitudinal strain and tricuspid annular peak systolic excursion have all demonstrated to be valid parameters for assessing RV systolic function and might be considered for RR evaluation.

The Impact of PAH-Specific Therapies on RV Reverse Remodeling

Although RV function is the major determinant of symptoms and outcome in PAH patients [4], therapies targeting directly the RV are still not available. Approved therapies largely rely on RV afterload reduction targeting the pulmonary circulation to allow reverse structural remodeling of the right heart (Fig. 16.1).

The effects of targeted therapies on echocardiographic indices of RV structure and function of PAH patients have been scarcely reported previously as substudies of randomized controlled trials. Hinderliter et al. [44] reported improved LV-EIs and RV end-diastolic volume in patients treated with intravenous epoprostenol in the randomized controlled trial which established the efficacy of this treatment [45]. Galiè et al. [46] showed an improvement in LV-EI and in the ratio of RV to LV surface areas in the group of patients treated with bosentan in the randomized controlled trial that established the efficacy of this drug [47]. Observational studies have further reported on improved CMR imaging-determined RV ejection fraction in PAH patients with various targeted therapies [48, 49].

However, treatments shown to be effective in randomized controlled trials are associated with only limited changes in PVR with consequent trivial improvement in RV size and function.

It has to be emphasized that most studies focusing on right-heart imaging metrics under targeted therapies were compliant to guidelines published in 2009 [50], providing monotherapy indication in clinical practice and being less insistent with more aggressive earlier combinations of drugs as currently recommended [51].

Notably, a small-size but long-term observational study showed that progressively increased RV dimension in spite of optimized targeted therapy regimen was associated with an increased mortality in PAH [52]. The relative dissociation between the evolution of functional class, six-minute walk distance and RV dimensions, and changes on patients' risk assessment is further illustrated in Fig. 16.2. In fact, as shown in panel a, the probability of clinical worsening will remain high unless a significant reduction in RV size is achieved. Additionally, panel b emphasizes how low- and intermediate-risk status is not necessarily associated with RV improvement in size.

In accordance with the pathophysiological model of afterload mismatch, important decrease of PVR brings in turn a profound reduction of RV size and a recovery of systolic function. In fact, the likelihood of decreased RV dimensions and associated improvement in afterload-dependent systolic function parameters is strongly correlated to the decrease in PVR after institution of targeted therapies [53].

Nevertheless, the optimal therapeutic strategy to reverse RV remodeling in severe PAH remains to be defined. Available data strongly suggest that drugs targeting the pulmonary circulation are to be combined to decrease PVR by at least 50%, and that the best results are obtained with incorporation of parenteral prostacyclins [54]. Impressive improvement in hemodynamics, in the range of 70–90% reduction of PVR, is potentially achieved with initial triple combination employing either intravenous epoprostenol or subcutaneous treprostinil [55], associated with dramatic reversal of right-heart remodeling [56].

Mild decrease in PVR, as occurs with less aggressive treatment strategies, is associated with the lack of or insufficient RV reverse remodeling

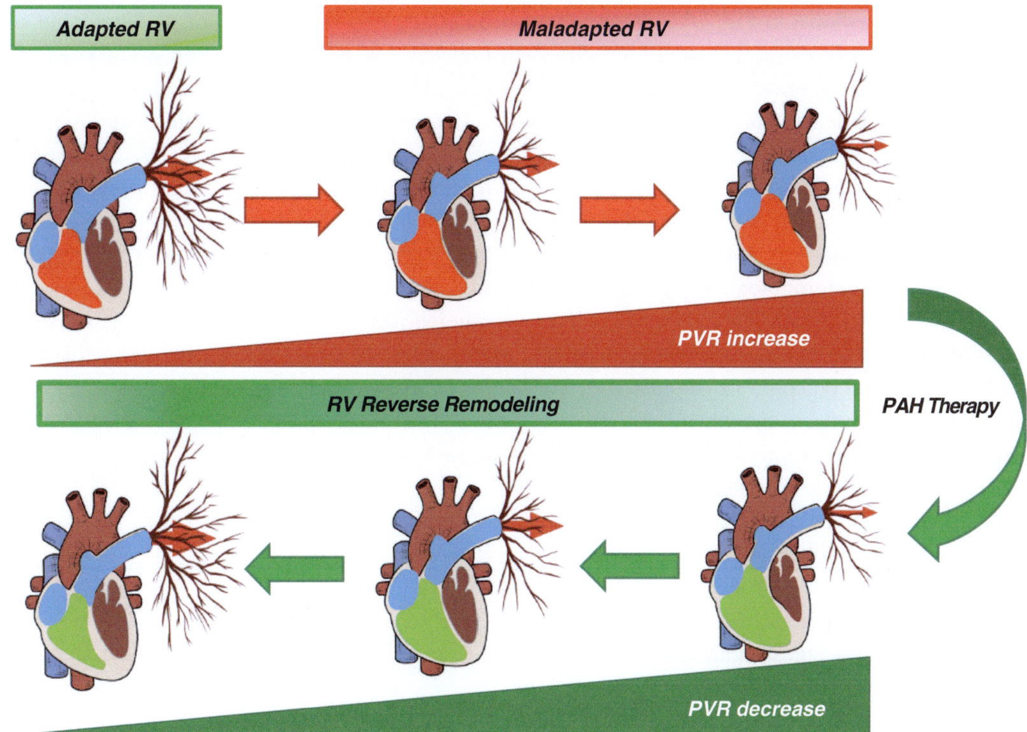

Fig. 16.1 The right ventricle remodeling and its reverse with PAH therapeutic strategies

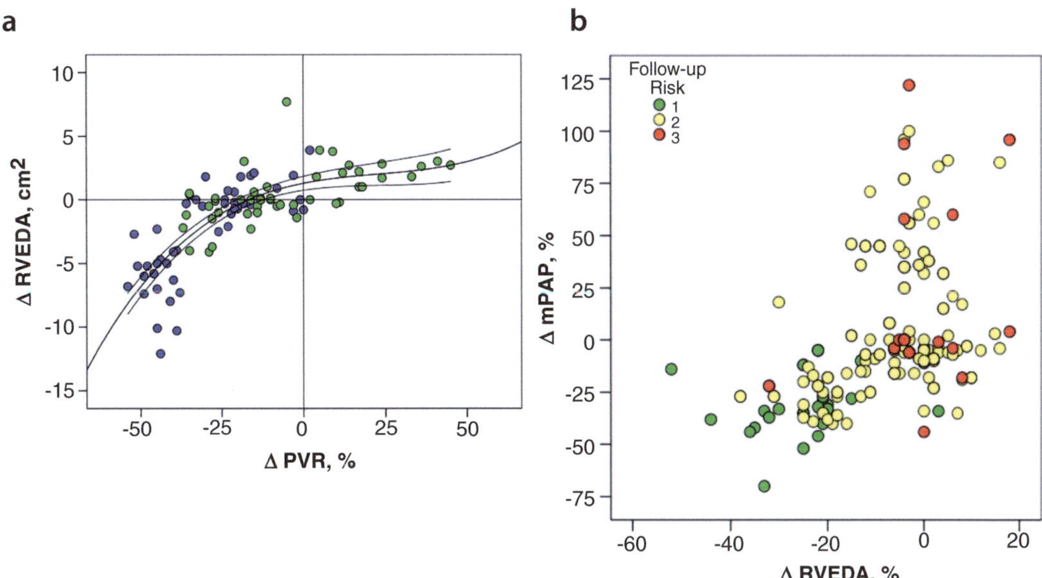

Fig. 16.2 Panel **(a)**: Correlations between the changes in RVEDA, RA area, LV-EIs, and PVR at 1-year assessment. Patients with and without clinical worsening are reported in the same scatterplot (green circles and blue circles, respectively). (Figure from Badagliacca R et al. J Heart Lung Transplant. 2017 Oct 2:S1053-2498(17)32041-7. doi: https://doi.org/10.1016/j.healun.2017.09.026). Panel **(b)**: Relationship between RVEDA and changes in mean pulmonary arterial pressure after targeted therapy according to the patient's risk profile at follow-up (figure from Badagliacca R et al. Int J Cardiol 2020; 301: 183–189). Legend: *RVEDA* right ventricular end-diastolic area, *RA area* right atrial area, *LV-EIs* left ventricular systolic eccentricity index, *PVR* pulmonary vascular resistance

[48, 57–61]. As shown in Fig. 16.3, the relationship between likelihood of reversal of RV dimensions and fall in PVR is sigmoid and very steep in the range of efficiency, so that small additional decrease in PVR above 50% results in marked reversal of RV dimensions to normal [62].

Recently, reversal of right-heart dimensions after 1 year of treatment, assessed as significant improvements in morphological parameters such as RV end-diastolic area, LV eccentricity index, and right atrial area, has been definitely associated with an improved outcome in patients with PAH [62, 63]. Interestingly, the extent of RV end-diastolic area decrease at 1-year follow-up that emerged as prognostically significant is approximately more than 10% from baseline evaluation, a value that is similar to the decrease in size observed in the failing LV when clinically significant reverse remodeling has been achieved after medical treatments [64]. This suggests that the definition of right-heart reverse remodeling recently adopted in PAH [63], for such a degree of reduction in RV size, might be consistent with the definition of reverse remodeling already applied in a number of studies for left-heart failure.

This observation makes the case for imaging-monitored intensification of therapy whenever possible and tolerated by the patients. For this purpose, the advantage of combining targeted

therapies has a strong rationale. Available data indicate that parenteral prostacyclins have to be part of this therapeutic optimization.

Nowadays, bedside echocardiography is widely available and effective in assessing RV function adaptation to afterload in PAH. The use of CMR is also expanding among referral centers. Both imaging modalities allow for the quantification of RV remodeling and its reversal by efficient therapeutic interventions. More studies are needed to strengthen the evidence that imaging is an essential component of risk assessment, but the clinical and pathophysiological rationale to favor it is strong.

References

1. Cohn JN, Ferrari R, Sharpe N. Cardiac remodeling—concepts and clinical implications: a consensus paper from an international forum on cardiac remodeling. Behalf of an International Forum on Cardiac Remodeling. J Am Coll Cardiol. 2000;35(3):569–82. https://doi.org/10.1016/s0735-1097(99)00630-0.
2. Saraon T, Katz SD. Reverse remodeling in systolic heart failure. Cardiol Rev. 2015;23(4):173–81. https://doi.org/10.1097/CRD.0000000000000068.
3. Konstam MA, Kramer DG, Patel AR, Maron MS, Udelson JE. Left ventricular remodeling in heart failure: current concepts in clinical significance and assessment. JACC Cardiovasc Imaging. 2011;4(1):98–108. https://doi.org/10.1016/j.jcmg.2010.10.008.
4. Vonk Noordegraaf A, Chin KM, Haddad F, Hassoun PM, Hemnes AR, Hopkins SR, Kawut SM, Langleben D, Lumens J, Naeije R. Pathophysiology of the right ventricle and of the pulmonary circulation in pulmonary hypertension: an update. Eur Respir J. 2019;53(1):1801900. https://doi.org/10.1183/13993003.01900-2018.
5. Naeije R, Vanderpool R, Peacock A, Badagliacca R. The right heart-pulmonary circulation unit: physiopathology. Heart Fail Clin. 2018;14(3):237–45. https://doi.org/10.1016/j.hfc.2018.02.001.
6. Sanz J, Sánchez-Quintana D, Bossone E, Bogaard HJ, Naeije R. Anatomy, function, and dysfunction of the right ventricle: state-of-the-art review. J Am Coll Cardiol. 2019;73:1463–82.
7. Badagliacca R, Poscia R, Pezzuto B, Nocioni M, Mezzapesa M, Francone M, et al. Right ventricular remodeling in idiopathic pulmonary arterial hypertension: adaptive versus maladaptive morphology. J Heart Lung Transplant. 2015;34(3):395–403. https://doi.org/10.1016/j.healun.2014.11.002. Epub 2014 Nov 8.
8. Badagliacca R, Poscia R, Pezzuto B, Papa S, Pesce F, Manzi G, et al. Right ventricular concentric hyper-

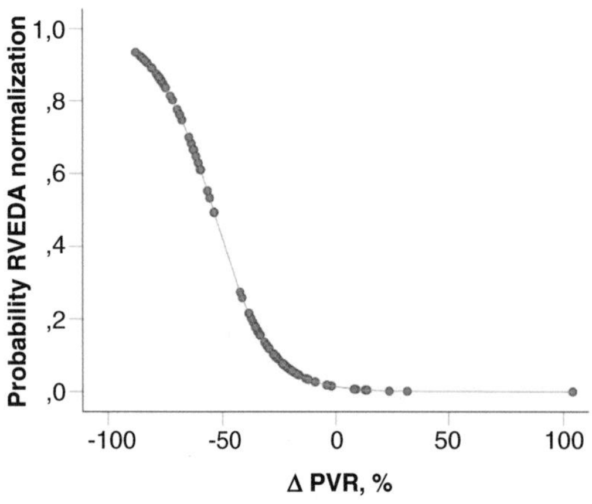

Fig. 16.3 Logistic probability of RVEDA normalization for any given PVR reduction. (Figure from Badagliacca R et al. JACC Cardiovasc Imaging. 2020; 13: 2054–2056). Legend: See Fig. 16.2

trophy and clinical worsening in idiopathic pulmonary arterial hypertension. J Heart Lung Transplant. 2016;35(11):1321–9. https://doi.org/10.1016/j.healun.2016.04.006. Epub 2016 May 6.

9. Waring AA, Litwin SE. Redefining reverse remodeling: can echocardiography refine our ability to assess response to heart failure treatments? J Am Coll Cardiol. 2016;68(12):1277–80. https://doi.org/10.1016/j.jacc.2016.07.718.

10. Pieske B. Reverse remodeling in heart failure—fact or fiction? Eur Heart J Suppl. 2004;6(Suppl_D):D66–78. https://doi.org/10.1016/j.ehjsup.2004.05.019.

11. Groenning BA, Nilsson JC, Sondergaard L, Fritz-Hansen T, Larsson HB, Hildebrandt PR. Antiremodeling effects on the left ventricle during beta-blockade with metoprolol in the treatment of chronic heart failure. J Am Coll Cardiol. 2000;36(7):2072–80. https://doi.org/10.1016/s0735-1097(00)01006-8.

12. Olsen SL, Gilbert EM, Renlund DG, Taylor DO, Yanowitz FD, Bristow MR. Carvedilol improves left ventricular function and symptoms in chronic heart failure: a double-blind randomized study. J Am Coll Cardiol. 1995;25:1225–31.

13. Dubach P, Myers J, Bonetti P, Schertler T, Froelicher V, Wagner D, et al. Effects of bisoprolol fumarate on left ventricular size, function, and exercise capacity in patients with heart failure: analysis with magnetic resonance myocardial tagging. Am Heart J. 2002;143(4):676–83. https://doi.org/10.1067/mhj.2002.121269.

14. Sutton MG, Plappert T, Hilpisch KE, Abraham WT, Hayes DL, Chinchoy E. Sustained reverse left ventricular structural remodeling with cardiac resynchronization at one year is a function of etiology: quantitative Doppler echocardiographic evidence from the Multicenter InSync Randomized Clinical Evaluation (MIRACLE). Circulation. 2006;113(2):266–72. https://doi.org/10.1161/CIRCULATIONAHA.104.520817. Epub 2006 Jan 9.

15. Maruo T, Seo Y, Yamada S, Arita T, Ishizu T, Shiga T, et al. The speckle tracking imaging for the assessment of cardiac resynchronization therapy (START) study. Circ J. 2015;79(3):613–22. https://doi.org/10.1253/circj.CJ-14-0842. Epub 2014 Dec 27.

16. Seo Y, Ito H, Nakatani S, Takami M, Naito S, Shiga T, et al., J-CRT Investigators. The role of echocardiography in predicting responders to cardiac resynchronization therapy. Circ J. 2011;75(5):1156–63. doi: https://doi.org/10.1253/circj.cj-10-0861. Epub 2011 Mar 4.

17. Chung ES, Leon AR, Tavazzi L, Sun JP, Nihoyannopoulos P, Merlino J, et al. Results of the predictors of response to CRT (PROSPECT) trial. Circulation. 2008;117(20):2608–16. https://doi.org/10.1161/CIRCULATIONAHA.107.743120. Epub 2008 May 5.

18. Levin HR, Oz MC, Chen JM, Packer M, Rose EA, Burkhoff D. Reversal of chronic ventricular dilation in patients with end-stage cardiomyopathy by prolonged mechanical unloading. Circulation. 1995;91(11):2717–20. https://doi.org/10.1161/01.cir.91.11.2717.

19. Ambardekar AV, Buttrick PM. Reverse remodeling with left ventricular assist devices: a review of clinical, cellular, and molecular effects. Circ Heart Fail. 2011;4(2):224–33. https://doi.org/10.1161/CIRCHEARTFAILURE.110.959684.

20. Wohlschlaeger J, Schmitz KJ, Schmid C, Schmid KW, Keul P, Takeda A, et al. Reverse remodeling following insertion of left ventricular assist devices (LVAD): a review of the morphological and molecular changes. Cardiovasc Res. 2005;68(3):376–86. https://doi.org/10.1016/j.cardiores.2005.06.030. Epub 2005 Jul 18.

21. Maybaum S, Mancini D, Xydas S, Starling RC, Aaronson K, Pagani FD, et al., LVAD Working Group. Cardiac improvement during mechanical circulatory support: a prospective multicenter study of the LVAD Working Group. Circulation. 2007;115(19):2497–505. doi: https://doi.org/10.1161/CIRCULATIONAHA.106.633180. Epub 2007 May 7.

22. Kent RL, Uboh CE, Thompson EW, Gordon SS, Marino TA, Hoober JK, Cooper G 4th. Biochemical and structural correlates in unloaded and reloaded cat myocardium. J Mol Cell Cardiol. 1985;17(2):153–65. https://doi.org/10.1016/s0022-2828(85)80018-3.

23. Ikeda Y, Inomata T, Iida Y, Iwamoto-Ishida M, Nabeta T, Ishii S, et al. Time course of left ventricular reverse remodeling in response to pharmacotherapy: clinical implication for heart failure prognosis in patients with idiopathic dilated cardiomyopathy. Heart Vessel. 2016;31(4):545–54. https://doi.org/10.1007/s00380-015-0648-2. Epub 2015 Feb 17.

24. Amorim S, Campelo M, Martins E, Moura B, Sousa A, Pinho T, Silva-Cardoso J, Maciel MJ. Prevalence, predictors and prognosis of ventricular reverse remodeling in idiopathic dilated cardiomyopathy. Rev Port Cardiol. 2016;35(5):253–60. English, Portuguese. https://doi.org/10.1016/j.repc.2015.11.014. Epub 2016 Apr 23. Erratum in: Rev Port Cardiol. 2017 Mar;36(3):231.

25. Hoshikawa E, Matsumura Y, Kubo T, Okawa M, Yamasaki N, Kitaoka H, Furuno T, Takata J, Doi YL. Effect of left ventricular reverse remodeling on long-term prognosis after therapy with angiotensin-converting enzyme inhibitors or angiotensin II receptor blockers and β blockers in patients with idiopathic dilated cardiomyopathy. Am J Cardiol. 2011;107(7):1065–70. https://doi.org/10.1016/j.amjcard.2010.11.033. Epub 2011 Feb 4.

26. Kubanek M, Sramko M, Maluskova J, Kautznerova D, Weichet J, Lupinek P, et al. Novel predictors of left ventricular reverse remodeling in individuals with recent-onset dilated cardiomyopathy. J Am Coll Cardiol. 2013;61(1):54–63. https://doi.org/10.1016/j.jacc.2012.07.072.

27. Merlo M, Pyxaras SA, Pinamonti B, Barbati G, Di Lenarda A, Sinagra G. Prevalence and prognostic

significance of left ventricular reverse remodeling in dilated cardiomyopathy receiving tailored medical treatment. J Am Coll Cardiol. 2011;57(13):1468–76. https://doi.org/10.1016/j.jacc.2010.11.030.

28. Yu CM, Bleeker GB, Fung JW, Schalij MJ, Zhang Q, van der Wall EE, et al. Left ventricular reverse remodeling but not clinical improvement predicts long-term survival after cardiac resynchronization therapy. Circulation. 2005;112(11):1580–6. https://doi.org/10.1161/CIRCULATIONAHA.105.538272. Epub 2005 Sep 6.

29. Sarashina T, Nakamura K, Akagi S, Oto T, Oe H, Ejiri K, et al. Reverse right ventricular remodeling after lung transplantation in patients with pulmonary arterial hypertension under combination therapy of targeted medical drugs. Circ J. 2017;81(3):383–90. https://doi.org/10.1253/circj.CJ-16-0838. Epub 2017 Jan 18.

30. Kasimir MT, Seebacher G, Jaksch P, Winkler G, Schmid K, Marta GM, et al. Reverse cardiac remodelling in patients with primary pulmonary hypertension after isolated lung transplantation. Eur J Cardiothorac Surg. 2004;26(4):776–81. https://doi.org/10.1016/j.ejcts.2004.05.057.

31. Reesink HJ, Marcus JT, Tulevski II, Jamieson S, Kloek JJ, Vonk Noordegraaf A, Bresser P. Reverse right ventricular remodeling after pulmonary endarterectomy in patients with chronic thromboembolic pulmonary hypertension: utility of magnetic resonance imaging to demonstrate restoration of the right ventricle. J Thorac Cardiovasc Surg. 2007;133(1):58–64. https://doi.org/10.1016/j.jtcvs.2006.09.032.

32. Berman M, Gopalan D, Sharples L, Screaton N, Maccan C, Sheares K, et al. Right ventricular reverse remodeling after pulmonary endarterectomy: magnetic resonance imaging and clinical and right heart catheterization assessment. Pulm Circ. 2014;4(1):36–44. https://doi.org/10.1086/674884.

33. D'Armini AM, Zanotti G, Ghio S, Magrini G, Pozzi M, Scelsi L, et al. Reverse right ventricular remodeling after pulmonary endarterectomy. J Thorac Cardiovasc Surg. 2007;133(1):162–8. https://doi.org/10.1016/j.jtcvs.2006.08.059. Epub 2006 Nov 30.

34. Fukui S, Ogo T, Morita Y, Tsuji A, Tateishi E, Ozaki K, et al. Right ventricular reverse remodelling after balloon pulmonary angioplasty. Eur Respir J. 2014;43(5):1394–402. https://doi.org/10.1183/09031936.00012914. Epub 2014 Mar 13.

35. Sumimoto K, Tanaka H, Mukai J, Yamashita K, Tanaka Y, Shono A, et al. Effects of balloon pulmonary angioplasty for chronic thromboembolic pulmonary hypertension on remodeling in right-sided heart. Int J Cardiovasc Imaging. 2020;36(6):1053–60. https://doi.org/10.1007/s10554-020-01798-5. Epub 2020 Feb 21.

36. McLure LE, Peacock AJ. Cardiac magnetic resonance imaging for the assessment of the heart and pulmonary circulation in pulmonary hypertension. Eur Respir J. 2009;33(6):1454–66. https://doi.org/10.1183/09031936.00139907.

37. Grothues F, Moon JC, Bellenger NG, Smith GS, Klein HU, Pennell DJ. Interstudy reproducibility of right ventricular volumes, function, and mass with cardiovascular magnetic resonance. Am Heart J. 2004;147(2):218–23. https://doi.org/10.1016/j.ahj.2003.10.005.

38. Wessels JN, de Man FS, Vonk Noordegraaf A. The use of magnetic resonance imaging in pulmonary hypertension: why are we still waiting? Eur Respir Rev. 2020;29(156):200139. https://doi.org/10.1183/16000617.0139-2020.

39. Mertens LL, Friedberg MK. Imaging the right ventricle-current state of the art. Nat Rev Cardiol. 2010;7(10):551–63. https://doi.org/10.1038/nrcardio.2010.118. Epub 2010 Aug 10.

40. Pavlicek M, Wahl A, Rutz T, de Marchi SF, Hille R, Wustmann K, et al. Right ventricular systolic function assessment: rank of echocardiographic methods vs. cardiac magnetic resonance imaging. Eur J Echocardiogr. 2011;12(11):871–80. https://doi.org/10.1093/ejechocard/jer138. Epub 2011 Sep 6.

41. Focardi M, Cameli M, Carbone SF, Massoni A, De Vito R, Lisi M, Mondillo S. Traditional and innovative echocardiographic parameters for the analysis of right ventricular performance in comparison with cardiac magnetic resonance. Eur Heart J Cardiovasc Imaging. 2015;16(1):47–52. https://doi.org/10.1093/ehjci/jeu156. Epub 2014 Sep 3.

42. Lang RM, Badano LP, Mor-Avi V, Afilalo J, Armstrong A, Ernande L, et al. Recommendations for cardiac chamber quantification by echocardiography in adults: an update from the American Society of Echocardiography and the European Association of Cardiovascular Imaging. J Am Soc Echocardiogr. 2015;28(1):1–39.e14. https://doi.org/10.1016/j.echo.2014.10.003.

43. Lee JH, Park JH. Strain analysis of the right ventricle using two-dimensional echocardiography. J Cardiovasc Imaging. 2018;26(3):111–24. https://doi.org/10.4250/jcvi.2018.26.e11. Epub 2018 Aug 29.

44. Hinderliter AL, Willis PW 4th, Barst RJ, Rich S, Rubin LJ, Badesch DB, et al. Effects of long-term infusion of prostacyclin (epoprostenol) on echocardiographic measures of right ventricular structure and function in primary pulmonary hypertension. Primary Pulmonary Hypertension Study Group. Circulation. 1997;95(6):1479–86. https://doi.org/10.1161/01.cir.95.6.1479.

45. Barst RJ, Rubin LJ, Long WA, McGoon MD, Rich S, Badesch DB. et al. Primary pulmonary hypertension study group. A comparison of continuous intravenous epoprostenol (prostacyclin) with conventional therapy for primary pulmonary hypertension. N Engl J Med. 1996;334(5):296–301. https://doi.org/10.1056/NEJM199602013340504.

46. Galiè N, Hinderliter AL, Torbicki A, Fourme T, Simonneau G, Pulido T, et al. Effects of the oral endothelin-receptor antagonist bosentan on echocardiographic and doppler measures in patients with pulmonary arterial hypertension. J Am Coll Cardiol. 2003;41(8):1380–6. https://doi.org/10.1016/s0735-1097(03)00121-9.

47. Rubin LJ, Badesch DB, Barst RJ, Galie N, Black CM, Keogh A, et al. Bosentan therapy for pulmonary arterial hypertension. N Engl J Med. 2002;346(12):896–903. https://doi.org/10.1056/NEJMoa012212. Erratum in: N Engl J Med 2002 Apr 18;346(16):1258.

48. Peacock AJ, Crawley S, McLure L, Blyth KG, Vizza CD, Poscia R, et al. Changes in right ventricular function measured by cardiac magnetic resonance imaging in patients receiving pulmonary arterial hypertension-targeted therapy: the EURO-MR study. Circ Cardiovasc Imaging. 2014;7(1):107–14. https://doi.org/10.1161/CIRCIMAGING.113.000629. Epub 2013 Oct 30. Erratum in: Circ Cardiovasc Imaging. 2017 Feb;10(2).

49. van de Veerdonk MC, Kind T, Marcus JT, Mauritz GJ, Heymans MW, Bogaard HJ, et al. Progressive right ventricular dysfunction in patients with pulmonary arterial hypertension responding to therapy. J Am Coll Cardiol. 2011;58(24):2511–9. https://doi.org/10.1016/j.jacc.2011.06.068.

50. Galiè N, Hoeper MM, Humbert M, Torbicki A, Vachiery JL, Barbera JA, et al., ESC Committee for Practice Guidelines (CPG). Guidelines for the diagnosis and treatment of pulmonary hypertension: the Task Force for the Diagnosis and Treatment of Pulmonary Hypertension of the European Society of Cardiology (ESC) and the European Respiratory Society (ERS), endorsed by the International Society of Heart and Lung Transplantation (ISHLT). Eur Heart J. 2009;30(20):2493–537. https://doi.org/10.1093/eurheartj/ehp297. Epub 2009 Aug 27. Erratum in: Eur Heart J. 2011 Apr;32(8):926.

51. Galiè N, Humbert M, Vachiery JL, Gibbs S, Lang I, Torbicki A, et al., ESC Scientific Document Group. 2015 ESC/ERS guidelines for the diagnosis and treatment of pulmonary hypertension: the Joint Task Force for the Diagnosis and Treatment of Pulmonary Hypertension of the European Society of Cardiology (ESC) and the European Respiratory Society (ERS): Endorsed by: Association for European Paediatric and Congenital Cardiology (AEPC), International Society for Heart and Lung Transplantation (ISHLT). Eur Heart J. 2016;37(1):67–119. https://doi.org/10.1093/eurheartj/ehv317. Epub 2015 Aug 29.

52. van de Veerdonk MC, Marcus JT, Westerhof N, de Man FS, Boonstra A, Heymans MW, et al. Signs of right ventricular deterioration in clinically stable patients with pulmonary arterial hypertension. Chest. 2015;147(4):1063–71. https://doi.org/10.1378/chest.14-0701.

53. Badagliacca R, Papa S, Matsubara H, Lang IM, Poscia R, Manzi G, Vizza CD. The importance of right ventricular evaluation in risk assessment and therapeutic strategies: raising the bar in pulmonary arterial hypertension. Int J Cardiol. 2020;301:183–9.

54. Badagliacca R, Raina A, Ghio S, D'Alto M, Confalonieri M, Correale M, et al. Influence of various therapeutic strategies on right ventricular morphology, function and hemodynamics in pulmonary arterial hypertension. J Heart Lung Transplant. 2018;37(3):365–75. https://doi.org/10.1016/j.healun.2017.08.009. Epub 2017 Aug 26.

55. Sitbon O, Jaïs X, Savale L, et al. Upfront triple combination therapy in pulmonary arterial hypertension: a pilot study. Eur Respir J. 2014;43:1691–7.

56. D'Alto M, Badagliacca R, Argiento P, Romeo E, Farro A, Papa S, et al. Risk reduction and right heart reverse remodeling by upfront triple combination therapy in pulmonary arterial hypertension. Chest. 2020;157(2):376–83.

57. van de Veerdonk MC, Huis In T Veld AE, Marcus JT, Westerhof N, Heymans MW, Bogaard HJ, Vonk-Noordegraaf A. Upfront combination therapy reduces right ventricular volumes in pulmonary arterial hypertension. Eur Respir J. 2017;49(6):1700007. https://doi.org/10.1183/13993003.00007-2017.

58. Sitbon O, Sattler C, Bertoletti L, Savale L, Cottin V, Jaïs X, et al. Initial dual oral combination therapy in pulmonary arterial hypertension. Eur Respir J. 2016;47(6):1727–36. https://doi.org/10.1183/13993003.02043-2015. Epub 2016 Mar 17.

59. D'Alto M, Romeo E, Argiento P, Paciocco G, Prediletto R, Ghio S, et al. Initial tadalafil and ambrisentan combination therapy in pulmonary arterial hypertension: cLinical and haemodYnamic long-term efficacy (ITALY study). J Cardiovasc Med (Hagerstown). 2018;19(1):12–7. https://doi.org/10.2459/JCM.0000000000000590.

60. Badagliacca R, D'Alto M, Ghio S, Argiento P, Bellomo V, Brunetti ND, et al. Risk reduction and hemodynamics with initial combination therapy in pulmonary arterial hypertension. Am J Respir Crit Care Med. 2020; https://doi.org/10.1164/rccm.202004-1006OC.

61. D'Alto M, Badagliacca R, Lo Giudice F, Argiento P, Casu G, Corda M, et al. Hemodynamics and risk assessment 2 years after the initiation of upfront ambrisentan–tadalafil in pulmonary arterial hypertension. J Heart Lung Transplant. 2020. pii: S1053-2498(20)31706-X; https://doi.org/10.1016/j.healun.2020.08.016.

62. Badagliacca R, Papa S, Manzi G, Miotti C, Luongo F, Sciomer S, et al. Usefulness of adding echocardiography of the right heart to risk assessment scores in prostanoid-treated pulmonary arterial hypertension. JACC Cardiovasc Imaging. 2020;13:2054–6.

63. Badagliacca R, Poscia R, Pezzuto B, Papa S, Reali M, Pesce F, et al. Prognostic relevance of right heart reverse remodeling in idiopathic pulmonary arterial hypertension. J Heart Lung Transplant. 2017. pii: S1053-2498(17)32041-7; https://doi.org/10.1016/j.healun.2017.09.026.

64. Braunwald E. Heart failure. JACC Heart Fail. 2013;1(1):1–20. https://doi.org/10.1016/j.jchf.2012.10.002. Epub 2013 Feb 4.

Laurent Savale, Athénaïs Boucly, Jérémie Pichon,
Anne Roche, and Marc Humbert

Introduction

Precapillary pulmonary hypertension (PH) defines a group of disorders characterized by a progressive increase in pulmonary vascular resistance (PVR) that develops as a result of abnormal remodeling of the pulmonary microvasculature [1, 2]. Improved understanding of the pathophysiology of precapillary pulmonary hypertension has led to the development of several medications that primarily target endothelial dysfunction [3]. Despite these major advances, pulmonary hypertension remains a progressive and fatal disease leading to right ventricular dysfunction and death [4, 5]. The function of the right ventricle is of great clinical importance in end-stage pulmonary hypertension since it determines the prognosis of patients [4]. The ability of the right ventricle to adapt to the progressive increase in afterload is closely linked to the outcome of the disease. Impaired cardiac output (CO) and elevation in central venous pressure are associated with functional deterioration, onset of congestive signs, and ultimately mortality in patients with advanced pulmonary hypertension [6, 7].

The prognostic importance of right ventricular function has been a renewed interest in recent years in the analysis of the pathophysiology of right ventricular remodeling and dysfunction [4]. End-stage pulmonary hypertension is associated with a high risk of acute right-heart failure (RHF), which has been defined as a rapidly progressive syndrome with systemic congestion resulting from impaired right ventricular filling and/or reduced right ventricular flow output [8]. The occurrence of acute RHF remains the most frequent cause of death with a dismal prognosis over the short term, highlighting the need for earlier recognition and better management options. This chapter aims to provide a comprehensive review of the state of the art in acute decompensated pulmonary hypertension.

Pathophysiology of Right-Heart Failure

Various definitions have been proposed to define right ventricular failure (RVF) that is a complex clinical syndrome characterized by decreased right ventricular function that leads to insufficient blood flow and/or elevated filling pressures at rest or during physiologically demanding conditions [4, 9, 10]. RVF can occur as a consequence of alterations in preload, intrinsic changes in RV function, or increases in afterload. In case of acute

L. Savale (✉) · A. Boucly · J. Pichon · A. Roche
M. Humbert
Université Paris-Saclay, Faculty of Medicine,
Le Kremlin-Bicêtre, France

INSERM UMR_S 999, Le Kremlin-Bicêtre, France

AP-HP, Service de Pneumologie et soins intensifs respiratoires, Hôpital Bicêtre,
Le Kremlin-Bicêtre, France
e-mail: laurent.savale@aphp.fr

or progressive increases in afterload, the right ventricle's ability to adapt to this physiological condition is a major determinant of functional prognosis and outcomes. The right ventricle (RV) differs from the left ventricle (LV) by its thin wall and complex three-dimensional conformation adapted to the low pressure, low resistance, and high compliance of the pulmonary circulation. Acute obstruction of less than 50% of the pulmonary circulation is generally well tolerated by a healthy RV, with the recruitment and vasodilation properties of the pulmonary vascular bed mitigating an increase in pulmonary vascular resistance (PVR). Beyond this level of obstruction, the RV responds to the acute rise in PVR by increasing its end-diastolic volume in order to restore the contractile properties of the RV myocardium via the Frank–Starling mechanism. However, this immediate adaptation is rapidly limited by the deleterious effect of the increased RV wall tension on right coronary flow and by the LV/RV interdependency and desynchronization caused by RV dilatation. Ultimately, reduction in the CO due to the RV dysfunction and impaired LV filling leads to hemodynamic instability [11].

The pathophysiological mechanisms of RVF in patients with chronic pulmonary hypertension are different due to chronic conformational adaptation of the RV to progressive increased afterload. The capacity of the RV to adapt to the progressive increases in afterload varies considerably from one individual to another leading to a continuum between an adapted RV and a maladapted ventricle. These adaptation capacities can be influenced by many factors like gender [12], genetic mutation [13–15], and the etiology of PAH [16]. The first conformational adaptation of the RV is a concentric myocardial hypertrophy combined with a slight dilatation which aims to normalize the imposed wall stress. Secondly, the RV expands in response to increased pressures. Eccentric hypertrophy combined with excessive dilation of the right cavities most often reflects a less favorable adaptive phenomenon leading to reduced SV and increased filling pressures. At this stage, we observe a severe alteration of the systolic and diastolic function of the RV combined with an alteration of the diastolic function of the left ventricle (LV) by mechanisms of RV/LV interdependence (Fig. 17.1). This phenotype corresponds to the final phase of PH which is characterized by the onset of NYHA functional class III or IV symptoms of dyspnea, the appearance of congestive signs, a risk of syncope, and hemodynamically a chronic rise in right atrial pressure and decreased CO [17]. All these parameters are closely correlated with a poor prognosis and result from a severe alteration of the ventriculoarterial coupling characterized by an inefficient transfer of myocardial energy from the RV to the downstream pulmonary arterial circulation [4, 9].

The modifications of the RV are the results of complex molecular and metabolomic mechanisms as well as cellular changes that have been more recently studied in experimental models and human tissue. The RV remodeling seems to be the result of an increase in both protein synthesis (collagen fibers in the extracellular matrix) and myocardial cell population [18–20]. Moreover, the cellular damage leading to a decrease in RV performance is promoted by multiple molecular mechanisms including changes in the neurohormonal system [21], inflammation oxidative stress and apoptosis [22], and metabolomic disorders characterized by reduced fatty acid oxidation in addition to increased glycolysis [23, 24].

Acute Right-Heart Failure Decompensation

Patients with end-stage precapillary PH are at high risk for developing acute right-heart decompensation. This clinical situation corresponds to an disturbance of the adaptive phenomena of the RV leading to an acute worsening of the symptoms, generally associated with circulatory failure and in the most severe cases with multiple-organ failure [8, 17]. Acute RHF can be precipitated by an external trigger or worsening factor or it can be the consequence of disease worsening. Most often, right-sided heart failure requiring treatment in the intensive care unit presents as combined systolic and diastolic heart failure. Diastolic failure promotes worsening

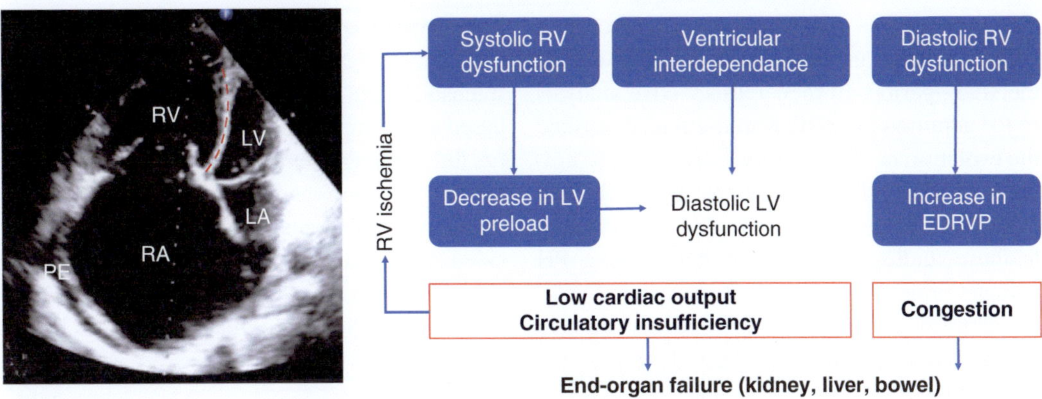

Fig. 17.1 Key factors contributing to acute right-heart failure in pulmonary hypertension. Abbreviations: *EDRVP* end-diastolic right ventricular pressure, *LA* left atrium, *LV* left ventricle, *PE* pericardial effusion, *RA* right atrium, *RV* right ventricle

congestive signs. Right ventricular systolic failure results in a sharp decrease in LV preload and a decrease in cardiac output followed by low peripheral perfusion pressure. The fall in cardiac output and the resulting acute circulatory failure may favor ischemia of the right ventricle by compromising the systolic component of coronary perfusion (Fig. 17.1).

Severe right-sided heart failure can promote the sudden development of multiple-organ failure. In the ICU setting, the consequences for the liver, kidneys, and gut are often most relevant. The pathophysiological mechanisms of acute renal dysfunction are probably similar to those observed in type I cardiorenal syndrome [25]. Acute worsening of renal function in the context of decompensated pulmonary hypertension has been strongly related to outcomes [26–29]. As in left-heart failure, the renin-angiotensin-aldosterone and the sympathetic nervous systems are stimulated, leading to a worsening of peripheral vascular resistance and sodium and water retention. Moreover, significant stimulation of antidiuretic hormone promotes excessive retention of free water, leading to volume overload and hyponatremia. These phenomena contribute to a decrease in renal perfusion due to both arterial vasoconstriction and venous congestion [25]. Malperfusion and congestion alter bowel wall permeability and may cause translocation of bacteria and endotoxins from the bowel into the cir-

culation resulting in a systemic inflammatory response or sepsis.

Epidemiology of Acute Decompensated Pulmonary Hypertension and Prognosis

Short-term outcome of acute decompensated RHF is very poor and remains the first cause of mortality in PAH. Few data are available on the epidemiology and management of acute PH decompensation. A US study analyzed the circumstances of death in a cohort of 84 PAH patients who died over a 4-year period. PH was determined to be the direct cause of death (right-heart failure or sudden death) in 37 (44%) patients; PH contributed to but did not directly cause death in 37 (44%) patients, and the death was not related to PH in the remaining cases ($n = 7$; 8.3%). It was underlined that death occurred in ICU in 80% of patients. Furthermore, half of the cohort received catecholamines during the hospital stay [30]. Similar results were reported in a Belgium database that analyzed the cause of death in 99 PAH patients [31].

The annual incidence of acute decompensation in a population of PAH patients has never been clearly studied. Huynh et al. also reported the outcome of 99 PH patients admitted in ICU for acute RHF over a 5-year period [32]. More than 900 patients with pulmonary hypertension (PH) were seen in the outpatient setting during the study period. In their retrospective analysis of PH admitted for RHF, Kurzina et al. described the evolution of 37 patients experiencing 60 episodes of RHF, while 172 patients were followed during the 3 years of study period [33]. According to these studies, incidence of RHF among PH patients ranges between 2.2% and 7.2%. Incidence of acute RHF in PH patients can also be estimated in trials on PAH drugs. In the GRIPHON study, 86 (15%) and 123 (21.1%) patients, respectively, in the selexipag and placebo group were admitted for acute RHF over a 3-year period [34]. In the AMBITION trial testing a combination of ambrisentan and tadalafil, Galie et al. described 10 (4%) and 30 (12%) of patients with acute RHF, respectively, in the combination and pooled monotherapy group over a 1.4-year study period [35]. Last, the SERAPHIN investigators testing the macitentan also found between 8.8% and 17.7% of patients according to groups affected by acute decompensated PH, syncope, or hemodynamic impairment, over 3 years [36]. Therefore, though limited by the absence of dedicated studies and limits pertaining to the design of investigational trials, it can be estimated from the aforementioned data that the annual incidence of acute RHF in PH patients probably ranges between 2% and 9%.

Prognosis of acute decompensated RHF in pulmonary hypertension has been mainly described by the retrospective cohort of patients with a limited number of patients and relative heterogeneity of the population studied, in terms of severity at admission. However, all these clinical studies have demonstrated the very strong impact of acute pulmonary hypertension decompensation on short-term prognosis. Depending on the type of population studied, in-hospital mortality varies from 14% to 100% [26–28, 32, 33, 37]. The prognostic factors identified in these studies are cardiac biomarkers, low systemic arterial pressures, inflammation, and reflective of multiple-organ failure induced by cardiac and circulatory insufficiency.

Treatment of RHF in ICU

Intensive care of acute decompensated PH is based on the treatment of triggering factors, careful fluid management, and strategies to improve cardiac function and reduce right ventricular afterload [8]. Patients with PH with severe right-sided heart failure decompensation requiring ICU admission should be treated at expert centers able to offer all modern treatment options if possible (Fig. 17.2).

Identification and Management of Triggering Factors

Chronic diseases are characterized by a delicate balance between persistent functional impairment and adaptation factors. In most chronic diseases, identification of a triggering factor for the exacerbation is one of the key points of the therapeutic strategy. Treatable precipitants of right-sided heart failure are diverse but must be systematically identified and managed.

Among them, supraventricular arrhythmias (tachyarrhythmia, atrial fibrillation, or atrial flutter) are frequently observed during PAH [38]. The loss of atrial function in patients with PAH may contribute to the impairment of RV function and precipitate acute right ventricular decompensation. In this context, some specificities on the management of arrhythmias should be known. Regarding the use of antiarrhythmic treatments, beta-blockers and calcium channel blockers should be avoided in these patients because of their deleterious negative inotropic effect in a period of right cardiac decompensation or more generally in all patients with precapillary PH. The use of digoxin is preferred to reduce the heart rate. Rapid restoration of sinus rhythm should be attempted by amiodarone and/or cardioversion if the clinical condition of the patient so permits. In the event of atrial flutter or persistent atrial tachycardia, radiofrequency ablation is preferred.

Infection is another important contributor to death in patients with right-sided heart failure. The source of infection is not always identified

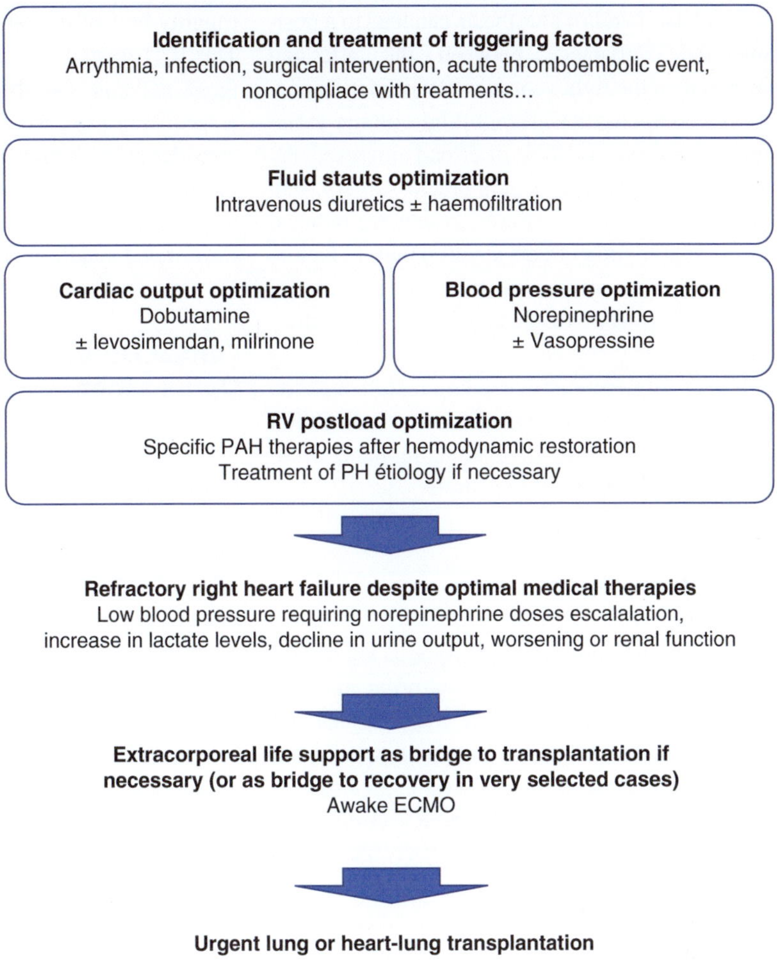

Fig. 17.2 Management of acute RHF in chronic pulmonary hypertension

> **Identification and treatment of triggering factors**
> Arrythmia, infection, surgical intervention, acute thromboembolic event, noncompliace with treatments…

> **Fluid stauts optimization**
> Intravenous diuretics ± haemofiltration

> **Cardiac output optimization**
> Dobutamine
> ± levosimendan, milrinone

> **Blood pressure optimization**
> Norepinephrine
> ± Vasopressine

> **RV postload optimization**
> Specific PAH therapies after hemodynamic restoration
> Treatment of PH étiology if necessary

Refractory right heart failure despite optimal medical therapies
Low blood pressure requiring norepinephrine doses escalalation,
increase in lactate levels, decline in urine output, worsening or renal function

**Extracorporeal life support as bridge to transplantation if
necessary (or as bridge to recovery in very selected cases)**
Awake ECMO

Urgent lung or heart-lung transplantation

and may correspond in some patients to a bacterial translocation precipitated by the low cardiac output and increased venous pressure. In patients treated with intravenous epoprostenol, a tunneling catheter infection must be excluded. The management of an infectious factor triggering or worsening a picture of right ventricular failure must not suffer from any delay in management. If the source of infection is not obvious, broad-spectrum antibiotics should be considered [8].

Exceptionally, right ventricular failure is accompanied by a picture of acute respiratory distress. Some patients may present with profound hypoxemia due to an opening of the foramen ovale, or in certain particular forms of PAH such as Eisenmenger syndrome or veno-occlusive disease. Most often, severe hypoxemia is rela-

tively well tolerated by the patient, with ventilatory mechanics being preserved. This hypoxemia should be corrected as best as possible by spontaneous ventilation to maintain a peripheral oxygen saturation >90%. In specific cases, high-flow oxygenation should be considered although no specific study has evaluated the tolerance and efficacy of this support in the specific setting of acute decompensated PH. In the event of acute respiratory distress related to a cause other than PAH such as infectious pneumonia, the use of invasive ventilation should be avoided as much as possible as it may lead to worsening of the RVF and then to postintubation collapse.

Surgical procedures are a well-known trigger of acute right-heart failure in patients with chronic pulmonary hypertension (PH) [39]. Various physiological disturbances induced by surgery itself and/or anesthesia can lead to a postoperative imbalance between the afterload imposed on the right ventricle (RV) and its capacity for compensation. Rapid fluid volume variations, increase in RV afterload imposed by mechanical ventilation or thoracic surgery, and decrease in systemic vascular resistance induced by anesthetic drug effects are all potential factors involved in postoperative ventriculoarterial uncoupling, RV distension, and circulatory insufficiency.

Other triggering or worsening factors must be checked like thromboembolic events, deviation from the salt-free diet, or noncompliance with specific PH therapies for example.

Fluid Status Optimization

Because both hypo- and hypervolemia are deleterious for RV function in PH, monitoring and optimization of volume status are major issues and can be sufficient to regain a state of equilibrium in less severe patients. In the physiological condition, the high compliance of the RV ensures the maintenance of a low right atrial pressure, which maintains systemic venous return and thus preserves the cardiac output. In PH, cardiac performance is closely linked to the RV preload. RV diastolic dysfunction promotes sodium and water retention, which may be exacerbated in the setting of acute decompensated RHF. Intravenous diuretics are used as a first-line treatment in order to reduce RV dilation and to improve right–left ventricular interdependence and thus improve left ventricular diastolic function, reduce tricuspid insufficiency, and reduce organ congestion.

Hemofiltration has also been suggested in case of fluid overload insufficiently treated with diuretics. However, the short- and long-term benefit of renal replacement therapy (RRT) in PH patients has never been properly evaluated. In a retrospective study, our group analyzed the benefit/risk ratio of RRT in PH patients with acute RHF. This work analyzed 36 continuous and 32 intermittent RRT sessions in 14 patients over an 11-year period. Significant systemic hypotension requiring a therapeutic intervention occurred in

roughly half of the sessions for both modalities. The ICU-related, 1-, and 3-month mortality of these patients was 46.7%, 66.7%, and 73.3%, respectively [28]. Regarding the poor outcomes, consideration should be given to extracorporeal life support (ECLS) and urgent lung or heart-lung transplantation in eligible patients with severe cardiorenal syndrome (see below).

Cardiac Output and Blood Pressure Optimization

Low CO induced by RV failure, LV preload disturbance, and ventricular interdependence contributes to hemodynamic instability. Use of inotropic agents to improve contractility and CO may be required (Table 17.1). β1-Adrenergic agonist remains the inotropic agent of choice. Dobutamine improved ventriculoarterial coupling in experimental models of acute occlusion of the pulmonary artery [40]. Low doses (2.5 µg/kg/min) must be initiated with a progressive up-titration in case of persistent signs of low CO. However, the dose of dobutamine must not exceed 5–7.5 µg/kg/min because of deleterious effects at higher doses: the precipitation of a decrease in systemic vascular resistance without improving CO. Inodilating agents, including levosimendan and milrinone, could alternatively be considered, however, the clinical effects of these drugs have been mainly studied in postcapillary PH after cardiac surgery. Levosimendan is a calcium-sensitizing agent with inotropic, pulmonary vasodilatory, and cardioprotective properties [41]. Experimental data suggested a better effect than dobutamine for improving ventriculoarterial coupling [42]. Data in pulmonary arterial hypertension are mainly limited to clinical cases. Initial infusion of 0.1 µg/kg/min without a bolus, for 24 h, could be recommended. This dose can be reduced to 0.05 µg/kg/min or increased to 0.2 µg/kg/min, according to the hemodynamic tolerance [41]. Milrinone, a selective PDE-3 inhibitor, has been shown to improve cardiac function in many preclinical studies without deleterious effects on PVR. Similar to levosimendan, milrinone is preferentially used in group 2 PH after cardiac surgery at a dose of

Table 17.1 Characteristics of inotropic and vasopressor drugs used for RVF failure management in PH patients (adapted from [8]). Reproduced with permission of the © ERS 2021: European Respiratory Journal Jan 2019, 53 (1) 1801906; DOI: https://doi.org/10.1183/13993003.01906-2018

Drug	Pharmacological properties	Beneficial hemodynamic effects	Side effects	Recommended doses	Clinical experience
Inotropic drugs					
Dobutamine	β1-Agonist catecholamine	– Increase in CO – Decrease in PVR – Improved V-A coupling	– Decrease in SVR – Tachycardia/arrhythmia (dose dependent)	2.5–10 µg/kg/min	– Large clinical experience in acute PH decompensation
Levosimendan	Calcium-sensitizing agent	– Increase in CO – Decrease in PVR – Improved V-A coupling	– Decrease in SVR – Tachycardia/arrhythmia (++)	0.05–0.2 µg/kg/min without bolus	– Mainly studied in postcapillary PH after cardiac surgery or transplantation – Limited data in PAH
Milrinone	Selective PDE-3 inhibitor	– Increase in CO – Decrease in PVR – Improved V-A coupling	– Decrease in SVR – Tachycardia/arrhythmia (+++)	50 µg/kg over 10 min, then 0.375–0.75 µg/kg/min infusion	
Dopamine	Agonist action on beta-adrenoceptors	– Increase in CO – Increase in SVR	– Tachycardia/arrhythmia	2–10 µg/kg/min	Increase in renal blood flow Few clinical data in PH
Vasopressor drugs					
Norepinephrine	α-Agonist ß-Agonist (high dose)	– Increase in SVR – Increase in CO	– Tachycardia/arrhythmia – Increase in PVR at high dose	0.1–5 mg/h	First-line vasopressor agent
Vasopressin		– Decrease in PVR – Increase in SVR	– Tachycardia/arrhythmia	0.01–0.04 U/min	Limited clinical data

Abbreviations: *CO* cardiac output, *PAH* pulmonary arterial hypertension, *PDE* phosphodiesterase, *PH* pulmonary hypertension, *PVR* pulmonary vascular resistance, *SVR* systemic vascular resistance, *V-A* ventriculoarterial

50 µg/kg over 10 min and then 0.375–0.75 µg/kg/min infusion. Inodilating agents, such as dobutamine, can cause arrhythmias and precipitate systemic vasodilatation requiring concomitant use of vasopressors. An alternative administration option for levosimendan and milrinone is by nebulization, which has also been studied to reduce the effect on systemic hypotension and V/Q mismatching [43, 44]. Finally, dopamine could be a potential alternative of dobutamine, due to its additional natriuretic properties. However, its use is limited by higher risk of arrhythmic events [45]. Epinephrine is not a drug of choice in the postoperative period due to its high risk of tachycardia and lactic disorders.

Patients with a low systemic vascular resistance need additional vasopressor treatment to restore blood pressure and another organ perfusion (Table 17.1). Prompt maintenance of aortic pressure is a critical point to protect right coronary perfusion and thereby prevent RV ischemia. Norepinephrine (NE) is generally used as a first-line vasopressor agent. In addition to its effect on systemic blood pressure, NE could contribute to improving RV function and ventriculoarterial coupling as well as reducing the PVR/SVR ratio. However, activation of alpha-1 adrenoreceptor by NE can lead to pulmonary vasoconstriction and increase in PVR at high doses [40]. Vasopressin could be an interesting alternative or additional option as it has pulmonary vasodilatory effects and fewer tachyarrhythmias in comparison with NE [46]. However, the clinical relevance of this pulmonary hemodynamic effect is unknown. Low doses of vasopressin (0.01–0.04 U/min) must be used to avoid the risk of bowel ischemia at higher doses [47]. Phenylephrine has been shown to induce potential paradoxical effects, leading to an increase in PVR, a decrease in cardiac output, and reflex bradycardia. The use of this drug is not recommended in the management of acute PH decompensation [48].

RV Postload Optimization

The most important intervention to restore a durable equilibrium status is to minimize the afterload of the RV as much as possible. The means and possibilities to achieve this will depend on the type of pulmonary hypertension and the therapeutic margins still available in the patient admitted for right ventricular failure.

For group 1 PAHs, the reduction in RV afterload is essentially based on the use of specific PAH treatments targeted at endothelial dysfunction. However, initiation of PAH-specific therapies must not be considered as emergency medications. The potential systemic hypotensive effects of PAH-targeted therapies can be deleterious in unstable patients with heart failure, low CO, and hypotension if they are introduced before hemodynamic restoration. In patients in whom RVF is the first diagnosis of PAH with NYHA functional class IV symptoms and dyspnea, it is now recommended to use the different therapeutic classes available in combination as the first line, including a prostacyclin analogue [5]. The introduction of this type of treatment requires expertise and must therefore be done in a center specializing in the management of PAH. For patients already treated for PAH, the possibility of strengthening the specific treatment for PAH will be considered on a case-by-case basis. In a retrospective analysis, Kurzyna et al. found that the addition of a therapy aimed at decreasing pulmonary vascular resistance during an episode of acute heart failure was associated with a favorable outcome [33].

In the specific case of newly diagnosed PH at the time of acute RHF, a postembolic origin of pulmonary hypertension must be systematically screened since it is the only form possibly accessible to surgical treatment (pulmonary endarterectomy) which can be discussed in an emergency or semi-emergency. The decision of a surgical intervention must take into account the anatomical location of the postembolic sequelae which must be accessible to surgery. For more distal lesions, the risk of failure and therefore of postoperative mortality becomes too high, especially in patients with right ventricular failure with very high levels of pulmonary vascular resistance [49].

It is also important to known the specific cases of PAH associated with lupus or mixed connective tissue disease. Pulmonary vascular involvement may be inaugural with a rapid onset of right-heart failure possibly associated with pericardial effusion related to the severity of PAH and favored by autoimmune pathology. The immunological assessment must therefore be systematic in the etiological assessment of an inaugural RVF. The initiation of an immuno-suppressive treatment combining corticosteroid therapy and cyclophosphamide bolus with specific PAH therapies can be useful to obtain, in some patients, spectacular results or even a reversibility of the pulmonary vascular involvement [50, 51].

The usefulness of continuous inhaled nitric oxide (NO) in the management of acute RHF has been suggested in many studies more specifically in PH due to ARDS. In acute decompensated PAH, NO inhalation seems to be safe but the efficacy has never been properly evaluated. In a cohort of 28 patients who were candidates for lung transplantation, a hemodynamic study showed that iNO and dobutamine have complementary effects on pulmonary circulation. Their association leads to an increase in the cardiac index without mean pulmonary arterial pressure modification and an increase in PaO_2 [52].

Management of Refractory Right-Heart Failure

The medical strategy is not always sufficient to restore a long-lasting balance between the afterload imposed on the right ventricle and its capacity for compensation. In case of refractory RHF despite maximal medical treatment, the use of mechanical support should now be considered in selected candidates for lung transplantation, or less commonly as a bridge to recovery in patients with a treatable cause of right-sided heart failure [8]. This strategy, combined with changes in organ allocation rules to prioritize patients with a short-term life-threatening condition, should contribute to improving the survival of eligible patients with end-stage pulmonary arterial hypertension.

Urgent Lung and Heart-Lung Transplantation in Pulmonary Hypertension

Urgent lung or heart-lung transplantation remains an important option in patients with severe RHF refractory to maximal medical therapy [8]. The frequent occurrence of acute right-heart decompensation in patients with PAH translates to a trend of a higher death rate on the transplant waiting list. Moreover, it has been reported that primary graft dysfunction and 1-year mortality rates after transplantation were higher in PAH than in other indications for lung transplantation [53].

To decrease waiting-list deaths, most countries have developed and refined lung allocation scores in order to prioritize the most severe patients at the time of listing and therefore reduce the risk of death on the waiting list. In the USA, a lung allocation score was implemented in May 2005 [54], which was followed by improved survival in patients with idiopathic PAH [53]. Nevertheless, the main parameters used in the lung allocation score did not correlate with the severity of right ventricular dysfunction. Modified lung allocation scores were proposed, including a mean right atrial pressure ≥ 14 mmHg and a 6-min walking distance ≤ 300 m, in order to improve the relative weighting of PAH severity at the time of listing [55]. A system of allocation score at the time of listing has also been adopted in some European countries such as Germany. In addition, an exceptional Eurotransplant lung allocation score has been proposed for patients with severe right-heart failure, in order to reduce the risk of mortality on list [56]. In other countries, such as France, another system based on a high-priority allocation program has been developed, rather than an initial score at the time of listing. In cases of life-threatening conditions such as acute decompensated pulmonary hypertension requiring the use of catecholamines, a national priority access to transplantation can be obtained for a period of 8 days, which is renewable once if necessary. The possibility to offer high-priority lung transplantation to PAH patients with refractory RHF has led to a major reduction of the waiting time and, by inference, reduced the risks of pre- and postoperative complications [57].

Extracorporeal Life Support in Acute Decompensated Pulmonary Hypertension

Extracorporeal life support (ECLS) is another major advance in the management of refractory right-heart failure due to decompensated pulmonary hypertension [8]. In case of refractory RHF despite maximal medical treatment, the use of mechanical support should now be considered in selected candidates for lung transplantation, or less commonly as a bridge to recovery in patients with a treatable cause of right-sided heart failure.

The indications for ECLS in the context of refractory RHF should be discussed preferably in an expert center with a multidisciplinary team able to offer all modern treatment options including all novel medical, instrumental, and surgical management of RHF. Because of potentially serious complications, the use of circulatory support must be reserved only for selected patients at high risk of imminent death despite optimal medical treatment with a plan for lung transplantation. Venoarterial extracorporeal membrane oxygenation (ECMO) is the most widely used technique in decompensated PAH. The main advantage of this system is the possibility of initiating it without general anesthesia in awake patients. Venous and arterial cannulas are introduced most often in femoral vessels but upper body approaches have also been proposed. ECMO leads to an immediate reduction in right ventricular afterload and restores systemic arterial pressure, thereby improving organ perfusion. ECMO flows of 2.5–4 L/min are appropriate for PAH patients who have been accustomed to lower CO. This flow rate is enough to allow unloading of the right ventricle, preservation of pulmonary blood flow, and adequate systemic oxygen delivery while avoiding overload of the left heart that may have secondary dysfunction in patients with severe right ventricular failure. The circulatory output is maintained by a pump, which necessitates the use of anticoagulation. Therefore, the major complications of ECMO are

the risk of bleeding, but also lower limb ischemia and systemic infection. For these reasons, time under ECMO must be optimized and systematically combined with a plan for urgent transplantation, or exceptionally with rapid recovery of right ventricular function [8].

Pumpless membrane oxygenators inserted between the pulmonary artery and the pulmonary veins or left atrium (Novalung, Hechingen, Germany) have also been used as a bridge to transplantation in decompensated pulmonary hypertension. With this system, no pump is needed, reducing the risk of bleeding. Because of PVR elevation in pulmonary hypertension, blood ejected by the right ventricle is preferentially redirected into the device, immediately reducing the afterload of the right ventricle [58]. The physiological effect of this device on left ventricular function is probably more interesting than ECMO, because it restores the left ventricular preload which is largely impaired in pulmonary hypertension. The major disadvantage of the Novalung system is the need for sternotomy under general anesthesia. In our practice, we have mainly used this system in patients who failed pulmonary endarterectomy with severe persistent pulmonary hypertension that precluded weaning from cardiopulmonary bypass [59].

The best timing for setting the indication for the establishment of an ECMO is not clearly established. ECLS should be initiated when the clinical course suggests that terminal right-heart failure and/or secondary organ failure is imminent despite optimized medical therapy [8]. The worsening of multiple-organ failure despite the inotropic and vasopressor supports should discuss circulatory assistance in a short time to allow rapid recovery of vital functions before transplantation. At the last world congress, a decline in S_{cvO2} accompanied by an increase in lactate and a decline in urine output have been listed as biomarkers of refractory RHF [8].

The use of ECMO as a bridge to recovery is much more exceptional and is only supported by very rare cases in the literature. This approach could be discussed in selected patients if there is the possibility to introduce combination PAH therapies and to treat a rapidly reversible cause of

PAH decompensation. Future feedback from expert centers will be essential to analyze the failure and success rate of this approach in order to improve the selection of candidates for such a therapeutic approach.

Sudden decrease in PVR after graft perfusion leads to a sudden elevation of left ventricular preload and a higher risk of primary graft dysfunction. For these reasons, the use of ECMO has been proposed in selected patients during a 48–72-h postoperative period until the end of the period of primary graft dysfunction (i.e., ischemia-reperfusion lung injuries) [60–62]. This approach seems to have contributed to decrease the risk of postoperative mortality. Interestingly, a progressive reversibility of the myocardial remodeling leading to a recovery of a normal right ventricular function was observed after double-lung transplantation, even in cases of end-stage right ventricular failure at the time of listing. This observation allowed the reduction in the indication for heart-lung transplantation. The determinants of time to right ventricular recovery after double-lung transplantation remain to be determined.

Monitoring of Acute RHF in PH Patients

The appropriate monitoring for this specific subset of patients remains a matter of uncertainty. An ideal tool should monitor cardiac variables that are the targets of treatments (RV preload, CO, and pulmonary vascular resistance) and not be associated with adverse effects such as arrhythmias or infections. Such a tool should also be able to evaluate the adequacy of initiated treatments on peripheral organ function. Ideally, the monitoring equipment should be easy to set up and repeatable over time.

Clinical Monitoring

The clinical assessment of the severity of the acute decompensated PH episode can be subtle in some patients. Indeed, the clinical presentation can be falsely reassuring at rest. Systemic arterial pressure at admission has been identified as a prognostic factor [27]. However, a majority of patients are able to maintain a normal level of systemic vascular resistance for a long time. A fall in systemic vascular resistance under diuretic and/or inotropic support treatment appears to be a determining prognostic factor in ICU as well as the necessity of introducing norepinephrine to maintain the systemic pressure. Similarly, clinical signs of low CO, such as encephalopathy, digestive intolerance, and recurrent syncope appear very late in the end-stage period. The occurrence of low urine output despite medical therapy is a major sign of cardiorenal syndrome that is clearly associated with a poor outcome in short term. Monitoring of diuresis and weight in order to assess daily water balance is a determinant clinical parameter.

Circulating Biomarkers

Markers of myocardial injury (troponin) and right ventricular dysfunction (BNP or NT-proBNP) were both identified as potential prognostic factors in PAH at stable condition but also during acute episode of decompensation [27, 63, 64]. Cardiac troponin T is a highly sensitive and specific marker of myocardial cell injury that can increase in RHF irrespective of the presence or absence of coronary artery disease. Release of cardiac troponin from myocardium results from impaired coronary blood flow leading to RV ischemia. Short-term outcome and right ventricular dysfunction in acute pulmonary embolism are associated with elevated serum level of troponin [52]. Prognosis value of troponin levels in acute decompensation needs to be further studied.

Several prospective studies and meta-analyses have demonstrated an association between high concentrations of BNP or NT-proBNP and clinical deterioration or survival in patients with PAH [63]. In the specific setting of acute decompensated PAH, retrospective studies reported a link between the level of BNP or NT-proBNP and outcomes [27]. Other dynamic studies are needed to investigate the prognosis value of BNP or

NT-proBNP not only at the time of admission but also after initiation of medical treatment in ICU. Growth differentiation factor 15 (GDF-15) is another cytokine induced in the heart after ischemia or pressure overload. The prognostic value of GDF-15 has been already investigated in PAH but its prognostic value in acute RHF needs to be studied [65].

Because cardiorenal syndrome is a major prognostic factor in right cardiac decompensation, biomarkers assessing renal function are of great importance in the follow-up of patients in ICU. In all studies, high levels of creatinine and hyponatremia are associated with poor prognosis in short term. Elevated C-reactive protein (CRP) plasma levels may be in favor of an infectious background in PAH patients displaying acute heart failure. In our experience, high CRP levels are indeed predictors of poor prognosis in acute worsening of PAH, even without evidence of infection, raising the potential involvement of inflammation among several pathophysiological injuries [4].

Noninvasive Hemodynamic Evaluation

Many echocardiographic parameters are useful to monitor right ventricular preload, right and left ventricular function, and right ventricular afterload. Some variables evaluating right ventricular contractile function, like tricuspid annular systolic excursion (TAPSE) or velocities (s′) or right cavity dimensions, have shown to be prognostic factors in PAH in the stable condition. Nevertheless, precise assessment of right ventricular function remains a challenge and very few data support its reliability in the setting of acute right-heart failure. Haddad et al. reported that tricuspid regurgitation severity was the only parameter associated with a worse prognosis in the setting of acute decompensated PH [26]. However, it was found that neither right-heart chamber size nor right atrial pressure estimation was associated with the outcome. Additional studies are necessary to evaluate precisely the accuracy of each echocardiographic parameter in

this specific setting and their impact on prognosis at admission but also after medical therapies' initiation.

Alternative noninvasive or minimally invasive techniques have been developed in order to reduce adverse events and provide continuous CO and fluid responsiveness variables in real time. However, these techniques have been mainly studied in sedated patients under mechanical ventilation. In contrast, very few data are available on the performance of these hemodynamic monitoring tools in awake patients admitted in ICU for right-heart failure. Many new systems have been developed to monitor the CO indirectly, with a continuous analysis of the arterial pressure waveform [66]. These techniques, combined with right ventricular preload estimation with central venous pressure, could be an interesting option in patients with acute decompensated pulmonary hypertension, but remain to be prospectively evaluated.

Invasive Hemodynamic Monitoring

In patients with a central venous line, it is useful to monitor the central venous pressure in order to assess right ventricular preload and improve management of fluid balance. In addition, measurement of central venous oxygen saturation is recommended to appreciate tissue oxygenation. Right hemodynamic monitoring by right cardiac catheterization remains the most effective tool in the evaluation of right ventricular preload, right ventricle afterload, and cardiac function in pulmonary hypertension. Right atrial pressure and CO are the main altered parameters in acute decompensation, and have been demonstrated to be major prognostic factors in PAH. However, invasive hemodynamic monitoring in the ICU is not widely used in routine practice, due to a risk of infection and arrhythmia, which may be considered too great in these fragile patients. Ultimately, right-heart catheterization preferably with continuous CO measurement should be considered in severe and complex cases after assessing the benefit-to-risk ratio [8].

Transpulmonary thermodilution-based methods to determine CO have generated great interest in the ICU population. This technology provides information regarding numerous physiological variables including systemic arterial pressure, CO, or stroke volume. This method has never been formally validated in right-heart failure. Moreover, right ventricular dilatation and tricuspid regurgitation are major limitations of the reliability of the device.

Conclusion

Acute decompensation of PAH remains a devastating life-threatening condition in the current management era. However, recent improvements combining implementation of novel medical, instrumental, and surgical management of RHF should translate to improvements in long-term survival of patients. Management of such patients requires expert centers with multidisciplinary teams able to offer all modern treatment options. Despite increasing knowledge on physiological features involved in RHF, many questions remain unclear on key cellular and molecular mechanisms and their clinical implications. There remains a considerable need for further research in this field.

References

1. Humbert M, Guignabert C, Bonnet S, Dorfmüller P, Klinger JR, Nicolls MR, Olschewski AJ, Pullamsetti SS, Schermuly RT, Stenmark KR, Rabinovitch M. Pathology and pathobiology of pulmonary hypertension: state of the art and research perspectives. Eur Respir J. 2019;53:1801887.
2. Simonneau G, Montani D, Celermajer DS, Denton CP, Gatzoulis MA, Krowka M, Williams PG, Souza R. Haemodynamic definitions and updated clinical classification of pulmonary hypertension. Eur Respir J. 2019;53:1801913.
3. Humbert M, Lau EMT, Montani D, Jaïs X, Sitbon O, Simonneau G. Advances in therapeutic interventions for patients with pulmonary arterial hypertension. Circulation. 2014;130:2189–208.
4. Vonk Noordegraaf A, Chin KM, Haddad F, Hassoun PM, Hemnes AR, Hopkins SR, Kawut SM, Langleben D, Lumens J, Naeije R. Pathophysiology of the right ventricle and of the pulmonary circulation in pulmonary hypertension: an update. Eur Respir J. 2019;53:1801900.
5. Galiè N, Channick RN, Frantz RP, Grünig E, Jing ZC, Moiseeva O, Preston IR, Pulido T, Safdar Z, Tamura Y, McLaughlin VV. Risk stratification and medical therapy of pulmonary arterial hypertension. Eur Respir J. 2019;53:1801889.
6. Humbert M, Sitbon O, Chaouat A, Bertocchi M, Habib G, Gressin V, Yaïci A, Weitzenblum E, Cordier J-F, Chabot F, Dromer C, Pison C, Reynaud-Gaubert M, Haloun A, Laurent M, Hachulla E, Cottin V, Degano B, Jaïs X, Montani D, Souza R, Simonneau G. Survival in patients with idiopathic, familial, and anorexigen-associated pulmonary arterial hypertension in the modern management era. Circulation. 2010;122:156–63.
7. Weatherald J, Boucly A, Chemla D, Savale L, Peng M, Jevnikar M, Jaïs X, Taniguchi Y, O'Connell C, Parent F, Sattler C, Hervé P, Simonneau G, Montani D, Humbert M, Adir Y, Sitbon O. Prognostic value of follow-up hemodynamic variables after initial management in pulmonary arterial hypertension. Circulation. 2018;137:693–704.
8. Hoeper MM, Benza RL, Corris P, de Perrot M, Fadel E, Keogh AM, Kühn C, Savale L, Klepetko W. Intensive care, right ventricular support and lung transplantation in patients with pulmonary hypertension. Eur Respir J. 2019;53:1801906.
9. Lahm T, Douglas IS, Archer SL, Bogaard HJ, Chesler NC, Haddad F, Hemnes AR, Kawut SM, Kline JA, Kolb TM, Mathai SC, Mercier O, Michelakis ED, Naeije R, Tuder RM, Ventetuolo CE, Vieillard-Baron A, Voelkel NF, Vonk-Noordegraaf A, Hassoun PM, American Thoracic Society Assembly on Pulmonary Circulation. Assessment of right ventricular function in the research setting: knowledge gaps and pathways forward. An Official American Thoracic Society Research Statement. Am J Respir Crit Care Med. 2018;198:e15–43.
10. Harjola V-P, Mebazaa A, Čelutkienė J, Bettex D, Bueno H, Chioncel O, Crespo-Leiro MG, Falk V, Filippatos G, Gibbs S, Leite-Moreira A, Lassus J, Masip J, Mueller C, Mullens W, Naeije R, Nordegraaf AV, Parissis J, Riley JP, Ristic A, Rosano G, Rudiger A, Ruschitzka F, Seferovic P, Sztrymf B, Vieillard-Baron A, Yilmaz MB, Konstantinides S. Contemporary management of acute right ventricular failure: a statement from the Heart Failure Association and the Working Group on Pulmonary Circulation and Right Ventricular Function of the European Society of Cardiology. Eur J Heart Fail. 2016;18:226–41.
11. Konstantinides SV, Meyer G, Becattini C, Bueno H, Geersing G-J, Harjola V-P, Huisman MV, Humbert M, Jennings CS, Jiménez D, Kucher N, Lang IM, Lankeit M, Lorusso R, Mazzolai L, Meneveau N, Áinle FN, Prandoni P, Pruszczyk P, Righini M, Torbicki A, Van Belle E, Zamorano JL, The Task Force for the Diagnosis and Management of Acute Pulmonary Embolism of the European Society of Cardiology

(ESC). 2019 ESC guidelines for the diagnosis and management of acute pulmonary embolism developed in collaboration with the European Respiratory Society (ERS): the Task Force for the diagnosis and management of acute pulmonary embolism of the European Society of Cardiology (ESC). Eur Respir J. 2019;54:1901647.

12. Jacobs W, van de Veerdonk MC, Trip P, de Man F, Heymans MW, Marcus JT, Kawut SM, Bogaard H-J, Boonstra A, Vonk NA. The right ventricle explains sex differences in survival in idiopathic pulmonary arterial hypertension. Chest. 2014;145:1230–6.

13. van der Bruggen CE, Happé CM, Dorfmüller P, Trip P, Spruijt OA, Rol N, Hoevenaars FP, Houweling AC, Girerd B, Marcus JT, Mercier O, Humbert M, Handoko ML, van der Velden J, Vonk Noordegraaf A, Bogaard HJ, Goumans M-J, de Man FS. Bone morphogenetic protein receptor type 2 mutation in pulmonary arterial hypertension: a view on the right ventricle. Circulation. 2016;133:1747–60.

14. Talati MH, Brittain EL, Fessel JP, Penner N, Atkinson J, Funke M, Grueter C, Jerome WG, Freeman M, Newman JH, West J, Hemnes AR. Mechanisms of lipid accumulation in the bone morphogenetic protein receptor type 2 mutant right ventricle. Am J Respir Crit Care Med. 2016;194:719–28.

15. Evans JDW, Girerd B, Montani D, Wang X-J, Galiè N, Austin ED, Elliott G, Asano K, Grünig E, Yan Y, Jing Z-C, Manes A, Palazzini M, Wheeler LA, Nakayama I, Satoh T, Eichstaedt C, Hinderhofer K, Wolf M, Rosenzweig EB, Chung WK, Soubrier F, Simonneau G, Sitbon O, Gräf S, Kaptoge S, Di Angelantonio E, Humbert M, Morrell NW. BMPR2 mutations and survival in pulmonary arterial hypertension: an individual participant data meta-analysis. Lancet Respir Med. 2016;4:129–37.

16. Giusca S, Popa E, Amzulescu MS, Ghiorghiu I, Coman IM, Popescu BA, Delcroix M, Voigt J-U, Ginghina C, Jurcut R. Is right ventricular remodeling in pulmonary hypertension dependent on etiology? An echocardiographic study. Echocardiography. 2016;33:546–54.

17. Savale L, Weatherald J, Jaïs X, Vuillard C, Boucly A, Jevnikar M, Montani D, Mercier O, Simonneau G, Fadel E, Sitbon O, Humbert M. Acute decompensated pulmonary hypertension. Eur Respir Rev. 2017;26:170092.

18. Hsu S, Kokkonen-Simon KM, Kirk JA, Kolb TM, Damico RL, Mathai SC, Mukherjee M, Shah AA, Wigley FM, Margulies KB, Hassoun PM, Halushka MK, Tedford RJ, Kass DA. Right ventricular myofilament functional differences in humans with systemic sclerosis-associated versus idiopathic pulmonary arterial hypertension. Circulation. 2018;137:2360–70.

19. Bogaard HJ, Abe K, Vonk Noordegraaf A, Voelkel NF. The right ventricle under pressure: cellular and molecular mechanisms of right-heart failure in pulmonary hypertension. Chest. 2009;135:794–804.

20. Rain S, Andersen S, Najafi A, Gammelgaard Schultz J, da Silva Gonçalves Bós D, Handoko ML, Bogaard H-J, Vonk-Noordegraaf A, Andersen A, van der Velden J, Ottenheijm CAC, de Man FS. Right ventricular myocardial stiffness in experimental pulmonary arterial hypertension: relative contribution of fibrosis and myofibril stiffness. Circ Heart Fail. 2016;9:e002636.

21. de Man FS, Tu L, Handoko ML, Rain S, Ruiter G, François C, Schalij I, Dorfmüller P, Simonneau G, Fadel E, Perros F, Boonstra A, Postmus PE, van der Velden J, Vonk-Noordegraaf A, Humbert M, Eddahibi S, Guignabert C. Dysregulated renin-angiotensin-aldosterone system contributes to pulmonary arterial hypertension. Am J Respir Crit Care Med. 2012;186:780–9.

22. Giordano FJ. Oxygen, oxidative stress, hypoxia, and heart failure. J Clin Invest. 2005;115:500–8.

23. Brittain EL, Talati M, Fessel JP, Zhu H, Penner N, Calcutt MW, West JD, Funke M, Lewis GD, Gerszten RE, Hamid R, Pugh ME, Austin ED, Newman JH, Hemnes AR. Fatty acid metabolic defects and right ventricular lipotoxicity in human pulmonary arterial hypertension. Circulation. 2016;133:1936–44.

24. Graham BB, Kumar R, Mickael C, Sanders L, Gebreab L, Huber KM, Perez M, Smith-Jones P, Serkova NJ, Tuder RM. Severe pulmonary hypertension is associated with altered right ventricle metabolic substrate uptake. Am J Physiol Lung Cell Mol Physiol. 2015;309:L435–40.

25. Ronco C, McCullough P, Anker SD, Anand I, Aspromonte N, Bagshaw SM, Bellomo R, Berl T, Bobek I, Cruz DN, Daliento L, Davenport A, Haapio M, Hillege H, House AA, Katz N, Maisel A, Mankad S, Zanco P, Mebazaa A, Palazzuoli A, Ronco F, Shaw A, Sheinfeld G, Soni S, Vescovo G, Zamperetti N, Ponikowski P. Acute Dialysis Quality Initiative (ADQI) consensus group. Cardio-renal syndromes: report from the consensus conference of the acute dialysis quality initiative. Eur Heart J. 2010;31:703–11.

26. Haddad F, Peterson T, Fuh E, Kudelko KT, de Jesus PV, Skhiri M, Vagelos R, Schnittger I, Denault AY, Rosenthal DN, Doyle RL, Zamanian RT. Characteristics and outcome after hospitalization for acute right heart failure in patients with pulmonary arterial hypertension. Circ Heart Fail. 2011;4:692–9.

27. Sztrymf B, Souza R, Bertoletti L, Jaïs X, Sitbon O, Price LC, Simonneau G, Humbert M. Prognostic factors of acute heart failure in patients with pulmonary arterial hypertension. Eur Respir J. 2010;35:1286–93.

28. Sztrymf B, Prat D, Jacobs FM, Brivet FG, O'Callaghan DS, Price LC, Jais X, Sitbon O, Simonneau G, Humbert M. Renal replacement therapy in patients with severe precapillary pulmonary hypertension with acute right heart failure. Respiration. 2013;85:464–70.

29. Shah SJ, Thenappan T, Rich S, Tian L, Archer SL, Gomberg-Maitland M. Association of serum creatinine with abnormal hemodynamics and mortality in pulmonary arterial hypertension. Circulation. 2008;117:2475–83.

30. Tonelli AR, Arelli V, Minai OA, Newman J, Bair N, Heresi GA, Dweik RA. Causes and circumstances of

death in pulmonary arterial hypertension. Am J Respir Crit Care Med. 2013;188:365–9.

31. Delcroix M, Naeije R. Optimising the management of pulmonary arterial hypertension patients: emergency treatments. Eur Respir Rev. 2010;19:204–11.

32. Huynh TN, Weigt SS, Sugar CA, Shapiro S, Kleerup EC. Prognostic factors and outcomes of patients with pulmonary hypertension admitted to the intensive care unit. J Crit Care. 2012;27:739.e7–13.

33. Kurzyna M, Zyłkowska J, Fijałkowska A, Florczyk M, Wieteska M, Kacprzak A, Burakowski J, Szturmowicz M, Wawrzyńska L, Torbicki A. Characteristics and prognosis of patients with decompensated right ventricular failure during the course of pulmonary hypertension. Kardiol Pol. 2008;66:1033–9; discussion 1040–1

34. Sitbon O, Channick R, Chin KM, Frey A, Gaine S, Galiè N, Ghofrani H-A, Hoeper MM, Lang IM, Preiss R, Rubin LJ, Di Scala L, Tapson V, Adzerikho I, Liu J, Moiseeva O, Zeng X, Simonneau G, McLaughlin VV, GRIPHON Investigators. Selexipag for the treatment of pulmonary arterial hypertension. N Engl J Med. 2015;373:2522–33.

35. Galiè N, Barberà JA, Frost AE, Ghofrani H-A, Hoeper MM, McLaughlin VV, Peacock AJ, Simonneau G, Vachiery J-L, Grünig E, Oudiz RJ, Vonk-Noordegraaf A, White RJ, Blair C, Gillies H, Miller KL, Harris JHN, Langley J, Rubin LJ, AMBITION Investigators. Initial use of ambrisentan plus tadalafil in pulmonary arterial hypertension. N Engl J Med. 2015;373:834–44.

36. Pulido T, Adzerikho I, Channick RN, Delcroix M, Galiè N, Ghofrani H-A, Jansa P, Jing Z-C, Le Brun F-O, Mehta S, Mittelholzer CM, Perchenet L, Sastry BKS, Sitbon O, Souza R, Torbicki A, Zeng X, Rubin LJ, Simonneau G, SERAPHIN Investigators. Macitentan and morbidity and mortality in pulmonary arterial hypertension. N Engl J Med. 2013;369:809–18.

37. Jiang R, Ai Z-S, Jiang X, Yuan P, Liu D, Zhao Q-H, He J, Wang L, Gomberg-Maitland M, Jing Z-C. Intravenous fasudil improves in-hospital mortality of patients with right heart failure in severe pulmonary hypertension. Hypertens Res. 2015;38:539–44.

38. Fingrova Z, Ambroz D, Jansa P, Kuchar J, Lindner J, Kunstyr J, Aschermann M, Linhart A, Havranek S. The prevalence and clinical outcome of supraventricular tachycardia in different etiologies of pulmonary hypertension. PLoS One. 2021;16:e0245752.

39. Hoeper MM, Granton J. Intensive care unit management of patients with severe pulmonary hypertension and right heart failure. Am J Respir Crit Care Med. 2011;184:1114–24.

40. Kerbaul F, Rondelet B, Motte S, Fesler P, Hubloue I, Ewalenko P, Naeije R, Brimioulle S. Effects of norepinephrine and dobutamine on pressure load-induced right ventricular failure. Crit Care Med. 2004;32:1035–40.

41. Hansen MS, Andersen A, Nielsen-Kudsk JE. Levosimendan in pulmonary hypertension and right heart failure. Pulm Circ. 2018;8:2045894018790905.

42. Vildbrad MD, Andersen A, Holmboe S, Ringgaard S, Nielsen JM, Nielsen-Kudsk JE. Acute effects of levosimendan in experimental models of right ventricular hypertrophy and failure. Pulm Circ. 2014;4:511–9.

43. Kundra TS, Prabhakar V, Kaur P, Manjunatha N, Gandham R. The effect of inhaled milrinone versus inhaled levosimendan in pulmonary hypertension patients undergoing mitral valve surgery—a pilot randomized double-blind study. J Cardiothorac Vasc Anesth. 2018;32:2123–9.

44. Buckley MS, Feldman JP. Nebulized milrinone use in a pulmonary hypertensive crisis. Pharmacotherapy. 2007;27:1763–6.

45. Price LC, Wort SJ, Finney SJ, Marino PS, Brett SJ. Pulmonary vascular and right ventricular dysfunction in adult critical care: current and emerging options for management: a systematic literature review. Crit Care. 2010;14:R169.

46. Tayama E, Ueda T, Shojima T, Akasu K, Oda T, Fukunaga S, Akashi H, Aoyagi S. Arginine vasopressin is an ideal drug after cardiac surgery for the management of low systemic vascular resistant hypotension concomitant with pulmonary hypertension. Interact Cardiovasc Thorac Surg. 2007;6:715–9.

47. Price LC, Dimopoulos K, Marino P, Alonso-Gonzalez R, McCabe C, Kemnpy A, Swan L, Boutsikou M, Al Zahrani A, Coghlan GJ, Schreiber BE, Howard LS, Davies R, Toshner M, Pepke-Zaba J, Church AC, Peacock A, Corris PA, Lordan JL, Gaine S, Condliffe R, Kiely DG, Wort SJ. The CRASH report: emergency management dilemmas facing acute physicians in patients with pulmonary arterial hypertension. Thorax. 2017;72:1035–45.

48. Kwak YL, Lee CS, Park YH, Hong YW. The effect of phenylephrine and norepinephrine in patients with chronic pulmonary hypertension. Anaesthesia. 2002;57:9–14.

49. Kim NH, Delcroix M, Jais X, Madani MM, Matsubara H, Mayer E, Ogo T, Tapson VF, Ghofrani H-A, Jenkins DP. Chronic thromboembolic pulmonary hypertension. Eur Respir J. 2019;53:1801915.

50. Jais X, Launay D, Yaici A, Le Pavec J, Tchérakian C, Sitbon O, Simonneau G, Humbert M. Immunosuppressive therapy in lupus and mixed connective tissue disease-associated pulmonary arterial hypertension: a retrospective analysis of twenty-three cases. Arthritis Rheum. 2008;58:521–31.

51. Chen Y, Guo L, Li Y, Chen G-L, Chen X-X, Ye S. Severe pulmonary arterial hypertension secondary to lupus in the emergency department: proactive intense care associated with a better short-term survival. Int J Rheum Dis. 2015;18:331–5.

52. Vizza CD, Rocca GD, Roma AD, Iacoboni C, Pierconti F, Venuta F, Rendina E, Schmid G, Pietropaoli P, Fedele F. Acute hemodynamic effects of inhaled nitric oxide, dobutamine and a combination of the two in patients with mild to moderate secondary pulmonary hypertension. Crit Care. 2001;5:355–61.

53. Schaffer JM, Singh SK, Joyce DL, Reitz BA, Robbins RC, Zamanian RT, Mallidi HR. Transplantation for

idiopathic pulmonary arterial hypertension: improvement in the lung allocation score era. Circulation. 2013;127:2503–13.

54. Davis SQ, Garrity ER. Organ allocation in lung transplant. Chest. 2007;132:1646–51.

55. Benza RL, Gomberg-Maitland M, Elliott CG, Farber HW, Foreman AJ, Frost AE, McGoon MD, Pasta DJ, Selej M, Burger CD, Frantz RP. Predicting survival in patients with pulmonary arterial hypertension: the REVEAL risk score calculator 2.0 and comparison with ESC/ERS-based risk assessment strategies. Chest. 2019;156:323–37.

56. Gottlieb J, Greer M, Sommerwerck U, Deuse T, Witt C, Schramm R, Hagl C, Strueber M, Smits JM. Introduction of the lung allocation score in Germany. Am J Transplant. 2014;14:1318–27.

57. Savale L, Le Pavec J, Mercier O, Mussot S, Jaïs X, Fabre D, O'Connell C, Montani D, Stephan F, Sitbon O, Simonneau G, Dartevelle P, Humbert M, Fadel E. Impact of high-priority allocation on lung and heart-lung transplantation for pulmonary hypertension. Ann Thorac Surg. 2017;104:404–11.

58. Strueber M, Hoeper MM, Fischer S, Cypel M, Warnecke G, Gottlieb J, Pierre A, Welte T, Haverich A, Simon AR, Keshavjee S. Bridge to thoracic organ transplantation in patients with pulmonary arterial hypertension using a pumpless lung assist device. Am J Transplant. 2009;9:853–7.

59. Boulate D, Mercier O, Mussot S, Fabre D, Stephan F, Haddad F, Jaïs X, Dartevelle P, Fadel E. Extracorporeal life support after pulmonary endarterectomy as a bridge to recovery or transplantation: lessons from 31 consecutive patients. Ann Thorac Surg. 2016;102:260–8.

60. Kortchinsky T, Mussot S, Rezaiguia S, Artiguenave M, Fadel E, Stephan F. Extracorporeal life support in lung and heart-lung transplantation for pulmonary hypertension in adults. Clin Transpl. 2016;30:1152–8.

61. Tudorache I, Sommer W, Kühn C, Wiesner O, Hadem J, Fühner T, Ius F, Avsar M, Schwerk N, Böthig D, Gottlieb J, Welte T, Bara C, Haverich A, Hoeper MM, Warnecke G. Lung transplantation for severe pulmonary hypertension–awake extracorporeal membrane oxygenation for postoperative left ventricular remodelling. Transplantation. 2015;99:451–8.

62. Moser B, Jaksch P, Taghavi S, Muraközy G, Lang G, Hager H, Krenn C, Roth G, Faybik P, Bacher A, Aigner C, Matilla JR, Hoetzenecker K, Hacker P, Lang I, Klepetko W. Lung transplantation for idiopathic pulmonary arterial hypertension on intraoperative and postoperatively prolonged extracorporeal membrane oxygenation provides optimally controlled reperfusion and excellent outcome. Eur J Cardiothorac Surg. 2018;53:178–85.

63. Lewis RA, Durrington C, Condliffe R, Kiely DG. BNP/NT-proBNP in pulmonary arterial hypertension: time for point-of-care testing? Eur Respir Rev. 2020;29:200009.

64. Heresi GA, Tang WHW, Aytekin M, Hammel J, Hazen SL, Dweik RA. Sensitive cardiac troponin I predicts poor outcomes in pulmonary arterial hypertension. Eur Respir J. 2012;39:939–44.

65. Nickel N, Kempf T, Tapken H, Tongers J, Laenger F, Lehmann U, Golpon H, Olsson K, Wilkins MR, Gibbs JSR, Hoeper MM, Wollert KC. Growth differentiation factor-15 in idiopathic pulmonary arterial hypertension. Am J Respir Crit Care Med. 2008;178:534–41.

66. Marik PE. Noninvasive cardiac output monitors: a state-of the-art review. J Cardiothorac Vasc Anesth. 2013;27:121–34.

Cardiac and Lung Transplantation and the Right Heart

18

Robert P. Frantz

Abbreviations

ARDS	Acute respiratory distress syndrome
ASD	Atrial septal defect
COPD	Chronic obstructive pulmonary disease
CPB	Cardiopulmonary bypass
DLCO	Diffusion capacity for carbon monoxide
dPpa	Diastolic pulmonary artery pressure
ECMO	Extracorporeal membrane oxygenation
IPF	Idiopathic pulmonary fibrosis
ISHLT	International Society for Heart and Lung Transplantation
LAS	Lung Allocation Score
LV	Left ventricle
mPpa	Mean pulmonary artery pressure
PAH	Pulmonary arterial hypertension
PH	Pulmonary hypertension
Ppw	Pulmonary capillary wedge pressure
PVR	Pulmonary vascular resistance
RV	Right ventricle
RVAD	Right ventricular assist device
SRTR	Scientific Registry of Transplant Recipients
TPG	Transpulmonary gradient
UNOS	United National Organ System
VSD	Ventricular septal defect

R. P. Frantz (✉)
Department of Cardiovascular Diseases, Mayo Clinic, Rochester, MN, USA
e-mail: frantz.robert@mayo.edu

Introduction

The right heart is a consistent source of consternation in patients being considered for, and undergoing, cardiac or lung transplantation. Donor right ventricular failure is a feared complication in cardiac transplantation. Mechanical circulatory support strategies in advanced cardiac failure depend heavily on the judgment of adequacy of right ventricular function. Decisions regarding the timing of lung transplantation in pulmonary arterial hypertension, and whether to perform lung or combined heart-lung transplant, often revolve around considerations of right-heart failure and whether it can be successfully managed. Cardiac failure in patients with multiple forms of pulmonary hypertension undergoing lung transplantation can contribute to lung allograft failure, multiorgan failure, and perioperative death. This chapter discusses these varied dilemmas that hinge on a common theme: right ventricular (RV) failure.

Donor Right Ventricular Failure in Cardiac Transplantation

The presence of pulmonary hypertension in patients with left ventricular (LV) failure is associated with a worse prognosis [1]. A study of patients with LV systolic failure who had ambulatory right ventricular pressure monitors implanted demonstrated that those patients who had subsequent clinical events had higher pulmonary artery systolic pressures, estimated pulmonary artery diastolic pressures, and right ventricular end-diastolic pressures [2]. Accordingly it is common that patients being considered for cardiac transplantation have significant pulmonary hypertension, and often substantial right ventricular failure. In the process of evaluating the prospective cardiac transplant candidate, it is incumbent upon the transplant team to make a determination regarding the risk of donor right ventricular failure following transplantation. The risk of RV failure following cardiac transplantation has multiple components that are summarized in Table 18.1. These include factors related to contractile state of the freshly transplanted heart, donor/recipient size discrepancies, and recipient preload and afterload properties, which are highly dynamic in the immediate postoperative period. We will focus on the aspects of the prediction of risk of RV failure in the cardiac transplant candidate.

Prediction of Risk of RV Failure in a Cardiac Transplant Candidate

This process essentially involves a mind game: "If this patient went to the operating room today for a heart transplant, what would the pulmonary hemodynamics look like immediately following the operation?" This question can be addressed via a process that may involve several steps, contingent upon initial observations. Firstly, the initial hemodynamics at the time of transplant referral are assessed. Secondly, an acute effort to modulate the hemodynamics may be made, essentially in an effort to mimic the immediate posttransplant state. Thirdly, subacute manipulation of hemodynamics while maintaining a pulmonary artery catheter to guide interventions can be performed. This may include use of diuretic, inotropes, vasodilators, and if necessary support devices such as an intra-aortic balloon pump or Impella™. All of these are in an effort to optimize hemodynamics in order to predict the posttransplant state, and also potentially serving to maintain the patient in stable condition while

Table 18.1 Factors influencing the risk of donor RV failure following cardiac transplantation

Afterload	Persistence of elevated pulmonary vascular resistance and impaired pulmonary artery compliance
	Pulmonary vasculopathy
	Hypoxemia
	Acidosis
	Positive-pressure ventilation
	Possible elevation of LV filling pressures
	Volume expansion
	Myocardial stunning
	Donor heart diastolic dysfunction (e.g., left ventricular hypertrophy)
Preload	Insufficient preload
	Bleeding for which inadequate volume is provided
	Excessive preload
	Intraoperative transfusion requirements (redo surgery, VAD removal, coagulopathy)
	Recipient vasoplegia for which excess volume expansion may be administered (preferred approach is vasoconstrictor administration)
	Perioperative renal failure
Contractile dysfunction	Ischemic time
	Adequacy of donor heart preservation
	RV contusion
	Myocardial stunning
	Catecholamine surge from donor brain death
	Inotropic requirements of the donor
	Donor-recipient size mismatch
	Female donor
	Donor age

awaiting transplant. Fourthly, longer term mechanical circulatory support devices may be implanted as a "bridge to decision." We will discuss these elements in sequential fashion.

Interpretation of Initial Hemodynamics

Hemodynamics must be performed and interpreted by physicians who are experts in this regard. Relatively common errors include failure to visually inspect the tracings to avoid confounders such as respiratory variability, and failure to achieve a true representation of the pulmonary capillary wedge pressure (Ppw). Such errors can cause major inaccuracy of the pressure measurements, leading to serious misinterpretation. Historically, the pulmonary artery pressure, the transpulmonary gradient (TPG) defined as the mean pulmonary artery pressure (mPpa) − Ppw, and the pulmonary vascular resistance (PVR) defined as (PAm − Ppw)/cardiac output have been the most widely used parameters for consideration of the risk for RV failure with transplantation [3]. In the 2012 ISHLT Registry, preoperative pulmonary artery pressure and serum bilirubin were among the independent predictors of 1-year posttransplant mortality. A mean pulmonary artery pressure of <27 mmHg was associated with somewhat superior outcome (Fig. 18.1a).

The mean pulmonary vascular resistance in patients undergoing cardiac transplantation was 2.1 Wood units, with the 95th percentile equal to 5.4 Wood units. Survival was somewhat superior for patients with PVR of 1–<3 Wood units compared to those with PVR of 3–5 Wood units, with most of the difference occurring in the early postoperative period (Fig. 18.1b). Pulmonary vascular resistance and bilirubin were among predictors of 5-year survival (Fig. 18.1c), with a completely normal pretransplant PVR being protective of outcome [4]. A pretransplant transpulmonary gradient of less than 9 mmHg was associated with somewhat superior 5-year survival contingent upon 1-year survival. This transpulmonary gradient relationship was confirmed utilizing data extending to June 2013 [5].

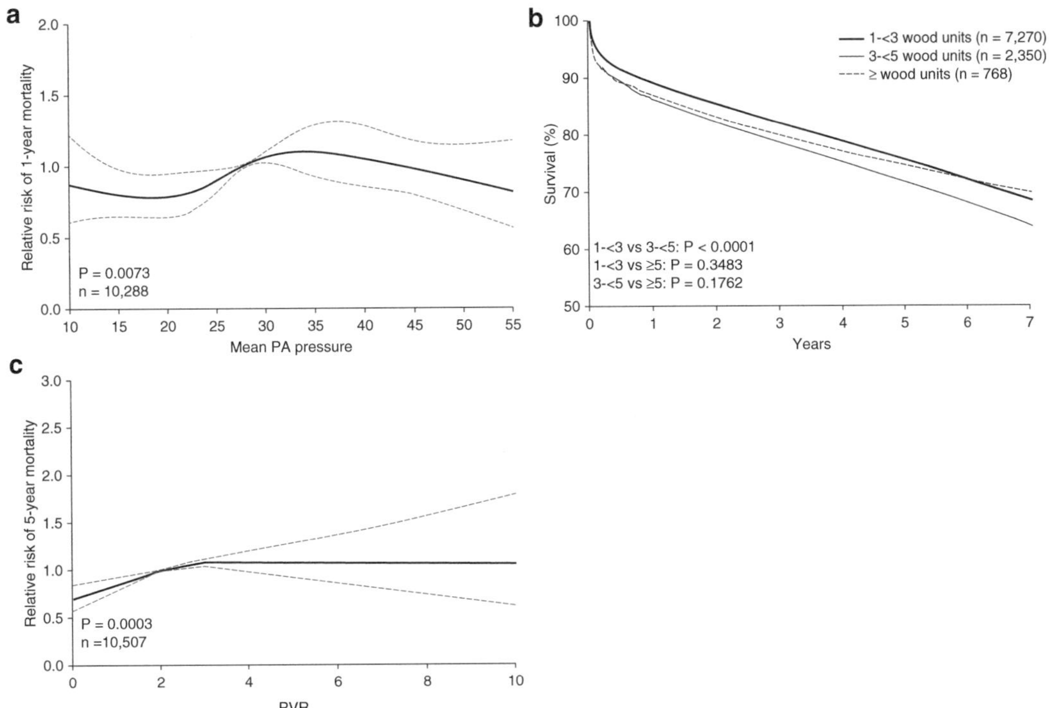

Fig. 18.1 (**a**) Relationship between pretransplant mean pulmonary artery pressure and risk of 1-year mortality in adult heart-transplant recipients in ISHLT Registry between 2005 and June 2010. *Dashed lines* represent 95% confidence intervals. (**b**) Kaplan-Meier survival curves based upon pretransplant PVR for adult heart-transplant recipients in ISHLT Registry between 2003 and June 2010. (**c**) Relative risk of mortality by preoperative pulmonary vascular resistance for adult heart-transplant recipients in ISHLT Registry between 2005 and 2010

Pulmonary Artery Diastolic Pressure to Pulmonary Capillary Wedge Gradient

The concept of utilizing the diastolic pulmonary artery pressure (dPpa) to Ppw gradient as a marker of pulmonary vasculopathy is not new, but has recently been discussed with renewed enthusiasm [6]. This parameter has advantages over transpulmonary gradient since it may be more informative across a range of cardiac outputs including high output states, although that aspect is less relevant in the context of candidates for cardiac transplantation where cardiac output is generally low. However, even in the setting of a low cardiac output, if the Ppw is elevated, it may disproportionately elevate the mPpa and accordingly transpulmonary gradient. This is because elevation in Ppw will increase pulmonary artery stiffening (reduced compliance) [7]. A dPpa to Ppw gradient >7 mmHg performs better than TPG >12 mmHg in predicting the outcome of heart failure in patients with elevated left-heart filling pressures [8], consistent with the concept that it may be a superior marker of pulmonary arteriopathy. However, when pre-heart transplant dPpa was examined utilizing the United National Organ Sharing database, there was no association of elevated dPpa with the outcome following cardiac transplantation [9]. It is possible that this in part reflects the difficulty of accurate measurement impacting the data that is entered into such databases. In a subsequent multivariate analysis of preoperative risk factors for greater than 30-day hospital stay following cardiac transplantation, a pulmonary artery diastolic pressure of >25 mmHg was among the variables maintaining significance [10].

Acute Modulation of Hemodynamics

Acute Vasoreactivity Testing

Acute vasoreactivity testing with nitroprusside is often effective in dropping the pulmonary artery pressure and pulmonary capillary wedge, increas-ing cardiac output, and improving the pulmonary vascular resistance, particularly in patients with LV systolic failure [1]. If the pulmonary vascular resistance can be lowered to less than 2.5 Wood units, this has been associated with a low risk of donor RV failure at the time of transplant.

Subacute Efforts to Improve Pulmonary Hemodynamics

Transferring a patient to the intensive care unit, administering diuretics and inotropes, and if necessary placing an intra-aortic balloon pump or temporary left ventricular support systems such as an Impella™ can be useful in improving hemodynamics and assessing reversibility of pulmonary hypertension. This may be especially true in patients with hypotension and low cardiac output, and/or restrictive cardiomyopathy for whom vasodilator modulation of wedge pressure can be challenging.

Left Ventricular Assist Devices to Improve Pulmonary Hemodynamics

In the presence of intractable concern about pulmonary hypertension, placement of a left ventricular assist device as a "bridge to decision" about candidacy for heart transplant is often a reasonable approach. Frequently the pulmonary artery pressure improves within 24 h, but sometimes several months may be necessary in order to presumably allow for pulmonary vascular reverse remodeling to occur [11].

In patients with persistent elevation of pulmonary vascular resistance following LVAD implantation, pulmonary vasodilators can be considered, though data in this regard is largely limited to case series. The concept here is that with LV unloading normalization of the pulmonary capillary wedge pressure should occur, so these patients effectively convert to a precapillary PH phenotype. Phosphodiesterase-5 inhibitors are the most commonly utilized, though they may cause hypotension and accordingly alter renal perfusion pressure and increase the need for inotropic or pressor support. Furthermore, a propensity-matched analysis of the INTERMACS registry of patients receiving preoperative PDE5i found no benefit and a suggestion of harm, with PDE5i-treated patients more likely to suffer early severe right-heart failure [12]. The SOPRANO (Macitentan in pulmonary hypertenSiOn Post-left ventRiculAr assist device implantation) study of the endothelin receptor antagonist macitentan in patients with pulmonary vascular resistance >3 Wood units and Ppw ≤18 mmHg following LVAD implantation, with primary endpoint of pulmonary vascular resistance at 16 weeks, has been completed; publication of results is expected in 2021 (NCT02554903).

Lung and Heart-Lung Transplantation in Pulmonary Hypertension

Pulmonary arterial hypertension (PAH) patients being considered for lung transplantation often have an advanced stage of cardiac dysfunction. This is inevitable given the young age of these patients, availability of PAH therapy that has substantially improved outcome, concern regarding perioperative risk, and uncertainty regarding whether a patient has truly reached a point where transplantation is likely to result in a better outcome than persisting with medical therapy. Three-month mortality in PAH patients undergoing lung transplantation as reported in the International Society for Heart and Lung Transplantation (ISHLT) Registry is 23%, compared with 9% for patients with chronic obstructive pulmonary disease (COPD), despite the much younger age of the PAH patients. In the ISHLT Registry, median survival of PAH patients undergoing lung transplant is only 5.0 years, with greater hazard for perioperative death than most other diagnoses. Nonetheless, conditional survival (assuming survival to 1 year) is among the very best, with a half-life of 10.0 years versus 6.8 years for COPD or idiopathic pulmonary fibrosis (IPF) [13] (Fig. 18.2a, b). This stark contrast encapsulates the need to better understand and manage this perioperative risk. In this sec-

tion, we will discuss factors that impact transplant waiting time, perioperative decision-making, management, and outcome of these compelling patients.

The advanced stage of right ventricular dysfunction in PAH patients undergoing transplantation in the United States is driven in part by a United Network for Organ Sharing (UNOS) Lung Allocation Scoring (LAS) system, implemented in 2005. This scoring system does not yield scores likely to result in donor offers in the absence of profound cardiac failure despite maximal PAH therapy including iv prostanoids. However, PH patients, with factors such as a high oxygen requirement, can see their score driven by this, and indeed may not have classical PAH in any case. Implementation of the LAS resulted in improved wait list mortality for all diagnostic groups except PAH [14]. In addition, the higher wait list mortality for PAH was despite having lower lung allocation scores than patients in other diagnostic groups, suggesting that the LAS system is not adequately capturing prognostic factors relevant to PAH. The impact of the LAS system on the phenotype of patients being listed under the PH category is well demonstrated in a recent analysis of temporal trends captured within the UNOS Scientific Registry of Transplant Recipients (SRTR) database of PH patients listed and undergoing transplantation in the United States [15]. Since the implementation of the LAS system, patients listed for transplantation under the PH category have had more severely abnormal pulmonary function tests, greater oxygen requirements, shorter 6-min walk distances, and better preserved cardiac output. This likely largely reflects the parameters that result in a high lung allocation score, and may be skewing the PH category toward patients with more parenchymal lung disease than is generally seen in PAH. While these patients undoubtedly are in need of transplant, those patients with severely deranged hemodynamics are not readily receiving LAS that will facilitate transplantation. For PAH patients whose pathophysiology primarily revolves around impaired hemodynamics, and awaiting transplant in the United States, the LAS score will be usually too low to obtain

Fig. 18.2 (**a**) Kaplan-Meier survival curves for lung-transplant recipients by diagnosis as reported to ISHLT Registry between January 1990 and June 2010. Note the disproportionate early mortality in the pulmonary hypertension cohort. (**b**) Kaplan-Meier survival curves for lung-transplant recipients contingent on 1-year survival by diagnosis as reported to ISHLT Registry between January 1990 and June 2010. Note that the contingent survival for the pulmonary hypertension cohort is among the best of all diagnostic categories

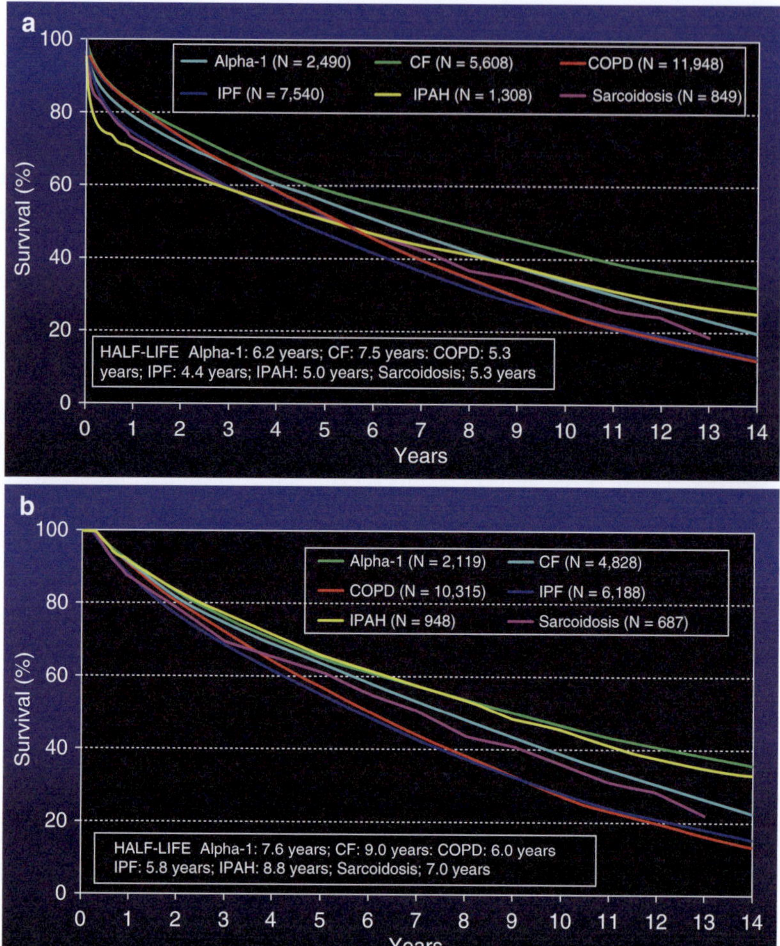

organs, unless the patient receives a waiver from the UNOS Thoracic Organ Allocation Committee. This requires that the right atrial pressure be greater than 15 mmHg or the cardiac index be less than 1.8 L/min/m^2 despite maximal medical therapy, which is usually understood to include parenteral prostanoid therapy. Such parameters create a situation of worrisome risk for death while waiting, and may result in increased perioperative risk and increased hazard of requiring extracorporeal membrane oxygenation (ECMO) support as a shaky bridge to transplant.

Patient and, at times, physician preference to avoid lung transplant as long as possible may also play a role in the delay of transplant referral and listing. Such patients are often young, and hope to live decades. Given that the long-term survival of lung-transplant recipients remains uncertain, it is often tempting to delay transplant until such advanced disease is present that survival to transplant, and recovery thereafter, becomes more problematic.

Double-lung transplant has clearly been associated with superior outcome to single-lung transplant, so it is definitely preferred. Nonetheless, lung transplantation in patients with advanced PAH has historically been associated with greater perioperative mortality than lung transplantation performed for other indications [13]. This has resulted in debate regarding the relative role of combined heart-lung transplant and double-lung transplant. Traditionally heart-lung blocks were often utilized in patients with pulmonary hypertension, and the hearts from such recipients were then used in domino fashion in patients requiring heart transplant who had elevated pulmonary vascular resistance [16, 17]. The hearts being used in domino fashion were hypertrophied and generally had well-preserved function, but it appears less common in the current era that pulmonary arterial hypertension patients undergo transplant at a time when their right ventricles are still functioning well, so this option of domino transplant is less relevant.

Registries and case series have generally not shown a mortality difference in outcome between double-lung and heart-lung transplant operations for pulmonary hypertension, but differing patient selection (e.g., potentially a decision to perform heart-lung in those patients with the most severe right ventricular failure) and variability in center expertise may obscure such differences. It is generally accepted that the perioperative course is less fraught with heart-lung transplantation, but proof of superior outcome is lacking, heart-lung organ blocks are quite scarce, and double-lung transplantation will surely remain a much more common transplant operation for PAH.

Cardiac and Noncardiac Pathophysiology of the Advanced PAH Patient

Transplantation for PH patients for whom transplant is actively considered most often falls under two different scenarios:

1. Gradually progressive RV failure despite chronic therapy with vasodilators
2. Abrupt deterioration precipitated by an acute insult in an otherwise previously compensated patient

In the first instance, the patient may have adapted over a prolonged period to quite low cardiac output, and have developed severe right ventricular dilation, often accompanied by moderate-to-severe tricuspid regurgitation. These patients may finally reach a point where exertional intolerance is severe, manifested by dyspnea, chest tightness, and syncope or near syncope. The peri-transplant period in such a setting involves a complex interplay of patient, procedural, and provider-specific factors that ultimately determine the outcome, as illustrated in Fig. 18.3. Hemodynamics typically include

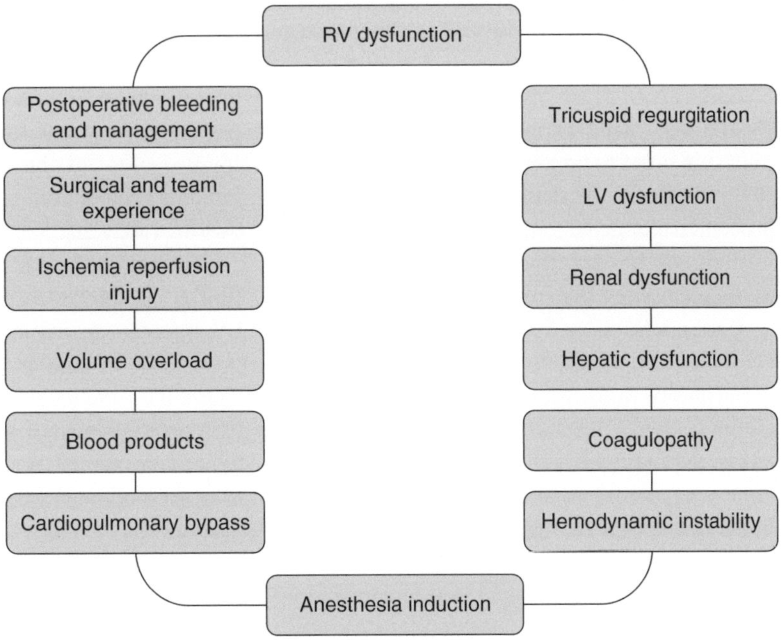

Fig. 18.3 Multiple factors influencing the outcome of lung transplantation in pulmonary hypertension

elevation of right atrial pressure and low cardiac index. Systemic saturation may also be low, reflecting impaired gas exchange and/or opening of a patent foramen ovale as right atrial pressure rises. End-organ function may become compromised due to a combination of inadequate oxygen delivery and impaired perfusion. The impaired perfusion may represent a combination of systemic hypotension, low cardiac output, and elevated venous pressure. Ascites with increased intra-abdominal pressure can further compromise renal perfusion. Hepatic dysfunction with elevated transaminases and bilirubin further compounds the picture. For PH patients on warfarin, labile prothrombin times are common, with the risk of hemorrhage either while awaiting transplantation or at the time of transplantation. Utilization of warfarin in PAH has become less common as recent retrospective studies have cast doubt on its utility [18]. Efforts to support cardiac output with inotropes can be useful, but also predisposed to arrhythmia, or, in the case of milrinone, possible exacerbation of hypotension or aggravation of prostanoid-related thrombocytopenia. Induction of anesthesia and potential for worsening hypoxemia, hypoventilation, acidosis, and hemodynamic effects of positive-pressure ventilation can make the induction period hazardous [19, 20]. Rapid requirement for institution of cardiopulmonary bypass may prolong cardiopulmonary bypass duration in the context of complex donor organ logistics.

The very need to institute cardiopulmonary bypass in order to proceed with lung transplant in PH immediately increases the complexity of the procedure compared to lung transplant performed for lung conditions without substantial accompanying pulmonary hypertension [21].

Cardiopulmonary bypass results in release of cytokines that increase the potential for vascular permeability in the transplanted lung, leading to allograft injury, hypoxemia, and increased ventilatory requirements [22–24]. The wide-ranging effects of cardiopulmonary bypass are nicely illustrated in Fig. 18.4 [24]. Intraoperative bleeding risk is exacerbated by preexisting thrombocytopenia, platelet dysfunction related to prostanoid

use, acquired von Willebrand disease related to shear stress in the pulmonary vasculature [25], effects of cardiopulmonary bypass, and coagulopathy related to preoperative warfarin use and hepatopathy. Cessation of anticoagulation at the time of transplant listing should be considered in order to reduce perioperative bleeding risk. In patients with PAH related to prior VSD or ASD who have had prior cardiac surgery, scarring in the chest further complicates operative complexity, duration, and bleeding risk. Volume overload related to administration of blood products and crystalloid in response to hypotension and bleeding, in the context of renal dysfunction reflecting preoperative factors, further exacerbates congestion and dysfunction of the allograft. Adding this scenario to a severely dysfunctional right ventricle makes it easy to understand why perioperative risk is higher in PAH patients undergoing transplant compared to, e.g., a pulmonary fibrosis patient without coagulopathy, hepatic dysfunction, RV failure, renal dysfunction, or need for cardiopulmonary bypass.

Surgical expertise in the management of such a patient may also play a role. Lung transplant most commonly does not involve cardiopulmonary bypass, and transplant for PAH remains relatively uncommon. In the context of thoracic transplant surgeons, the need for cardiopulmonary bypass may also be an uncommon part of their practice. Center-specific outcomes vary, and to some extent reflect the number of transplants performed [13]. Anesthesiology awareness of the fragile nature of the PAH patient and need for judicious induction and avoidance of volume overload may also be variable.

Distention of the RV by the volume excess can further compromise LV filling by virtue of RV/LV interaction, impaired RV performance, and persistence of tricuspid regurgitation. In contexts where RV function is better preserved at the time of transplant, which seems increasingly rare, a hyper-contractile right ventricle "suicide RV" may develop, aggravated by perioperative use of inotropes.

The left ventricle also has an important role to play in perioperative hazards [26, 27]. Given the

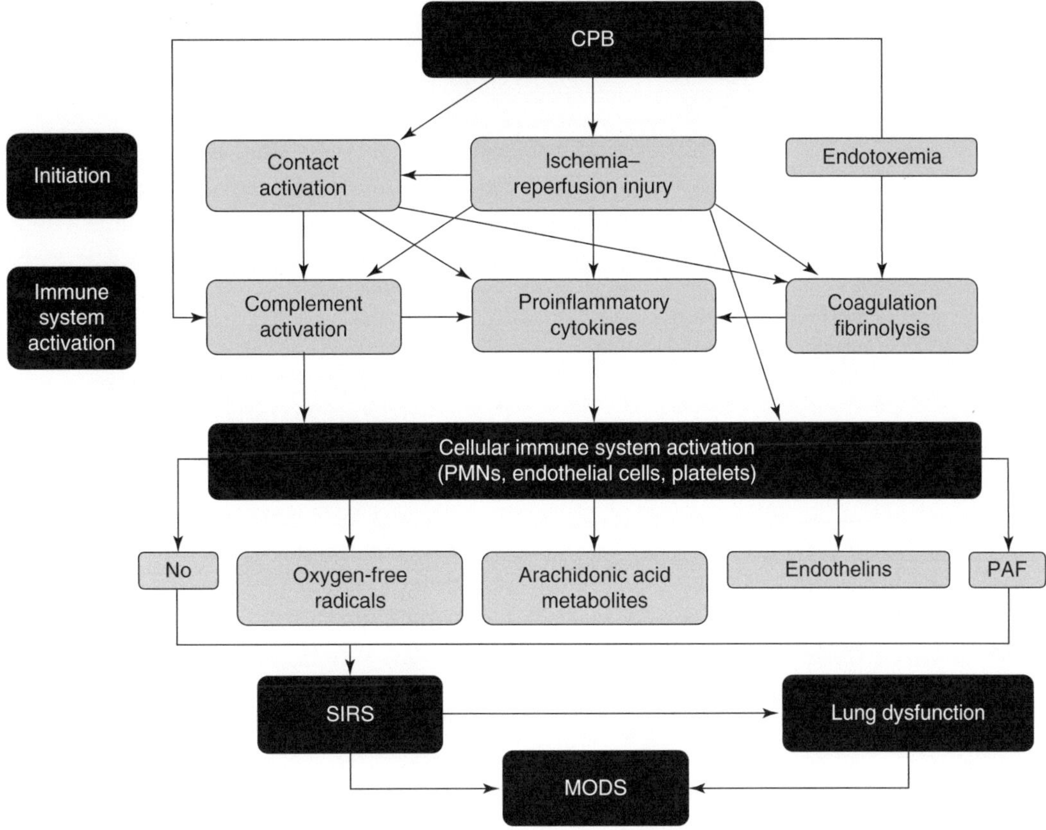

Fig. 18.4 A schematic representation by which cardiopulmonary (*CPB*) may lead to systemic inflammatory response syndrome (*SIRS*), lung dysfunction, and multiple-organ dysfunction syndrome (*MODS*). *PMNs* polymorphonuclear cells, *NO* nitric oxide, *PAF* platelet-activating factor. (Reprinted from Apostolakis et al. [24]. With permission from John Wiley & Sons, Inc.)

typically very low cardiac output state of the PAH patient at the time of transplant, the LV has been chronically underfilled, becomes small in size, and possesses diastolic filling abnormalities [28]. If the RV is severely dysfunctional in the immediate postoperative phase, septal shift and pericardial constraint may contribute to the difficulty that the LV faces in adapting to an abrupt increase in LV filling when coming off cardiopulmonary bypass. This may result in a rise in left atrial pressure, which will aggravate tendency toward edema of the recently ischemic, cytokine-stressed, freshly transplanted lung. Monitoring of the pulmonary capillary wedge pressure or placement of a left atrial pressure monitoring line at the time of lung transplant may be helpful in avoiding excess

rise in left atrial pressure following the transplant, by facilitating more aggressive volume management if LA pressure begins to rise. Utilization of ECMO with appropriate left heart venting and with gradual weaning following transplantation may facilitate avoidance of rise in LA pressure and accompanying lung allograft congestion that can seriously compromise the freshly transplanted lungs [29]. In some cases, continuous venovenous hemodialysis or ultrafiltration can be useful to facilitate volume management in the face of inadequate urine output despite diuretics. Occasionally, LV systolic failure is observed, and may improve with appropriate supportive measures. These complex, interacting processes are summarized in Table 18.2.

Table 18.2 Factors influencing the outcome of lung transplantation in pulmonary hypertension

Right-heart issues	Contractile dysfunction
	Tricuspid regurgitation
	Pulmonic regurgitation
	Distention related to volume overload
Left-heart issues	Chronically underfilled
	Diastolic dysfunction
	RV/LV interaction
	Pericardial constraint
	Volume overload
Renal issues	Preexisting renal dysfunction
	Elevated venous pressure
	Systemic hypotension reducing perfusion pressure
	Compromised cardiac output
	Ascites with renal vein compression
	Impact of vasoconstrictors
Coagulation issues	Preoperative warfarin
	Preoperative thrombocytopenia
	Platelet dysfunction (prostanoids, aspirin, cardiopulmonary bypass)
	Hepatic dysfunction
Anesthesia and intraoperative issues	Risk of hemodynamic collapse with induction
	Hemodynamic effects of positive-pressure ventilation
	Low systemic pressure and resistance when coming off bypass
	Potential for metabolic acidosis related to hemodynamic compromise after bypass weaning
	Atrial arrhythmias
	Surgical and team experience
Lung allograft issues	Cytokine effects secondary to cardiopulmonary bypass
	Vascular permeability related to above and ischemia
	Impact of elevated LV filling pressures with sudden filling of chronically underfilled LV
	Effects of blood product administration (volume, transfusion-related acute lung injury TRALI)

Timing of Lung Transplantation in PAH1

Ideally, lung transplantation should occur electively prior to the development of end-stage RV failure and ensuing end-organ dysfunction and while the patient still has reasonable peripheral muscle preservation. Unfortunately there are multiple barriers to this timing. In the United States, the most severe barrier is the current LAS system. Utilization of the LAS waiver for patients with elevated right atrial pressure or severely reduced cardiac index is commonly employed when the patient reaches this level of deterioration. Further revision of this system is under active consideration.

Factors Relevant to a Previously Compensated Patient Who Suffers Abrupt Deterioration

Compensated PAH patients can rapidly decompensate in the face of a variety of stressors. These include sepsis related to indwelling lines or other factors, pneumonia, pulmonary hemorrhage, GI hemorrhage related to anticoagulation, intra-abdominal processes, and trauma. Detailed discussion of the management of these varied scenarios is beyond the scope of this document. Advanced RV failure despite maximal vasodilator therapy can sometimes be mitigated by use of inotropes. Dopamine, milrinone, or norepinephrine may be of some benefit but there is risk of tachyarrhythmia, which is often poorly tolerated, and milrinone can cause hypotension or aggravate thrombocytopenia. Phenylephrine can help support systemic pressure. Atrial septostomy is sometimes utilized as a way to improve systemic blood flow, thereby delivering more oxygen to peripheral tissue, at the expense of systemic hypoxemia, and can be used as a bridge to lung transplantation [30–32]. This has the benefit of improving LV filling which may facilitate LV adaptation at the time of transplantation. However, atrial septostomy is best performed prior to the development of end-stage RV failure, since marked right atrial pressure elevation and markedly reduced cardiac output are risk factors for mortality with the septostomy procedure [33]. Patients with advanced RV failure can in principle be managed with mechanical circulatory support either as a bridge to recovery or a as bridge to transplantation [34]. The wisdom of such an approach depends on the probability of recovery for non-transplant candidates, and on the probability that organs will be identified within an acceptable time frame in order to avoid the support approach being a stressful bridge to nowhere. Options for circulatory support theoretically include right ventricular assist devices (RVADs) and ECMO. RVADs have generally not been successful, since the sudden high flow into the pulmonary hypertensive pulmonary bed poses a risk of intrapulmonary hemorrhage or edema. Development of RVADs with more readily titratable flow characteristics would be a useful advance but issues of the markedly elevated PVR may limit success of such an approach. Case reports of successful biventricular bridging in patients with biventricular failure with devices such as the HeartWare™ are available [35]. Advances in ECMO technology have created both new opportunity and new dilemmas for critically ill PAH patients. Veno-venous ECMO with right internal jugular vein cannulation can mitigate issues of hypoxemia in the event of pneumonia, intrapulmonary hemorrhage, acute respiratory distress syndrome (ARDS), or other forms of acute lung injury. In the event of hemodynamic instability, which is a more common scenario in PAH, venoarterial ECMO can be employed, utilizing a variety of support systems and cannulation sites [36]. Avoidance of femoral cannulation is important in situations where support is expected to be prolonged, since the impact of immobility, and risk of line-related infection, can rapidly lead to an unsustainable scenario. Right internal jugular vein cannulation and right subclavian or axillary arterial cannulation can be successful, generally employing a cut-down to the artery with the use of a chimney graft. This allows patient mobilization, and has been successfully utilized as a bridge to transplant or recovery in a variety of situations. However, there is significant risk of injury to the brachial plexus, posing the risk of long-standing upper extremity problems.

Central cannulation with the arterial return coming back to the aorta, and use of an oxygenator and a centrifugal pump, has allowed mobilization and successful bridge to transplant [37]. This leaves the left ventricle potentially under-filled, which may compromise its adjustment at the time of transplant. Leaving the patient on ECMO for a few days post-lung transplant, with gradual reduction in ECMO flows, can facilitate LV adaptation to the normalization of cardiac output [29]. An alternative is the Novalung™ system, connecting from the pulmonary artery to the left atrium, and utilizing the patient's own RV as the pump, which has been remarkably successful [38–41]. The unloaded RV will improve its function and geometry, a potential advantage at the time of transplant. This system also has the advantage of avoiding the need for a centrifugal pump with its attendant issues, and allows the LV to become accommodated to at least a somewhat higher cardiac output, potentially facilitating the perioperative hemodynamic course. A Quadrox™ system can also be utilized in such a fashion; the Quadrox iD™ system can be utilized for neonatal support [42].

Use of support systems as a bridge to lung transplant is dependent on waiting times that are not excessively long, and careful assessment of probability of survival if lung transplant is undertaken [43]. With the advent of support systems that allow patient mobilization, support for months is possible, but is an enormous commitment of resources, fraught with risks of sepsis, bleeding, coagulation issues such as thrombocytopenia related to the support system or related to the prolonged use of heparin, and an emotional roller coaster for all involved.

Conclusions

Pulmonary hypertension is extremely common in patients with advanced cardiac failure, and has substantial prognostic and management implications. Pulmonary hypertension in patients being considered for cardiac transplantation requires careful evaluation with regard to reversibility. A consistent, stepwise approach will optimize the ability to assess the risk of postoperative RV failure, and to take steps to mitigate that risk.

Lung transplantation in pulmonary hypertension patients is more complex than for most other lung-transplant candidates, related to the wide range of issues described in this manuscript. A successful transplant requires a well-functioning team with expertise in identifying proper timing of transplant, proactively preparing the patient for transplant, bridging to transplant as needed with inotropes, atrial septostomy, or ECMO, optimal anesthesia support, skilled surgical teams fully comfortable with cardiopulmonary bypass and complex hemodynamic management. Judicious postoperative ventilatory, volume, renal, coagulation, and hemodynamic management including possible use of ECMO for a few days following transplant to allow the heart to adapt may be useful. In skilled hands, pulmonary hypertension patients can do very well with transplant, and, once clear of the perioperative period, have some of the best intermediate- and long-term outcomes of any of the indications for lung transplantation.

References

1. Miller WL, Grill DE, Borlaug BA. Clinical features, hemodynamics, and outcomes of pulmonary hypertension due to chronic heart failure with reduced ejection fraction pulmonary hypertension and heart failure. JACC. 2013;1(4):290–9.
2. Adamson PB, Gold MR, Bennett T, Bourge RC, Stevenson LW, Trupp R, et al. Continuous hemodynamic monitoring in patients with mild to moderate heart failure: results of the Reducing Decompensation Events Utilizing Intracardiac Pressures in Patients with Chronic Heart Failure (REDUCEhf) Trial. Congest Heart Fail. 2011;17(5):248–54.
3. Goland S, Czer LSC, Kass RM, De Robertis MA, Mirocha J, Coleman B, et al. Pre-existing pulmonary hypertension in patients with end-stage heart failure: impact on clinical outcome and hemodynamic follow-up after orthotopic heart transplantation. J Heart Lung Transplant. 2007;26(4):312–8.
4. Stehlik J, Edwards LB, Kucheryavaya AY, Benden C, Christie JD, Dipchand AI, et al. The Registry of the International Society for Heart and Lung Transplantation: 29th official adult heart transplant report—2012. J Heart Lung Transplant. 2012;31(10):1052–64.
5. Hayes D Jr, Cherikh WS, Chambers DC, et al. The International Thoracic Organ Transplant Registry of the International Society for Heart and Lung Transplantation: twenty-second pediatric lung and heart-lung transplantation report-2019; focus theme: donor and recipient size match. J Heart Lung Transplant. 2019;38(10):1015–27.
6. Naeije R, Vachiery J-L, Yerly P, Vanderpool R. The transpulmonary pressure gradient for the diagnosis of pulmonary vascular disease. Eur Respir J. 2013;41(1):217–23.
7. Tedford RJ, Hassoun PM, Mathai SC, Girgis RE, Russell SD, Thiemann DR, et al. Pulmonary capillary wedge pressure augments right ventricular pulsatile loading. Circulation. 2012;125(2):289–97.
8. Gerges C, Gerges M, Lang MB, Zhang Y, Jakowitsch J, Probst P, et al. Diastolic pulmonary vascular pressure gradient: a predictor of prognosis in "out-of-proportion" pulmonary hypertension. Chest. 2013;143(3):758–66.
9. Tedford RJ, Beaty CA, Mathai SC, et al. Prognostic value of the pre-transplant diastolic pulmonary artery pressure-to-pulmonary capillary wedge pressure gradient in cardiac transplant recipients with pulmonary hypertension. J Heart Lung Transplant. 2014;33(3):289–97.
10. Crawford TC, Magruder JT, Grimm JC, et al. A comprehensive risk score to predict prolonged hospital length of stay after heart transplantation. Ann Thorac Surg. 2018;105(1):83–90.
11. Nair PK, Kormos RL, Teuteberg JJ, Mathier MA, Bermudez CA, Toyoda Y, et al. Pulsatile left ventricular assist device support as a bridge to decision in patients with end-stage heart failure complicated by pulmonary hypertension. J Heart Lung Transplant. 2010;29(2):201–8.
12. Gulati G, Grandin EW, Kennedy K, et al. Preimplant phosphodiesterase-5 inhibitor use is associated with higher rates of severe early right heart failure after left ventricular assist device implantation. Circ Heart Fail. 2019;12(6):e005537.
13. Christie JD, Edwards LB, Kucheryavaya AY, Benden C, Dipchand AI, Dobbels F, et al. The Registry of the International Society for Heart and Lung Transplantation: 29th adult lung and heart-lung transplant report—2012. J Heart Lung Transplant. 2012;31(10):1073–86.
14. Chen H, Shiboski SC, Golden JA, Gould MK, Hays SR, Hoopes CW, et al. Impact of the lung allocation score on lung transplantation for pulmonary arterial hypertension. Am J Respir Crit Care Med. 2009;180(5):468–74.
15. Gomberg-Maitland M, Glassner-Kolmin C, Watson S, Frantz R, Park M, Frost A, et al. Survival in pulmonary arterial hypertension patients awaiting lung transplantation. J Heart Lung Transplant. 2013;32(12):1179–86.
16. Birks EJ, Yacoub MH, Anyanwu A, Smith RR, Banner NR, Khaghani A. Transplantation using hearts from primary pulmonary hypertensive donors for recipients with a high pulmonary vascular resistance. J Heart Lung Transplant. 2004;23(12):1339–44.
17. Mikhail G, al-Kattan K, Banner N, Mitchell A, Radley-Smith R, Khaghani A, et al. Long-term results of heart-lung transplantation for pulmonary hypertension. Transplant Proc. 1997;29(1–2):633.

18. Frantz RP. Whither anticoagulation in pulmonary arterial hypertension? Conflicting evidence REVEALed. Circulation. 2015;132(25):2360–2.
19. Pritts CD, Pearl RG. Anesthesia for patients with pulmonary hypertension. Curr Opin Anaesthesiol. 2010;23(3):411–6.
20. McGlothlin D, Ivascu N, Heerdt PM. Anesthesia and pulmonary hypertension. Prog Cardiovasc Dis. 2012;55(2):199–217.
21. Diso D, Venuta F, Anile M, De Giacomo T, Ruberto F, Pugliese F, et al. Extracorporeal circulatory support for lung transplantation: institutional experience. Transplant Proc. 2010;42(4):1281–2.
22. Denizot Y, Nathan N. Interleukin-6 and -10 as master predictive mediators of the postcardiopulmonary bypass inflammatory response. J Thorac Cardiovasc Surg. 2012;144(3):743.
23. Wang JF, Bian JJ, Wan XJ, Zhu KM, Sun ZZ, Lu AD. Association between inflammatory genetic polymorphism and acute lung injury after cardiac surgery with cardiopulmonary bypass. Med Sci Monit. 2010;16(5):CR260–5.
24. Apostolakis E, Filos KS, Koletsis E, Dougenis D. Lung dysfunction following cardiopulmonary bypass. J Card Surg. 2010;25(1):47–55.
25. Sokkary NA, Dietrich JE, Venkateswaran L. Idiopathic pulmonary hypertension causing acquired von Willebrand disease and menorrhagia. J Pediatr Adolesc Gynecol. 2011;24(5):e107–9.
26. Verbelen T, Van Cromphaut S, Rega F, Meyns B. Acute left ventricular failure after bilateral lung transplantation for idiopathic pulmonary arterial hypertension. J Thorac Cardiovasc Surg. 2013;145(1):e7–9.
27. Bîrsan T, Kranz A, Mares P, Artemiou O, Taghavi S, Zuckermann A, et al. Transient left ventricular failure following bilateral lung transplantation for pulmonary hypertension. J Heart Lung Transplant. 1999;18(4):304–9.
28. Forfia PR, Vachiéry J-L. Echocardiography in pulmonary arterial hypertension. Am J Cardiol. 2012;110(6, Supplement):S16–24.
29. Ius F, Tudorache I, Warnecke G. Extracorporeal support, during and after lung transplantation: the history of an idea. J Thorac Dis. 2018;10(8):5131–48.
30. Hayden AM. Balloon atrial septostomy increases cardiac index and may reduce mortality among pulmonary hypertension patients awaiting lung transplantation. J Transpl Coord. 1997;7(3):131–3.
31. Lordan JL, Corris PA. Pulmonary arterial hypertension and lung transplantation. Expert Rev Respir Med. 2011;5(3):441–54.
32. Rothman A, Sklansky MS, Lucas VW, Kashani IA, Shaughnessy RD, Channick RN, et al. Atrial septostomy as a bridge to lung transplantation in patients with severe pulmonary hypertension. Am J Cardiol. 1999;84(6):682–6.
33. Sandoval J, Gaspar J, Peña H, Santos LE, Córdova J, del Valle K, et al. Effect of atrial septostomy on the survival of patients with severe pulmonary arterial hypertension. Eur Respir J. 2011;38(6):1343–8.
34. Camboni D, Akay B, Pohlmann JR, Koch KL, Haft JW, Bartlett RH, et al. Veno-venous extracorporeal membrane oxygenation with interatrial shunting: a novel approach to lung transplantation for patients in right ventricular failure. J Thorac Cardiovasc Surg. 2011;141(2):537.e1–42.
35. Strueber M, Meyer AL, Malehsa D, Haverich A. Successful use of the HeartWare HVAD rotary blood pump for biventricular support. J Thorac Cardiovasc Surg. 2010;140(4):936–7.
36. Strueber M. Bridges to lung transplantation. Curr Opin Organ Transplant. 2011;16(5):458–61. https://doi.org/10.1097/MOT.0b013e32834ac7ec.
37. Olsson KM, Simon A, Strueber M, Hadem J, Wiesner O, Gottlieb J, et al. Extracorporeal membrane oxygenation in nonintubated patients as bridge to lung transplantation. Am J Transplant. 2010;10(9):2173–8.
38. Strueber M, Hoeper MM, Fischer S, Cypel M, Warnecke G, Gottlieb J, et al. Bridge to thoracic organ transplantation in patients with pulmonary arterial hypertension using a pumpless lung assist device. Am J Transplant. 2009;9(4):853–7.
39. de Perrot M, Granton JT, McRae K, Cypel M, Pierre A, Waddell TK, et al. Impact of extracorporeal life support on outcome in patients with idiopathic pulmonary arterial hypertension awaiting lung transplantation. J Heart Lung Transplant. 2011;30(9):997–1002.
40. de Perrot M, Granton JT, McRae K, Pierre AF, Singer LG, Waddell TK, et al. Outcome of patients with pulmonary arterial hypertension referred for lung transplantation: a 14-year single-center experience. J Thorac Cardiovasc Surg. 2012;143(4):910–8.
41. de Perrot M, Chaparro C, McRae K, Waddell TK, Hadjiliadis D, Singer LG, et al. Twenty-year experience of lung transplantation at a single center: influence of recipient diagnosis on long-term survival. J Thorac Cardiovasc Surg. 2004;127(5):1493–501.
42. Hoganson DM, Gazit AZ, Sweet SC, Grady RM, Huddleston CB, Eghtesady P. Neonatal paracorporeal lung assist device for respiratory failure. Ann Thorac Surg. 2013;95(2):692–4.
43. Gottlieb J, Warnecke G, Hadem J, Dierich M, Wiesner O, Fühner T, et al. Outcome of critically ill lung transplant candidates on invasive respiratory support. Intensive Care Med. 2012;38(6):968–75.

Arrhythmias in Right-Heart Failure due to Pulmonary Hypertension

Michele D'Alto and Andrea Farro

Abbreviations

^{123}I-MIBG	Iodine-123-metaiodobenzylguanidine
6MWD	Six-minute walk distance
AF	Atrial fibrillation
AFl	Atrial flutter
APD	Action potential duration
AVNRT	Atrioventricular nodal reentry tachycardia
CPR	Cardiopulmonary resuscitation
CTEPH	Chronic thromboembolic pulmonary hypertension
CTI	Cavo-tricuspid isthmus
ECG	Electrocardiogram
HRV	Heart rate variability
I_{to}	Transient outward potassium current
LV	Left ventricle
NCX	Na^+-Ca^{2+} exchanger
PAH	Pulmonary arterial hypertension
QTc	Corrected QT interval
RV	Right ventricle
SCD	Sudden cardiac death
SR	Sinus rhythm
SSc	Systemic sclerosis
SVT	Supraventricular tachycardia
VF	Ventricular fibrillation
VT	Ventricular tachycardia

M. D'Alto (✉) · A. Farro
Department of Cardiology, Monaldi Hospital—
University "L. Vanvitelli", Naples, Italy

Introduction

The term *"cor pulmonale"* classically refers to the associated hypertrophic and/or dilated remodeling of the right ventricle that may accompany a variety of chronic respiratory diseases [1]. Right-heart failure occurs in many diseases associated with the dysfunction of the pulmonary circulation [2–4], including pulmonary arterial hypertension (PAH) [2] and chronic lung diseases such as chronic obstructive pulmonary disease [5, 6]. In particular, right ventricle (RV) failure, that is the major cause of death in PAH [2], is associated with RV electrical remodeling [7, 8] and a higher risk of arrhythmias [9, 10].

Pathophysiology

Remodeling of the right ventricle and right atrium in response to long-standing pressure and volume overload is responsible for the underlying arrhythmogenic substrate in patients with right-heart failure. Different electrophysiological changes predispose to arrhythmias in right-heart failure and rely on the underlying heart disease. These include alterations in Ca^{2+} handling, remodeling of the extracellular matrix and ion channels, presence of scars and fibrosis, activation of the sympathetic nervous and renin–angiotensin–aldosterone systems, dilatation and stretch, and delayed cardiac repolarization, all of which result in enhanced QT dispersion [11]. In addition, insufficient blood supply associated with heart failure may also affect the heart, leading to acute myocardial ischemia that has its own arrhythmogenic mechanisms [12].

Modulation of autonomic activity plays a key role in predisposing to cardiac arrhythmias. Folino et al. [9] assessed the arrhythmic profile in nine patients with PAH and its correlation with autonomic features, echocardiographic indexes, and pulmonary function. PAH patients showed increased sympathetic activity (reduced heart rate variability) that correlated with higher RV systolic pressure at echocardiography. Premature ventricular beats were more frequent in subjects with higher adrenergic drive and lower oxygen saturation. Moreover, patients with episodes of syncope showed a relatively higher vagal activity, and effective mechanisms of adjustment in blood oxygenation during effort. In addition to reduced heart rate variability, elevated levels of plasma norepinephrine and selective downregulation of beta-adrenergic receptors in the right ventricle in PAH patients were indicators of increased sympathetic activity affecting the right ventricle. The increased sympathetic activity correlated positively with right-heart failure severity [13]. Thus, the increase in pulmonary pressure and subsequent reduction in cardiac output may induce changes in autonomic activity resulting in increased sympathetic drive, well known for its pro-arrhythmic effects [14].

Iodine-123-metaiodobenzylguanidine (^{123}I-MIBG) myocardial imaging has been used to evaluate cardiac sympathetic nervous activity using single-photon emission computed tomography (SPECT). Uptake of ^{123}I-MIBG occurs via the same mechanism that normally uptakes norepinephrine. Therefore, by comparing the ^{123}I-MIBG activity at 3-h scans to those at 30 min, it is possible to assess the washout of the ^{123}I-MIBG, which is a measure of the retained norepinephrine within sympathetic neurons. When the sympathetic system is activated there occurs a reduction of norepinephrine uptake, manifest as lower retention of ^{123}I-MIBG. Increasing mean pulmonary arterial pressure is associated with decreased ^{123}I-MIBG activity in the RV, indicative of increased RV sympathetic activity. This decreased ^{123}I-MIBG activity correlates with worse survival in PAH [15–17].

Another important factor involved in RV electrical remodeling is delayed cardiac repolarization that leads to enhanced QT dispersion. The latter has been shown to be a precursor of arrhythmias and a predictor of all-cause mortality [18]. In a study of 201 patients with PAH, mean heart rate-corrected QT (QTc) and QTc dispersion positively correlated with mean pulmonary arterial pressure and were significantly increased in patients with severe PAH [19].

Finally, RV myocardial ischemia has been suggested as a mechanism of ventricular arrhythmias in patients with PAH. This may be due to a number of factors, including RV subendocardial ischemia due to changes in large epicardial coronary branches (reduced perfusion pressure in the right coronary artery due to elevated right ventricular systolic pressure [20], left main coronary artery compression [21], intramyocardial arteriolar compromise, impaired angiogenesis with capillary rarefaction related to decreased angiogenic gene expression) [22–24], decreased perfusion pressure gradient, and increased myocardial oxygen demand as a result of RV pressure overload [12, 14].

Secondary ischemia-related metabolic changes may perpetuate the vicious cycle of ischemia in the maladaptive RV [24].

Electro-anatomical remodeling in failing ventricular myocytes plays a key role in determining life-threatening arrhythmias. This has been intensively studied in the clinical setting of left-heart failure [25–30]. Prolongation of the ventricular action potential is a hallmark of heart failure. Studies in animal models and in humans with heart failure have consistently revealed action potential duration (APD) prolongation due to functional downregulation of transient outward potassium current (I_{to}) [31, 32], functional upregulation of inward Ca^{2+} current and changes in Ca^{2+} current inactivation [33, 34], or increases in late sodium currents [35, 36]. APD prolongation may prolong Ca^{2+} channel opening and thereby contribute to preservation of contractile force. However, it also increases the risk of Ca^{2+} overload, which may contribute to abnormal triggered impulses and perturbed signaling events. Although all myocardial cell layers exhibit significant APD prolongation in heart failure, such prolongation is typically heterogeneous. In a mouse model of pressure-overload heart failure, Wang et al. [37] found that APD was more prolonged in subepicardial than in subendocardial myocytes due to a more significant reduction in transient outward potassium currents. The dispersion and heterogeneous prolongation of repolarization between cell types across the ventricular wall represent an electrophysiological mechanism for unidirectional block, reentry, and arrhythmogenicity.

The Na^+-Ca^{2+} exchanger (NCX) is a surface membrane protein that transports one Ca^{2+} ion in exchange for three Na^+ ions. Its activity is said to be "forward" when Na^+ is transported into the cell and Ca^{2+} is extruded outwards, and "reverse" when ions are transported in the opposite directions. Most studies from hypertrophied and failing human hearts have demonstrated an increase in both NCX mRNA and protein levels [38–41], which has been posited to preserve diastolic extrusion of cytosolic Ca^{2+}. At the same time, increased NCX activity may impair systolic function by favoring transport of Ca^{2+} out of the cell rather than back into intracellular stores.

I_{to}, a major determinant of the early phase of action potential repolarization, also plays a key role in modulating action potential plateau and repolarization profiles. In fact, downregulation in I_{to} contributes to changes in action potential morphology observed in many forms of heart disease [42–44].

Further, APD prolongation and abnormal handling of intracellular Ca^{2+} promote abnormal increases in focal activity and automaticity. In addition, heterogeneous APD prolongation within the ventricular wall amplifies dispersion of repolarization, an established mechanism contributing to reentry. Finally, spatially different changes in I_{to} across the ventricular wall in heart failure alter cellular coupling current.

Taken together, these changes, along with the alteration of gap junctions and tissue alignment, lead to significant changes in electrical conduc-

tivity and sequence, which are important mechanisms underlying the increased propensity to ventricular arrhythmia and sudden cardiac death (SCD) in heart failure.

Therefore, right-heart failure is not characterized by a single set of electrophysiological changes.

Three possible electrophysiological mechanisms are involved in the development of cardiac arrhythmias in the presence of right-heart failure: (a) increased automaticity, (b) triggered activity, and (c) reentry phenomena around an anatomical obstacle. *Automaticity* is the property of cardiac cells to undergo spontaneous diastolic depolarization and initiate an electrical impulse in the absence of external electrical stimulation [45]. *Triggered activity* is a term used to describe impulse initiation in cardiac fibers that is dependent on after-depolarizations. These are oscillations in the membrane potential that follow the upstroke of an action potential [45, 46]. The fundamental requirements for *reentry* are unidirectional conduction block, a core of unexcitable tissue around which the wave front propagates, and maintenance of excitable tissue ahead of the propagating wave front (an excitable gap) that is facilitated by either slowing of conduction, shortening of the refractory period, or both [46].

Awareness of arrhythmias in patients with PAH and/or right-heart failure has occurred for a long time. In 1962, James [47] first described autopsy findings of sinoatrial and atrioventricular nodal artery disease in three patients with severe PAH and syncope who died suddenly. In 1979, Kanemoto and Sasamoto [48] assessed 171 electrocardiograms (ECGs) from 101 patients with PAH and found arrhythmias in 27% of the considered patients. The main types of arrhythmias were sinus tachycardia, sinus bradycardia, and first-degree atrioventricular block, which accounted for 70% of the total, whereas ventricular arrhythmias were very rare.

Although the primary cause of death in PAH is right-heart failure, approximately 50% of patients die from another cause, with PAH as a contributing factor [49–51]. Arrhythmias have been recognized as serious, end-stage complications of PAH reflecting the maladaptive response of the right heart to the increased afterload.

Supraventricular Arrhythmias

Baseline characteristics do not consistently predict which PAH patients will develop supraventricular tachycardias (SVTs) [52]. However, the findings that most correlated with the development of SVTs include serological (NT-proBNP) or hemodynamic (right atrial pressure, cardiac index) markers of overall cardiac dysfunction. RV failure and SVTs, in particular atrial flutter (AFl) (Fig. 19.1) and atrial fibrillation (AF), may be part of a vicious circle. From one side, SVTs are mainly due to structural changes in the right atrium secondary to chronic pressure overload and alterations in autonomic tone. In fact, they are more often present in advanced stages of right-heart failure or PAH. From the other side, the occurrence of SVT may compromise cardiac function and worsen the prognosis of PAH. Actually, the observation that sinus rhythm restoration was followed by marked and rapid clinical improvement suggests some degree of causal role of SVTs in precipitating and/or worsening RV failure. Such clinical deterioration appeared to be related to the deleterious hemodynamic effects of the loss of atrial transport mechanism and/or compromise in diastolic filling time resulting from rapid heart rates in the presence of ventricular dysfunction. In particular AFl, but also AF, almost invariably leads to further clinical deterioration [53]. In these patients, RV function is a main determinant of clinical stability and outcome and SVTs constitute a relevant problem. Data about SVT incidence and clinical role are based on a small number of retrospective studies.

In a retrospective single-center analysis involving 231 consecutive patients with PAH or inoperable chronic thromboembolic pulmonary hypertension (CTEPH), Tongers et al. [54] observed that the cumulative incidence for SVT was 11.7% (annual risk 2.8% per patient), including AFl, AF, and atrioventricular nodal reentry tachycardia (AVNRT). SVT onset was almost invariably associated with marked clinical deterioration and RV failure (84% of SVT episodes). The outcome was strongly associated with the type of SVT and restoration of sinus rhythm

(SR). In fact, cumulative mortality was lower when SR was restored (all cases of AVNRT and AFl). In contrast, the vast majority of patients with permanent AF (9/11) died from RV failure at 1-year follow-up. In this study, the average interval between diagnosis of pulmonary hypertension and onset of SVT was 3.5 years, suggesting that these arrhythmias are mostly manifestations of long-standing pulmonary hypertension.

In another retrospective single-center analysis [55] involving 281 patients with PAH, the average interval between PAH diagnosis and SVT onset was 60.3 ± 55.9 months. The cumulative incidence of SVT, consistent with Tongers' study [54], was 10%. The type of arrhythmia distribution was AF in 42.8%, "uncommon" AFl in 25%, "common" AFl in 17.8%, and AVNRT in 14.2%. AF and AFl occurred in older patients compared with AVNRT. Most episodes of SVT (82%) were symptomatic with clinical worsening or RV failure. In particular, the mean distance at the 6-min walk test (6MWD) decreased after SVT onset (423.7 ± 74.6 vs. 252.1 ± 145.8 m; $p < 0.001$). Patients with AFl presented the most marked decrease in 6MWD. Restoration of SR was associated with clinical improvement in all patients, with an average increase in 6MWD of 196 ± 163 m. After a first episode of SVT, and despite restoration of SR or adequate control of ventricular rate, 46.4% of patients needed an increase in PAH-specific therapy due to progressive clinical deterioration or right-heart failure. The average time between SVT onset and death or transplantation was 17.8 months.

Olsson et al. [56] in a 5-year prospective study, involving 157 patients with PAH and 82 patients with inoperable CTEPH, observed that the cumulative incidence of new-onset AFl and AF was 25.1% (95% confidence interval, 13.8–35.4%). The development of these arrhythmias was frequently accompanied by clinical worsening (80%) and signs of right-heart failure (30%). Stable sinus rhythm was successfully re-established in 21/24 (88%) of patients initially presenting with AFl and in 16/24 (67%) of patients initially presenting with AF. New-onset

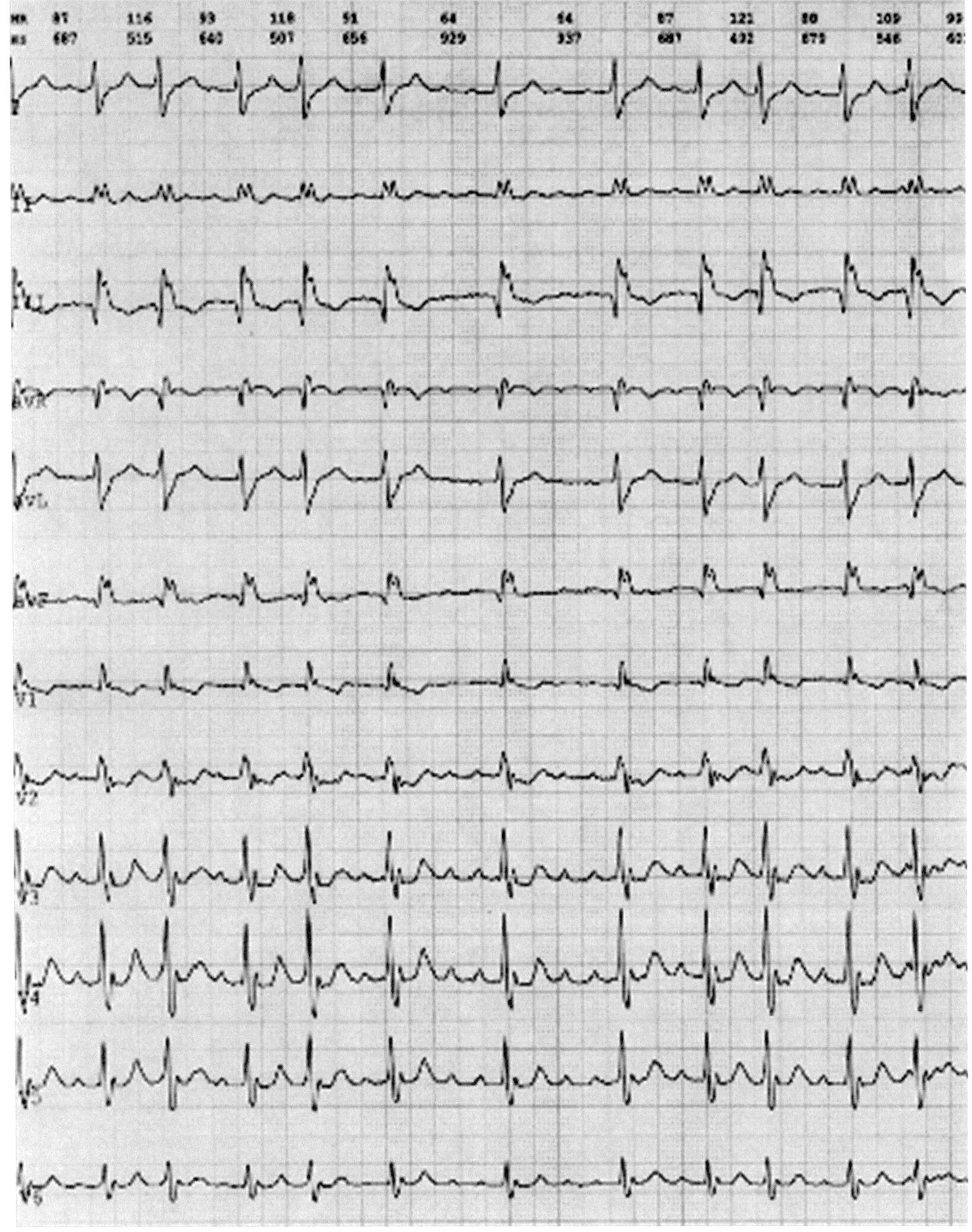

Fig. 19.1 Uncommon form of typical atrial flutter due to clockwise rotation within the right atrial reentrant circuit

AFl and AF were an independent risk factor of death ($p = 0.04$, simple Cox regression analysis) with a higher mortality in patients with persistent AF when compared to patients in whom sinus rhythm was restored (estimated survival at 1, 2, and 3 years 64%, 55%, and 27% versus 97%, 80%, and 57%, respectively; $p = 0.01$, log rank analysis).

Medi et al. [57] evaluated atrial electrical and structural remodeling in 8 patients with long-standing PAH compared to 16 controls. PAH patients showed prolongation of corrected sinus node recovery time without significant changes in atrial effective refractory period and an increase in AF inducibility. PAH was associated with lower tissue voltage, increased low-voltage areas, and presence of electrically silent areas. Conduction velocities were slower and fractionated electrograms and double potentials were more prevalent in PAH patients compared with controls, respectively. Taking these data together, they concluded that PAH is associated with right atrial electro-anatomical remodeling, characterized by generalized conduction slowing with marked regional abnormalities, reduced tissue voltage, and regions of electrical silence. These changes provide important insights into the isolated effects of PAH, fundamental to a range of clinical conditions associated with AF.

In a 6-year prospective multicenter study [58] involving 280 patients with idiopathic PAH, the cumulative 6-year incidence of SVTs was 15.8%. The most common types were AF ($n = 16$) and AFl ($n = 13$), followed by ectopic atrial tachycardia ($n = 11$). SVTs had clinical relevance for the prognosis of patients with idiopathic PAH. In fact, the majority of SVTs were associated with clinical deterioration and right-heart failure. Sinus rhythm was successfully restored in most patients, resulting in clinical recovery. SVTs predicted a higher risk of mortality in a stepwise forward Cox analysis (hazard ratio of 4.757, 95% confidence interval 2.695–8.397, $p < 0.001$). Kaplan-Meier survival curves showed that patients with SVTs, mainly permanent SVTs, had a lower survival rate ($p = 0.008$).

Recent data reinforce the concept that the new onset of SVTs reflects clinical worsening predicting adverse outcome. Cannillo et al. [59] observed that 17/77 (22%) PAH patients experienced new-onset SVTs during a median follow-up of 35 months. The development of SVTs was associated with worsening of prognostic parameters at the follow-up: increasing of WHO functional class ($p = 0.005$) and NT-proBNP ($p = 0.018$) and reduction of 6MWD ($p = 0.048$), tricuspid annular plane systolic excursion ($p = 0.041$), and diffusing capacity of the lung for carbon monoxide ($p = 0.025$). A composite primary endpoint of all-cause mortality and hospitalization occurred in 76% in the SVT group compared with 37% in the group without SVTs ($p = 0.004$), whereas 53% among those with SVTs died during the follow-up compared with 13% among those without ($p = 0.001$). At multivariate analysis, development of SVTs was independently associated with an increased risk of all-cause mortality and hospitalization (hazard ratio of 2.13; 95% confidence interval 1.07–4.34; $p = 0.031$).

A validated method to evaluate cardiac autonomic system dysfunction is the heart rate variability (HRV). A decrease in HRV is predictive of arrhythmic events, particularly in left ventricular diseases. Witte et al. [60] evaluated the clinical relevance of HRV assessed by 24-h Holter electrocardiogram in 64 patients with different forms of PH (25 PAH, 11 CTEPH, and 28 lung disease-induced PH). Compared to healthy controls, PAH patients showed significant reduction of HRV with an increase of ventricular arrhythmic burden, indicating a high risk for malignant arrhythmic events. Differently, in CTEPH patients only the amount of premature ventricular contractions differed from controls.

A retrospective analysis from 167 patients with different types of PH (Group 1: 59 patients, Group 2: 28 patients, Group 3: 39 patients, Group 4: 41 patients) [61] showed that 30 patients (18%) had AF at baseline evaluation, and 13 (8%) developed new-onset AF during a long-term follow-up. Patients with baseline AF showed higher atrial diameters and higher right atrial pressure. Atrial fibrillation predicted adverse prognosis in the whole PH population. In fact, the mean survival times were 79 ± 5 months for patients in sinus rhythm, 64 ± 13 months for patients with baseline AF, and 59 ± 9 months for those with newly onset AF during follow-up. Patients with P-wave duration >110 ms had shorter survival.

Recently, Mercurio et al. [62] in a prospective cohort study collected baseline data from 317 patients (201 with systemic sclerosis [SSc]-related PAH and 116 with idiopathic PAH) enrolled in the Johns Hopkins Pulmonary

Hypertension Registry. The authors found that 42 patients developed SVT during the follow-up: 19 AF, 10 flutter-fibrillation, 9 AFl, and 4 atrial ectopic tachycardia, with a 13.2% cumulative incidence. Patients with SVTs had higher right atrial pressure, pulmonary artery wedge pressure (both $p < 0.005$), NT-proBNP ($p < 0.05$), and thyroid disease prevalence defined as hypo- or hyperthyroidism, or radiographic thyroid nodules ($p < 0.005$). The worst prognosis was observed in patients who developed SVT that was not related to thyroid dysfunction. These results suggest that SVTs associated with thyroid dysfunction may be considered a relatively benign condition, while on the contrary, SVTs unrelated to thyroid dysfunction reflect a more advanced disease and may adversely affect prognosis in PAH patients. Furthermore, SSc-PAH with SVTs had the worst prognosis and idiopathic PAH with SVTs and SSc-PAH without SVTs had a similar long-term mortality.

Therapy

Given the detrimental hemodynamic effects of SVT on clinical outcome, restoration and maintenance of SR represent a paramount in the management of PAH patients [53].

Many studies have reported different treatment strategies, highlighting the heterogeneity in real-world approach and outcomes (different drugs, eventual use of catheter ablation, different success rate) [52]. A variety of drugs have been used for SVTs in PAH patients, but their efficacy is limited from the severity of the underlying disease (electro-anatomical right-heart remodeling in response to long-standing pressure and volume overload with increased wall stretch, fibrosis, delayed cardiac repolarization, ischemia, increased sympathetic activity), the potential adverse effects, and the possible drug–drug interactions between antiarrhythmic and PAH-specific drugs.

Similarly to AF in the setting of left-heart disease (i.e., systemic hypertension, mitral or aortic valve disease, left ventricle [LV] systolic or diastolic dysfunction), "non-antiarrhythmic" therapy must be optimized. This means that background therapy (such as warfarin, diuretics, digoxin if necessary) and PAH-specific therapy (endothelin receptor antagonists, phosphodiesterase-5 inhibitors, stimulators of soluble guanylate cyclase, and prostacyclin analogues) have to be individually adjusted and personalized. Following optimization of PAH-specific therapy, treatment options for SVT may include rate control (i.e., digoxin, calcium channel blockers) or rhythm control (i.e., antiarrhythmic agents or non-pharmacological treatment).

The need for systemic anticoagulation should be considered in all patients with AF/AFl [63].

The 2015 ESC/ERS guidelines on pulmonary hypertension [53] give a weak recommendation to anticoagulated patients with idiopathic, heritable, or anorexigen-induced PAH (grade of recommendation IIb, level of evidence C) and consider oral anticoagulation harmful in patients with associated PAH. Registry and RCT data appear to be heterogeneous and inconclusive [64–66] regarding the effects of anticoagulants in PAH. Likely, the guidelines' recommendations should change in the event of permanent atrial fibrillation or flutter considering a wider and stronger recommendation for the use of anticoagulation. Finally, it is unknown if the current risk stratification models (such as CHA_2DS_2-VASc score) are valid also in patients with PAH [67].

With regard to atrioventricular nodal active drugs in patients with AF, the Atrial Fibrillation Follow-up Investigation of Rhythm Management (AFFIRM) trial [68] randomized 4060 patients with AF at high risk of stroke or death to a rate control vs. rhythm control strategy. In the rate control arm, different therapies were allowed to achieve adequate heart rate control, including digoxin, beta-blockers, calcium channel blockers (verapamil and diltiazem), or combinations of these drugs. In the rhythm control arm, antiarrhythmic drugs included amiodarone, disopyramide, flecainide, moricizine, procainamide, propafenone, quinidine, sotalol, or combinations of these drugs. The strategy of rate control vs. rhythm control was randomized, whereas the choice of specific agents used was left to the discretion of the treating physician in both arms. During a mean follow-up of 3.5 years, there were 356 deaths (23.8%) in the rhythm control group vs. 310 deaths (21.3%) in the rate control group, a directionally but not significantly lower mortality with rate control ($p = 0.08$). Two reports from the AFFIRM trial [69, 70] explored the association of digoxin use with mortality among patients with AF, reaching conflicting conclusions: one reported that digoxin use was associated with a significant increase in all-cause mortality [69] and the other documented no association of digoxin use with mortality [70]. Several factors contributed to these different conclusions. Given the non-randomized, observational design of both studies, these findings should be considered "hypothesis generating," and not even the most sophisticated statistical methods, such as propensity-matched analysis, can replace randomization [71].

Digoxin has been traditionally largely used in the setting of chronic obstructive pulmonary disease also in patients with SR [72, 73]. In a single open-label study [39], digoxin was shown to improve ventricular function only if LV function was reduced and despite the improvement in ventricular function, digoxin has failed to improve pulmonary function, cardiopulmonary response to exercise, or general feeling of well-being. Moreover, at present the role of digoxin in patients with pulmonary hypertension and AF/AFl is not well established. Current guidelines on pulmonary hypertension [53] suggest that digoxin may be considered in patients with PAH who develop atrial tachyarrhythmias to slow ventricular rate.

Calcium channel blockers are commonly used as part of the PAH treatment regimen for "vasoreactive" patients. The use of verapamil or diltiazem for arrhythmia management may be challenging because the effects of these drugs in "non-vasoreactive" patients are not known and because of their negative inotropic activity. As a consequence, no specific recommendations can be given at this time.

Beta-blocker therapy, often used in patients with portal hypertension to reduce the risk of variceal bleeding, has been shown to worsen hemodynamics and exercise capacity in portopulmonary PAH patients [74]. Thus, the use of beta-blockers for the treatment of SVT in patients with PAH is currently discouraged because of their negative inotropic effects [53].

The use of many antiarrhythmic agents in the PAH population is limited due to the significant side effect profile and lack of data. For instance, in patients with structural heart disease and/or heart failure, class IC antiarrhythmic agents (i.e., sodium channel blockers such as propafenone and flecainide) are not recommended because of increased risk of premature death [75].

The class III antiarrhythmic agent sotalol prolongs the QT interval and possesses negative inotropic effects due to its beta-blocker action.

In the absence of more effective pharmacological options, the need to restore SR using antiarrhythmic agents with no negative inotropic effects makes amiodarone an ideal drug in the acute setting for controlling hemodynamically significant arrhythmias. Nevertheless, the role of chronic prophylactic administration of amiodarone in maintaining SR remains uncertain, given significant potential side effects, such as development of pneumonitis/fibrosis, and its potential drug-drug interaction with PAH-specific drugs. Moreover, amiodarone is a CYP2C9 inhibitor and may cause a significant increase in plasma bosentan levels [53].

The safety and efficacy profiles of newer antiarrhythmics, such as ivabradine and dronedarone, have not been well established yet.

A reliable alternative approach to SVT, in particular AVNRT [54, 55] and AFl [54, 55, 76–78], is percutaneous catheter ablation (Figs. 19.2, 19.3, and 19.4). Data from a retrospective analysis of 22 patients with AFl and PAH or CTEPH [76] showed that cavo-tricuspid isthmus (CTI) ablation can be performed successfully without complications, leading to a significant clinical improvement in terms of functional class. In addition, the absence of changes in echocardiographic parameters after catheter ablation suggested that acute improvement in clinical status was secondary to SR restoration rather than cardiac remodeling. In a retrospective single-center

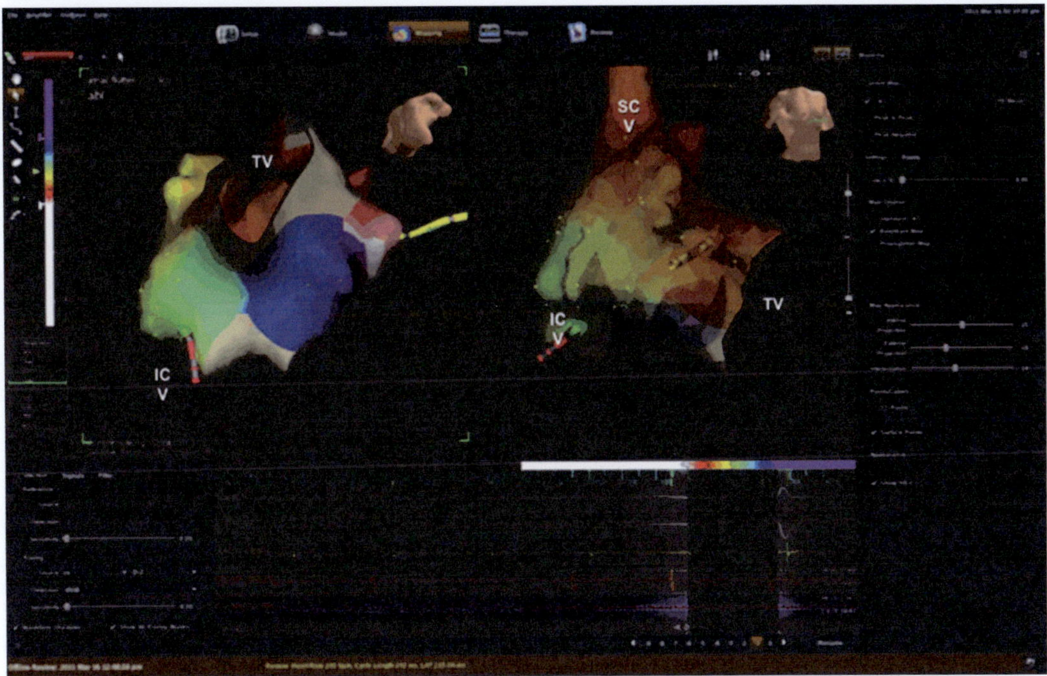

Fig. 19.2 Electro-anatomical reconstruction of typical right atrial flutter. *SCV* superior cava vein, *ICV* inferior cava vein, *TV* tricuspid valve

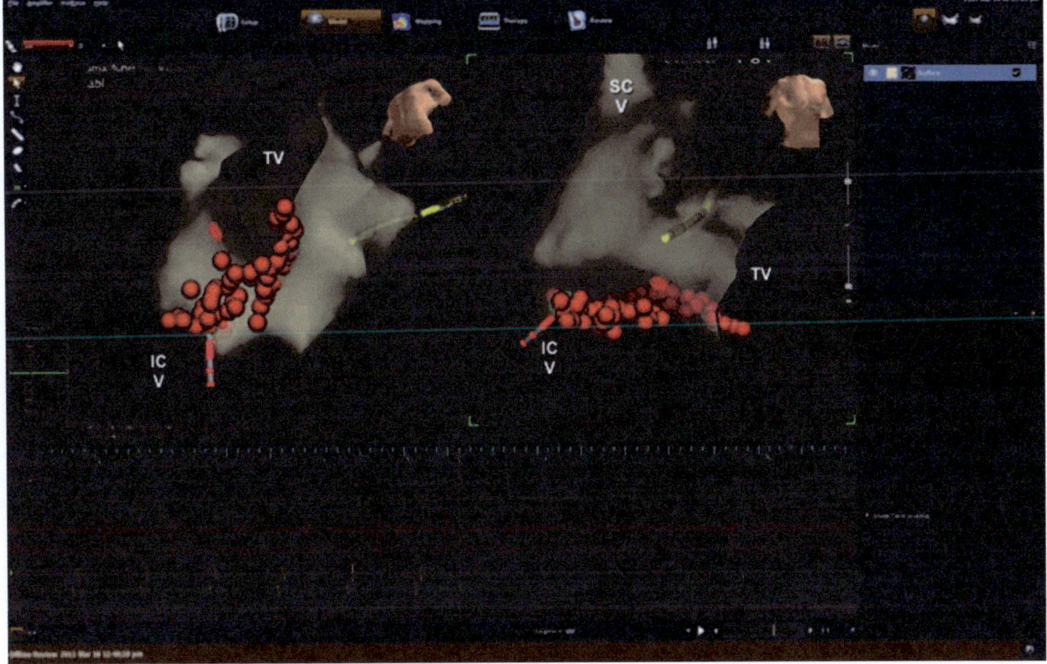

Fig. 19.3 Ablation lines of typical right atrial flutter. Abbreviation: see Fig. 19.2

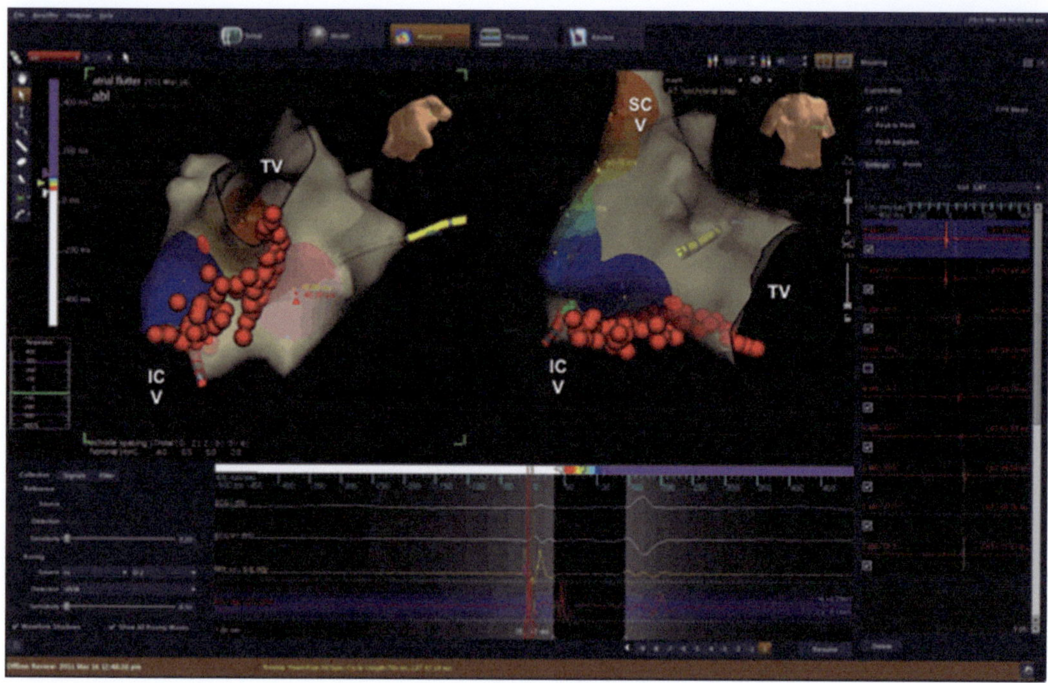

Fig. 19.4 Validation of ablation lines showing bidirectional block. Abbreviation: see Fig. 19.2

study [77] involving 38 PAH patients with CTI-dependent AFl undergoing an ablation procedure, a bidirectional block of the CTI was achieved in all patients. Nevertheless, patients with severe PAH had a significantly longer procedure, longer ablation time, and a greater amount of cumulative tissue lesions than patients without PAH. Finally, in another single-center retrospective study, catheter ablation was performed in 12 PAH patients with AFl resistant to medical management. Acute success was obtained in 86% of procedures. After catheter ablation, echocardiographic estimated pulmonary artery systolic pressure decreased from 114 ± 44 to 82 ± 38 mmHg ($p = 0.004$) and B-type natriuretic peptide levels were lower (787 ± 832 vs. 522 ± 745 pg/mL, $p = 0.02$). A total of 80% of patients were free from AFl at 3-month follow-up and 75% at 1 year.

Thus, according to available limited data [54, 55, 76–78], treatment of AFl or AVNRT by catheter ablation is feasible, safe, and effective in patients with PAH.

Ventricular Arrhythmias

A prolonged QRS duration (>120 ms) is common in patients with left-sided heart failure and is associated with more advanced myocardial disease, worse LV function and prognosis, and higher all-cause mortality compared with patients with a narrow QRS complex [79–82]. QRS prolongation results in systolic ventricular dyssynchrony, which can further decrease cardiac output of the left side of the heart.

Ventricular arrhythmias (Fig. 19.5) are less common in PAH patients compared with patients with left-heart diseases. Although previous studies have demonstrated interventricular dyssynchrony also in patients with PAH [83], only limited data on the prevalence of QRS prolongation across the spectrum of idiopathic PAH are available at present. In a recent retrospective study including 212 consecutive patients with idiopathic PAH [84], 35 patients (16.5%) had a prolonged QRS duration (>120 ms). QRS duration was positively correlated with right atrial

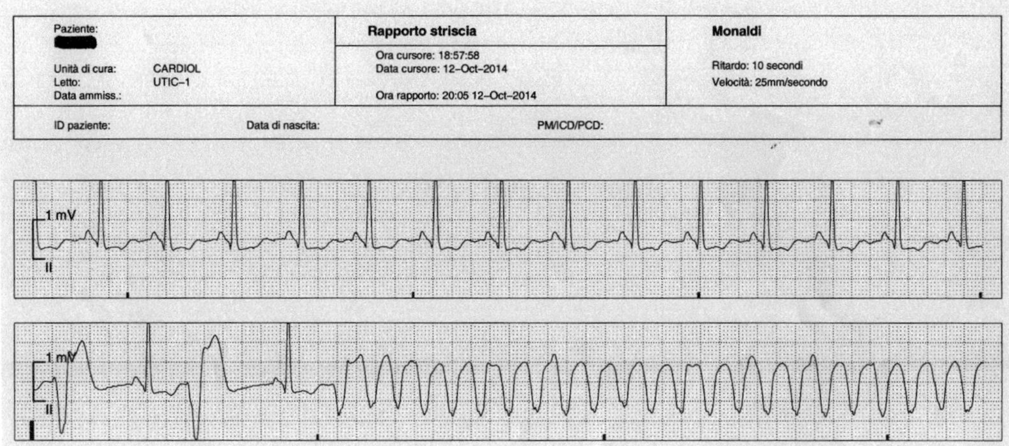

Fig. 19.5 Premature ventricular beats inducing life-threatening ventricular tachycardia

and RV dimensions, suggesting a possible role of RV overload in its pathogenesis. Interestingly, QRS prolongation was associated with a worse WHO functional class and 6MWD and higher serum uric acid when compared with patients with normal QRS duration ($p < 0.05$). Moreover, QRS prolongation was an independent predictor of mortality and was associated with a 2.5-fold increased risk of death ($p = 0.024$). Therefore, QRS duration >120 ms may be considered a new predictor of adverse outcome in patients with idiopathic PAH, and screening for prolonged QRS duration should be part of the routine assessment of patients with idiopathic PAH for risk stratification and treatment.

An experimental study on male Wistar rats receiving monocrotaline to induce either RV hypertrophy or failure investigated the electro-anatomical ventricular remodeling and the possible mechanisms responsible for the pro-arrhythmic state [85]. Failing hearts showed greater fiber angle disarray that correlated with APD. Failing myocytes had reduced sarcoplasmic reticular Ca^{2+}-ATPase activity, increased sarcoplasmic reticular Ca^{2+} release fraction, and increased Ca^{2+} spark leak. Moreover, in hypertrophied hearts and myocytes, dysfunctional adaptation had begun but alternans did not develop. The authors concluded that increased electrical and structural heterogeneity and dysfunctional sarco-plasmic reticular Ca^{2+} handling increase the probability of alternans, a pro-arrhythmic predictor of SCD. These mechanisms are potential therapeutic targets for the correction of arrhythmias in hypertensive, failing right ventricles.

The clinical course of pulmonary hypertension and PAH is one of progressive deterioration combined with episodes of acute heart failure [53]. RV failure and SCD are the most common causes of death in PAH.

Nowadays, RV failure (36%) and SCD (28%) together account for the majority of deaths in patients with PAH [86, 87]. However, in contrast to patients with advanced left-heart disease, life-threatening arrhythmias such as ventricular tachycardia (VT) and ventricular fibrillation (VF) are relatively rare in patients with PAH. Conversely, patients with PAH may often show bradycardia as pulseless electrical activity. The major determinant of prognosis in PAH patients is RV function and SCD is more likely to occur in such patients with severe hypoxia [88]. Less common "non-arrhythmogenic" causes of SCD should also be considered, including rare cases of dissection or rupture of the pulmonary artery [89] or left main extrinsic compression by dilated pulmonary artery [90–92].

In a study [51] evaluating a total of 84 PAH patients (mean age 58 ± 14 years, 73% female) who died between June 2008 and May 2012,

PAH was the direct cause of death (for right-heart failure or SCD) in 37 (44%) and PAH contributed but did not directly cause death in 37 (44%) patients. Moreover, 50% of all patients with PAH and 75.7% of those who died of right-heart failure received parenteral prostanoid therapy and less than half of patients had advanced healthcare directives.

Recently, a retrospective study [93] explored the role of non-sustained VT and its prognostic relevance in a population of 55 PAH and 23 CTEPH patients who underwent 24-h Holter ECG. Twenty-one patients died during follow-up. In patients with non-sustained VT, tricuspid annular plane systolic excursion was lower ($p = 0.001$). Nevertheless, the mean survival of patients with vs. without non-sustained VT was not different (146 ± 21 vs. 155 ± 8 months; $p = 0.690$). Age, gender, 6MWD, or arterial hypertension did not affect the association between arrhythmias and survival.

A retrospective multicenter study [50] on the frequency and results of cardiopulmonary resuscitation (CPR) in patients with PAH considered a total of 3130 patients with PAH treated between 1997 and 2000 in 17 referral centers in Europe and in the United States. During this 3-year period, 513 (16%) patients had circulatory arrest and CPR was attempted in 132 (26%) of them. Although 96% of the CPR attempts took place in hospitalized patients (74% in intensive care units or equally equipped facilities) and although there was only minimal delay between collapse and initiation of CPR, resuscitation efforts were primarily unsuccessful in 104 patients (79%). Only 8 patients (6%) survived for more than 90 days. The initial ECGs at the time of CPR showed bradycardia in 58 cases (45%), electromechanical dissociation in 37 cases (28%), asystole in 19 cases (15%), VF in 10 cases (8%), and other rhythms in 6 cases (4%). The initial ECG rhythm was unknown in 2 cases. Data from right-heart catheterization within 3 months before CPR were available for 80 patients (61%). The hemodynamic variables confirmed the presence of severe PAH in these patients but did not show any significant differences between survivors and non-survivors. Except for one patient, all long-term survivors had identifiable causes of circulatory arrest that were rapidly reversible. Moreover, in approximately 50% of the patients in this study, an intercurrent illness contributed to death. These conditions were often minor abnormalities such as respiratory or gastrointestinal tract infections, which underscores the notion that patients with PAH are clinically fragile with little or no compensatory reserve in the setting of concomitant illnesses. The authors hypothesized that poor results of CPR in patients with PAH may be explained by the underlying hemodynamic condition. In fact, the mean pulmonary vascular resistance in the study population was 1694 dynes s/cm^5, which is more than eight times above the upper normal limit of 200 dynes s/cm^5. Under these conditions, it is extremely difficult to achieve effective pulmonary blood flow and LV filling with chest compression. These data indicate that CPR for circulatory arrest in patients with PAH is rarely successful unless the cause of cardiopulmonary decompensation can be corrected.

On the basis of these pathophysiological considerations, measures to improve the results of CPR in PAH patients should aim at optimizing PAH-specific therapy to lower pulmonary vascular resistance. In this context, it is noteworthy that three of the successful CPR attempts included the intravenous bolus administration of iloprost, a prostacyclin analogue.

Given the lower incidence of VT/VF in patients experiencing cardiac arrest in the setting of PAH compared to patients with advanced left-heart disease, the clinical role of implantable cardioverter-defibrillators in PAH patients remains unclear. Furthermore, the relative paucity of patients with such end-stage arrhythmias in the field of PAH makes systematic research difficult to track.

At present, no prospective clinical trial has been conducted to establish the true incidence of SCD in different subgroups of PAH. Prophylactic antiarrhythmic therapy is not indicated for primary prevention of SCD in patients with PAH [94]. In the absence of clinical trials showing the benefit of prophylactic antiarrhythmic therapy in these patients, a "tailored therapy" based on clinical judgment may be considered in the management of asymptomatic arrhythmias such as non-sustained VT, taking into account the pros and cons of antiarrhythmic agents (antiarrhythmic benefit vs. potential pro-arrhythmic risk and side effects). Otherwise, implantable cardioverter-defibrillators should be offered as a treatment option to PAH patients who manifest either syncope or cardiac arrest in the setting of documented VT/VF.

The role of pacing in PAH patients for relative bradycardia is not well established, highlighting the intrinsic difficulty in the clinical management of PAH patients during cardiac arrest.

At present, there are not enough data supporting the role of cardiac resynchronization therapy in this setting. From a pathophysiological viewpoint, it is known that RV pressure overload may induce electrophysiological remodeling, with conduction slowing and APD prolongation, contributing to the loss of left and right ventricular synchrony. Moreover, delayed left ventricle-to-right ventricle peak shortening results in decreased cardiac output in patients with CTEPH and PAH.

Right-heart failure in PAH is associated with mechanical ventricular dyssynchrony, which leads to impaired RV function and, by adverse diastolic interaction, to impaired LV function as well. However, therapies aiming to restore synchrony by pacing are currently not available and the role of cardiac resynchronization therapy in these patients remains undefined.

In an experimental model of PAH and right-heart failure induced in rats by injection of monocrotaline, Handoko et al. [95] found that preexcitation of the RV free wall obtained by RV pacing improved RV function and reduced adverse LV diastolic interaction.

Hardziyenka et al. [96] conducted epicardial mapping during pulmonary endarterectomy placing a multielectrode grid on the epicardium of the RV free wall and LV lateral wall in 26 patients with CTEPH and compared these findings with clinical, hemodynamic, and echocardiographic variables. They found that the onset of diastolic relaxation of RV free wall with respect to LV lateral wall (diastolic interventricular delay) was delayed by 38 ± 31 ms in patients with CTEPH vs. −12 ± 13 ms in control subjects ($p < 0.001$), because in patients with CTEPH the right ventricle completed electrical activation later than the left ventricle (65 ± 20 vs. 44 ± 7 ms, $p < 0.001$) and epicardial APD duration, as assessed by activation-recovery interval measurement, was longer in RV free wall than in LV lateral wall (253 ± 29 vs. 240 ± 22 ms, $p < 0.001$). They concluded that additive effects of electrophysiological changes in the right ventricle, in particular conduction slowing and APD prolongation as assessed by epicardial activation-recovery interval, may contribute to diastolic interventricular delay in patients with CTEPH.

The same group [97] evaluated 14 CTEPH patients with right-heart failure and significant ventricular dyssynchrony ($\geq$60 ms right-to-left ventricle delay in the onset of diastolic relaxation), showing that resynchronization therapy acutely reduced ventricular dyssynchrony and enhanced RV contractility, LV diastolic filling, and stroke volume. These findings provide a strong rationale for further investigations on cardiac resynchronization therapy and RV pacing as a novel treatment for right-heart failure secondary to PAH.

An algorithm for tachyarrhythmia treatment in pulmonary arterial hypertension is reported in Fig. 19.6.

Conclusion

Electro-anatomical remodeling of the right ventricle and right atrium in response to long-standing pressure and volume overload, due to altered autonomics, repolarization abnormalities, ischemia, and scar, may be the underlying substrate predisposing to enhanced arrhythmogenicity in patients with right-heart failure and PAH.

Supraventricular arrhythmias, namely AFl and AF, are common findings in patients with PAH, and are often associated with worsening heart failure and a decline in patient clinical status. Given the significant potential side effects of antiarrhythmic drugs, percutaneous catheter ablation represents a safe and reliable alternative

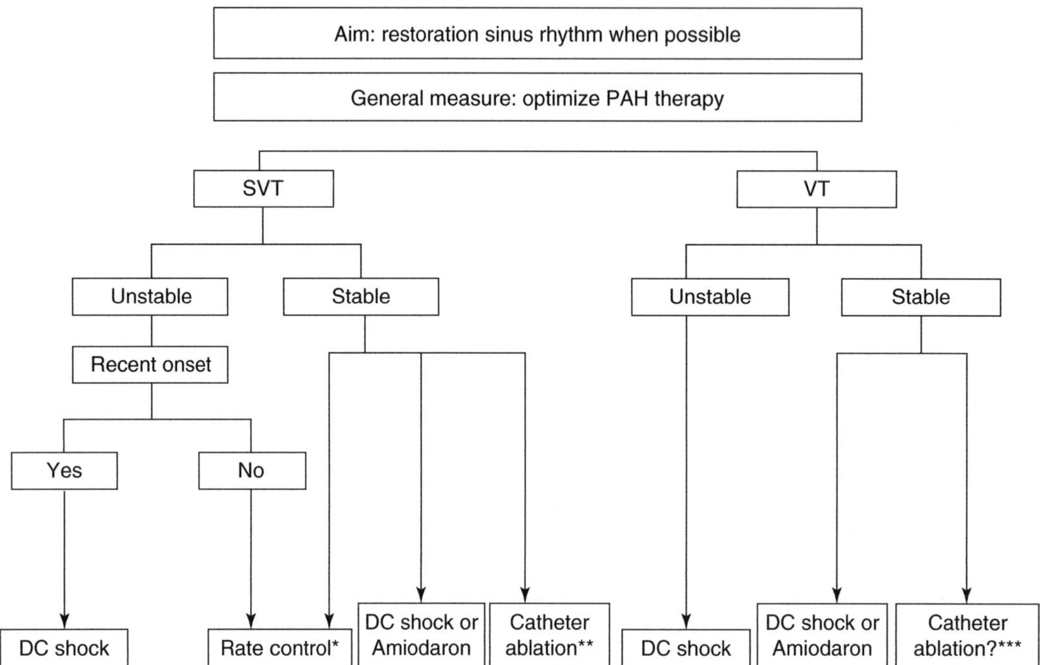

Fig. 19.6 Algorithm for tachyarrhythmia treatment in pulmonary arterial hypertension

approach in this patient population. VT is less common, and relative bradycardia is a threatening sign, with bradyarrhythmias frequently observed in the setting of cardiopulmonary arrest. The role of pacing in PAH patients for relative bradycardia is not well established, highlighting the intrinsic difficulty in the clinical management of PAH patients during cardiac arrest. Finally, the exact role of cardiac resynchronization therapy in these patients remains to be elucidated.

Acknowledgements Declaration: Authors declare that there is no grant support or any potential conflicts of interest, including related consultancies, shareholdings, and funding grants.

References

1. Fishman AP. State of the art: chronic cor pulmonale. Am Rev Respir Dis. 1976;114:775–94.
2. Bogaard HJ, Abe K, Vonk NA, Voelkel NF. The right ventricle under pressure: cellular and molecular mechanisms of right-heart failure in pulmonary hypertension. Chest. 2009;135:794–804.
3. Haddad F, Doyle R, Murphy DJ, Hunt SA. Right ventricular function in cardiovascular disease, part II: pathophysiology, clinical importance, and management of right ventricular failure. Circulation. 2008;117:1717–31.
4. Voelkel NF, Quaife RA, Leinwand LA, Barst RJ, McGoon MD, Meldrum DR, et al. Right ventricular 670 function and failure: report of a National Heart, Lung, and Blood Institute working group on cellular and molecular mechanisms of right heart failure. Circulation. 2006;114:1883–91.
5. Anand IS, Chandrashekhar Y, Ferrari R, Sarma R, Guleria R, Jindal SK, et al. Pathogenesis of congestive state in chronic obstructive pulmonary disease. Studies of body water and sodium, renal function, hemodynamics, and plasma hormones during edema and after recovery. Circulation. 1992;86:12–21.
6. Farber MO, Roberts LR, Weinberger MH, Robertson GL, Fineberg NS, Manfredi F. Abnormalities of sodium and H2O handling in chronic obstructive lung disease. Arch Intern Med. 1982;142:1326–30.
7. Henkens IR, Mouchaers KT, Vonk-Noordegraaf A, Boonstra A, Swenne CA, Maan AC, et al. Improved ECG detection of presence and severity of right ventricular pressure load validated with cardiac magnetic

resonance imaging. Am J Physiol Heart Circ Physiol. 2008;294:2150–7.

8. Hlaing T, Guo D, Zhao X, DiMino T, Greenspon L, Kowey PR, et al. The QT and Tp-e intervals in left and right chest leads: comparison between patients with systemic and pulmonary hypertension. J Electrocardiol. 2005;38:154–8.

9. Folino AF, Bobbo F, Schiraldi C, Tona F, Romano S, Buja G, et al. Ventricular arrhythmias and autonomic profile in patients with primary pulmonary hypertension. Lung. 2003;181:321–8.

10. Coronel R, Wilders R, Verkerk AO, Wiegerinck RF, Benoist D, Bernus O. Electrophysiological changes in heart failure and their implications for arrhythmogenesis. Biochim Biophys Acta. 2013 [Epub ahead of print].

11. Janse MJ, van Capelle FJ, Morsink H, Kléber AG, Wilms-Schopman F, Cardinal R, et al. Flow of "injury" current and patterns of excitation during early ventricular arrhythmias in acute regional myocardial ischemia in isolated porcine and canine hearts. Evidence for two different arrhythmogenic mechanisms. Circ Res. 1980;47:151–65.

12. Fontaine G, Aouate P, Fontaliran F. Repolarization and the genesis of cardiac arrhythmias. Role of body surface mapping. Circulation. 1997;95:2600–2.

13. Schrier RW, Bansal S. Pulmonary hypertension, right ventricular failure, and kidney: different from left ventricular failure? Clin J Am Soc Nephrol. 2008;3:1232–7.

14. Rajdev A, Garan H, Biviano A. Arrhythmias in pulmonary arterial hypertension. Prog Cardiovasc Dis. 2012;55:180–6.

15. Morimitsu T, Miyahara Y, Sinboku H, et al. Iodine-123-metaiodobenzylguanidine myocardial imaging in patients with right ventricular pressure overload. J Nucl Med. 1996;37:1343–6.

16. Sakamaki F, Satoh T, Nagaya N, et al. Correlation between severity of pulmonary arterial hypertension and 123I-metaiodobenzylguanidine left ventricular imaging. J Nucl Med. 2000;41:1127–33.

17. Maron BA, Leopold JA. Emerging concepts in the molecular basis of pulmonary arterial hypertension: part II: neurohormonal signaling contributes to the pulmonary vascular and right ventricular pathophenotype of pulmonary arterial hypertension. Circulation. 2015;131:2079–91.

18. Algra A, Tijssen JG, Roelandt JR, Pool J, Lubsen J. QTc prolongation measured by standard 12-lead electrocardiography is an independent risk factor for sudden death due to cardiac arrest. Circulation. 1991;83:1888–94.

19. Hong-liang Z, Qin L, Zhi-hong L, Zhi-hui Z, Chang-ming X, Xin-hai N, et al. Heart rate-corrected QT interval and QT dispersion in patients with pulmonary hypertension. Wien Klin Wochenschr. 2009;121:330–3.

20. van Wolferen SA, Marcus JT, Westerhof N, et al. Right coronary artery flow impairment in patients with pulmonary hypertension. Eur Heart J. 2008;29:120–7.

21. Galiè N, Saia F, Palazzini M, et al. Left main coronary artery compression in patients with pulmonary arterial hypertension and angina. J Am Coll Cardiol. 2017;69:2808–17.

22. Bogaard HJ, Abe K, Vonk Noordegraaf A, Voelkel NF. The right ventricle under pressure: cellular and molecular mechanisms of right-heart failure in pulmonary hypertension. Chest. 2009;135:794–804.

23. Bogaard HJ, Natarajan R, Henderson SC, et al. Chronic pulmonary artery pressure elevation is insufficient to explain right heart failure. Circulation. 2009;120:1951–60.

24. Archer SL, Fang Y-H, Ryan JJ, Piao L. Metabolism and bioenergetics in the right ventricle and pulmonary vasculature in pulmonary hypertension. Pulm Circ. 2013;3:144–52.

25. Tomaselli GF, Zipes DP. What causes sudden death in heart failure? Circ Res. 2004;95:754–63.

26. Nattel S, Maguy A, Le Bouter S, Yeh YH. Arrhythmogenic ion-channel remodeling in the heart: heart failure, myocardial infarction, and atrial fibrillation. Physiol Rev. 2007;87:425–56.

27. Nass RD, Aiba T, Tomaselli GF, Akar FG. Mechanisms of disease: ion channel remodeling in the failing ventricle. Nat Clin Pract Cardiovasc Med. 2008;5:196–207.

28. Akar FG, Tomaselli GF. Ion channels as novel therapeutic targets in heart failure. Ann Med. 2005;37:44–54.

29. Cutler MJ, Rosenbaum DS, Dunlap ME. Structural and electrical remodeling as therapeutic targets in heart failure. J Electrocardiol. 2007;40(6 Suppl):S1–7.

30. Wang Y, Hill JA. Electrophysiological remodeling in heart failure. J Mol Cell Cardiol. 2010;48:619–32.

31. Kääb S, Nuss HB, Chiamvimonvat N, O'Rourke B, Pak PH, Kass DA, et al. Ionic mechanism of action potential prolongation in ventricular myocytes from dogs with pacing-induced heart failure. Circ Res. 1996;78:262–73.

32. Kaab S, Dixon J, Duc J, Ashen D, Nabauer M, Beuckelmann DJ, et al. Molecular basis of transient outward potassium current downregulation in human heart failure: a decrease in Kv4.3 mRNA correlates with a reduction in current density. Circulation. 1998;98:1383–93.

33. O'Rourke B, Kass DA, Tomaselli GF, Kaab S, Tunin R, Marban E. Mechanisms of altered excitation-contraction coupling in canine tachycardia-induced heart failure, I: experimental studies. Circ Res. 1999;84:562–70.

34. Houser SR, Piacentino V 3rd, Weisser J. Abnormalities of calcium cycling in the hypertrophied and failing heart. J Mol Cell Cardiol. 2000;32:1595–607.

35. Wang Y, Tandan S, Cheng J, Yang C, Nguyen L, Sugianto J, et al. Ca^{2+}/calmodulin-dependent protein kinase II-dependent remodeling of Ca^{2+} current in pressure overload heart failure. J Biol Chem. 2008;283:25524–32.

36. Undrovinas AI, Maltsev VA, Sabbah HN. Repolarization abnormalities in cardiomyocytes

of dogs with chronic heart failure: role of sustained inward current. Cell Mol Life Sci. 1999;55:494–505.

37. Wang Y, Cheng J, Joyner RW, Wagner MB, Hill JA. Remodeling of early-phase repolarization: a mechanism of abnormal impulse conduction in heart failure. Circulation. 2006;113:1849–56.

38. Studer R, Reinecke H, Bilger J, Eschenhagen T, Bohm M, Hasenfuss G, et al. Gene expression of the cardiac Na$^+$-Ca^{2+} exchanger in end-stage human heart failure. Circ Res. 1994;75:443–53.

39. Flesch M, Schwinger RH, Schiffer F, Frank K, Sudkamp M, Kuhn-Regnier F, et al. Evidence for functional relevance of an enhanced expression of the Na$^+$-Ca^{2+} exchanger in failing human myocardium. Circulation. 1996;94:992–1002.

40. Reinecke H, Studer R, Vetter R, Holtz J, Drexler H. Cardiac Na$^+$/Ca^{2+} exchange activity in patients with end-stage heart failure. Cardiovasc Res. 1996;31:48–54.

41. Wang Z, Nolan B, Kutschke W, Hill JA. Na$^+$-Ca^{2+} exchanger remodeling in pressure overload cardiac hypertrophy. J Biol Chem. 2001;276:17706–11.

42. Yue L, Feng J, Gaspo R, Li GR, Wang Z, Nattel S. Ionic remodeling underlying action potential changes in a canine model of atrial fibrillation. Circ Res. 1997;81:512–25.

43. Beuckelmann DJ, Nabauer M, Erdmann E. Alterations of K$^+$ currents in isolated human ventricular myocytes from patients with terminal heart failure. Circ Res. 1993;73:379–85.

44. Wang HS, Dixon JE, McKinnon D. Unexpected and differential effects of Cl$^-$ channel blockers on the Kv4.3 and Kv4.2 K$^+$ channels. Implications for the study of the I$_{to2}$ current. Circ Res. 1997;81:711–8.

45. Zipes DP, Jalife J. Arrhythmogenic mechanisms: automaticity, triggered activity, and reentry. In: Zipes DP, Jalife J, editors. Cardiac electrophysiology. From cell to bedside. 3rd ed. Philadelphia: WB Saunders; 2000. p. 345–56.

46. Cranefield PF. Action potentials, after potentials and arrhythmias. Circ Res. 1977;41:415–25.

47. James TN. On the cause of syncope and sudden death in primary pulmonary hypertension. Ann Intern Med. 1962;56:252–64.

48. Kanemoto N, Sasamoto H. Arrhythmias in primary pulmonary hypertension. Jpn Heart J. 1979;20:765–75.

49. Demerouti EA, Manginas AN, Athanassopoulos GD, Karatasakis GT. Complications leading to sudden cardiac death in pulmonary arterial hypertension. Respir Care. 2013;58:1246–54.

50. Hoeper MM, Galiè N, Murali S, Olschewski H, Rubenfire M, Robbins IM, et al. Outcome after cardiopulmonary resuscitation in patients with pulmonary arterial hypertension. Am J Respir Crit Care Med. 2002;165:341–4.

51. Tonelli AR, Arelli V, Minai OA, Newman J, Bair N, Heresi GA, et al. Causes and circumstances of death in pulmonary arterial hypertension. Am J Respir Crit Care Med. 2013;188:365–9.

52. Cirulis MM, Ryan JJ, Archer SL. Pathophysiology, incidence, management, and consequences of cardiac arrhythmia in pulmonary arterial hypertension and chronic thromboembolic pulmonary hypertension. Pulm Circ. 2019;9(1):2045894019834890.

53. Galie N, Humbert M, Vachiery JL, Gibbs S, Lang I, Torbicki A, et al. 2015 ESC/ERS guidelines for the diagnosis and treatment of pulmonary hypertension: The Joint Task Force for the Diagnosis and Treatment of Pulmonary Hypertension of the European Society of Cardiology (ESC) and the European Respiratory Society (ERS): Endorsed by: Association for European Paediatric and Congenital Cardiology (AEPC), International Society for Heart and Lung Transplantation (ISHLT). Eur Heart J. 2016;37:67–119.

54. Tongers J, Schwerdtfeger B, Klein G, Kempf T, Schaefer A, Knapp JM, et al. Incidence and clinical relevance of supraventricular tachyarrhythmias in pulmonary hypertension. Am Heart J. 2007;153:127–32.

55. Ruiz-Cano MJ, Gonzalez-Mansilla A, Escribano P, et al. Clinical implications of supraventricular arrhythmias in patients with severe pulmonary arterial hypertension. Int J Cardiol. 2011;146:105–6.

56. Olsson KM, Nickel NP, Tongers J, Hoeper MM. Atrial flutter and fibrillation in patients with pulmonary hypertension. Int J Cardiol. 2013;167:2300–5.

57. Medi C, Kalman JM, Ling LH, Teh AW, Lee G, Lee G, et al. Atrial electrical and structural remodeling associated with longstanding pulmonary hypertension and right ventricular hypertrophy in humans. Cardiovasc Electrophysiol. 2012;23:614–20.

58. Wen L, Sun ML, An P, Jang X, Sun K, Zheng L, et al. Frequency of supraventricular arrhythmias in patients with idiopathic pulmonary arterial hypertension. Am J Cardiol. 2014;114(9):1420–5.

59. Cannillo M, Grosso Marra W, Gili S, D'Ascenzo F, Morello M, Mercante L, et al. Supraventricular arrhythmias in patients with pulmonary arterial hypertension. Am J Cardiol. 2015;116:1883–9.

60. Witte C, Meyer Zur Heide Genannt Meyer-Arend JU, Andrié R, Schrickel JW, Hammerstingl C, Schwab JO, et al. Heart rate variability and arrhythmic burden in pulmonary hypertension. Adv Exp Med Biol. 2016;934:9–22.

61. Bandorski D, Bogossian H, Ecke A, Wiedenroth C, Gruenig E, Benjamin N, et al. Evaluation of the prognostic value of electrocardiography parameters and heart rhythm in patients with pulmonary hypertension. Cardiol J. 2016;23(4):465–72.

62. Mercurio V, Peloquin G, Bourji KI, Diab N, Sato T, Enobun B, et al. Pulmonary arterial hypertension and atrial arrhythmias: incidence, risk factors, and clinical impact. Pulm Circ. 2018;8:2045894018769874.

63. Epstein AE, DiMarco JP, Ellenbogen KA, Estes NA 3rd, Freedman RA, Gettes LS, et al. 2012 ACCF/AHA/HRS focused update incorporated into the ACCF/AHA/HRS 2008 guidelines for device-based therapy of cardiac rhythm abnormalities: a report of the American College of Cardiology Foundation/

American Heart Association Task Force on Practice Guidelines and the Heart Rhythm Society. Circulation. 2013;127(3):e283–352.

64. Olsson KM, Delcroix M, Ghofrani HA, Tiede H, Huscher D, Speich R, et al. Anticoagulation and survival in pulmonary arterial hypertension: results from the Comparative, Prospective Registry of Newly Initiated Therapies for Pulmonary Hypertension (COMPERA). Circulation. 2014;129:57–65.

65. Galiè N, Delcroix M, Ghofrani A, Jansa P, Minai OA, Perchenet L, et al. Anticoagulant therapy does not influence long-term outcomes in patients with pulmonary arterial hypertension (PAH): insights from the randomised controlled SERAPHIN trial of macitentan. Eur Heart J. 2014;35:10.

66. Preston RJ, Roberts KE, Miller DP, Sen GP, Selej M, Benton WW, et al. Effect of warfarin treatment on survival of patients with pulmonary arterial hypertension (PAH) in the Registry to Evaluate Early and Long-Term PAH Disease Management (REVEAL). Circulation. 2015;132(25):2403–11.

67. Lip GYH, Nieuwlaat R, Pisters R, Lane DA, Crijns HJ. Refining clinical risk stratification for predicting stroke and thromboembolism in atrial fibrillation using a novel risk factor-based approach: the euro heart survey on atrial fibrillation. Chest. 2010;137:263–72.

68. Wyse DG, Waldo AL, DiMarco JP, Domanski MJ, Rosenberg Y, Schron EB, et al., Atrial Fibrillation Follow-up Investigation of Rhythm Management (AFFIRM) Investigators. A comparison of rate control and rhythm control in patients with atrial fibrillation. N Engl J Med. 2002;347:1825–33.

69. Whitbeck MG, Charnigo RJ, Khairy P, Ziada K, Bailey AL, Zegarra MM, et al. Increased mortality among patients taking digoxin—analysis from the AFFIRM study. Eur Heart J. 2013;34:1481–98.

70. Gheorghiade M, Fonarow GC, van Veldhuisen DJ, Cleland JG, Butler J, Epstein AE, et al. Lack of evidence of increased mortality among patients with atrial fibrillation taking digoxin: findings from post hoc propensity-matched analysis of the AFFIRM trial. Eur Heart J. 2013;34:1489–97.

71. Murphy SA. When 'digoxin use' is not the same as 'digoxin use': lessons from the AFFIRM trial. Eur Heart J. 2013;34:1465–7.

72. Mathur PN, Powles P, Pugsley SO, McEwan MP, Campbell EJ. Effect of digoxin on right ventricular function in severe chronic airflow obstruction. A controlled clinical trial. Ann Intern Med. 1981;95:283–8.

73. Mathur PN, Powles AC, Pugsley SO, McEwan MP, Campbell EJ. Effect of long-term administration of digoxin on exercise performance in chronic airflow obstruction. Eur J Respir Dis. 1985;66:273–83.

74. Provencher S, Herve P, Jais X, Lebrec D, Humbert M, Simonneau G, et al. Deleterious effects of beta-blockers on exercise capacity and hemodynamics in patients with portopulmonary hypertension. Gastroenterology. 2006;130:120–6.

75. Echt DS, Liebson PR, Mitchell LB, Peters RW, Obias-Manno D, Barker AH, et al., CAST Investigators. Mortality and morbidity in patients receiving encainide, flecainide, or placebo. The Cardiac Arrhythmia Suppression Trial. N Engl J Med. 1991;324:781–8.

76. Showkathali R, Tayebjee MH, Grapsa J, Alzetani M, Nihoyannopoulos P, Howard LS, et al. Right atrial flutter isthmus ablation is feasible and results in acute clinical improvement in patients with persistent atrial flutter and severe pulmonary arterial hypertension. Int J Cardiol. 2011;149:279–80.

77. Luesebrink U, Fischer D, Gezgin F, Duncker D, Koenig T, Oswald H, et al. Ablation of typical right atrial flutter in patients with pulmonary hypertension. Heart Lung Circ. 2012;21:695–9.

78. Bradfield J, Shapiro S, Finch W, Tung R, Boyle NG, Buch E, et al. Catheter ablation of typical atrial flutter in severe pulmonary hypertension. J Cardiovasc Electrophysiol. 2012;23:1185–90.

79. Murkofsky RL, Dangas G, Diamond JA, Mehta D, Schaffer A, Ambrose JA. A prolonged QRS duration on surface electrocardiogram is a specific indicator of left ventricular dysfunction. J Am Coll Cardiol. 1998;32:476–82.

80. Iuliano S, Fisher SG, Karasik PE, Fletcher RD, Singh SN, Department of Veterans Affairs Survival Trial of Antiarrhythmic Therapy in Congestive Heart Failure. QRS duration and mortality in patients with congestive heart failure. Am Heart J. 2002;143:1085–91.

81. Shenkman H, Pampati V, Khandelwal AK, McKinnon J, Nori D, Kaatz S, et al. Congestive heart failure and QRS duration: establishing prognosis study. Chest. 2002;122:528–34.

82. Baldasseroni S, Gentile A, Gorini M, Marchionni N, Marini M, Masotti G, et al., Italian Network on Congestive Heart Failure Investigators. Intraventricular conduction defects in patients with congestive heart failure: left but not right bundle branch block is an independent predictor of prognosis. A report from the Italian Network on Congestive Heart Failure (IN-CHF database). Ital Heart J 2003;4:607–613.

83. Marcus JT, Gan CT, Zwanenburg JJ, Boonstra A, Allaart CP, Gotte MJ, et al. Interventricular mechanical asynchrony in pulmonary arterial hypertension: left-to-right delay in peak shortening is related to right ventricular overload and left ventricular underfilling. J Am Coll Cardiol. 2008;51:750–7.

84. Sun PY, Jiang X, Gomberg-Maitland M, Zhao QH, He J, Yuan P, et al. Prolonged QRS duration: a new predictor of adverse outcome in idiopathic pulmonary arterial hypertension. Chest. 2012;141:374–80.

85. Benoist D, Stones R, Drinkhill MJ, Benson AP, Yang Z, Cassan C, et al. Cardiac arrhythmia mechanisms in rats with heart failure induced by pulmonary hypertension. Am J Physiol Heart Circ Physiol. 2012;302:H2381–95.

86. Tateno S, Niwa K, Nakazawa M, Iwamoto M, Yokota M, Nagashima M, et al. Risk factors for arrhythmia and late death in patients with right ventricle to pulmonary artery conduit repair—Japanese multicenter study. Int J Cardiol. 2006;106:373–81.

87. Humbert M. A critical analysis of survival in idiopathic pulmonary arterial hypertension. Presse Med. 2010;39(Suppl 1):1S41–5.

88. McLaughlin VV. Looking to the future: a new decade of pulmonary arterial hypertension therapy. Eur Respir Rev. 2011;20:262–9.

89. Arena V, De Giorgio F, Abbate A, Capelli A, De Mercurio D, Carbone A. Fatal pulmonary arterial dissection and sudden death as initial manifestation of primary pulmonary hypertension: a case report. Cardiovasc Pathol. 2004;13:230–2.

90. Salhab KF, Al Kindi AH, Ellis SG, Lad N, Svensson LG. Percutaneous coronary intervention of the left main coronary artery in a patient with extrinsic compression caused by massive pulmonary artery enlargement. J Thorac Cardiovasc Surg. 2012;144:1517–8.

91. Doyen D, Moceri P, Moschietto S, Cerboni P, Ferrari E. Left main coronary artery compression associated with primary pulmonary hypertension. J Am Coll Cardiol. 2012;60:559.

92. Lee MS, Oyama J, Bhatia R, Kim YH, Park SJ. Left main coronary artery compression from pulmonary artery enlargement due to pulmonary hypertension: a contemporary review and argument for percutaneous revascularization. Catheter Cardiovasc Interv. 2010;76:543–50.

93. Bandorski D, Bogossian H, Stempfl J, Seeger W, Hecker M, Ghofrani A, et al. Prognostic relevance of nonsustained ventricular tachycardia in patients with pulmonary hypertension. Biomed Res Int. 2016;2016:1327265.

94. Zipes DP, Camm AJ, Borggrefe M, Buxton AE, Chaitman B, Fromer M, et al. ACC/AHA/ESC 2006 guidelines for management of patients with ventricular arrhythmias and the prevention of sudden cardiac death: a report of the American College of Cardiology/American Heart Association Task Force and the European Society of Cardiology Committee for Practice Guidelines (writing committee to develop Guidelines for Management of Patients With Ventricular Arrhythmias and the Prevention of Sudden Cardiac Death): developed in collaboration with the European Heart Rhythm Association and the Heart Rhythm Society. Circulation. 2006;114:e385–484.

95. Handoko ML, Lamberts RR, Redout EM, de Man FS, Boer C, Simonides WS, et al. Right ventricular pacing improves right heart function in experimental pulmonary arterial hypertension: a study in the isolated heart. Am J Physiol Heart Circ Physiol. 2009;297:H1752–9.

96. Hardziyenka M, Campian ME, Bouma BJ, Linnenbank AC, de Bruin-Bon HA, Kloek JJ, et al. Right-to-left ventricular diastolic delay in chronic thromboembolic pulmonary hypertension is associated with activation delay and action potential prolongation in right ventricle. Circ Arrhythm Electrophysiol. 2009;2:555–61.

97. Hardziyenka M, Surie S, de Groot JR, de Bruin-Bon HA, Knops RE, Remmelink M, et al. Right ventricular pacing improves haemodynamics in right ventricular failure from pressure overload: an open observational proof-of-principle study in patients with chronic thromboembolic pulmonary hypertension. Europace. 2011;13:1753–9.

Atrial Septostomy

Adam Torbicki, Marcin Kurzyna, and Julio Sandoval

Introduction

Lowering pulmonary input impedance is the obvious therapeutic target in right ventricular failure (RVF), if RVF has been caused by increased afterload. However, potential clinical gain can also be expected from attempts to unload the right heart by redistribution of blood to underfilled left-heart chambers or directly to the aorta. Atrial septostomy and pulmonary-aortic shunt (Potts anastomosis) represent clinically recognized methods serving this purpose at a cost of systemic desaturation. A more instrumentalized but physiologically appealing way of achieving similar hemodynamic goal, but with enriching the shunted blood with oxygen, is represented by venous-arterial extracorporeal membrane oxygenators. This chapter presents the physiological background and clinical value of atrial septostomy in the context of current management algorithms for patients with pulmonary hypertension.

A. Torbicki (✉) · M. Kurzyna
Department of Pulmonary Hypertension and Thromboembolic Diseases, Center of Postgraduate Medical Education, ECZ-Otwock, Otwock, Poland
e-mail: adam.torbicki@ecz-otwock.pl; marcin.kurzyna@ecz-otwock.pl

J. Sandoval
National Institute of Cardiology of Mexico, Mexico, DF, Mexico

Rationale

Right ventricular systolic failure is the leading cause of death in patients with pulmonary arterial hypertension (PAH) and chronic thromboembolic pulmonary hypertension (CTEPH): two pulmonary vascular diseases characterized by progressive increase in RV afterload. There is convincing evidence that absolute RV elastance, reflecting its contractility, is increasing in PAH. However, the progression of pulmonary vascular disease (PVD) usually is too fast to be matched by appropriate functional remodeling of the RV. Moreover, although there is an initially beneficial stretch of the RV wall resulting in compensatory increase of RV performance—known as the Frank-Starling effect—this initiates a chain of unfavorable morphological and functional consequences starting a vicious circle, leading to uncoupling of the RV and pulmonary arterial bed. This, in turn, leads to progressive functional deterioration and ultimately to death. Indeed, the natural history of patients with PAH or CTEPH and chronic RV failure evidenced by a cardiac index (CI) below 2.0 L/min/m^2, and/or mean right atrial pressure (RAP) above 20 mmHg, is grim [1]. Moreover, any additional "second hit" leading to exacerbation of chronic RV dysfunction represents a life-threatening situation with in-hospital mortality of 25–60% despite advanced ICU management. Taken together, RV failure is responsible for about 3/4th of deaths

S. P. Gaine et al. (eds.), *The Right Heart*, https://doi.org/10.1007/978-3-030-78255-9_20

within the 10% annual mortality among PAH and non-operable CTEPH patients.

All this clearly suggests an urgent need for effective and safe prevention of end-stage RV failure, if necessary, using interventional methods suitable for clinical application.

Theoretical Background

Atrial septostomy has been proposed as a treatment of RV failure secondary to pulmonary hypertension based on the reasoning derived from comparison of the outcome of two subgroups of PAH patients: with idiopathic PAH and those in whom PAH was associated with congenital shunts ultimately resulting in Eisenmenger syndrome.

Despite similar elevation of pulmonary artery pressure and resistance the patients with Eisenmenger syndrome were found to have much better life expectancy than those with idiopathic PAH [2, 3] (Fig. 20.1). Not only was overall mortality lower, but also in 30–55% it was due to sudden death and not end-stage RV failure [4–6].

Indeed, in most patients with Eisenmenger syndrome RV function and systemic perfusion are preserved, as evidenced by near-normal RA pressures and systemic cardiac output found at right-heart catheterization (Fig. 20.2). If the mechanisms of such adaptation of the cardiovascular system to extremely elevated RV afterload could be understood this might offer the chance of using them as new therapeutic approaches for patients with other forms of PAH.

Out of several adaptive mechanisms which have been suggested, including

- preservation of a "fetal" phenotype of RV myocytes
- appropriate RV hypertrophy
- preserved, more dense RV coronary network
- reversed shunt feeding the systemic circuit through a persisting defect

the latter could potentially be reproduced in non-Eisenmenger patients suffering from PAH. Opening a shunt between the atria has been practiced since the times of Rashkind, though for other indications.

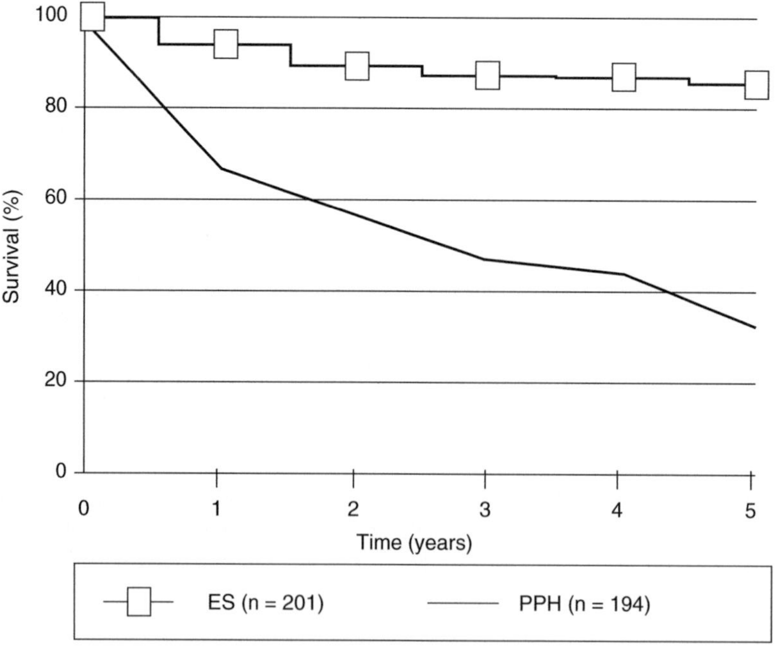

Fig. 20.1 Comparison of survival of patients with idiopathic pulmonary arterial hypertension and Eisenmenger syndrome. *ES* patients with Eisenmenger syndrome, *PPH* patients with idiopathic pulmonary arterial hypertension. (Based on data from Ref. [2])

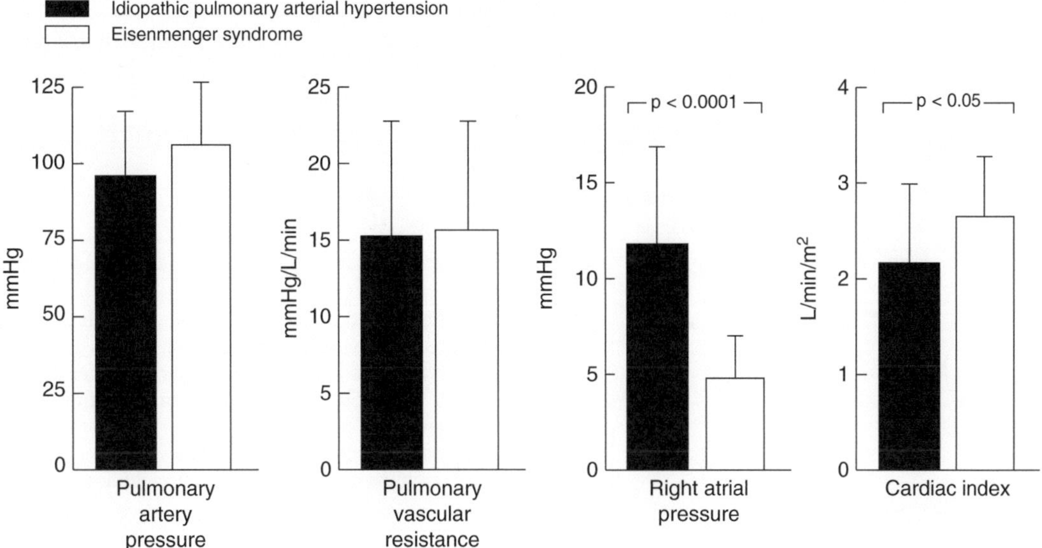

Fig. 20.2 Comparison of the hemodynamics of adults with severe idiopathic pulmonary arterial hypertension and Eisenmenger syndrome. (Based on data from Ref. [2])

Shunting blood from the right to left heart at the level of interatrial septum (Fig. 20.3) could potentially result in increase in systemic output by improving LV filling and in decompression of the RV alleviating its failure, with further improvements, e.g., better right ventricular coronary perfusion, less tendency for RV remodeling and functional tricuspid regurgitation, decreased kidney congestion, and their improved perfusion.

A price to pay would be systemic oxygen desaturation, particularly on exercise, with an unclear net result regarding tissue oxygen delivery and utilization.

Even more importantly, it is not clear whether and to what extent atrial septostomy alone would improve clinical outcome of patients with PAH if not accompanied by other adaptive mechanisms operating in patients born with congenital heart disease and steadily developing Eisenmenger syndrome. The evidence, that such an isolated shunt at the atrial level could be beneficial even if functionally opened only after development of PAH in the adult life, is based on a higher prevalence of patent foramen ovale in long-term survivors of PAH as reported by Rozkovec et al. [8] (Table 20.1).

Computational Models

Mathematical modeling of the effects of complex hemodynamic interventions, such as atrial septostomy in a setting of chronic PH, is tempting, particularly with increasing availability of advanced computational hardware and software. In a recent trial of Koeken et al., a Dutch group involving biomedical engineers assessed consequences of atrial septostomy with a multiscale computational model of cardiovascular system [7]. They suggested that atrial septostomy could improve symptoms of right-heart failure in patients with severe PH if net right-to-left shunt flow occurs during exercise. While their model confirmed that septostomy improves left ventricular filling and stroke volume (Fig. 20.4) and stabilizes systemic blood pressure, the expected beneficial effect on peripheral tissue oxygen delivery could not be found. The increase in systemic oxygen delivery after atrial septostomy has

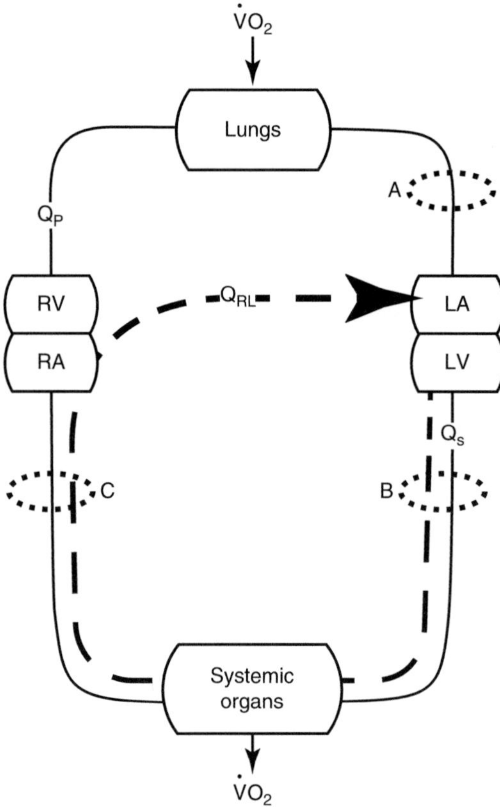

Fig. 20.3 Schematic representation of circulation with a right-to-left shunt through atrial septostomy. *LA* left atrium, *RA* right atrium, *RV* right ventricle, *Qs* systemic blood flow, *Qp* pulmonary blood flow, *QRL* right-to-left shunt through atrial septostomy, *VO₂* total oxygen consumption by the body. In contrast to carbon dioxide removal and oxygen delivery that are determined by the effective Qp (*location A*) the delivery of nutrients (*location B*) and the removal of waste products (*location C*) are determined by systemic flow. Part of the venous return is redirected through atrial septostomy directly to the LA, thereby bypassing the pulmonary circulation. (Modified from Koeken et al. [7]. With permission from The American Physiological Society)

been examined by computer modeling, suggesting that the clinically observed beneficial effects of atrial septostomy may be more related to improved flow rather than oxygen delivery to perfused tissues [9].

Table 20.1 Factors predicting life expectancy in primary pulmonary hypertension, including the presence of patent foramen ovale (PFO)

	Survival		
	<5 years ($n =$)	>5 years ($n =$)	p
Family	1	1	NS
CTD	3	0	NS
Pregnancy	0	5	<0.02
PFO	0	4	<0.05
RHF any	18	10	<0.05

According to Rozkovec et al. [8]. (Reprinted from Rozkovec A, Montanes P, Oakley CM. Factors that influence the outcome of primary pulmonary hypertension. Br Heart J 1986;55:449–58. With permission from BMJ Publishing Ltd.)
CTD connective tissue disease, *Pregnancy* disease diagnosed during or after pregnancy, *RHF* right-heart failure

Experimental Models

Experimental evidence suggesting that atrial septostomy may be beneficial in chronic PH dates back to the work of Austen et al. [10] (Fig. 20.5). After inducing chronic RV pressure overload by pulmonary artery banding ten dogs were submitted to a second surgical intervention. Five had an ASD and the remaining five had a sham operation. Dogs with ASD were able to perform moderate and severe exercise on a treadmill, whereas dogs who had the sham operation could not tolerate it.

Other authors have also shown beneficial effects of similar interventions in canine models [11, 12].

The effect of an interatrial shunt on right atrial (RA) and right ventricular mechanics was reassessed by Zierer et al. [11]. After banding the pulmonary artery they used an 8 mm cannula to connect both atria. The model permitted controlled closing and opening of the shunt to assess potential hemodynamic effects of septostomy. Also, by changing the venous return two levels of shunting could be compared—15% and 30% of the total cardiac output, respectively. Comprehensive analysis based on the assessment of ventricular and atrial pressure/volume loops revealed that after "septostomy" RV and RA contractility did not change. Some changes were found in compliance of the right atrium, which

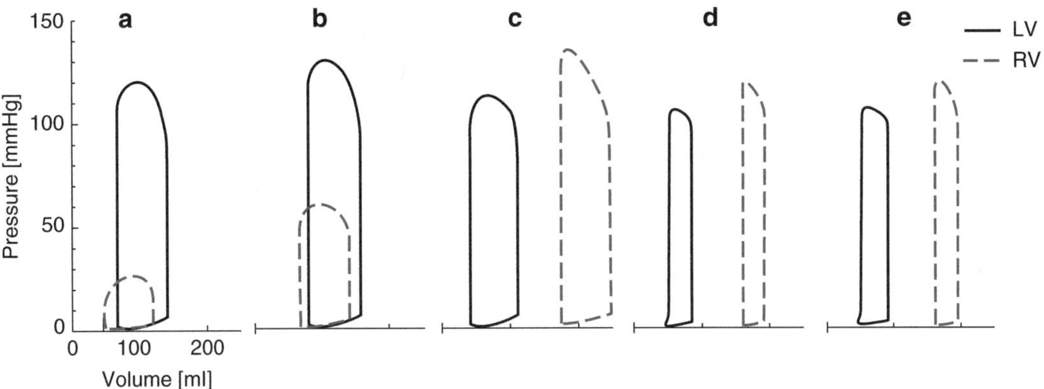

Fig. 20.4 Pressure-volume loops of the right (*dashed lines*) and left (*solid lines*) ventricles. *a* normal, *b* compensated pulmonary hypertension, *c* decompensated pulmonary hypertension, *d* severely decompensated pulmonary hypertension with decreased cardiac output, *e* same as *d* but after atrial septostomy of 14 mm in diameter. Note increased stroke volume of the left ventricle compared to *d*. (Modified from Koeken et al. [7]. With permission from The American Physiological Society)

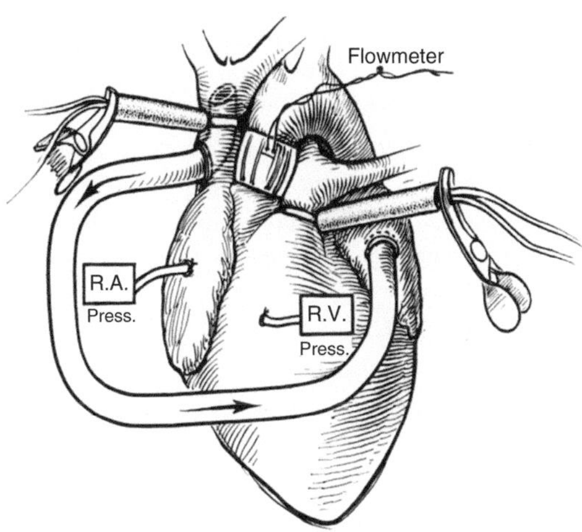

Fig. 20.5 Animal model used for assessing the acute effects of right-to-left atrial shunting, as described by Austen et al. in 1964. *RA* right atrium, *LV* left ventricle. *Arrow* indicates pulmonary artery banding used to chronically increase right ventricular afterload

increased especially at lower shunt flows. There was also a significant shift from the reservoir to the conduit function ratio in this chamber. While the experiment confirmed that cardiac output and systemic oxygen delivery increased after septostomy, this effect was present only with right-to-left shunting corresponding to 15% of cardiac output. At higher shunt flow beneficial effects on systemic oxygen delivery were lost.

Similar message was conveyed by Weimar et al. [12], who found a right-to-left shunt flow of 11% of baseline cardiac output at the atrial level to be an optimal therapeutic target in severe RV pressure overload. The authors suggested that atrial septostomy was not of significant hemodynamic benefit in moderate RV pressure overload. However, in contrast to previously discussed models, in the latter trial banding was done acutely, and thus the results and conclusions may not be fully representative for chronic pulmonary hypertension.

Clinical Evidence

The evidence regarding hemodynamic effects of atrial septostomy in patients with right ventricular dysfunction caused by increased RV afterload is limited, when compared to data regarding pharmacological treatment of pulmonary arterial hypertension. This limitation is a consequence of relatively low number of patients submitted so far to AS as well as to the insufficient quality of data due to the design of trials. At best the information comes from short case series. At present published series provide data on about 350 procedures performed in over 300 patients [13–32]. No randomized trials have ever been performed to assess the long-term effects of AS. In some reports the outcome was compared to that of matched historical controls followed earlier by the same clinical team. The dynamic changes in medical care and availability of pharmacological therapy of PAH over time make such comparisons questionable.

Nevertheless, the published evidence, as well as our personal observations, permits analysis of hemodynamic effects, clinical benefits, and safety of AS. To allow generally applicable conclusions we decided to exclude single case reports from such analyses, which are more likely to be affected by favorable publication bias.

Characteristics of Patients Submitted to Atrial Septostomy

Out of 304 patients in whom AS was performed at least once, 76 were pediatric patients, 201 (71.6%) were female, and 277 (91%) suffered from PAH. All the patients were either in third or in fourth WHO functional class with almost 50% reporting syncope [13–32].

In a vast majority of cases balloon atrial septostomy was performed (see below for explanation). Out of 79 procedures in which blade balloon septostomy was used as either the main or the contributing method, 32 were performed before the year 2000 and others performed afterwards—were almost entirely (41/42) in young children.

Safety, Clinical and Hemodynamic Effects of Atrial Septostomy

There were 24 deaths within the first 24 h after the procedure, resulting in 6.8% periprocedural mortality. Cumulative mortality at 1 month was 10.8%. Interestingly, 11.5% (35/304) of patients could be transplanted.

Hemodynamic effects of AS could be analyzed for 104 procedures for which complete hemodynamic data sets were available. In order to provide some practical guidance regarding indication for AS in various stages of RV dys-

function we report the results according to the level of mean right atrial pressure before the procedure (Table 20.2).

Based on this analysis AS appears to result in immediate improvement of left-heart filling, and systemic flow regardless of the baseline level of RA pressure. In patients with RAP elevated at baseline its significant decrease immediately after the procedure was noted. Those beneficial effects occurred at a cost of fall of systemic oxygen saturation, most marked in patients with RAP >20 mmHg at baseline (Table 20.3). Despite clinically relevant increase in systemic CI (from 1.6 to 2.2 L/min/m^2, i.e., 37%) the periprocedural mortality in this subgroup was very high, with 11 deaths after 26 procedures (42%) contrasting with 2 periprocedural deaths in patients with RAP below 20 mmHg (2.5%) (Table 20.3).

In a recently published systematic review and meta-analysis by Khan et al. [33], the acute hemodynamic effects of atrial septostomy were confirmed. The review included 16 studies comprising 204 patients (mean age, 35.8 years; 73.1% women). Meta-analysis revealed significant and beneficial changes in two of the hemodynamic variables associated with survival in PAH, namely a decrease in right atrial pressure (−2.77 mmHg [95% CI, −3.50, −2.04]; $p < 0.001$) and an increase in cardiac index (0.62 L/min/m^2 [95% CI, 0.48, 0.75]; $p < 0.001$) following BAS, along with a significant reduction in arterial oxygen saturation (−8.45% [95% CI, −9.93, −6.97]; $p < 0.001$). In this analysis, the pooled incidence of procedure-related (48 h), short-term (<30 days), and long-term (>30 days) mortality was 4.8% (1.7–9.0%), 14.6% (8.6–21.5%), and 37.7% (27.9–47.9%), respectively. Spontaneous closure of the orifice due to elastic recoil occurred in 23.8% of cases. The authors concluded that this analysis suggests that BAS is relatively safe in advanced PAH, with beneficial hemodynamic effects. They considered relatively high postprocedural and short-term survival contrasting with less impressive long-term outcomes as a suggestion of suitability of BAS as a bridge to lung transplantation.

There is hardly any information on hemodynamic effects of septostomy during exercise.

Table 20.2 Hemodynamic effects of atrial septostomy according to the level of right atrial pressure prior to the procedure [13–32]

Variable	Baseline RAP < 10 mmHg ($N = 27$)		$p <$	Baseline RAP 10–20 mmHg ($N = 51$)		$p <$	Baseline RAP > 20 mmHg ($N = 26$)		$p <$
	Before	After		Before	After		Before	After	
RAP, mmHg	5.8 ± 1.96	5.48 ± 3.1	NS	14.1 ± 3.2	11.4 ± 3.8	0.001	25.8 ± 4.9	19.2 ± 4.4	0.001
LAP, mmHg	4.9 ± 2.47	6.5 ± 2.5	0.05	5.3 ± 3.6	7.9 ± 4.2	0.001	7.9 ± 3	10.4 ± 3.7	0.02
R-L atrial pressure, mmHg	1.17 ± 3.2	-1.32 ± 3.2	0.02	8.4 ± 4.1	3.3 ± 5.5	0.001	17.3 ± 5	7.7 ± 5.3	0.001
Mean PAP, mmHg	62.8 ± 17	64 ± 19.6	NS	64.9 ± 16.7	65.6 ± 16.7	NS	64.8 ± 23	69.9 ± 24.7	NS
Cardiac index, L/min/m^2	2.37 ± 0.61	2.80 ± 0.7	0.001	2.10 ± 0.70	2.7 ± 0.9	0.001	1.6 ± 0.5	2.2 ± 0.6	0.001
SaO$_2$%	93.5 ± 4.1	87.2 ± 7.4	0.001	92.9 ± 4.1	82.8 ± 7.4	0.001	92.2 ± 4.5	78.3 ± 9.7	0.001

RAP mean right atrial pressure, *LAP* mean left atrial pressure, *R-L* right to left, *SaO$_2$* systemic oxygen saturation

Table 20.3 Clinical characteristics and procedure-related mortality according to right atrial pressure before the operation

	Baseline RAP < 10 mmHg ($N = 27$)	Baseline RAP 10–20 mmHg ($N = 51$)	Baseline RAP > 20 mmHg ($N = 26$)
Age, years	23 ± 14	28 ± 14	27.5 ± 12
Syncope (%)	73.9	66.7	36
RVF (%)	34.7	73.8	88
Procedure-related mortality 1 month	0/27 (0%)	2/51 (4%)	11/26 (42.3%)

RAP mean right atrial pressure, *RVF* right ventricular failure

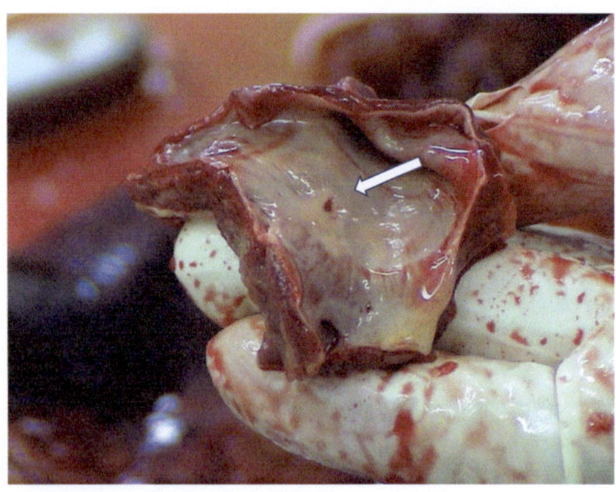

Fig. 20.6 Residual, hemodynamically noneffective orifice (arrow) seen postmortem at the interatrial septum 6 months after initially successful atrial septostomy

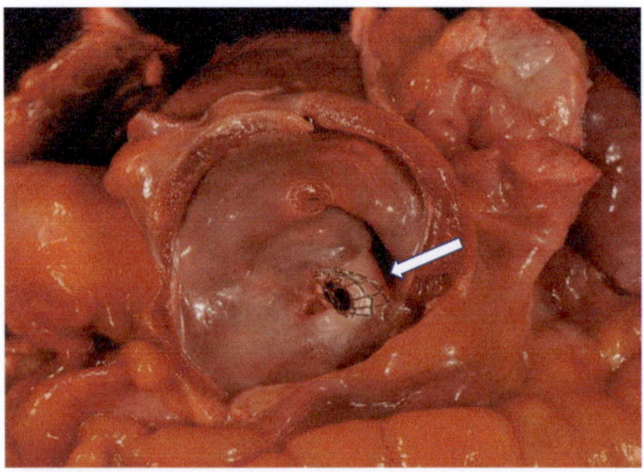

Fig. 20.7 Stent-protected septostomy orifice found fully patent at autopsy performed 5 years after intervention. (From Ref. [34] with permission)

While many series reported increased exercise tolerance [19, 24, 31], particularly increased distance covered during 6-min walk test, it is diffi-cult to judge the contribution of psychological factor in patients who were submitted to septostomy. The assessment of long-term effects of septostomy on exercise capacity is complicated by common tendency of the created orifice to shrink or close (Fig. 20.6).

Recently a largest-ever series of 68 BAS protected with stents from elastic recoil has been reported suggesting excellent chronic patency of creating orifices [34] (Fig. 20.7). Together with 39 earlier reported cases a total of 107 stented BAS seem to suggest this strategy as being safer and more hemodynamically and clinically effective in long term than oversized septostomy orifices or repeated procedures performed after reocclusion occurs. Studies aiming to further improve long-term BAS patency, such as cryoplasty to freeze the margins of the newly created atrial defect, are ongoing (PROPHET trial: *https://clinicaltrials.gov/ct2/show/NCT03022851*).

Late Effects of Septostomy on Right Ventricular Function

Improved left ventricular filling and reduced pre-load of the right ventricle in patients in whom it had been severely increased before septostomy should lead to improved right ventricular function and—hopefully—its reversed remodeling. Indeed, better LV filling may improve RV systolic performance by direct support through interventricular septum. Also, reduced RV wall stress could mitigate increased RV myocardial oxygen demand and potential ischemia, particularly during exercise. Decrease in BNP plasma levels reported after septostomy support reduced diastolic wall stretch and reduced RV afterload [29]. Moreover, in some reports improvement in hemodynamics after septostomy, as evidenced by RAP and CI, was even more marked at long-term follow-up than immediately after the procedure [15, 28]. Also echocardiographic follow-up demonstrated reduction of RA and RV dimensions up to 6 months after septostomy suggesting persistent beneficial effects of this intervention on right-heart remodeling [35].

Such effects may also be induced by restoration of more physiological autonomic system balance. It has been demonstrated that sympathetic overdrive may be one of the mechanisms involved in the pathophysiology of RV failure in patients with PAH. Ciarka and coworkers showed a significant decrease in initially elevated muscle sympathetic nerve activity after the procedure [27]. Less sympathetic drive can reduce myocardial oxygen demand, ischemia, and tendency to arrhythmia. Of note, heart rate did not increase despite a significant systemic oxygen desaturation following septostomy.

Effects on Blood Gases and Oxygen Transport

The effects of septostomy on systemic oxygen transport (SOT) and its tissue delivery are unclear. An increase in SOT resulting from the increase in CI despite the drop in $SaO_2\%$ has been suggested in some clinical studies [36] but seems unlikely and has not been confirmed when tested in recently developed computational models addressing this issue [7, 9]. Whether better perfusion of peripheral tissues improve local utilization of oxygen even if delivered in similar quantities remains unclear.

A potential adverse effect induced by acute systemic desaturation on pulmonary hemodynamic has been suggested by Kurzyna et al. Within an hour after successful septostomy and despite initially stable and well-controlled degree of SaO_2 they noticed unexpected "secondary" significant drop in oxygen saturation [26]. It occurred in patients who were not receiving chronic targeted therapy and could be effectively reversed by inhalation of a prostanoid (iloprost). The authors linked this observation with an increase in PVR seen in some of their patients soon after completion of atrial septostomy [26]. This increase correlated in turn with the degree of desaturation of mixed venous blood entering pulmonary arterial bed, which was a direct consequence of acutely reduced systemic SaO_2. Hypoxemic constriction of pulmonary arterioles as a reaction to profound sudden reduction in SvO_2 despite alveolar normoxia has been suggested, but could not be proved. We generally think that it is alveolar hypoxia rather than hypoxemia that causes pulmonary vasoconstriction so this is a surprising conclusion. Interestingly, the hemodynamic data collected from 104 patients indeed show a trend towards increase of PAP after septostomy (Table 20.2). An alternative explanation of such a trend might however come from improved RV output supported through interventricular septum by a better filled LV. In view of protection of patients from potential pulmonary hypoxic/hypoxemic vasoconstriction by powerful vasodilating drugs the clinical relevance of this potential side effect of septostomy was abrogated [32].

Risks and Limitation of Atrial Septostomy

Atrial septostomy is not an easy procedure. There is an important difference between puncturing interatrial septum to perform mitral annuloplasty or ablation in the left heart and atrial septostomy in severe pulmonary hypertension. The remodeling of the heart, and particularly reduced distance between interatrial septum and left atrial free wall as well as disturbed topography of the ascending aorta, increases the risk of perforation with potentially immediate fatal consequences. Fluoroscopy alone is used to guide the procedure in some experienced centers. However, with less experience more comprehensive imaging is needed to monitor the procedure. Parallel use of fluoroscopy and transesophageal imaging of the interatrial septum are probably the best choice.

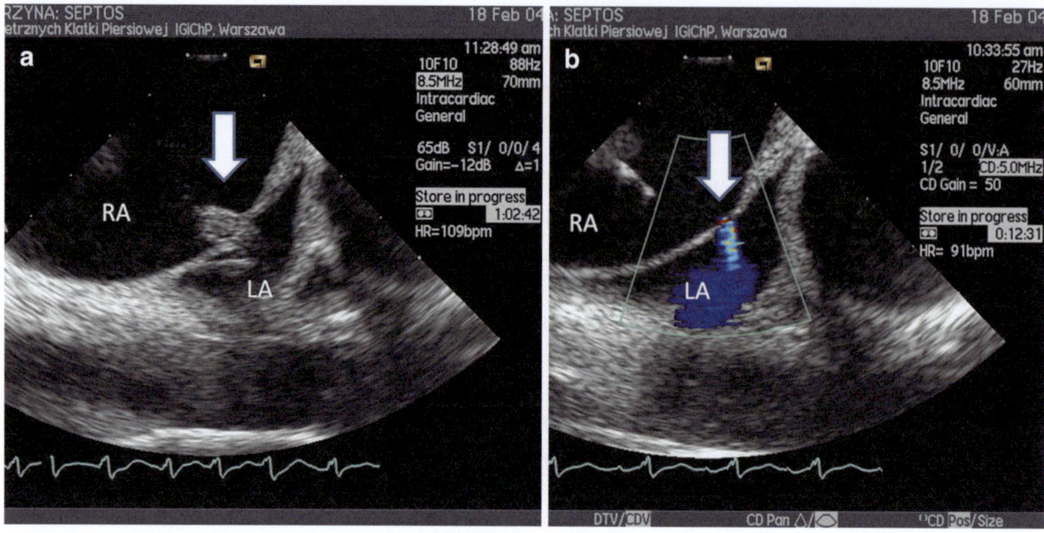

Fig. 20.8 Intracardiac echocardiographic monitoring of (**a**) balloon inflation (*arrow*) and (**b**) right-to-left shunt after puncturing interatrial septum. *RA* right atrium, *LA* left atrium. The intracardiac echocardiographic transducer is introduced via jugular vein and placed in high right atrium

Prolonged insertion of TEE probe however requires general anesthesia, which is not without risks in severe pulmonary hypertension. Good collaboration of anesthesiologist, interventionist, and PAH expert is crucial to avoid problems. Transthoracic echocardiography offers some support during the procedure but is far less informative than TEE. Intracardiac ultrasound is an acceptable alternative (Fig. 20.8). While not as versatile as TEE, it can be performed without discomfort to the patient without anesthesia.

Once the septum is punctured the next important step is to select the optimal orifice size. This is difficult with the blade balloon technique, which has been gradually abandoned because of the risk of creating tears in the septum which may result in oversized shunts with uncontrollable and life-threatening hypoxemia. Stepwise balloon technique is now used by most active centers. It allows precise control over the size of created orifice.

As an example, the procedure used in the Institute of Cardiology in Mexico is the following: baseline right and left-heart pressures are recorded simultaneously with a pigtail catheter in the ascending aorta just over the aortic valve to serve as an additional marker lowering the risk of aortic puncture. Cardiac output is calculated by the Fick method. Following transseptal puncture using standard technique, the septostomy orifice is balloon-dilated in a carefully graded step-by-step approach, beginning at a diameter of 4 mm, and followed by 6, 8, 12, and 16 mm dilatations, as appropriate. Between each step and after 3 min allowed for stabilization of hemodynamics, left ventricular end-diastolic pressure (LVEDP) recordings and arterial oxygen saturation (SaO_2) are obtained. The final size of the defect is individualized in each patient and limited by the time at which any of the following first occurred: (1) an LVEDP increase of ≥ 18 mmHg; (2) a SaO_2 reduction to 80%; or (3) a 10% SaO_2 decrease from baseline. Follow-up of the patients is done in the intensive care area for the first 48 h, where continuous supplementary oxygen is administrated and appropriate anticoagulation is started. All patients are followed at outpatient clinic with particular care to maintain correct oral anticoagulation and appropriate hemoglobin levels [32].

The stepwise approach is safer but tedious, time consuming, and expensive, as many balloons have to be used. Moreover, balloon dilation does not protect from elastic recoil and closure (Fig. 20.6). Therefore, some teams aim at a predefined single-size orifice but protected from closure with a butterfly stent [37, 38] or fenestrated occluding device [25]. However, follow-up revealed occlusion of this device in four out of nine patients despite chronic anticoagulation or antiplatelet therapy [30] making such approach questionable. Butterfly stents seem to be more effective, but they have to be prepared and positioned on a septostomy balloon on-site by the operator during the procedure. This again significantly increases procedural time, and requires dedicated personnel and a long time slot of the hemodynamic laboratory. Recently a new concept of cryoablation to septostomy borders has also been applied with a good long-term result after the second septostomy, which was performed because the first one closed (J. Sandoval, personal communication, 2014). In our experience and not unexpectedly the small orifices closed most often suggesting that septostomies should be made earlier—in patients with no more than mildly elevated RAP—but larger.

Closing of septostomy can be suspected if at pulse oximetry checkups SaO_2 gradually returns towards baseline values. In such a case an attempt to push the leader across a still patent orifice avoiding risky puncture and limiting the procedure to balloon dilatation is tempting. However finding the residual hole may be very difficult and usually a new puncture is needed.

Atrial Septostomy and Therapeutic Strategy in Pulmonary Hypertension

Based on the available evidence as well as our personal experience regarding the efficacy and safety of atrial septostomy it seems that this procedure has both a place and—even more importantly—a potential to play a more prominent role in the management of patients with PAH and right ventricular dysfunction. This is justified by

- Sound pathophysiological background
- Experimental and computational evidence consistent with clinical findings
- Convincing data on increased systemic output due to improved left ventricular preload and resulting in clinical improvement
- Lack of clinically significant consequences of systemic desaturation
- Better understanding of periprocedural risk and optimal patient selection

These characteristics permit considering atrial septostomy particularly in patients who are suboptimally controlled by modern medical therapy. Syncope and fluid retention may be relieved by septostomy and time can be gained increasing the chance to survive on the lung transplantation list. If septostomy is considered in a patient it is of paramount importance not to miss the optimal moment characterized by still preserved acceptable oxygen saturation without prohibitive levels of RAP.

Septostomy may be particularly useful in countries/centers who have suboptimal access to lung transplantation programs or to expensive double- and triple-targeted therapy.

Following actions are urgently needed:

- Identification and implementation of the best method to prevent reocclusion of atrial septostomy
- Designation of referral septostomy teams with appropriate experience and perspectives to create a high-volume/high-quality environment with appropriate quality monitoring
- Preparation of a properly designed interactive registry offering standardized management suggestions and at the same time collecting evidence with a goal of using the results for future optimization of patient selection and methodology of procedure. Such registry—if extended to centers not performing septostomy—would also allow comparison of long-term outcome between matched groups of patients to whom septostomy was or was not offered.

To optimize the risk/benefit ratio of atrial septostomy as well as introduce this procedure as a preventive measure which delays failure of the right ventricle despite progressive pulmonary vascular disease new data are needed. This includes a prospective trial to verify whether atrial septostomy may be effective in the setting of moderate right ventricular hypertension.

Such an early intervention has been recently suggested by a clinical retrospective study but seems not to be supported by experimental data [12, 32].

In view of great achievements regarding assessment of efficacy and safety of modern pharmacotherapy of PAH and continuing problems with availability of donors for lung transplantation programs the community caring for patients with PH and the patients themselves have to mobilize resources and enthusiasm to arrange a landmark trial identifying optimal positioning of atrial septostomy in the future management strategy. New technical developments, including remote-controlled devices with modifiable shunt fractions and preventing from reocclusion of the septostomy orifice, should encourage the industry to support our efforts, hopefully in the near future. This may be facilitated by a recently emerging interest in using atrial septostomy in another much more prevalent indication, indirectly confirming the clinical benefits of creating and regulating intraatrial shunt.

Atrial Septostomy Plus Dedicated Devices for the Management of HF with Preserved Ejection Fraction

In the last few years there has been a conceptual transfer of the use of atrial septostomy plus dedicated devices to treat heart failure with preserved ejection fraction as that seen in group 2 of pulmonary hypertension, which appears an appealing concept given the lack of an effective treatment in this group. Elevated left atrial (LA) filling pressure leading to pulmonary congestion is the common final pathway in decompensated HF. This provides the basis for creating a left-to-right shunt for reducing LA pressures, and relieving volume excess from the left atrium, thus improving symptoms (particularly during exercise) and functional class and reducing rehospitalizations [39–43]. The rationale for this proposal is based on several clinical observations: (1) It has been recognized that patients with the rare combination of an atrial septal defect and mitral stenosis

(Lutembacher's syndrome) do better and are less symptomatic than patients with isolated mitral stenosis, presumably because the shunt allows for LA decompression [39–42]. (2) Increase in left atrial pressure and acute pulmonary edema has been described after closure of congenital atrial septal defects, particularly in patients with preexisting or unrecognized left ventricular dysfunction [44]. (3) Balloon atrial septostomy or placement of a transseptal cannula has been associated with ventricular recovery in patients who could not be weaned from extracorporeal membrane oxygenation for intractable pulmonary edema [45]. (4) It has been reported that a residual communication after percutaneous mitral valve repair (using a MitraClip device through a 22F guiding catheter) resulted in a volume and pressure relief of the left atrium [46].

Atrial septostomy with shunt device placement in the setting of HF with preserved ejection fraction may be superior to exclusive static balloon dilatation of the interatrial septum [41]. Devices used for this purpose include InterAtrial Shunt Device (IASD®, Corvia Medical Inc., Tewksbury, MA, USA), V-Wave device (V-Wave, Caesarea, Israel), Second-generation (valveless) V-Wave device (V-Wave, Caesarea, Israel), and ROOT device (Edwards Lifesciences) [43]. Besides its use, in PAH patients [47] the future application of the atrial flow regulator (Occlutech) device may also be extended to other heart failure populations. Implantation of this device may permit left-heart decompression via fenestration. Further clinical trials are still required.

Current evidence for interatrial shunting alone or with dedicated devices is based on observational studies and small randomized trials showing the feasibility, safety, and preliminary efficacy in patients with PH and left HF [43]. These data seem to be insufficient to modify current clinical practice but support the use of interatrial shunting as a palliative therapy in selected patients with PH or left HF that remain symptomatic despite optimal treatment based on current guidelines. Several ongoing randomized trials will provide definite evidence about the exact role of this therapy for the treatment of HF patients [43]. If the results are positively associated with improved clinical outcomes, device-mediated left-to-right atrial shunting might become an important new approach to the treatment of this population.

It must be emphasized that the creation of an atrial communication is a palliative not a curative approach. The restrictive character of a generated shunt makes this mechanical therapeutic measure a helpful, low-risk treatment. However, an oversized atrial communication with shunt-dependent pressure equalizing between both atria should be avoided [41]. Overall, shunt device size in HF patients has ranged from 5 to 8 mm. In a validated cardiovascular simulation model, it has been shown that with a shunt of 8–9 mm there is no increase in right atrial and pulmonary artery pressures [48]. However, further studies are needed to determine the optimal shunt size for patients with left HF. Also, because of the introduction of a left-to-right shunt, patients with evident right ventricular dysfunction or significant pulmonary arterial hypertension (PA systolic >60 mmHg) should be excluded [39, 49]. However, milder cases of postcapillary pulmonary hypertension due to left ventricular failure with its preserved systolic function may potentially benefit from a bidirectional interatrial shunt dynamically regulating filling of both ventricles.

References

1. D'Alonzo GE, Barst RJ, Ayres SM, Bergofsky EH, Brundage BH, Detre KM, Fishman AP, Goldring RM, Groves BM, Kernis JT, et al. Survival in patients with primary pulmonary hypertension. Results from a national prospective registry. Ann Intern Med. 1991;115:343–9.
2. Hopkins WE, Ochoa LL, Richardson GW, Trulock EP. Comparison of the hemodynamics and survival of adults with severe primary pulmonary hypertension or Eisenmenger syndrome. J Heart Lung Transplant. 1996;15:100–5.
3. Hopkins WE, Waggoner AD. Severe pulmonary hypertension without right ventricular failure: the unique hearts of patients with Eisenmenger syndrome. Am J Cardiol. 2002;89:34–8.
4. Saha A, Balakrishnan KG, Jaiswal PK, Venkitachalam CG, Tharakan J, Titus T, Kutty R. Prognosis for patients with Eisenmenger syndrome of various aetiology. Int J Cardiol. 1994;45:199–207.
5. Oya H, Nagaya N, Uematsu M, Satoh T, Sakamaki F, Kyotani S, Sato N, Nakanishi N, Miyatake K. Poor prognosis and related factors in adults with Eisenmenger syndrome. Am Heart J. 2002;143:739–44.
6. Diller GP, Dimopoulos K, Broberg CS, Kaya MG, Naghotra US, Uebing A, Harries C, Goktekin O, Gibbs JS, Gatzoulis MA. Presentation, survival prospects, and predictors of death in Eisenmenger syndrome: a combined retrospective and case-control study. Eur Heart J. 2006;27:1737–42.
7. Koeken Y, Kuijpers NH, Lumens J, Arts T, Delhaas T. Atrial septostomy benefits severe pulmonary hypertension patients by increase of left ventricular preload reserve. Am J Physiol Heart Circ Physiol. 2012;302:H2654–62.
8. Rozkovec A, Montanes P, Oakley CM. Factors that influence the outcome of primary pulmonary hypertension. Br Heart J. 1986;55:449–58.
9. Diller GP, Lammers AE, Haworth SG, Dimopoulos K, Derrick G, Bonhoeffer P, Gatzoulis MA, Francis DP. A modelling study of atrial septostomy for pulmonary arterial hypertension, and its effect on the state of tissue oxygenation and systemic blood flow. Cardiol Young. 2010;20:25–32.
10. Austen WG, Morrow AG, Berry WB. Experimental studies of the surgical treatment of primary pulmonary hypertension. J Thorac Cardiovasc Surg. 1964;48:448–55.
11. Zierer A, Melby SJ, Voeller RK, Moon MR. Interatrial shunt for chronic pulmonary hypertension: differential impact of low-flow vs. high-flow shunting. Am J Physiol Heart Circ Physiol. 2009;296:H639–44.
12. Weimar T, Watanabe Y, Kazui T, Lee US, Montecalvo A, Schuessler RB, Moon MR. Impact of differential right-to-left shunting on systemic perfusion in pulmonary arterial hypertension. Catheter Cardiovasc Interv. 2013;81:888–95.
13. Nihill MR, O'Laughlin MP, Mullins CE. Effects of atrial septostomy in patients with terminal cor pulmonale due to pulmonary vascular disease. Catheter Cardiovasc Diagn. 1991;24:166–72.
14. Sobrino N, Frutos A, Calvo L, Casamayor LM, Arcas R. Palliative interatrial septostomy in severe pulmonary hypertension. Rev Esp Cardiol. 1993;46:125–8.
15. Kerstein D, Levy PS, Hsu DT, Hordof AJ, Gersony WM, Barst RJ. Blade balloon atrial septostomy in patients with severe primary pulmonary hypertension. Circulation. 1995;91:2028–35.
16. Rich S, Dodin E, McLaughlin VV. Usefulness of atrial septostomy as a treatment for primary pulmonary hypertension and guidelines for its application. Am J Cardiol. 1997;80:369–71.
17. Thanopoulos BD, Georgakopoulos D, Tsaousis GS, Simeunovic S. Percutaneous balloon dilatation of the atrial septum: immediate and midterm results. Heart. 1996;76:502–6.
18. Hayden AM. Balloon atrial septostomy increases cardiac index and may reduce mortality among pulmonary hypertension patients awaiting lung transplantation. J Transpl Coord. 1997;7:131–3.
19. Sandoval J, Gaspar J, Pulido T, Bautista E, Martinez-Guerra ML, Zeballos M, Palomar A, Gomez

A. Graded balloon dilation atrial septostomy in severe primary pulmonary hypertension. A therapeutic alternative for patients nonresponsive to vasodilator treatment. J Am Coll Cardiol. 1998;32:297–304.

20. Rothman A, Sklansky MS, Lucas VW, Kashani IA, Shaughnessy RD, Channick RN, Auger WR, Fedullo PF, Smith CM, Kriett JM, Jamieson SW. Atrial septostomy as a bridge to lung transplantation in patients with severe pulmonary hypertension. Am J Cardiol. 1999;84:682–6.

21. Kothari SS, Yusuf A, Juneja R, Yadav R, Naik N. Graded balloon atrial septostomy in severe pulmonary hypertension. Indian Heart J. 2002;54:164–9.

22. Reichenberger F, Pepke-Zaba J, McNeil K, Parameshwar J, Shapiro LM. Atrial septostomy in the treatment of severe pulmonary arterial hypertension. Thorax. 2003;58:797–800.

23. Kurzyna M, Dabrowski M, Torbicki A, Burakowski J, Kuca P, Fijalkowska A, Sikora J. Atrial septostomy for severe primary pulmonary hypertension—report on two cases. Kardiol Pol. 2003;58:27–33.

24. Allcock RJ, O'Sullivan JJ, Corris PA. Atrial septostomy for pulmonary arterial hypertension. Heart. 2003;89:1344–7.

25. Micheletti A, Hislop AA, Lammers A, Bonhoeffer P, Derrick G, Rees P, Haworth SG. Role of atrial septostomy in the treatment of children with pulmonary arterial hypertension. Heart. 2006;92:969–72.

26. Kurzyna M, Dabrowski M, Bielecki D, Fijalkowska A, Pruszczyk P, Opolski G, Burakowski J, Florczyk M, Tomkowski WZ, Wawrzynska L, Szturmowicz M, Torbicki A. Atrial septostomy in treatment of end-stage right heart failure in patients with pulmonary hypertension. Chest. 2007;131:977–83.

27. Ciarka A, Vachiery JL, Houssiere A, Gujic M, Stoupel E, Velez-Roa S, Naeije R, van de Borne P. Atrial septostomy decreases sympathetic overactivity in pulmonary arterial hypertension. Chest. 2007;131:1831–7.

28. Law MA, Grifka RG, Mullins CE, Nihill MR. Atrial septostomy improves survival in select patients with pulmonary hypertension. Am Heart J. 2007;153:779–84.

29. O'Byrne ML, Rosenzweig ES, Barst RJ. The effect of atrial septostomy on the concentration of brain-type natriuretic peptide in patients with idiopathic pulmonary arterial hypertension. Cardiol Young. 2007;17:557–9.

30. Lammers AE, Derrick G, Haworth SG, Bonhoeffer P, Yates R. Efficacy and long-term patency of fenestrated amplatzer devices in children. Catheter Cardiovasc Interv. 2007;70:578–84.

31. Troost E, Delcroix M, Gewillig M, Van DK, Budts W. A modified technique of stent fenestration of the interatrial septum improves patients with pulmonary hypertension. Catheter Cardiovasc Interv. 2009;73:173–9.

32. Sandoval J, Gaspar J, Pena H, Santos LE, Cordova J, del Valle K, Rodriguez A, Pulido T. Effect of atrial septostomy on the survival of patients with severe pulmonary arterial hypertension. Eur Respir J. 2011;38:1343–8.

33. Khan MS, Memon MM, Amin E, Yamani N, Khan SU, Figueredo VM, Deo S, Rich JD, Benza RL, Krasuski RA. Use of balloon atrial septostomy in patients with advanced pulmonary arterial hypertension. A systematic review and meta-analysis. Chest. 2019;156(1):53–63.

34. Gorbachevsky SV, Shmalts AA, Dadabaev GM, Nishonov NA, Pursanov MG, Shvartz VA, Zaets SB. Outcomes of atrioseptostomy with stenting in patients with pulmonary arterial hypertension from a large single-institution cohort. Diagnostics. 2020;10(9):725.

35. Espinola-Zavaleta N, Vargas-Barron J, Tazar JI, Casanova JM, Keirns C, Cardenas AR, Gaspar J, Sandoval J. Echocardiographic evaluation of patients with primary pulmonary hypertension before and after atrial septostomy. Echocardiography. 1999;16:625–34.

36. Sandoval J, Rothman A, Pulido T. Atrial septostomy for pulmonary hypertension. Clin Chest Med. 2001;22:547–60.

37. Prieto LR, Latson LA, Jennings C. Atrial septostomy using a butterfly stent in a patient with severe pulmonary arterial hypertension. Catheter Cardiovasc Interv. 2006;68:642–7.

38. Roy AK, Gaine SP, Walsh KP. Percutaneous atrial septostomy with modified butterfly stent and intracardiac echocardiographic guidance in a patient with syncope and refractory pulmonary arterial hypertension. Heart Lung Circ. 2013;22:668–71.

39. Borlaug BA. The shunt for better breathing in heart failure with preserved ejection fraction. Eur J Heart Fail. 2014;16:709–11.

40. Søndergaard L, Reddy V, Kaye D, Malek F, Walton A, Mates M, Franzen O, Neuzil P, Ihlemann N, Gustafsson F. Transcatheter treatment of heart failure with preserved or mildly reduced ejection fraction using a novel interatrial implant to lower left atrial pressure. Eur J Heart Fail. 2014;16:796–801.

41. Bauer A, et al. Creation of a restrictive atrial communication in heart failure with preserved and mid-range ejection fraction. Clin Res Cardiol. 2018;107:845–57.

42. Feldman T, Komtebedde J, Burkhoff D, Massaro J, Maurer MS, Leon MB, et al. Transcatheter interatrial shunt device for the treatment of heart failure. Rationale and design of the randomized trial to REDUCE Elevated Left Atrial Pressure in Heart Failure (REDUCE LAP-HF I). Circ Heart Fail. 2016;9:e003025. https://doi.org/10.1161/CIRCHEARTFAILURE.116.003025.

43. Guimaraes L, Lindenfeld J, Sandoval J, Bayés-Genis A, Bernier M, Provencher S, Rodés-Cabau J. Interatrial shunting for heart failure current evidence and future perspectives. EuroIntervention. 2019; https://doi.org/10.4244/EIJ-D-18-01211.

44. Ewert P, Berger F, Nagdyman N, Kretschmar O, Dittrich S, Abdul-Khaliq H, Lange P. Masked left ventricular restriction in elderly patients with atrial septal defects: a contraindication for closure? Catheter Cardiovasc Interv. 2001;52:177–80.

45. Seib PM, Faulkner SC, Erickson CC, et al. Blade and balloon atrial septostomy for left heart decompression in patients with severe ventricular dysfunction on extracorporeal membrane oxygenation. Catheter Cardiovasc Interv. 1999;46:179–86.

46. Hoffmann R, Altiok E, Reith S, Brehmer K, Almalla M. Functional effect of new atrial septal defect after percutaneous mitral valve repair using the MitraClip device. Am J Cardiol. 2014;113:1228–33.

47. Rajeshkumar R, Pavithran S, Sivakumar K, Vettukattil JJ. Atrial septostomy with a predefined diameter using a novel Occlutech atrial flow regulator improves symptoms and cardiac index in patients with severe pulmonary arterial hypertension. Catheter Cardiovasc Interv. 2017;90:1145–53.

48. Kaye D, Shah SJ, Borlaug BA, Gustafsson F, Komtebedde J, Kubo S, Magnin C, Maurer MS, Feldman T, Burkhoff D. Effects of an interatrial shunt on rest and exercise hemodynamics: results of a computer simulation in heart failure. J Card Fail. 2014;20:212–21.

49. Del Trigo M, Bergeron S, Bernier M, Amat-Santos IJ, Puri R, Campelo-Parada F, et al. Unidirectional left-to-right interatrial shunting for treatment of patients with heart failure with reduced ejection fraction: a safety and proof-of-principle cohort study. Lancet. 2016;387:1290–7.

Part V

Future Perspectives

Norbert F. Voelkel, Dietmar Schranz, Liza Botros, and Harm Jan Bogaard

The rationale for the assessment of the root causes of right ventricular failure simply lies in the acknowledged fact that patients with severe and chronic pulmonary hypertension die from right heart failure. During the last two decades, we have witnessed several paradigm shifts in the research of pulmonary hypertension. The first shift occurred when investigators recognized that pulmonary vascular tone and vessel constriction were insufficient to explain the pathobiology of severe forms of pulmonary hypertension. A more recent shift occurred when investigators began to consider the RV as a specific participant in the pathobiology of pulmonary hypertension and part of the sick lung circulation right heart failure axis, both of which are considered as treatment targets [1].

Introduction

It has been widely accepted that a significant reduction in the pulmonary artery pressure will unload the stressed right ventricle, "the RV under pressure" [2]. A "significant" reduction in pulmonary artery pressure unfortunately cannot be achieved presently for all patients and, as Van de Veerdonk et al. [3] have showed, patients that do not achieve an improvement of their right ventricular ejection fraction on therapy deteriorate

N. F. Voelkel (✉) · L. Botros · H. J. Bogaard
Pulmonary Department, University of Amsterdam Medical Centers, Vrije Universiteit, Amsterdam, The Netherlands

D. Schranz
Pediatric Heart Center, Johann Wolfgang Goethe University, Frankfurt, Germany

and have a bad prognosis. Recent large cohort studies have focused on "risk assessment" and "risk calculators" have been developed and published [4, 5].

On the other hand, there are patients with severe pulmonary arterial hypertension that remain for a considerable length of time highly functional. These patients are in NYHA functional class I and early on there were reports of long-term survivors of primary pulmonary hypertension at a time when there was no targeted PH therapy [6]; see Fig. 21.1.

Taken together, one can frame the problem of the "at-risk" patient as the problem of a RV that cannot successfully adjust to the high pressure, and explain the "good fortune" of the patient in functional class I—who can run 5-km races—with a robust and appropriately hypertrophied and vascularized RV muscle.

While the secrets of the astonishingly functional RV in NYHA class I patients still remain secrets, presently the goal of supporting RV function and improving RV function can be accomplished in several different ways.

There are pharmacologic treatments which, in addition to being pulmonary vasodilators, *also* directly affect the RV function; then there are non-vasodilator drugs that impact RV function; and then there are procedures, catheter guided and surgical, resulting in a shunt, that are aiming to treat RV failure by reducing wall stress of the RV.

Although there have been—and still are—skeptics and self-pronounced nonbelievers, the

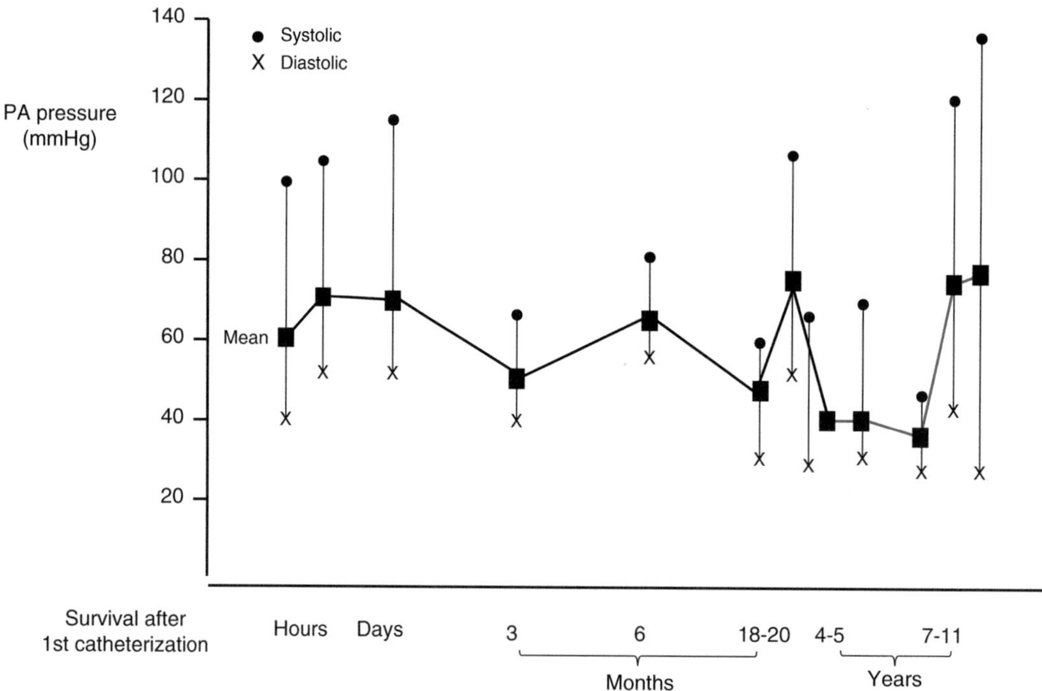

Fig. 21.1 The magnitude of pulmonary hypertension at the time of initial heart catheterization is not correlated with the duration of subsequent survival. (Voelkel & Reeves 1979, Redrawn and reproduced with the permission of the author [6])

very first treatment for severe PAH was a game-changer, because—as we believe—the continuous infusion of the very powerful vasodilator prostacyclin directly impacts the heart and in addition the systemic circulation both far beyond the pulmonary vasculature. After so many years it is worth to revisit the seminal report of the first successful treatment of a moribund 27-year-old woman with IPAH by Tim Higenbottam and associates in 1984 in Lancet [7]. Tim wrote:

Whilest the patient breathed air the pulmonary vascular resistance (PVR) was estimated by means of a flow-guided balloon catheter at between 25 and 30 units, An intravenous infusion of epoprostenol was then started and increased to 4 ng/kg/min. The PVR fell to 15 units and this was associated with an immediate improvement of oxygenation. The pulmonary blood flow, measured by thermodilution increased from 3.0 to 4.1 l/min.

At the time, in 1984, and still today, this finding was/is interpreted as follows: the powerful pulmonary vasodilator prostacyclin (PGI2) relaxed constricted pulmonary arterioles allowing more blood to flow through the lung vessels and a drop in the vascular resistance to blood flow *allowed* the cardiac output to increase. This explanation is entirely consistent with Ohm's law—and yet it is wanting because it did not (does not) consider that prostacyclin could perhaps also *directly* work on the myocardium—possibly both of the right and left ventricles.

We believe that not considering a direct effect on the heart was shortsighted. This dogmatic interpretation at the time stood in the way of the pursuit of a "prostacyclin-induced partially recovered myocardial function" hypothesis. Such a hypothesis should have been entertained.

Here is why.

Clinicians in the catheter lab have observed that there were unfortunate patients with severe PAH where the infusion of incremental prostacyclin doses does not increase the cardiac output. These are the high-risk patients that cannot increase their RVEF with any therapy [3]; these are the patients that die. In these patients one finds a decrease in the pulmonary arterial pressure that is not accompanied by an increase in the cardiac output. We suggest that in these patients the contractile myocardial machinery has become unresponsive to prostacyclin and its power to increase cellular cyclic AMP, or that the contractile machinery has become irreparably damaged.

Our concepts of RV failure have since then evolved; we are now accepting that the heart muscle, its contractile force, and its metabolism are—while not completely independent of the "sick lung circulation"—critically important determinants of overall PAH patients' outcome.

One of us observed a young woman that had been admitted with ascites and anasarca due to IPAH and terminal RV failure, and how continuous epoprostenol infusion caused a dramatic recovery *within 1 week* of treatment. The treatment of this patient had been inspired by Tim Higenbottam's case report [7], and was made possible by a speedy shipment of the prostacyclin by Burroughs Wellcome in England and a compassionate approval to use iv epoprostenol by the Colorado University Institutional Review Board.

This rapid clinical improvement was difficult to explain by prostacyclin causing a deremodeling of the obstructed pulmonary arterioles or a considerable anti-inflammatory response directed at the lung vessels.

The concept for explaining how this moribund patient was able to walk out of the hospital after 1 week of continuous epoprostenol treatment was that the failing right ventricle had recovered most of its function. The same young woman remained stable and functional for several years on this treatment until she developed a severe depressive illness. She insisted that the prostacyclin treatment should be stopped. After several months of counseling and psychiatric treatment—that had not changed the patient's mind—the patient was admitted to the hospital in order to slowly taper the prostacyclin infusion. This accomplished, the patient died 1 week later.

So much for anecdotes and observations, yet the lesson experienced was that the failing RV can recover and that the recovery was, without any doubt, the result of, and dependent on, continuous prostacyclin treatment.

How mechanistically prostacyclin can restore RV function remains largely unknown and we believe that the impact of prostacyclin treatment on the myocardial microcirculation, cells, and expressed genes and enzymatic activities needs to be investigated. In addition to its postulated cardiac and pulmonary circulatory effect, the impact of PGI2 on the systemic circulation with subsequent improved oxygen uptake and diminishing of the neurohumoral hyperactivity cannot be ruled out.

A first step in this direction would be a catheter- or cMRI-based study of RV-arterial coupling before prostacyclin and at various time points after the treatment has started.

Drugs Targeting Pulmonary Hypertension That Are Vasodilators and May Have a Pressure-Independent Effect on the Right Ventricle

In addition to prostacyclin [8], there are pulmonary vasodilator drugs which may also improve right ventricular function by impacting cellular and molecular alterations that characterize the failing heart. It is intuitive that a clean separation of a direct cardiac effect from the consequence of a drug's reduction in the RV afterload in patients with severe PAH is not possible. In animal model studies where an agent causes a significant drop in the pulmonary artery pressure one can usually observe a commensurate decrease in the RV hypertrophy, while there are few studies that evaluate the effect of drug treatment on the RV in models of pulmonary artery banding (PAB) where the remodeling of the RV is independent of pulmonary vasoconstriction.

A recent example illustrates the difficulty of demonstrating a direct myocardial effect of pulmonary hypertension drugs. Monzo et al. [9] evaluated 22 patients using right-heart catheterization and gated equilibrium blood pool single-photon emission computed tomography to assess RV function before and after 20 mg of iv sildenafil; the authors found a 20% acute increase in the RVEF which they explained by an improved RV-PA coupling due to a reduced RV load.

Ralph Schermuly's group in Giessen treated rats with pulmonary artery banding (PAB) for 2 weeks with 10 mg/kg of the endothelin receptor blocker macitentan and documented in this model a modest effect on RV remodeling which was not observed by sildenafil treatment (10 mg/kg for 2 weeks) of PAB rats [10].

The lipophilic dual-endothelin receptor blocker macitentan [11], developed by Actelion to replace bosentan, was studied in a rather large cohort trial of patients with PAH and shown in 2015 to decrease mortality [12]. Because patients with severe PAH die from RV failure, one would like to assume that the reduction in mortality in this SERAPHIN trial was because of macitentan stabilizing the RV or slowing down RV failure. Yet, while a study of patients of PH associated with thromboembolic pulmonary disease showed a hemodynamic improvement [13], a study of patients with left-heart disease-associated PH (12-week treatment of 31 patients with macitentan) showed an insignificant increase in the cardiac index and decrease in NT-proBNP [14]. The data from the REPAIR macitentan treatment trial have been published in abstract form [15]; briefly, 71 patients were enrolled in this study, 48% of the patients were in FC II, and 24% were studied on macitentan monotherapy, while the balance of patients received macitentan in combination with a PDEV inhibitor. While the abstract remains silent on the effect of macitentan treatment on the PA pressure, the primary endpoint of the study— an improvement of the right ventricular stroke volume (RVSV)—was met; for the entire study cohort, macitentan treatment increased the RVSV by 10.5% and RVEF by 10.6%. There was a reduction in the RV mass of 10.5%. The conservative interpretation of this first cMRI endpoint study is that the endothelin receptor blocker reduced the PVR which resulted over the treatment period in a moderate improvement of the RV function.

Riociguat is a soluble guanylate cyclase (GC) stimulator that has been approved for the treatment of inoperable thromboembolic disease-associated PAH [16, 17]. Several studies have showed that riociguat reduces the PA pressure and subsequently improves RV function [18]. The authors of one study of patients with PAH and PAH associated with chronic embolic disease suggest that riociguat improves RV contractile function, as evidenced by a decreased RV global longitudinal strain [19]. However measurements of cardiac contractility in piglets after acute administration of riociguat did not show increased contractility [20], while several preclinical studies support reduction of RV fibrosis after chronic riociguat treatment evaluated in PAB models and in a transaortic constriction mouse model [21]. One study in PAB mice showed that the GC stimulator Bay 41-2272 failed to prevent RV hypertrophy and also the development of RV failure [22]. Taken together, these data show that riociguat can reduce the PA pressure in patients with CTEPH to the degree that there is a recovery of RV function [23, 24], while the preclinical data in the aggregate are not strong in support of a direct RV contractility improving action.

Selexipag is an oral prostacyclin receptor agonist that acts as a vasodilator which is not specific for the lung circulation; systemic hypotension and headaches are dose limiting. The GRYPHON trial with the enrollment of 1156 patients, randomized 1:1 to placebo or selexipag, was the largest PAH cohort trial with the primary endpoint of all-cause death, hospitalization, transplantation, or worsening of PAH [25]. In this large cohort study (376 patients on ETR blocker and PDEV inhibitors), selexipag did not affect the overall mortality but had an effect on clinical worsening. The hemodynamic changes reported in the first proof-of-concept study of 43 patients [26] were modest: after 17 weeks of treatment the CI was 2.7 when compared to 2.3 in the placebo group and the mean PA pressure was 53 when compared with 46 mmHg in the placebo group. No study so far has addressed the question whether selexipag improves RV function [27, 28]. Examining the effect of the active selexipag metabolite in the Sugen/chronic hypoxia rat model of severe pulmonary arterial hypertension, Honda et al. [29] reported a profound reduction in the PA pressure, pulmonary vascular lumen obliteration, RV hypertrophy, and mortality. However, these results are based on a rather high drug dose of 30 mg/kg. This PGI2 receptor agonist affected hemodynamics, vascular remodeling, and RV hypertrophy displaying antihypertensive, antiproliferative, and antifibrotic actions. Whether such actions could modify the disease in human patients with severe PAH is unknown. Antifibrotic effects of the active selexipag metabolite have also been recently documented in in vitro *studies* [30].

Myocardial Capillaries and Fibrosis in Right Ventricular Failure

Alterations in the tissue of the failing right ventricle are found on the subcellular organelle level, and on the cellular and tissue level, and gene and protein expressions are reflective of these morphological changes. The energy metabolism is altered; there is evidence of inflammation and evidence for an oxidant/antioxidant imbalance [2]. While we do not yet understand the root cause of these alterations and imbalances, it is perhaps somewhat intuitive that capillary loss and myocardial fibrosis can be a consequence of impaired energy metabolism and oxidant stress— and that re-capillarization, improvement of endothelial cell function, and reversal of myocardial fibrosis could be strategic targets in the service of the overall goal of preserving the function of the pressure-overloaded RV [2]. One hypothesis of potentially reversible RV failure is that either a microvascular myocardial angiopathy coexists with myocardial fibrosis or a scarring of the tissue occurs because of the reduced tissue perfusion. Again, if we believe that it is important to explore these potentially important pathobiological connections, we need to develop techniques which allow us to characterize the quantity and quality of RV microvessels and/or techniques which assess impaired perfusion of the RV myocardial capillaries in vivo. We can call this technique perhaps "microvascular angiography" and "functional assessment of the RV microvascular endothelium."

As in the lung, the myocardial capillary endothelial cells represent a metabolically active surface area, and impaired myocardial endothelial metabolism conceptually should lead us to tracers which can give a quantitative readout of function and impairment.

One example, and the first step in such a direction, is experiments which have assessed the effects of carvedilol treatment in the Sugen/chronic hypoxia model of severe PAH [31]; see below. While the Sugen/chronic hypoxia rat model is characterized by capillary rarefaction of the RV and RV myocardial fibrosis, carvedilol treatment of rats with established severe PAH reversed capillary rarefaction and RV fibrosis. Because in this model carvedilol treatment did not cause a significant reduction in the RV afterload—mainly due to a failure of de-remodeling of the obliterated pulmonary vessels [31]—we can interpret the reversal of RV myocardial capillary rarefaction as a direct action of carvedilol. Indeed, follow-up studies with normal rats have documented that carvedilol induced the expression of a number of genes encoding proteins involved in angiogenesis (Fig. 21.2). Whether carvedilol can have such a pro-angiogenic effect on the RV of patients with chronic severe PAH is unknown.

A second example is studies conducted with rats subjected to the Sugen/chronic hypoxia protocol in order to generate severe PAH and examine the effect of inhaled stable prostacyclin analogue iloprost on the pathological alterations of the pressure-overloaded RV [32]. In these experiments it was shown that inhaled iloprost reversed RV fibrosis, but not capillary rarefaction.

Recently, Paul Schumacker and his group investigated in the chronic hypoxic mouse model of mild PAH the effects of cardiomyocyte HIF-1alpha and HIF-2alpha knockout and found that the knockout enhanced the RV hypertrophy induced by hypoxia, but the authors concluded that the loss of myocardial HIF did not cause a deterioration of RV function [33]. Yet, we need to point out that the knockout did not affect the myocardial endothelial cells and the authors did not examine RV microvessels. In the Sugen/

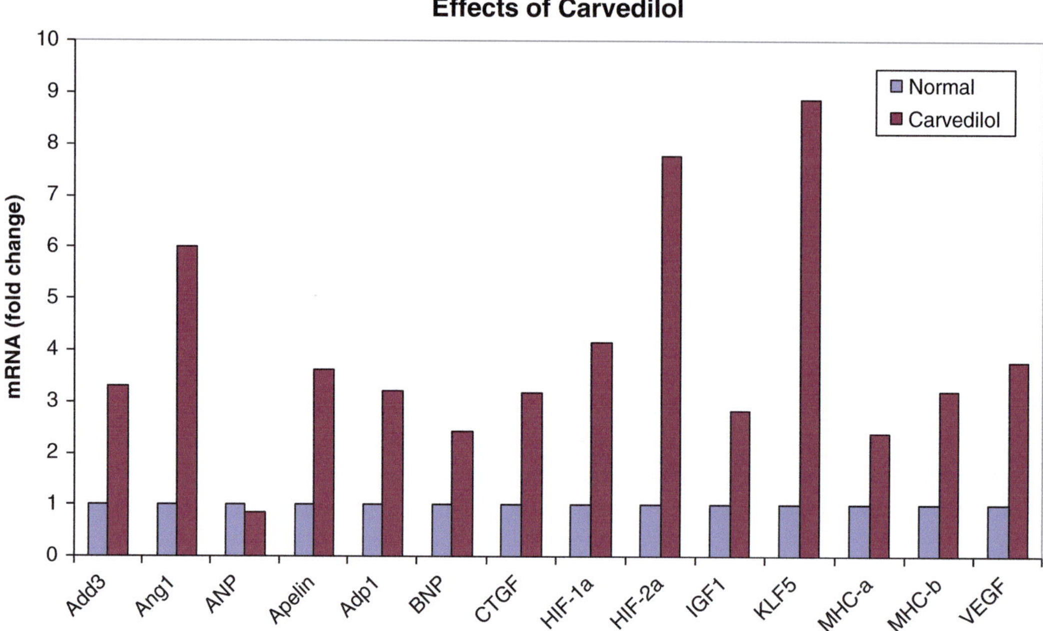

Fig. 21.2 Carvedilol treatment is associated with increased mRNA expression of angiogenic-associated genes (angiopoietin 1 = Ang1, apelin, aquaporin 1 = Aqp1, HIF-1alpha and HIF-2alpha, and VEGF) in healthy rats

chronic hypoxia model of severe PAH the capillary rarefaction of the RV myocardium is associated with a decreased expression of HIF-1alpha and RV failure [34]. Here we have emphasized the concept that RV function or failure in the presence of a chronic afterload and increased RV wall stress may depend on the myocardial capillarization and function of its endothelium.

Multiple interactions between the neurohormonal system and inflammation synergistically promote right-heart failure. As the overworked failing heart is damaged by sustained adrenergic stimulation, it evades this stimulation through phosphorylation of the adrenergic receptors by protein kinases A and C, which results in the desensitization of the receptors [35]. Subsequent to agonist binding, activated β-adrenergic receptors (βAR) are phosphorylated by G protein-coupled βAR kinases (BARK) leading to recruitment of β-arrestins with subsequent receptor internalization and ultimately desensitization. Indeed, heart failure is associated with increased BARK levels [36]. In right ventricular failure, the number of β1AR was reduced and tissue norepinephrine was depleted in the affected right ventricle [37] and the βAR density was reduced in PAH and this was associated with worse right ventricular function [38].

Heart rate reduction in animal models of pulmonary hypertension, and in the PAB model of RV stress, independent of beta-adrenergic receptor blockade has been shown to improve RV fibrosis [35]. Both carvedilol and ivabradine reduce heart rate in models of PAH, but it does not necessarily follow that the effect of ivabradine treatment (10 mg/kg/day) on the RV in the Sugen/chronic hypoxia and PAB rat models—the reduction of TGF beta-dependent fibrosis—was due to heart rate reduction, or that the carvedilol effects on the RV [36] (see above) can be explained by heart rate reduction.

Improved endothelial cell function and increased myocardial perfusion as a consequence of ivabradine have been reported [37–40].

Several preclinical studies showed favorable effects of β-blocker therapy; for example treatment with the selective β-blockers bisoprolol and carvedilol improved RHF as well as reduced RV inflammation in experimental PH, possibly by reducing the heart rate and RV wall stress [31, 39].

The β-blocker carvedilol is a β-arrestin-biased βAR ligand that preferentially activates β-arrestin-mediated pathways while having inverse agonism towards Gαs signaling [40]. Carvedilol treatment was associated with directional changes in gene expression controlling RV hypertrophy and RVF in the SuHx model [41]; see Fig. 21.2. By contrast, clinical reports showed no overall clinical benefit of β-blockers in PAH [39–42]. To understand this discrepancy, the effect of β-blocker therapy in RV sympathetic activity was studied using [11C]-hydroxyephedrine, a norepinephrine analogue tracer, in positron-emission tomography scanning, to determine the sympathetic innervation of the RV [42]. No alterations in local RV sympathetic activity or RV function in patients with PAH after bisoprolol treatment were observed [42]. As currently no clear demonstration of a favorable benefit-to-risk ratio is provided, the use of β-blockers is not recommended unless required by comorbidities (i.e., high blood pressure, coronary artery disease, or LHF) [43]. More data about the efficacy and safety of β-blocker treatment in left-sided heart disease PH are needed in addition to studies that evaluate the benefits of pulmonary artery and renal sympathetic denervation as treatment against chronic sympathetic nerve activation in PAH. Whether carvedilol can have a pro-angiogenic effect on the RV of patients with chronic severe PAH is unknown.

At last, the myocardial endothelial metabolism is also affected by the iron status as this is essential for the myocardial oxygen supply. Increased inflammatory mediators such as cytokines IL-1β, IL-6, and IL-22 have been implicated to increase the expression of hepcidin, which is essential for iron metabolism. Iron deficiency is common in patients with pulmonary arterial hypertension and is closely associated with poor survival and low exercise capacity [44]. Indeed, iron deficiency leads to deterioration of cardiac function [45], which is why several interventional studies have evaluated whether iron supplements improve RV function. So far cardiac magnetic resonance imaging has not shown improvements in right ventricular (RV) function [46].

Lessons Learned from Solving Hemodynamic Problems in Children with Congenital Cardiac Abnormalities

The pediatric experience gained from treating children of all ages with congenital heart diseases has led to the appreciation of the importance of the ventriculo-ventricular interactions (VVI), as they play a decisive role in the balance of cardiovascular function in health and disease [47, 48] (see also Chap. 4). Both sides of the heart are inextricably linked, morphologically through a shared ventricular septum, myofibers, and pericardial space, and a shared circulation [49], functionally through contraction relationships [50] and biologically because of age- and disease-dependent cardiac degenerative as well as regenerative processes [51–53]. The adverse effects of inappropriate ventricular-ventricular interactions (VVI) in heart failure still seem to be frequently ignored. Surprisingly, the knowledge of these chamber interactions is rarely harnessed therapeutically (see also Chap. 20). Yet, the knowledge and experience of the pediatric cardiologist provide an opportunity for the translation towards more generalized therapeutic concepts. They can be derived from the observation of the interactions between the right and left heart in patients with the persistent pulmonary hypertension of the newborn (PPHN) or congenital heart defects other than the Eisenmenger syndrome (see also R. Berger, M. Douwes). It is acknowledged that the right ventricle (RV) can work adequately for decades under systemic pressure. For example, neonates born with a congenitally corrected transposition of the great arteries (ccTGA) can live seven decades with a right ventricle that supplies the systemic circulation [54] especially when the subpulmonary left ventricle is inherently banded by a balanced obstruction of right ventricular outflow tract (RVOTO). Newborns with a borderline left ventricle (BLV) or the hypoplastic left-heart syndrome (HLHS) illustrate the relevance of a dominant or single right ventricle and the reliance on intra- and extracardiac communications [55]. It is apparent that a sufficient systemic cardiac output and an adequate oxygen supply can only be achieved when all cardiac structures are integrated through intra-cardiac and arterial communications. These are responsible for balancing the pulmonary and systemic circulation at similar vascular resistance levels. In addition, various congenital heart defects (CHD) show the importance of the *"best preload."* An optimal or "best preload" avoids congestive heart failure and guarantees an adequate cardiac output, and, in addition, leads in young patients to the growth or restoration of a moderately sized chamber [56, 57]. In extreme forms with duct-dependent systemic blood flow, the "best preload," also via precapillary pulmonary hypertension, supports the systemic circulation through a right-left-shunting arterial duct [58–60]. It was no accident that the reverse Potts shunt was developed by pediatric cardiac surgeons and cardiologists experienced in complex CHD, which illustrates how the left and right sides of the heart work together [61]. An artificially created arterial communication (reverse Potts shunt) between the (left) pulmonary artery and the descending aorta, resulting in a right-to-left shunt, continues to be valuable as a palliation for patients of all ages with various forms of pulmonary arterial hypertension (PAH) (Fig. 21.3).

The catheter-based atrial septostomy (AS) was introduced by William Rashkind in the 1960s [62]. Instead of generating an uncontrolled atrial septum serving the purpose of mixing of oxygenated and deoxygenated blood on the atrial level for patients with advanced PAH [63–67], CpcPH [68–70] or isolated postcapil-

lary pulmonary hypertension (IpcPH) caused by heart failure with reduced LV-ejection fraction (HFrEF) requires a well-defined atrial communication with restrictive pathophysiology [71]. A restrictive ASD is defined by a residual pressure gradient across the atrial septum or by a hole-septum ratio of less than 20% [72, 73]. The procedure can be surgically performed using a punched patch or by transcatheter techniques utilizing the Brockenbrough transseptal needle for atrial septum puncture followed by gradual balloon dilatation [66] as well as by device placement with a defined hole [62, 63]. For such a restrictive ASD there are two main indications in patients with PAH [66, 67]: children with PAH-related syncope and patients with acute or chronic right ventricular dysfunction with low systemic cardiac output and systemic vein congestion. Syncope occurs in young children with a low right atrial pressure at rest, during a sudden and rapid increase of RV and PH pressures (mostly caused by a neurohumoral storm followed by an acute low cardiac output) during a pulmonary hypertensive crisis [67]. The PH crisis occurs in the setting of a strong, well-muscularized right ventricle with a nearly competent tricuspid valve which acts suddenly against an extremely high pulmonary arterial resistance (Rp). A limited blood flow through the lungs with subsequent acute reduction of the LV pre-load leads to symptoms of intermittent acute ischemia-related "epileptic-like" convulsions. In this setting a restrictive atrial communication

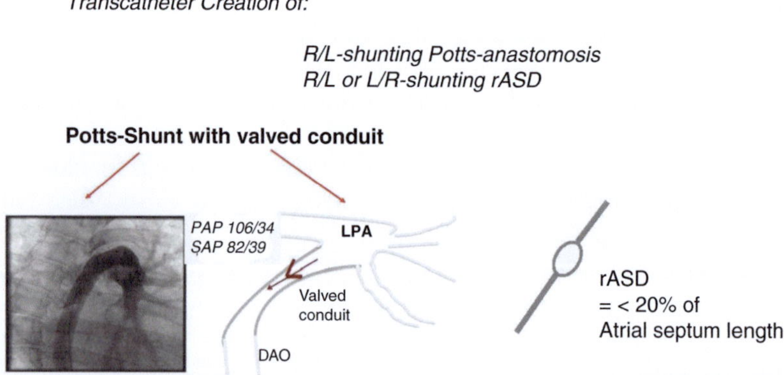

Fig. 21.3 Creation of a restrictive atrial septum defect (rASD). Abbreviations: *DAO* descending aorta, *L* left, *LPA* left pulmonary artery, *PAP* pulmonary artery pressure, *R* right, *rASD* restrictive atrial septum defect, *SAP* systemic atrial pressure

works *on demand* and avoids syncope and ischemic attacks.

These PH patients are different from adult patients suffering from a chronic low cardiac output and systemic vein congestion diagnosed by a high right atrial pressure (RAP). Depending on the imbalanced right-to-left ventricular compliance and the degree of tricuspid valve regurgitation, the RAP subsequently increases, being higher than the left atrial pressure (LAP). The generation of an interatrial communication with a right-to-left shunt leads to a decompression of the RA and an increased LV preload, and thus to an ASD-associated Eisenmenger syndrome. Despite lower arterial oxygen saturation, systemic oxygen transport will increase due to the increased cardiac output [67]. The creation of a restrictive ASD in patients with high RAP (>18 mmHg) must be done with caution [68]: in these patients already a 4 mm communication is sufficient to reduce the RAP significantly without inducing severe hypoxemia, while a larger shunt might be not tolerated due to severe hypoxemia and loss of a necessitating (best) right ventricular preload. Unfortunately, we lack randomized controlled trials and the role of AS in PH is still unclear. But AS in severe PH represents a useful treatment strategy in selected cases. A restrictive ASD should be considered in patients in the stages of advanced NYHA class III and IV associated with recurrent syncope or chronically low CO as a bridge to transplant [71].

In patients with left-heart-related CpcPH, or isolated postcapillary PH (IpcPH), congestion of left atrium and pulmonary veins is effectively treated by creation of a rASD and diuretics can be reduced or weaned [71, 72]. Left atrial congestion and hypertension are different entities and the degree of the LAP is not directly linked to congestive symptoms. A chronic restrictive left ventricular physiology as observed in restrictive cardiomyopathy (RCM) with a LAP of 25–30 mmHg is tolerated and not necessarily associated with pulmonary congestion at rest. Generating a rASD significantly reduces the atrial pressure and thus improves exercise capacity and reduces the incidence of atrial tachyarrhythmias. Reducing the LA pressure decreases the LV end-diastolic pressure, which in turn improves endocardial capillary perfusion and systolic/diastolic function. In patients with CpcPH a rASD improves exercise performance, provided that an adequate, that is, still increased, preload is guaranteed. According to single-center experience [71, 73, 74], the decision regarding the choice of heart (HTX) versus heart-lung transplantation (HLTx) in patients with associated CpcPH and a NYHA functional class IV HFpEF (heart failure with preserved ejection fraction) should optimally not be made unless a rASD has been created prior to performing the diagnostic heart catheter study including reactivity proofing. A diastolic pressure gradient (PAP-diastolic—LAP) of empirically less than 7 mmHg in adults and 12 mmHg in young children, estimated after creation of a rASD, favors HTX instead of a HLTx. This decision is independent of the level of the systolic pulmonary artery pressure, especially in children and young adults.

In patients with advanced heart failure, HFrEF (heart failure with reduced ejection fraction) defined by an increased LAP and reduced LV-EF and associated with a low cardiac output at rest or exercise, a restrictive ASD palliates congestive symptoms of left heart disease, but also reduces the risk of PAH-associated syncope and RV failure, independent of the level of pulmonary hypertension. A rASD can be created with low risk, and low mortality from infancy to advanced adulthood [71, 73, 74]. The efficacy of a rASD is demonstrable by an immediate and long-lasting improvement of the clinical functional class. The technique of gradual balloon dilatation has the advantage of subsequent adaption by gradually increasing the communication, if necessary. However, there is the disadvantage that the created atrial fenestration without a defined device might require repetitive interventions. In reported case series repetitive interventions became necessary in about 30% of transcatheter-treated patients.

Reverse Potts Shunt

Generation of an <u>arterial</u> communication resulting in a right-to-left shunt, the reverse Potts shunt

[75], is a novel surgical approach for palliating children with severe (idiopathic) pulmonary arterial hypertension and supra-systemic PH [61]. This procedure is a reasonable alternative strategy and an alternative to lung transplantation [76]. The reverse Potts shunt establishes a connection between the (left) pulmonary artery and the descending aorta allowing a right-to-left shunt which corresponds to patients with a patent ductus arteriosus-related Eisenmenger syndrome. Ideally, a reverse Potts shunt provides highly oxygenated blood for the perfusion of coronary arteries and the central nervous system and only a partially desaturated blood for the lower body. The risk of paradoxical embolisms is lower compared to a right-left shunt on the atrial level. In addition, the hemodynamic improvement because of the unloading of the RV pressure with a subsequent reduction of the ventricular septum shift from the right to left ventricle also improves the systolic and diastolic performance of the left heart [77]. The diameter of the interarterial communication has to be chosen in order to balance an improved systemic blood flow, but not at the expense of a sufficient pulmonary blood flow. In the absence of an atrial right-to-left shunt, a still properly filled left atrium correlates with a sufficient amount of oxygenated blood. The connection between the pulmonary artery and the descending aorta can be achieved surgically either by a direct side-by-side anastomosis or by using a synthetic graft tube/prosthesis [61, 76, 78] or by transcatheter techniques [79–81]. The size of the interarterial communication depends on the pathophysiological condition of the underlying disease and the type of connection, but in particular on the diameter of the descending aorta. Several modifications of the procedure have been recently published with the goal to reduce perioperative morbidity and mortality due to open-chest surgery [81, 82]. A further step towards a higher acceptance of establishing a Potts shunt physiology is the implementation of a unidirectional valved Potts anastomosis [83, 84].

Reversed Potts shunt placement has also been reported in patients with left-heart disease with severe and fixed PH [78]. The pathophysiology of those patients is different when compared with patients with PAH in which a Potts shunt is indicated. Patients with CpcPH benefit by the combination of a left-to-right shunting-restrictive ASD together with an arterial right-left shunt. The pathophysiology of the left-to-right shunt on the atrial level combined to right-to-left shunting arterial duct is similar to neonates with hypoplastic left-heart syndrome treated with a hybrid approach [58]. The atrial left-to-right shunt prevents severe deoxygenation of the lower body. Some patients treated in Giessen have survived for almost 10 years without any further complications.

Lessons Learned: Age- and Disease-Related RV Function

As pointed out above, the exact mechanisms leading to failure versus adaptation to right ventricular load and stress are still not fully understood [85]. In recent years it became evident that there is no such thing as THE right ventricle and it is also clear that even large cohort therapeutic studies will not address the situation of the individual patient. Personalized diagnostic approaches and therapy strategies that take into account age, phenotype, and genotype need to be developed. As myocardial biopsies are not popular for the assessment of the right ventricle in PAH patients, less invasive options need to be considered.

Yet, biopsy-based single-nuclei sequencing (snRNA-seq) of heart tissue could identify cellular gene expression signatures [86]. Only recently it was shown in pediatric DCM patients [87] that the cardiac cellular transcriptomes display remarkable age-dependent changes in the expression patterns of fibroblast and cardiomyocyte genes with less fibrotic and pro-regenerative signatures in infants. Genes coding for fibroblast activity and fibrillar collagens were more highly expressed in older children. In addition, the expression of genes in control of adrenergic signaling differed by age and disease allowing individualized drug (beta-adrenergic receptor blocker) therapy [87]. Recent studies [88] showed that human induced pluripotent stem cells (iPSCs) derived from patients with HLHS (single RV, in systemic position) are associated with impaired cardiac differentiation and intrinsic cardiomyocyte abnormalities, characterized by decreased contraction force and acceleration. Single-cell RNA sequencing unveiled downregulated expression of genes involved in mitochondrial function and metabolism. In addition, three sets of genes have been identified as molecular coordinators in heart failure. One of the findings confirmed decreased mitochondrial respiration and oxidative metabolism, reflected in a significantly reduced oxygen consumption rate in iPSC-CMs from HLHS with failed RV. Cells maintained in a medium with high fatty acid content improved contractility, and a drug such as istaroxime which acts by inhibiting Na+/K+-adenosine triphosphatase and stimulating the calcium ATPase isoform 2 of the sarco/endoplasmic reticulum, comparable to digoxin but with less narrow therapeutic-toxic window [88]. The importance to assess the quality of the heart tissue was further underlined by a study of Liu et al., where the beta-adrenergic receptor-controlled cytokinesis suggests a mechanism for regulating cardiomyocyte behavior [89]. Myocardial biopsies obtained from young children with tetralogy of Fallot (ToF) presenting with a hypertrophied right ventricle had significantly greater number of right ventricular cardiomyocytes with bi- or multi-nucleation. Katherine Yutzey summarized the clinical implications of these findings [90]. Independent of the high numbers of bi- or multiple-nucleated cells, animal studies indicated that the protein Ect2 (epithelial cell transforming 2, a regulator of intracellular signaling with effects on structural proteins important in cytoplasmic adhesion and motility) expression might be decreased in the cardiomyocytes from infants with ToF compared to control cardiomyocytes. Liu et al. [89] showed that inhibiting beta-adrenergic receptor signaling by using the nonselective β-blockers propranolol/alprenolol increased Ect2 levels and promoted cytokinesis of cardiomyocytes with a subsequent increase of the numbers of cardiomyocytes. Considering that ß-blockers are often used for the treatment of heart failure (see above), the research data underline the need for a differentiated therapy based on molecular knowledge. It also appears that the endogenous stem cell capacity-dependent cardiac regenerative potentials of infants with congenital diseases—when compared with acquired DCM—differ fundamentally. Beyond 1 year of age there was a marked reduction or absence of cardiac stem cell content [51], in particular in HLHS and DCM patients.

Additionally, the right ventricle in infants with HLHS exhibits a depleted stem cell number when compared with the hypoplastic left ventricle [51]. In this context, it has been shown that infants with HLHS benefit from exogenous stem cell therapy [58], while in young DCM patients the high endogenous regenerative capacity might be taken advantage of by applying stress and induction and protective medication [91–93]. These novel insights shed light on age-, disease-, and clinical functional class-related cellular and subcellular differences which may support the concept of a failure-prone and failure-resistant RV and the concept of a "responder to treatment" RV phenotype [94].

Conclusions and Outlook

The pathophysiology of RVF involves a complex interplay of neurohormonal activation, inflammation, apoptosis, insufficient coronary perfusion, and a variable degree of fibrosis and hypertrophy [95]. Reduced RV contractile function is associated with the activation of several inflammatory cascades. As all types of PAH are associated with increased circulating levels of cytokines that are known to give rise to cardiac fibrosis and remodeling, cardiac contractility will become further impaired (Fig. 21.4). The current management of RHF includes preload optimization and augmentation of contractility through optimization of the iron status and reduction of inflammation. However, we are still falling short of our goal to effectively treat RHF.

A recent review by Carlos Lopez-Otin and Guido Kroemer provides a novel concept of healthy organ function, as a compendium of organizational and dynamic features that maintain physiology [96]. Integrity of barriers and

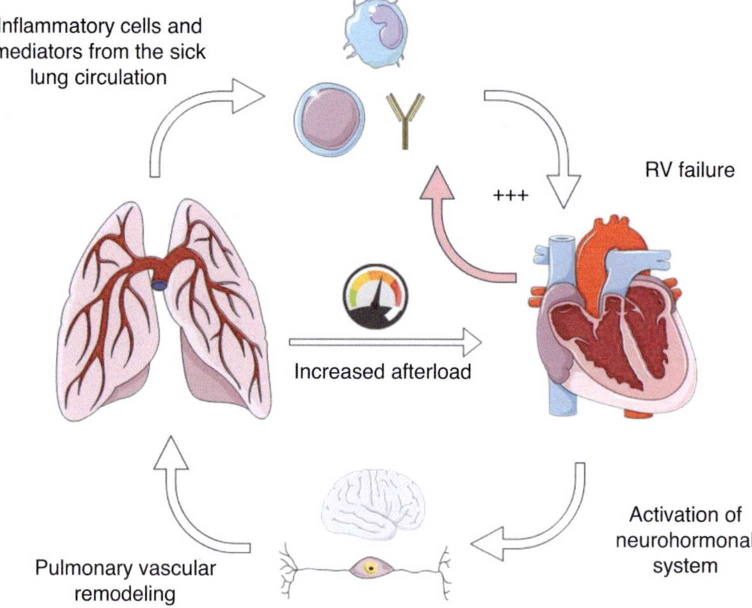

Fig. 21.4 The vicious circle of multiple mediators released from the sick lung circulation (inflammation, cells, vesicles, free DNA) that can lead to RV failure. RV failure itself further amplifies inflammation and leads to neurohormonal overdrive

containment of local perturbations, maintenance of homeostasis over time, and an array of adequate responses to stress, the so-called homeostatic resilience, are features of normal healthy organ function. Beyond the genetic background and specific gene mutations in PAH patients, other factors such as exogenous exposure to drugs and toxins, inflammation, hormones, and aging are all factors that influence repair and regeneration capacities of the heart. Mechanic, chemical, or physical trauma causes permanent loss of functional units and surpasses the capacity of the organ to repair the damage. In light of this concept, RHF becomes a problem that is based on damage and dysfunction of mitochondria, impaired proteostasis, impaired endothelial cell function, and deranged cell metabolism—all amplified by a neurohormonal overdrive. In addition, repair and regeneration mechanisms are not working as the heart is also receiving the "bad humor" released by a "sick lung circulation" [1]. Such a view puts the failing heart in the center of a system of multiple altered feed-forward and feedback loops resulting in a vicious cycle of mutually amplifying injuries. This leads to the conclusion that a strategy directly and highly focused on the right ventricle will likely fail. As pointed out above, homeostatic resilience cannot

Table 21.1 Research priorities: the low-hanging fruits

1. To investigate the PAH patients remaining stable in NYHA FC I
2. To investigate whether there is a role for anti-fibrotic and anti-inflammatory agents
3. To develop drug-targeting strategies
4. To determine the "best RV preload"
5. To develop methods to assess the RV microcirculation and its endothelial cell functions

be achieved when adaptive responses to the persistent stress of a high afterload, inflammation, and inadequate myocardial perfusion are impaired or lost.

Lopez-Otin and Kroemer point us in a different direction—which gets us to our starting point: the patient with severe PAH remaining for a long time in functional class I.

We need to learn from these patients. Longitudinal and multi-omics profiling of these individuals can now be done. We hypothesize that the "liquid biopsy," the blood proteome of the patients endowed with a resilient right ventricle, will provide the answers. By investigating the healthy RV of the pulmonary hypertensive patient we will arrive at a better understanding of the "medicine of disease."

Table 21.1 covers research priorities.

References

1. Voelkel NF, Gomez-Arroyo J, Abbate A, Bogaard HJ. Chapter 13: The pathobiology of chronic right heart failure. In: The right ventricle in health and disease. New York: Springer Science+Business Media; 2015.
2. Bogaard HJ, Abe K, Vonk Noordegraaf A, Voelkel NF. The right ventricle under pressure: cellular and molecular mechanisms of right-heart failure in pulmonary hypertension. Chest. 2009;135(3):794–804.
3. van de Veerdonk MC, Kind T, Marcus JT, Mauritz GJ, Heymans MW, Bogaard HJ, et al. Progressive right ventricular dysfunction in patients with pulmonary arterial hypertension responding to therapy. J Am Coll Cardiol. 2011;58(24):2511–9.
4. Benza RL, Gomberg-Maitland M, Elliott CG, Farber HW, Foreman AJ, Frost AE, et al. Predicting survival in patients with pulmonary arterial hypertension: the REVEAL risk score calculator 2.0 and comparison with ESC/ERS-based risk assessment strategies. Chest. 2019;156(2):323–37.
5. Galie N, Channick RN, Frantz RP, Grunig E, Jing ZC, Moiseeva O, et al. Risk stratification and medical therapy of pulmonary arterial hypertension. Eur Respir J. 2019;53(1):1801889.
6. Voelkel NRJ. Primary pulmonary hypertension in pulmonary vascular diseases. Lung Biol Health Dis. 1979;14:573–628.
7. Higenbottam T, Wheeldon D, Wells F, Wallwork J. Long-term treatment of primary pulmonary hypertension with continuous intravenous epoprostenol (prostacyclin). Lancet. 1984;1(8385):1046–7.
8. Gabrielli L, Ocaranza MP, Sitges M, Kanacri A, Saavedra R, Sepulveda P, et al. Acute effect of iloprost inhalation on right atrial function and ventricular dyssynchrony in patients with pulmonary artery hypertension. Echocardiography. 2017;34(1):53–60.
9. Monzo L, Reichenbach A, Al-Hiti H, Borlaug BA, Havlenova T, Solar N, et al. Acute unloading effects of sildenafil enhance right ventricular-pulmonary artery coupling in heart failure. J Card Fail. 2021;27:224–32.
10. Mamazhakypov A, Weiss A, Zukunft S, Sydykov A, Kojonazarov B, Wilhelm J, et al. Effects of macitentan and tadalafil monotherapy or their combination on the right ventricle and plasma metabolites in pulmonary hypertensive rats. Pulm Circ. 2020;10(4):2045894020947283.
11. Pulido T, Adzerikho I, Channick RN, Delcroix M, Galie N, Ghofrani HA, et al. Macitentan and morbidity and mortality in pulmonary arterial hypertension. N Engl J Med. 2013;369(9):809–18.
12. Belge C, Delcroix M. Treatment of pulmonary arterial hypertension with the dual endothelin receptor antagonist macitentan: clinical evidence and experience. Ther Adv Respir Dis. 2019;13:1753466618823440.
13. Ghofrani HA, Simonneau G, D'Armini AM, Fedullo P, Howard LS, Jais X, et al. Macitentan for the treatment of inoperable chronic thromboembolic pulmonary hypertension (MERIT-1): results from the multicentre, phase 2, randomised, double-blind, placebo-controlled study. Lancet Respir Med. 2017;5(10):785–94.
14. Vachiery JL, Delcroix M, Al-Hiti H, Efficace M, Hutyra M, Lack G, et al. Macitentan in pulmonary hypertension due to left ventricular dysfunction. Eur Respir J. 2018;51(2):1701886.
15. Vonk Noordegraaf ACR, Cottreel E, Kiely D, Martin N, Moiseeva O, Peacock A, Tawakol A, Torbicki A, Rosenkranz S, Galiè N. Results from the REPAIR study final analysis: effects of macitentan on right ventricular remodeling in pulmonary arterial hypertension. J Heart Lung Transplant. 2020;39(4S):S16–7.
16. Marra AM, Egenlauf B, Ehlken N, Fischer C, Eichstaedt C, Nagel C, et al. Change of right heart size and function by long-term therapy with riociguat in patients with pulmonary arterial hypertension and chronic thromboembolic pulmonary hypertension. Int J Cardiol. 2015;195:19–26.
17. Tsai CH, Wu CK, Kuo PH, Hsu HH, Chen ZW, Hwang JJ, et al. Riociguat improves pulmonary hemodynamics in patients with inoperable chronic thromboembolic pulmonary hypertension. Acta Cardiol Sin. 2020;36(1):64–71.
18. Ahmadi A, Thornhill RE, Pena E, Renaud JM, Promislow S, Chandy G, et al. Effects of riociguat on right ventricular remodelling in chronic thromboembolic pulmonary hypertension patients: a prospective study. Can J Cardiol. 2018;34(9):1137–44.
19. Murata M, Kawakami T, Kataoka M, Moriyama H, Hiraide T, Kimura M, et al. Clinical significance of guanylate cyclase stimulator, riociguat, on right ventricular functional improvement in patients with pulmonary hypertension. Cardiology. 2021;146:130–6.
20. Naesheim T, How OJ, Myrmel T. The effect of Riociguat on cardiovascular function and efficiency in healthy, juvenile pigs. Physiol Rep. 2020;8(17):e14562.
21. Rai N, Veeroju S, Schymura Y, Janssen W, Wietelmann A, Kojonazarov B, et al. Effect of riociguat and sildenafil on right heart remodeling and function in pressure overload induced model of pulmonary arterial banding. Biomed Res Int. 2018;2018:3293584.
22. Andersen A, Nielsen JM, Holmboe S, Vildbrad MD, Nielsen-Kudsk JE. The effects of cyclic guanylate cyclase stimulation on right ventricular hypertrophy and failure alone and in combination with phosphodiesterase-5 inhibition. J Cardiovasc Pharmacol. 2013;62(2):167–73.
23. Rudebusch J, Benkner A, Nath N, Fleuch L, Kaderali L, Grube K, et al. Stimulation of soluble guanylyl cyclase (sGC) by riociguat attenuates heart failure and pathological cardiac remodelling. Br J Pharmacol. 2020; https://doi.org/10.1111/bph.15333.
24. Ghofrani HA, Humbert M, Langleben D, Schermuly R, Stasch JP, Wilkins MR, et al. Riociguat: mode of action and clinical development in pulmonary hypertension. Chest. 2017;151(2):468–80.

25. Sitbon O, Channick R, Chin KM, Frey A, Gaine S, Galie N, et al. Selexipag for the treatment of pulmonary arterial hypertension. N Engl J Med. 2015;373(26):2522–33.

26. Asaki T, Kuwano K, Morrison K, Gatfield J, Hamamoto T, Clozel M. Selexipag: an oral and selective IP prostacyclin receptor agonist for the treatment of pulmonary arterial hypertension. J Med Chem. 2015;58(18):7128–37.

27. Coghlan JG, Picken C, Clapp LH. Selexipag in the management of pulmonary arterial hypertension: an update. Drug Healthc Patient Saf. 2019;11:55–64.

28. McLaughlin VV, Channick R, De Marco T, Farber HW, Gaine S, Galie N, et al. Results of an expert consensus survey on the treatment of pulmonary arterial hypertension with oral prostacyclin pathway agents. Chest. 2020;157(4):955–65.

29. Honda Y, Kosugi K, Fuchikami C, Kuramoto K, Numakura Y, Kuwano K. The selective PGI2 receptor agonist selexipag ameliorates Sugen 5416/hypoxia-induced pulmonary arterial hypertension in rats. PLoS One. 2020;15(10):e0240692.

30. Zmajkovicova K, Menyhart K, Bauer Y, Studer R, Renault B, Schnoebelen M, et al. The antifibrotic activity of prostacyclin receptor agonism is mediated through inhibition of YAP/TAZ. Am J Respir Cell Mol Biol. 2019;60(5):578–91.

31. Bogaard HJ, Natarajan R, Mizuno S, Abbate A, Chang PJ, Chau VQ, et al. Adrenergic receptor blockade reverses right heart remodeling and dysfunction in pulmonary hypertensive rats. Am J Respir Crit Care Med. 2010;182(5):652–60.

32. Gomez-Arroyo J, Sakagami M, Syed AA, Farkas L, Van Tassell B, Kraskauskas D, et al. Iloprost reverses established fibrosis in experimental right ventricular failure. Eur Respir J. 2015;45(2):449–62.

33. Smith KA, Waypa GB, Dudley VJ, Budinger GRS, Abdala-Valencia H, Bartom E, et al. Role of hypoxia-inducible factors in regulating right ventricular function and remodeling during chronic hypoxia-induced pulmonary hypertension. Am J Respir Cell Mol Biol. 2020;63(5):652–64.

34. Drake JI, Gomez-Arroyo J, Dumur CI, Kraskauskas D, Natarajan R, Bogaard HJ, et al. Chronic carvedilol treatment partially reverses the right ventricular failure transcriptional profile in experimental pulmonary hypertension. Physiol Genomics. 2013;45(12):449–61.

35. Wang J, Gareri C, Rockman HA. G-protein-coupled receptors in heart disease. Circ Res. 2018;123(6):716–35.

36. Ahmed A. Myocardial beta-1 adrenoceptor downregulation in aging and heart failure: implications for beta-blocker use in older adults with heart failure. Eur J Heart Fail. 2003;5(6):709–15.

37. Bristow MR, Minobe W, Rasmussen R, Larrabee P, Skerl L, Klein JW, et al. Beta-adrenergic neuroeffector abnormalities in the failing human heart are produced by local rather than systemic mechanisms. J Clin Invest. 1992;89(3):803–15.

38. Rose JA, Wanner N, Cheong HI, Queisser K, Barrett P, Park M, et al. Flow cytometric quantification of peripheral blood cell beta-adrenergic receptor density and urinary endothelial cell-derived microparticles in pulmonary arterial hypertension. PLoS One. 2016;11(6):e0156940.

39. de Man FS, Handoko ML, van Ballegoij JJ, Schalij I, Bogaards SJ, Postmus PE, et al. Bisoprolol delays progression towards right heart failure in experimental pulmonary hypertension. Circ Heart Fail. 2012;5(1):97–105.

40. Wang J, Hanada K, Staus DP, Makara MA, Dahal GR, Chen Q, et al. Galphai is required for carvedilol-induced beta-1 adrenergic receptor beta-arrestin biased signaling. Nat Commun. 2017;8(1):1706.

41. Drake JI, Bogaard HJ, Mizuno S, Clifton B, Xie B, Gao Y, et al. Molecular signature of a right heart failure program in chronic severe pulmonary hypertension. Am J Respir Cell Mol Biol. 2011;45(6):1239–47.

42. Rijnierse MT, Groeneveldt JA, van Campen J, de Boer K, van der Bruggen CEE, Harms HJ, et al. Bisoprolol therapy does not reduce right ventricular sympathetic activity in pulmonary arterial hypertension patients. Pulm Circ. 2020;10(2):2045894019873548.

43. Perros F, de Man FS, Bogaard HJ, Antigny F, Simonneau G, Bonnet S, et al. Use of beta-blockers in pulmonary hypertension. Circ Heart Fail. 2017;10(4):e003703.

44. Rhodes CJ, Howard LS, Busbridge M, Ashby D, Kondili E, Gibbs JS, et al. Iron deficiency and raised hepcidin in idiopathic pulmonary arterial hypertension: clinical prevalence, outcomes, and mechanistic insights. J Am Coll Cardiol. 2011;58(3):300–9.

45. Anker SD, Comin Colet J, Filippatos G, Willenheimer R, Dickstein K, Drexler H, et al. Ferric carboxymaltose in patients with heart failure and iron deficiency. N Engl J Med. 2009;361(25):2436–48.

46. Ruiter G, Manders E, Happe CM, Schalij I, Groepenhoff H, Howard LS, et al. Intravenous iron therapy in patients with idiopathic pulmonary arterial hypertension and iron deficiency. Pulm Circ. 2015;5(3):466–72.

47. Voelkel NSD. The right ventricle in health and disease. Heidelberg: Springer; 2015.

48. Burns KM, Byrne BJ, Gelb BD, Kuhn B, Leinwand LA, Mital S, et al. New mechanistic and therapeutic targets for pediatric heart failure: report from a National Heart, Lung, and Blood Institute working group. Circulation. 2014;130(1):79–86.

49. Sanchez-Quintana D, Anderson RH, Ho SY. Ventricular myoarchitecture in tetralogy of Fallot. Heart. 1996;76(3):280–6.

50. Damiano RJ Jr, La Follette P Jr, Cox JL, Lowe JE, Santamore WP. Significant left ventricular contribution to right ventricular systolic function. Am J Phys. 1991;261(5 Pt 2):H1514–24.

51. Traister A, Patel R, Huang A, Patel S, Plakhotnik J, Lee JE, et al. Cardiac regenerative capacity is age- and disease-dependent in childhood heart disease. PLoS One. 2018;13(7):e0200342.

52. Amir G, Ma X, Reddy VM, Hanley FL, Reinhartz O, Ramamoorthy C, et al. Dynamics of human myocardial progenitor cell populations in the neonatal period. Ann Thorac Surg. 2008;86(4):1311–9.
53. Mishra R, Vijayan K, Colletti EJ, Harrington DA, Matthiesen TS, Simpson D, et al. Characterization and functionality of cardiac progenitor cells in congenital heart patients. Circulation. 2011;123(4):364–73.
54. Prieto LR, Hordof AJ, Secic M, Rosenbaum MS, Gersony WM. Progressive tricuspid valve disease in patients with congenitally corrected transposition of the great arteries. Circulation. 1998;98(10):997–1005.
55. Corno AF. Borderline left ventricle. Eur J Cardiothorac Surg. 2005;27(1):67–73.
56. Emani SM, McElhinney DB, Tworetzky W, Myers PO, Schroeder B, Zurakowski D, et al. Staged left ventricular recruitment after single-ventricle palliation in patients with borderline left heart hypoplasia. J Am Coll Cardiol. 2012;60(19):1966–74.
57. Schranz D, Akintuerk H, Voelkel NF. 'End-stage' heart failure therapy: potential lessons from congenital heart disease: from pulmonary artery banding and interatrial communication to parallel circulation. Heart. 2017;103(4):262–7.
58. Michel-Behnke I, Akintuerk H, Marquardt I, Mueller M, Thul J, Bauer J, et al. Stenting of the ductus arteriosus and banding of the pulmonary arteries: basis for various surgical strategies in newborns with multiple left heart obstructive lesions. Heart. 2003;89(6):645–50.
59. Yerebakan C, Murray J, Valeske K, Thul J, Elmontaser H, Mueller M, et al. Long-term results of biventricular repair after initial Giessen hybrid approach for hypoplastic left heart variants. J Thorac Cardiovasc Surg. 2015;149(4):1112–20; discussion 20–2e2.
60. Ohye RG, Schranz D, D'Udekem Y. Current therapy for hypoplastic left heart syndrome and related single ventricle lesions. Circulation. 2016;134(17):1265–79.
61. Blanc J, Vouhe P, Bonnet D. Potts shunt in patients with pulmonary hypertension. N Engl J Med. 2004;350(6):623.
62. Watson H, Rashkind WJ. Creation of atrial septal defects by balloon catheter in babies with transposition of the great arteries. Lancet. 1967;1(7487):403–5.
63. Kerstein D, Levy PS, Hsu DT, Hordof AJ, Gersony WM, Barst RJ. Blade balloon atrial septostomy in patients with severe primary pulmonary hypertension. Circulation. 1995;91(7):2028–35.
64. Nihill MR, O'Laughlin MP, Mullins CE. Effects of atrial septostomy in patients with terminal cor pulmonale due to pulmonary vascular disease. Catheter Cardiovasc Diagn. 1991;24(3):166–72.
65. Sandoval J, Gaspar J, Pulido T, Bautista E, Martinez-Guerra ML, Zeballos M, et al. Graded balloon dilation atrial septostomy in severe primary pulmonary hypertension. A therapeutic alternative for patients nonresponsive to vasodilator treatment. J Am Coll Cardiol. 1998;32(2):297–304.
66. Micheletti A, Hislop AA, Lammers A, Bonhoeffer P, Derrick G, Rees P, et al. Role of atrial septostomy in the treatment of children with pulmonary arterial hypertension. Heart. 2006;92(7):969–72.
67. Keogh AM, Mayer E, Benza RL, Corris P, Dartevelle PG, Frost AE, et al. Interventional and surgical modalities of treatment in pulmonary hypertension. J Am Coll Cardiol. 2009;54(1 Suppl):S67–77.
68. Hoffmann R, Altiok E, Reith S, Brehmer K, Almalla M. Functional effect of new atrial septal defect after percutaneous mitral valve repair using the MitraClip device. Am J Cardiol. 2014;113(7):1228–33.
69. Del Trigo M, Bergeron S, Bernier M, Amat-Santos IJ, Puri R, Campelo-Parada F, et al. Unidirectional left-to-right interatrial shunting for treatment of patients with heart failure with reduced ejection fraction: a safety and proof-of-principle cohort study. Lancet. 2016;387(10025):1290–7.
70. Hasenfuss G, Hayward C, Burkhoff D, Silvestry FE, McKenzie S, Gustafsson F, et al. A transcatheter intracardiac shunt device for heart failure with preserved ejection fraction (REDUCE LAP-HF): a multicentre, open-label, single-arm, phase 1 trial. Lancet. 2016;387(10025):1298–304.
71. Bauer A, Khalil M, Ludemann M, Bauer J, Esmaeili A, De-Rosa R, et al. Creation of a restrictive atrial communication in heart failure with preserved and mid-range ejection fraction: effective palliation of left atrial hypertension and pulmonary congestion. Clin Res Cardiol. 2018;107(9):845–57.
72. Kaye D, Shah SJ, Borlaug BA, Gustafsson F, Komtebedde J, Kubo S, et al. Effects of an interatrial shunt on rest and exercise hemodynamics: results of a computer simulation in heart failure. J Card Fail. 2014;20(3):212–21.
73. Bauer A, Esmaeili A, de Rosa R, Voelkel NF, Schranz D. Restrictive atrial communication in right and left heart failure. Transl Pediatr. 2019;8(2):133–9.
74. Bauer A, Khalil M, Schmidt D, Recla S, Bauer J, Esmaeili A, et al. Transcatheter left atrial decompression in patients with dilated cardiomyopathy: bridging to cardiac transplantation or recovery. Cardiol Young. 2019;29(3):355–62.
75. Potts WJ, Smith S, Gibson S. Anastomosis of the aorta to a pulmonary artery; certain types in congenital heart disease. J Am Med Assoc. 1946;132(11):627–31.
76. Baruteau AE, Belli E, Boudjemline Y, Laux D, Levy M, Simonneau G, et al. Palliative Potts shunt for the treatment of children with drug-refractory pulmonary arterial hypertension: updated data from the first 24 patients. Eur J Cardiothorac Surg. 2015;47(3):e105–10.
77. Delhaas T, Koeken Y, Latus H, Apitz C, Schranz D. Potts shunt to be preferred above atrial septostomy in pediatric pulmonary arterial hypertension patients: a modeling study. Front Physiol. 2018;9:1252.
78. Latus H, Apitz C, Schmidt D, Jux C, Mueller M, Bauer J, et al. Potts shunt and atrial septostomy in pulmonary hypertension caused by left ventricular disease. Ann Thorac Surg. 2013;96(1):317–9.
79. Esch JJ, Shah PB, Cockrill BA, Farber HW, Landzberg MJ, Mehra MR, et al. Transcatheter Potts

shunt creation in patients with severe pulmonary arterial hypertension: initial clinical experience. J Heart Lung Transplant. 2013;32(4):381–7.

80. Schranz D, Kerst G, Menges T, Akinturk H, van Alversleben I, Ostermayer S, et al. Transcatheter creation of a reverse Potts shunt in a patient with severe pulmonary arterial hypertension associated with Moyamoya syndrome. EuroIntervention. 2015;11(1):121.

81. Boudjemline Y, Sizarov A, Malekzadeh-Milani S, Mirabile C, Lenoir M, Khraiche D, et al. Safety and feasibility of the transcatheter approach to create a reverse Potts shunt in children with idiopathic pulmonary arterial hypertension. Can J Cardiol. 2017;33(9):1188–96.

82. Latus H, Apitz C, Moysich A, Kerst G, Jux C, Bauer J, et al. Creation of a functional Potts shunt by stenting the persistent arterial duct in newborns and infants with suprasystemic pulmonary hypertension of various etiologies. J Heart Lung Transplant. 2014;33(5):542–6.

83. Bui MT, Grollmus O, Ly M, Mandache A, Fadel E, Decante B, et al. Surgical palliation of primary pulmonary arterial hypertension by a unidirectional valved Potts anastomosis in an animal model. J Thorac Cardiovasc Surg. 2011;142(5):1223–8.

84. Rosenzweig EB, Ankola A, Krishnan U, Middlesworth W, Bacha E, Bacchetta M. A novel unidirectional-valved shunt approach for end-stage pulmonary arterial hypertension: early experience in adolescents and adults. J Thorac Cardiovasc Surg. 2021;161:1438–1446.e2.

85. Lahm T, Douglas IS, Archer SL, Bogaard HJ, Chesler NC, Haddad F, et al. Assessment of right ventricular function in the research setting: knowledge gaps and pathways forward. An Official American Thoracic Society Research Statement. Am J Respir Crit Care Med. 2018;198(4):e15–43.

86. Litvinukova M, Talavera-Lopez C, Maatz H, Reichart D, Worth CL, Lindberg EL, et al. Cells of the adult human heart. Nature. 2020;588(7838):466–72.

87. Nicin LAW, Schänzer A, Sprengel A, John D, Mellentin H, Tombor L, Keuper M, Ullrich E, Klingel K, Dettmeyer RB, Hoffmann J, Akintuerk H, Jux C, Schranz D, Zeiher AM, Rupp S, Dimmeler S. Single nuclei sequencing reveals novel insights into the regulation of cellular signatures in children with dilated cardiomyopathy. Circulation. 2021;143:1704–19.

88. Paige SL, Galdos FX, Lee S, Chin ET, Ranjbarvaziri S, Feyen DAM, et al. Patient-specific induced pluripotent stem cells implicate intrinsic impaired contractility in hypoplastic left heart syndrome. Circulation. 2020;142(16):1605–8.

89. Liu H, Zhang CH, Ammanamanchi N, Suresh S, Lewarchik C, Rao K, et al. Control of cytokinesis by beta-adrenergic receptors indicates an approach for regulating cardiomyocyte endowment. Sci Transl Med. 2019;11(513):eaaw6419.

90. Yutzey KE. Cytokinesis, beta-blockers, and congenital heart disease. N Engl J Med. 2020;382(3):291–3.

91. Mollova M, Bersell K, Walsh S, Savla J, Das LT, Park SY, et al. Cardiomyocyte proliferation contributes to heart growth in young humans. Proc Natl Acad Sci U S A. 2013;110(4):1446–51.

92. Schranz D, Akintuerk H, Bailey L. Pulmonary artery banding for functional regeneration of end-stage dilated cardiomyopathy in young children: world network report. Circulation. 2018;137(13):1410–2.

93. Schranz D, Recla S, Malcic I, Kerst G, Mini N, Akintuerk H. Pulmonary artery banding in dilative cardiomyopathy of young children: review and protocol based on the current knowledge. Transl Pediatr. 2019;8(2):151–60.

94. Bogaard HJ, Voelkel NF. Is myocardial fibrosis impairing right heart function? Am J Respir Crit Care Med. 2019;199(12):1458–9.

95. Inampudi C, Tedford RJ, Hemnes AR, Hansmann G, Bogaard HJ, Koestenberger M, et al. Treatment of right ventricular dysfunction and heart failure in pulmonary arterial hypertension. Cardiovasc Diagn Ther. 2020;10(5):1659–74.

96. Lopez-Otin C, Kroemer G. Hallmarks of health. Cell. 2021;184(1):33–63.

Index

H

Healthy carriers, 273
Heart failure (HF), 88, 96, 97, 157
  drugs, 283
Heart failure and preserved ejection fraction (HFPEF), 97
  atrial septostomy for, 360, 361
Heart failure with preserved ejection fraction (HFpEF), 157
  causes of right heart dysfunction in, 159
Heart failure with reduced ejection fraction (HFrEF), 157, 375
  causes of right heart dysfunction in, 157, 158
Heart remodeling, 291
Heart transplant, 284
HeartWare™, 327
Heterometric adaptation, 291
High altitude
  as cause of increased RV afterload, 172–174
  definition of, 171
    hypoxic exposure exert negative inotropic effects, 174, 175
    right ventricle during hypoxic exercise, 175, 176
High-altitude induced right heart failure (HARHF), 171, 174, 176–178
Homeometric adaptation, 291
Hypertrophic cardiomyopathy (HCM), 284, 285
Hypoplastic left heart syndrome (HLHS), 195, 196, 373, 377
Hypoxemia, 305
Hypoxia inducible factor-1α, 149
Hypoxia-induced pulmonary hypertension, 33
Hypoxic exercise, 175, 176
Hypoxic pulmonary vasoconstriction (HPV), 172
Hypoxic vasoconstriction, 173

I

ICD implantation, 283
Idiopathic pulmonary arterial hypertension, RV-PA coupling in, 145
Induced pluripotent stem cells (iPSCs), 376–377
Intermittent hypoxia, 43
International Cooperative Pulmonary Embolism Registry (ICOPER), 220
Interventricular septum (IVS), 223, 225
Intravenous epoprostenol, 305
Invasive hemodynamic monitoring, 312, 313
Invasive pressure method, 78
Ipsi-lateral ventricular function, 57
Ischemia, 17, 18
Isovolumic relaxation time (IVRT), 110

L

Laminin, 271
Left (LV) and right (RV) ventricles interactions
  in congenital heart disease, 59, 60
  mechanical-molecular, in RV hypertension, 58
  molecular tissue, in RV hypertension, 59

physiology of, 53–55
RV hypertensive, 55–58
  at septal hinge-point regions, 58, 59
Left atrial pressure (LAP), 104
Left bundle branch block (LBBB) pattern, 278
Left ventricular assist devices (LVADs), 292
Left ventricular end-diastolic pressure (LVEDP), 358
Levosimendan, 306
Lung and heart-lung transplantation in pulmonary hypertension, 321–323
Lung cancer-associated PH, 43
Lung transplantation, 326
  abrupt deterioration, 326, 327
  in PAH, 326

M

Macitentan, 370
Macro- and micro-vascular ischemia, 17, 148
Massive pulmonary embolism, 165
McConnell's sign, 235, 238
Mean pulmonary artery pressures (mPAP), 104, 172, 173
Mechanical circulatory support strategies, 317
Metabolic shifts in RV myocardium, 149
Metabolic syndrome, 39, 150
Metabolomics approach, 22
Minimally invasive techniques, 312
Mitochondrial dysfunction, 20
Monocrotaline, 21
Monocrotaline (MCT)-induced PAH, 30–32
Monocrotaline (MCT) plus pneumonectomy, 32, 33
Multi-detector computed tomographic (MDCT) angiography, 225
Multivariate regression model, 222
Myocardial biopsies, 377
Myocardial capillaries and fibrosis in right ventricular failure, 371–373
Myocardial Infarction (MI), 37, 38
Myocardial ischemia, 21, 158
Myocardial mechanics, 223–225
Myocardial perfusion, 78
Myocardial scintigraphy, 17
Myocardial tagging and strain mapping, 72, 73
Myocyte contraction, 4
Myocyte hypertrophy, 138
Myocyte relaxation, 5

N

Na$^+$-Ca^{2+} exchanger (NCX), 333
Natriuretic peptide clearance receptor (NPRC), 22
Neurohormonal activation, 18, 19, 149, 150
Nitric oxide (NO), 309
Non-invasive hemodynamic evaluation, 312
Non-massive acute pulmonary embolism, 222
Nonthrombogenic State of Endothelial Surfaces, 211
Norepinephrine (NE), 308
Norepinephrine infusion, 167
Norwood procedure, 195

MIX
Papier aus verantwortungsvollen Quellen
Paper from responsible sources
FSC® C105338

If you have any concerns about our products,
you can contact us on
ProductSafety@springernature.com

In case Publisher is established outside the EU,
the EU authorized representative is:
Springer Nature Customer Service Center GmbH
Europaplatz 3, 69115 Heidelberg, Germany

Printed by Libri Plureos GmbH
in Hamburg, Germany